Instruments for Clinical Health-Care Research

Jones and Bartlett Series in Oncology

Instruments for Clinical Health-Care Research

Second Edition

Editors

Marilyn Frank-Stromborg, RN, EdD, FAAN, JD
Chair and Presidential Research Professor
School of Nursing
Northern Illinois University
DeKalb, Illinois

Sharon J. Olsen, RN, MS, AOCN
Instructor
The Johns Hopkins University
School of Nursing
Baltimore, Maryland

With Foreword by
Nola J. Pender, RN, PhD, FAAN

Jones and Bartlett Publishers
Sudbury, Massachusetts
Boston • London • Singapore

Editorial, Sales, and Customer Service Offices

Jones and Bartlett Publishers, Inc.
40 Tall Pine Drive
Sudbury, MA 01776
508-443-5000
800-832-0034
info@jbpub.com
http://www.jbpub.com

Jones and Bartlett Publishers International
Barb House, Barb Mews
London W6 7PA
UK

Library of Congress Cataloging-in Publication Data

Instruments for clinical health-care research / editors, Marilyn Frank-
  Stromborg, Sharon J. Olsen ; with foreword by Nola J. Pender . — 2nd ed.
      p.   cm. — (Jones and Bartlett series in oncology)
   Rev. ed. of: Instruments for clinical nursing research. c1988.
   Includes bibliographical references and index.
   ISBN 0-7637-0316-8
   1. Nursing assessment.   I. Frank-Stromborg, Marilyn.   II. Olsen,
Sharon J.   III. Instruments for clinical nursing research.
IV. Series.
   [DNLM: 1. Nursing.   2. Research—methods.   WY 20.5 I59 1997]
RT48.I57   1997
610.73'072—dc21
DNLM/DLC
for Library of Congress   97-3049
                                                              CIP

Production Editor: Marilyn E. Rash
Editorial Production Service: Tower Graphics
Typesetting: Publishers' Design and Production Services, Inc.
Cover Design: Hannus Design Associates
Printing and Binding: Hamilton Printing Company

Printed in the United States of America
01 00 99 98 97   10 9 8 7 6 5 4 3 2 1

Were there none who were discontented
with what they have, the world would
never reach anything better.
❧

Florence Nightingale

This book is dedicated to my mother, Rosanne Krcek-Frank, R.N., M.S., Professor Emeritus, School of Nursing, Northern Illinois University, DeKalb, Illinois. She taught nursing for 17 years at the NIU School of Nursing, and led the way toward advanced practice nursing years before the term had been coined. Striving for excellence was her creed in the classroom as well as in life.

Marilyn Frank-Stromborg

Contents

Foreword

Consumers' demand for accountability in health care has increased the need for relevant, reliable, and valid instruments for measuring the actual outcomes of care. Evaluating only the procedures that direct care or the processes through which care is provided will no longer suffice without also assessing whether the care given makes a difference in the lives of care recipients. In an era of cost consciousness and economic constraint, tools for assessing a wide array of nurse-sensitive biopsychosocial outcomes will be essential as attempts are made to document the impact of care delivered by a wide array of health professionals.

Databases must be put in place so that the data collected in the everyday activities of patient care, such as history taking or psychosocial and physical assessment, can be used in research as well as for collaborative decision making by the patient and health-care professionals. The patient's level of health, adequacy of functioning, health-promotion activities, and the presence or absence of clinical problems are areas that must be rigorously measured in comprehensive nursing assessment.

This book provides a rich compilation of research instruments for use in clinical research to measure phenomena of critical concern to nursing. An important feature of this second edition of *Instruments for Clinical Health-Care Research* is to focus on creating or adapting tools for use with vulnerable populations, such as the socioeconomically disadvantaged, children, and the elderly. Furthermore, a separate section focuses on assessing health-promotion activities, an area frequently neglected in other health measurement handbooks. A chapter on evaluating family outcomes expands measurement issues to address aggregates.

You will find this new edition a valuable resource for both the development and use of "state-of-the-science" instrumentation in nursing research and clinical practice. The roster of contributing experts is impressive. As nurses become increasingly responsible for delivering primary care and tertiary care in various settings, measuring the outcomes of care will be essential. This book will be one of the references you will turn to often to provide you with the latest information on measuring health parameters and the clinical status of individuals of all ages to whom you provide care.

Nola J. Pender, RN, PhD, FAAN
Professor and Associate Dean
for Academic Affairs and Research
School of Nursing
The University of Michigan

Preface

The overwhelmingly positive national response to the first edition, *Instruments for Clinical Nursing Research*, resulted in multiple printings. Health-care professionals demonstrated significant interest and need for information on research tools appropriate for use in the clinical setting. The goals of the first edition remain the goals of this second edition. They include: review of available clinical research instruments to measure select clinical phenomena, description of the psychometric properties of each tool, review of selected studies employing the tool, identification of instrument strengths and weaknesses, and discussion of the relevance of each instrument for nursing.

The first edition selectively addressed concepts that measured holistic dimensions of human functioning and client status associated with the most common clinical problems. The first edition provided new nurse researchers with one resource for identifying clinical research instruments, describing sample questions from the instruments, and accessing original tools. Responses from nurses and other health-care professionals in education, practice, and research settings affirmed that the first edition successfully served as such a resource.

This second edition has been significantly expanded. An additional 14 chapters have been added, and its size, as the loyal reader has noticed, has significantly increased. The goals of this second edition remain the same as the first. However, the title has been changed to *Instruments for Clinical Health-Care Research* to reflect the national emphasis on the new U.S. health-care agenda for the 1990s for a "team" approach to health care.

The purpose of Part I is to provide an overview of generic issues related to clinical research. Measurement issues unique to research with different levels of human development are addressed in two new chapters: Chapter 3, Measurement Issues with Children and Adolescents, and Chapter 4, Measurement Issues with the Elderly. This second edition also addresses research issues unique to the changing demographics of this country. Chapter 2 reviews tool adaptation for socioeconomically disadvantaged populations, and Chapter 5 explores measurement issues concerning linguistic translation. As opportunities to triangulate subjective and objective measures increasingly present themselves, we have added a new chapter on physiological measurement issues, Chapter 6.

Five new chapters have been added to Part II, Instruments for Assessing Health and Function. The new chapters are: Chapter 18, Measuring Sleep; Chapter 21, Measuring Family Outcomes; Chapter 22, Measuring Anxiety; and Chapter 23, Measuring Depression. A new topical area has been added, Part III, Instruments for Assessing Health-Promotion Activities. The two new chapters in this part are: Chapter 24, Measuring Healthy Lifestyle, and Chapter 26, Instruments for Measuring Breast Self-Examination. Four new chapters have been added to Part IV, Instruments for Assessing Clinical Problems: Chapter 30, Measuring Cardiac Parameters; Chapter 31, Measuring Physiologic Parameters in Obstetrics and Gynecology; Chapter 33, Measuring Fatigue; and Chapter 34, Measuring Mobility and Potential for Falls.

The *intended audience* of this book includes health-care professionals in educational, clinical, and research settings who are interested in conducting clinical research. The health-care professional with at least one beginning-level research course should have no difficulty understanding and utilizing the material in this book.

Organization of the Text

The primary focus of this book is on the measurement of concepts relevant to clinical research. We are currently living in an era where many professional groups are investing considerable time and energy into developing clinical practice guidelines. The outcome of which should be to assist the clinician in making decisions about clinical interventions that will be effective in producing desired clinical outcomes. Assessing the effect or outcome of a clinical intervention has not consistently been part of guideline development. However, it is the contention of both the editors and the authors that outcomes assessment and measurement are critical to documenting the effects of clinical intervention and imperative to guide cost-effective care. The chapters in this book provide the basis for clearly defining the outcome variable(s) of interest and for identifying appropriate instruments for measuring selected clinical outcome variables and concepts. The introductory chapters in Part I provide guides for rigorously assessing the appropriateness of the measure for the sample under study.

This book can be used in two different ways. The first way is to select a concept and read the related chapter. The second way is look in the index for a specific tool or a group of tools that measure the specific topic or identify one tool that measures multiple concepts. Some instruments (e.g., Sickness Impact Profile–SIP) are discussed in a number of chapters because they measure more than one concept. Historical experience has taught us that most readers select a specific chapter that describes the concept they are interested in studying.

The reader will notice that many of the chapters are authored by individuals who are prominent researchers in the area of interest they are writing about; thus, their chapters reflect both their scholarship and clinical research expertise. Tables are used throughout to highlight important aspects of instruments, and exemplar studies are used to illustrate various research studies that have been conducted with selected instruments.

The 39 chapters are subdivided into four parts. In Part I, six chapters are devoted to special issues related to the use of instruments in clinical research. The first chapter is devoted to research instrument evaluation and has been extensively expanded by Jacobson from the first edition. Weinrich and colleagues review important issues concerning the adaptation of instruments for socioeconomically disadvantaged populations. Health professionals working with children will profit from the chapter by Hymovich. Those who work with the elderly or include this group in their research sample, will equally profit from the chapter in this part by Rasin. Varricchio confronts problems encountered with instrument translation from one language to another. Finally, DeKeyser and Pugh examine the unique problems associated with physiologic measurement.

Part II has been significantly expanded to include the measurement of concepts that are essential to the assessment of health and function. Of the seventeen chapters in this part, six address new concepts. The opening chapter is by Richmond and McCorkle on assessing functional status. Foreman has significantly updated and enhanced the chapter on measuring cognitive status. Padilla and Frank-Stromborg discuss individual research tools for measuring quality of life, while Dean chronicles how tools can be combined to measure quality of life. Lindsey discusses the concept of social support and the multiple instruments the researcher can use to measure it. Tools that researchers can use to measure coping and hope are detailed. Wegmann and Stoner, respectively, artfully present the underlying theoretical concepts of coping and hope. Ellerhorst-Ryan presents the expanding knowledge base about tools that can be used to assess spirituality.

This part continues with a chapter on the multitude of methods for assessing body image by Robertson and Diekmann, including the latest audiovisual methods under development. Saunders and colleagues present a thoughtful discussion of the physiologic, psychologic, and relationship dimensions of various tools to measure sexuality. Stotts and Bergstrom provide ample tools for the researcher interested in measuring dietary intake and discuss the conceptual issues behind the measurement of this clinical parameter. F. Cohen's chapter on sleep is new, and the author provides the researcher interested in this area with an in-depth conceptual discussion. R. Cohen presents numerous tools that can be used singularly or together to measure attitudes toward chronic illness. Burns takes this one step further and presents research instruments that can be used to measure attitudes toward cancer. Another new chapter in this section is by Ferrell and Rhiner who discuss the issues in measuring family outcomes and the different tools that are being advocated to measure this area. Grimm introduces the issues involved in measuring anxiety and follows this with a critique of the various research tools available to the researcher desiring to measure this variable. Pasacreta also introduces the issues encountered when attempting to measure depression and then the tools that can be used by the researcher interested in assessing depression.

Part III is devoted to the issues involved in assessing health-promotion activities. New chapters, which include variables not presented in the first edition, have been added. Beginning this part is Berger's and Walker's chapter on measuring healthy lifestyles. Dodd follows this by presenting information on how researchers have proposed measuring self-care activities and the tools available for doing so. Champion's chapter on assessing breast self-examination (SBE) is one of the new chapters in this part and presents a thorough discussion of the universe of research tools available for measuring this preventive practice. Although there is debate about SBE and long-term survival, it is still recommended as an important cancer early-detection practice. Bagley-Burnett and Heppler conclude this part with an in-depth discussion of what constitutes information-seeking behaviors and decision-making preferences, and the available instruments for measuring these behaviors.

Part IV focuses on instruments for assessing clinical problems and four new chapters have been added. Strohl details the research tools and clinical methods that can be used to assess alterations in taste and smell. McMillan follows suit by discussing the clinical methods that can be used to measure bowel elimination. Quaal's chapter on measuring cardiac parameters is a new addition and provides valuable information for researchers interested in assessing this clinical entity. Lauderdale first presents the conceptual framework for appraising the physiologic variables that are essential when conducting research with obstetric and gynecologic clients, then the available clinical methods for measuring these physiologic variables are presented. Scott-Brown provides an extensive overview of what is involved in measuring dyspnea and the instruments available for doing so. Another new chapter, by Piper, assesses fatigue. She offers the reader a thought-provoking conceptualization of this clinical entity and the methods for judging it. Also new is Spellbring's and Ryan's chapter on assessing mobility and the potential for falls. With the graying of the U.S. population, this research area merits increasing importance and attention.

Part IV continues with the chapter on measuring nausea, vomiting, and retching by new authors Rhodes and McDaniel. They conducted a rigorous review of the literature in this area and offer the reader a concise, scholarly overview of the subject and tools available for assessing these variables. Hyland offers a thorough review of what instruments are available for the researcher who desires to assess the oral cavity. McGuire has extensively revamped the chapter on measuring pain and provides both the issues involved in assessing this variable clinically and the tools available to do so. Braden and Frantz provide valuable assistance to the reader measuring skin integrity and the issues that surround the measurement of this variable. Grant and Davidson conclude this part with their detailed discussion of assessing vaginitis and the clinical methods that can be used to determine it.

How to Use the Book

This book will be useful to both the novice and the experienced researcher, though each may use the information somewhat differently. For the novice, concepts are defined and historically situated. Many instruments are critiqued and sample populations are suggested. For the expert, this book offers a ready reference to the ever-expanding database of clinical instruments and their available psychometric testing qualities.

Clinical researchers often must balance clinical responsibilities, teaching, and research activities. We hope that *Instruments for Clinical Health-Care Research* will ease the burden of researching clinical concepts and variables of interest and enhance focus on linking clinical variable assessment with everyday measurement of everyday clinical interventions.

Contributors

Caroline Bagley-Burnett, RN, ScD
Clinical Associate Professor of Nursing, Clinical Scholar, Center for Clinical Bioethics, Georgetown University Medical Center, Washington, DC

Linda Bartkowski-Dodds, RN, MN

Ann Malone Berger, RNC, PhD
Clinical Nurse Specialist, Oncology, College of Nursing, University of Nebraska Medical Center, Omaha, Nebraska

Nancy Bergstrom, RN, PhD
College of Nursing, University of Nebraska Medical Center, Omaha, Nebraska

Marilyn D. Boyd, RN, PhD, CHES
Adjunct Associate Professor, Department of Health Promotion and Education, College of Nursing, University of South Carolina, Columbia, South Carolina

Barbara J. Braden, RN, PhD, FAAN
Professor, Graduate School of Nursing, Creighton University, Omaha, Nebraska

Nancy Burns, RN, PhD
Professor and Director, Center for Nursing Research, School of Nursing, University of Texas at Arlington, Arlington, Texas

Victoria Champion, RN, DNS, FAAN
Professor, Associate Dean for Research, School of Nursing, Center for Nursing Research, Indiana University, Indianapolis, Indiana

Felissa L. Cohen, RN, PhD, FACG, FAAN
Dean and Professor, School of Nursing, Southern Illinois University, Edwardsville, Illinois

Rebecca F. Cohen, RN, EdD, MPA, CPHQ
Associate Professor and Consultant, Health Care Management/UR/QI, Department of Nursing, Rockford College, Rockford, Illinois

Sue B. Davidson, RN, MS
Oregon Health Sciences University, Portland, Oregon

Hannah Dean, RN, PhD
Quality Assurance Coordinator, Northridge Hospital Medical Center, Northridge, California

Freda G. DeKeyser, RN, PhD
Hadassah Medical Organization, Kiryat Hadassah, Jerusalem, Israel

Judy M. Diekmann, RN, EdD, OCN
School of Nursing, Elmhurst College, Elmhurst, Illinois

Marilyn J. Dodd, RN, PhD
Professor, Department of Physiological Nursing, University of California at San Francisco, San Francisco, California

Jan M. Ellerhorst-Ryan, RN, MSN, CS
Vitas Hospice Group, Norwood Office, Cincinnati, Ohio

Jacqueline Fawcett, RN, PhD, FAAN
Professor, School of Nursing, University of Pennsylvania, Philadelphia, Pennsylvania

Betty R. Ferrell, RN, PhD, FAAN
Department of Nursing Research and Education, City of Hope National Medical Center, Duarte, California

Susan Gross Fisher, RN, PhD

Marquis D. Foreman, RN, PhD, FAAN
Associate Professor, Department of Medical-Surgical Nursing, College of Nursing, University of Illinois at Chicago, Chicago, Illinois

Marilyn Frank-Stromborg, RN, EdD, FAAN, JD
Chair and Presidential Research Professor, School of Nursing, Northern Illinois University, DeKalb, Illinois

Rita A. Frantz, RN, PhD
Associate Professor, College of Nursing, The University of Iowa, Iowa City, Iowa

Marcia M. Grant, RN, DNS, FAAN
Director and Associate Research Scientist, Department of Nursing Research and Education, City of Hope National Medical Center, Duarte, California

Patricia M. Grimm, RN, PhD, CS
Assistant Professor and American Cancer Society Professor of Oncology Nursing, School of Nursing, The Johns Hopkins University, Baltimore, Maryland

Bettyann Heppler, RN, BSN
Master's Candidate, School of Nursing, Georgetown University, Washington, DC

Sharon Ann Hyland, RN, MS, NP
Solid Tumor Division, Roswell Park Cancer Institute, Buffalo, New York

Debra P. Hymovich, RN, PhD
Professor, Department of Family Nursing and Director of Nursing Research, College of Nursing, University of North Carolina at Charlotte, Charlotte, North Carolina

Sharol F. Jacobson, RN, PhD, FAAN
Professor and Director, Nursing Research, College of Nursing, The University of Oklahoma Health and Sciences Center, Oklahoma City, Oklahoma

Susan Heame Kaempfer, RN, DNSc

Jana Lauderdale, RN, PhD
School of Nursing, Vanderbuilt University, Nashville, Tennessee

Ada M. Lindsey, RN, PhD, FAAN
Dean, College of Nursing, University of Nebraska Medical Center, Omaha, Nebraska

Ruth McCorkle, RN, PhD, FAAN
Professor, School of Nursing, University of Pennsylvania, Philadelphia, Pennsylvania

Roxanne W. McDaniel, RN, PhD
Associate Professor, School of Nursing, University of Missouri-Columbia, Columbia, Missouri

Deborah B. McGuire, RN, PhD, FAAN
Edith Folsom Honeycutt Chair, Oncology Nursing, Associate Professor, Nell Hodgson Woodruff School of Nursing, Emory University, Atlanta, Georgia

Susan C. McMillan, RN, PhD, FAAN
ACS Professor of Oncology Nursing, College of Nursing, University of South Florida, Tampa, Florida

Sharon J. Olsen, RN, MS, AOCN
Instructor, School of Nursing, The Johns Hopkins University, Baltimore, Maryland

Geraldine V. Padilla, RN, PhD
School of Nursing, University of California at Los Angeles, Los Angeles, California

Jeannie V. Pasacreta, RN, PhD
Project Director, School of Nursing and Psychiatric Consultation Liason Nurse for Inpatient Oncology, University of Pennsylvania, Philadelphia, Pennsylvania

Barbara F. Piper, RN, DNSc, OCN, FAAN
School of Nursing, University of Nebraska Medical Center, Omaha, Nebraska

Barbara D. Powe, RN, PhD, CCRN
Assistant Professor, College of Nursing, Medical Center, University of South Carolina, Charlestown, South Carolina

Linda C. Pugh, RNC, PhD
Director, Center for Nursing Research, Hershey Medical Center, Pennsylvania State University, Hershey, Pennsylvania

Susan J. Quaal, RN, PhD, CVS, CCRN
Cardiovascular Clinical Specialist, Department of Veterans Affairs Medical Center, Salt Lake City, Utah

Joyce H. Rasin, RN, PhD
Post Doctoral Fellow, School of Nursing-ORDU, Oregon Health Sciences University, Portland, Oregon

Michelle Rhiner, RN, MSN, NP
Clinical Specialist, Nurse Practitioner Supportive Care Services, City of Hope National Medical Center, Duarte, California

Verna A. Rhodes, RN, EdS
Associate Professor, School of Nursing, University of Missouri-Columbia, Columbia, Missouri

Therese Richmond, PhD, CCRN, FAAN
Lecturer, Interim Program Director, Tertiary Nurse Practitioner Program, School of Nursing, University of Pennsylvania, Philadelphia, Pennsylvania
Also: Research Associate, Division of Traumatology and Surgical Critical Care, Hospital of the University of Pennsylvania

Julie F. Robertson, RN, EdD
Associate Professor, School of Nursing, Northern Illinois University, DeKalb, Illinois

Judith W. Ryan, RN, PhD, CRNP
School of Nursing, University of Maryland, Baltimore, Maryland

Saundra E. Saunders, RN, PhD, MEd
University of Wisconsin Hospital and Clinics, Madison, Wisconsin

Mary L. Scott, RN, MS, OCN
Oncology Administrative Director, Columbia, Colorado Division, Denver, Colorado

Ann Marie Spellbring, RN, PhD
School of Nursing, University of Maryland, Baltimore, Maryland

Martha H. Stoner, RN, PhD
Associate Professor, Associate Director of Nursing Research, School of Nursing, University Hospital, University of Colorado Health Sciences Center, Denver, Colorado

Nancy A. Stotts, RN, EdD
Associate Professor and Vice Chair, Department of Physiological Nursing, University of California at San Francisco, San Francisco, California

Roberta Anne Strohl, RN, MN, OCN
Clinical Nurse Specialist, Department of Radiation Oncology, University of Maryland at Baltimore, Baltimore, Maryland

Lorraine Tulman, DNSc, FAAN
Associate Professor, School of Nursing, University of Pennsylvania, Philadelphia, Pennsylvania

Claudette G. Varricchio, RN, DSN, FAAN
Division of Cancer Prevention and Control, National Cancer Institute, Rockville, Maryland

Susan Noble Walker, RN, EdD, FAAN
Professor, College of Nursing, University of Nebraska Medical Center, Omaha, Nebraska

Jo Ann Wegmann, RN, PhD
Professor and Graduate Coordinator, Division of Nursing, Statewide Nursing Program, California State University Dominguez Hills, Southwest Region, San Marcos, California

Sally P. Weinrich, RNC, PhD
Associate Professor, College of Nursing, University of South Carolina, Columbia, South Carolina

I

Overview

1

Evaluating Instruments for Use in Clinical Nursing Research

Sharol F. Jacobson

This chapter provides a brief review of key concepts in measurement and a summary of current recommendations for the selection, use, and continued development of existing instruments in clinical nursing research. The emphasis is on practical information for decision making. The chapter is aimed at health-care professionals who have had at least one course in research methods and statistics but whose background in measurement and research may be neither extensive nor recent. It is not the purpose of the chapter to serve as a comprehensive research or measurement text. This chapter uses the terms *measure*, *tool*, *test*, and *instrument* interchangeably; the terms *concept* and *attribute* refer to what is being measured.

The State of the Art of Measurement in Nursing Research

A common error in selecting an instrument is to assume that it is sound if it has been published or widely used. Conceptualizations of measurement and standards for measurement adequacy change over time,[1-4] and journals vary in the rigor demanded to publish a report on instrument development.

In the early 1980s Waltz and Strickland[5,6] appraised the state of measurement in nursing research through a content analysis of articles published in major nursing research journals from 1980 to 1984. They found that conceptual frameworks were identified for only 20.2% of the measures. In almost half (44.6%) of these reports, the consistency of the tool and framework could not be determined, or the tool and framework were clearly inconsistent. In over one-half of the articles (57.6%), reviewers could not determine the measurement framework of the tools. No reliability data were reported for 38.4% of the measures. No validity data were reported for 58% of the measures. Reliability and validity data from both the current study and previous studies were provided in only 1.7% and 2.1% of the cases, respectively. Strickland and Waltz concluded that the state of measurement in nursing was not high and recommended that researchers, readers, and manuscript reviewers place more emphasis on measurement principles and practices.

Norbeck[3] also proposed standards for what constitutes a publishable report of instrument development. The necessary descriptive information about the instrument consists of the conceptual basis for the tool, the methods of item generation and refinement, sociodemographic characteristics for the intended respondents, details of administration, method of scoring, type of data obtained, and any other instrument-specific information. Variable means, standard deviations, and range of scores should be provided so that users may compare their study samples with others. An initial report also should provide examples of the tool format and sample items or a complete copy of the instrument in an appendix. She suggested that the minimal standard for publishing psychometric testing should include test–retest reliability, internal consistency reliability, and at least one type each of content- and construct- or criterion-related validity. Moreover, beginning work on instruments should be reported through papers or posters at research meetings. Results should not be published until all planned psychometric testing has been accomplished and all indicators meet the minimal acceptable levels as specified by measurement theory. If heeded, Norbeck's recommendations should improve the quality of articles on instrument development and reduce the need to search for fragmented reports. They also can serve the prospective tool user as a standard for evaluating the adequacy of an instrument's development.

Tool users should be aware that there is a relationship between the amount of relevant psychometric information provided by the developer or publisher of a tool and the quality of a tool. Missing data can be assumed to be negative.[7] They also should continue to review the literature *after* reading a report of a promising instrument. The literature is all too rich in accounts of the widespread use of instruments whose psychometric properties have been severely criticized. For example, the Holmes and Rahe Schedule of Recent Experiences was widely used even after a devastating critique and the development of superior instruments.[8]

The authors in the first edition of this book noted that a distressing number of tools were developed on very small samples. Small samples are, by nature, less representative of the population and more prone to sampling error (the tendency for statistics to fluctuate from one sample to another) than large samples.[9] Therefore, one cannot be as confident that a tool developed on a small sample will perform that way again.

Assessing the Conceptual Basis of Instruments

Instrument development, like other research, can be based on a conceptual or a theoretical model. Developers may select concepts and models from other disciplines that are compatible with nursing perspectives,[10] or they may design instruments to operationalize existing or original nursing perspectives.[11] For example, Jacobson[12] based her tools for assessing nurses' stress and coping on Lazarus's model because this mediated, transactional view was more compatible with nursing perspectives than Selye's more biochemical mechanistic approach. Kearney and Fleischer developed an instrument to measure the exercise of self-care agency based on Orem's model of nursing.[13]

Even when instruments are not based on an identifiable model, some assumptions, biases, and values can be detected in them. One must be particularly cautious with older instruments and with concepts from other fields. A tool developed in 1954 to assess female sex role adjustment may be based on now-untenable assumptions about the female destiny. Concepts from other fields may have definitions and dimensions not consistent with their use in nursing, as Ellis illustrated using the psychological phrase "regression in the service of the ego."[10]

Tool users should ascertain through extensive literature review or concept analysis or synthesis[14] that the tool's conceptual basis is at least compatible with, if not identical to, their individual and professional perspectives on the problem. Failure to do so is more than a mere philosophical matter. It may create a validity problem in that the findings obtained with a particular tool cannot be interpreted adequately.[14]

Measurement Frameworks

Two major frameworks guide the design and interpretation of measurement.[15] The *norm-referenced framework* discriminates among individuals and spreads people across a range of scores, ideally, normally distributed.[15] The majority of personality, affective, attitudinal, and cognitive constructs used in nursing employ this framework.[16]

The *criterion-referenced framework* determines what a person knows or can do in relation to a specified domain or fixed performance standard. How one person compares with others is irrelevant in this framework. Criterion-referenced measures (CRMs) produce classifications or judgments, such as satisfactory/unsatisfactory or met/not met. Scores from a CRM have a narrower range than those from a norm-referenced measure and are skewed (clustered) toward one end of the scale. Criterion-referenced measures often are useful in clinical research that requires measuring a process or attaining outcome variables.[15] For example, the Denver Developmental Screening Test and the National Cancer Institute's criteria for the proper performance of breast self-examination are useful CRMs. Space limitations do not permit further discussion of this measurement framework, but a comprehensive description can be found in Waltz et al.[15]

Choosing a Data-Collection Method

Every instrument uses one or more methods of data collection to operationalize the variables of interest. Each method has its own advantages and disadvantages for certain purposes and populations and its special reliability and validity problems. For example, because semantic differentials are rapid to complete, many items can be used. Q sorts are time-consuming and are best suited to intensive analysis of individuals or to small samples.[17] Tools whose items use identical response formats, such as Likert or numerical rating scales, are prone to response sets, in which subjects respond to items in characteristic ways regardless of the item content; such tendencies are threats to validity.[9]

Although it is beyond the scope of this chapter to describe the features of each data-collection method, tool users need this knowledge. Comprehensive research and measurement texts[9,15,17-19] provide basic information and helpful references, and current research literature and such journal research increasingly comment on the practical, as well as the theoretical, aspects of different data-collection methods.

Item Generation and Analysis

Reports of instrument development should contain some description of how items were developed and refined. Items can be generated by reviewing the literature, clinical observations and interviews, qualitative methodologies such as grounded theory, selection from existing instruments, or by combinations of these strategies. Some form of item analysis, which is an examination of the pattern of responses to each item to assess its effectiveness and provide guidelines for its revision, also should be described. The results of item analysis affect both reliability and validity by manipulating the variability of scores, eliminating the extraneous effects of very easy or very difficult items, and strengthening the relationship between items and an external criterion.[15]

Several statistical procedures are widely used in item development and analysis. Item intercorrelations (the correlation of each item with every other item) and item-total correlations (the correlation of each item with the total score for the entire scale) are very helpful in deciding which items to retain, revise, or delete. A common rule of thumb for such correlations is that they should be between 0.30 and 0.70. Those below 0.30 are not contributing much to measurement of the concept; those above 0.70 are probably redundant.[9]

Three item analysis procedures are useful in norm-referenced measurement. Although they are traditionally associated with the development of classroom tests, they can be used for any measure where responses indicative of a high level of some attribute can be identified or for measures intended to discriminate between two groups, such as expert or novice clinicians. Item difficulty (ID), also called "item p level," is the percentage of correct responses to the item. Item difficulty can range from 0 to 100. The closer it is to zero, the more difficult the item is.[15] Average item difficulties, around 50 or with a range of 30 to 70, are generally sought to promote variability of scores and, hence, reliability.[7]

The discrimination power or index (D) represents the degree to which an item distinguishes high and low achievers on the test or to which performance on any one item predicts performance on the entire test. D scores can range from –1.00 to +1.00. Positive D scores are desirable and indicate that the item is discriminating in the desired direction. Those who answered the item correctly tended to do well on the test or to have a large amount of the measured attribute. D scores near zero mean that the item is not discriminating and serves no useful purpose in the test. Negative D scores mean that respondents who answered the item correctly tended to do poorly on the total test. The latter items need major revision. D scores of +0.30 are generally accepted as adequate.[15]

Item response charts display the response patterns to items and allow the inspection, comparison, and chi-square testing of differences between high- and lower-scoring groups. An explanation of how to perform the various item analysis calculations can be found in Waltz et al.[15]

Psychometric Characteristics of Instruments

Theory of Measurement Error

In classic measurement theory, an observed score on any measure is seen as a combination of a true score (what the subject would get if the instrument were perfect) and random and systematic error. Random error results from chance variations in the test (the directions may not be clear), the subject (he or she may have a headache today), or the conditions of test administration (the room may be very hot, or not all administrators may use the same instructions). By sometimes raising and sometimes lowering the observed score, random error reduces the consistency of measurements and, indirectly, makes it difficult to know what exactly is being measured.

Systematic error results from the presence of some extraneous factor that affects all measurements made with the tool in the same way. For example, a scale that reads three pounds high is systematically upwardly biased. Systematic bias compromises validity, the extent to which an instrument measures what it is intended to measure. The aim of all reliability and validity measures is to minimize the portion of the observed score that is due to error and to maximize the portion that is true. The larger the portion of random error in a score, the lower the reliability coefficient of the tool. The lower the reliability coefficient, the lower the confidence that can be placed in any subsequent judgments or relationships using that tool.[7]

Reliability

The first characteristic that any instrument must possess is reliability. Concerns about reliability involve the consistency or repeatability of measurements made with the instrument. Reliability can be conceptualized in terms of stability, equivalence, or internal consistency. It often is possible and desirable to use more than one approach.[9] The most common estimate of reliability is a correlation coefficient. Theoretically, correlation coefficients may range between –1.00 and +1.00, but in reliability assessment, they usually fall between 0.0 and 1.0. The closer the correlation coefficient is to 1.00, the more reliable the tool.[9]

Reliability as Stability

Reliability as stability takes two forms. Test–retest reliability is the correlation between scores from the same subjects tested at two different times. The interval between testings should not be so short that subjects' recall of items can spuriously inflate the reliability coefficient or so long that one is studying the stability of the characteristic over time rather than the performance of the instrument.[20] Two to four weeks is a suitable interval for most uses of stability estimates. Test–retest reliability is more useful for measures of enduring attributes than for changeable states and for affective rather than cognitive measures.[15] For example, a test–retest correlation is better suited to a measure of introversion/extroversion (an enduring affective attribute) than to a measure of knowledge of the warning signals of cancer (a changeable cognitive state).

The second form of reliability as stability is intrarater reliability, the consistency with which one rater assigns scores to a single event on two different occasions. The correlation is calculated from the scores of the same observer at time 1 and time 2.[15]

Reliability as Equivalence

Reliability as equivalence has two forms. Parallel (or alternate) forms reliability requires the development of two different tests that measure the same trait in the same way. The correlation coefficient is based on the scores of the same individuals taking test A and test B sequentially. This procedure overcomes the problem of specific recall associated with the administration of a single test twice. Thus, parallel forms are useful for studies using repeated measures. The disadvantage is that parallel tests are very difficult to construct.[21] The chief application of parallel forms reliability has been with standardized tests in education; occasionally, one finds parallel forms for a psychological construct, such as Hoskins' Interpersonal Conflict Scale.[22]

The second form of reliability as equivalence, much more common in nursing research than parallel forms, is interrater (or interobserver) reliability. Here, two or more trained observers watch an event simultaneously and score it independently, using established scoring criteria.[15] Training raters to achieve adequate interrater reliability is considerably more complex than it may first appear. Washington and Moss[23] identified six essential aspects: (1) understanding the theoretical perspective; (2) familiarization of raters with the instrument; (3) selection of an adequate number of subjects (a minimum of 10 is recommended); (4) use of a set time frame for observations; (5) concern for interfering variables; and (6) completing scoring and discussion soon after the observation session. An excellent description of training raters to use an instrument for assessment of patient intensity can be found in Castorr et al.[24]

Various procedures besides the Pearson r (for interval data) are available for assessing intrarater and interrater reliability. For nominal dichotomous data, the percent of agreement is easy to compute and provides useful information, such as two raters agreed 90% of the time, but it is easily inflated by agreements as a result of chance.[9] Cohen's kappa controls for the amount of agreement that may have occurred by chance and can be extended to cases with more than two raters;[25] weighted kappa also allows assessment of the relative seriousness of disagreement among raters.[26] Because kappa controls for chance agreement, kappa reliabilities are likely to be lower than reliability based on other estimates. Topf[27] provides an example showing a kappa of 0.59 and a total percentage agreement of 80% for the same data.

Reliability as Internal Consistency

The third approach to reliability, internal consistency, is perhaps the most widely used today. Internal consistency is concerned with the degree to which a set of items designed to measure the same concept are intercorrelated. A tool is said to be internally consistent (or homogeneous) to the extent that all items demonstrate desirable intercorrelations, thus appearing to measure the concept of interest and nothing else.[15]

Historically, the oldest method of assessing internal consistency is the split-half technique. The items of a single test are divided into halves—usually odd- and even-numbered items—and scored separately. The correlation coefficient is calculated from the scores on each half of the test. Although splitting the test avoids the need to create two tests, it creates another problem. Because reliability is related to test length, a correlation coefficient based on split-halves systematically underestimates the reliability of the entire scale. A statistical correction known as the Spearman–Brown prophecy formula is used to adjust (prophecy) the split-half correlation coefficient for the full-length test. The chief disadvantage of the split-half technique is that different splits (e.g., odd–even, first half–second half) yield different reliability estimates.[9] Because of this problem, psychometricians have developed reliability coefficients that do not require item repetition or splitting.

The most widely used measure of internal consistency is the Cronbach coefficient alpha, called alpha hereafter. *Alpha*—not to be confused with alpha, the level of significance—measures the extent to which performance on any one item in an instrument indicates performance on any other item in that instrument.[15] Alpha can range from 0.00 to 1.00, indicating very low to very high internal consistency.[9] Alpha has many strengths as an indicator of internal consistency. It addresses the sampling of content, which is the major source of measurement error and also the sampling of the situational factors that accompany individual items. Because it is equal to the average of all possible split halves, it subsumes the Spearman–Brown prophecy formula.[28] Alternatives to alpha should be considered if the items are heterogeneous (i.e., have low intercorrelations) and when the number of items in the scale is small.[29]

The Kuder–Richardson formulas (KR 20 and KR 21) are two other measures of internal consistency. They are special cases of alpha developed for dichotomous responses.[15]

Interpretation of Reliability Coefficients

Reliability is a matter of degree rather than an all-or-nothing affair, and it is not a self-contained property of an instrument but of an instrument when administered to certain people under certain conditions. For all types of reliability, prospective users must ascertain the characteristics of the group on or for whom the tool was developed. The more similar the original group to the user's target group, the more likely that the tool will perform reliably for the new study. Reliability is increased by longer test length (up to a point), by speeded conditions in which all subjects do not finish, by heterogeneous samples, and by variability of scores on the total test.[29]

Other things being equal, the tool with the highest reliability is best,[9] subject to the caution that very high reliabilities may indicate redundant items. Because reliability coefficients are not automatically generalizable, they should be recalculated each time an instrument is used, particularly if used on a different population.[15]

"How high is high?" is a common question about reliability coefficients. There is no simple answer. The judgment depends on the nature of the trait being measured, the stage of development of the instrument, and the procedure used to estimate reliability. The reliability of physiologic measures often is expected to be 0.90 or more, whereas that of attitudinal measures may be acceptable at 0.70.[30] Pearson correlation coefficients for interrater reliabilities should be at least 0.80.[9] Acceptable standards for interrater reliability using percentage agreement range from 70% to 90%.[31] Standards for kappa reliabilities are: slight, 0.00–0.20; fair, 0.21–0.40; moderate, 0.41–0.60; substantial, 0.61–0.80; and almost perfect, 0.81–1.00.[32] Nunnally and Bernstein's guidelines[33] propose that an alpha coefficient of 0.70 is acceptable for an instrument in the early stages of development and a coefficient of 0.80 is adequate for a more developed instrument. If a tool contains subscales that are analyzed, the reliability of each subscale must be assessed, as well as that of the total tool. Because they are shorter, the reliability of subscales often is lower than that of the total tool.[7]

Generalizability Theory

Generalizability theory (G theory) is an extension and liberalization of classical measurement theory. Although classical theory recognizes that there are multiple sources of measurement error, it deals with them collectively. Generalizability theory, however, uses analysis of variance procedures to provide separate, simultaneous estimates of the effects of different sources of error[34] and, in the process, a summary coefficient reflecting the level of dependability of the instrument.[35] Although not yet common in the nursing measurement literature, use of this approach to assess measurement error is likely to increase.

Validity

The second characteristic of a measuring instrument is validity, commonly and briefly defined as whether a tool measures what it claims to measure. Tool users should be aware that the conceptualization of validity by measurement specialists always is evolving and that descriptions of validity in research reports do not always reflect the most current publications by educational psychologists and the standards of the American Psychological Association.[1]

The current view is that validity is a unitary construct, referring to the "degree to which empirical evidence and theoretical rationales support the adequacy and appropriateness of interpretations and actions based on test scores."[4,p13] As such, validation is a process of scientific inquiry, and any method of science may be used to evaluate it. Because of its emphasis on meaning and understanding, this definition also means that all validity ultimately is construct validity and that the previous "types" of validity are but forms or aspects of construct validity. The familiar terminology of face, content, criterion, and construct validity and the methods for assessing them are still used and will be discussed here, but readers are encouraged to consider them as supplements rather than alternatives to one another in understanding the full meaning of test scores and their uses.

Validity depends on reliability in that a tool must measure something consistently (be reliable) before one can determine what that something is. An instrument can be reliable without being valid, but an unreliable instrument cannot possibly be valid.[21]

Establishing validity is more difficult than establishing reliability for at least three reasons. First, many validity assessments are based on measures or outcomes external to the test and require evaluating the meaning of logical, but indirect, relationships. Second, because many logical relationships may need to be examined to establish validity, validation often requires the completion of several distinct studies. Third, validation often involves the use of more and more complex statistical procedures than does estimation of reliability.

Face Validity

Face validity is a judgment of what the tool appears to measure to the untrained eye. Although often discounted as validity in the strict sense of the term because it provides no evidence of what a tool really measures,[36] its presence or absence is sometimes important for public relations reasons. If a test appears irrelevant to the stated purpose, subjects may respond carelessly or not at all, and the user or the public may not readily accept the findings. Conversely, when it is necessary to disguise the true nature of a measure as in some cases of personality and attitude assessment, face validity would be undesirable.[4]

Content Validity

Although associated most with the development of tests of cognitive knowledge, content validity is necessary for all measures.[15] Traditionally content validity is concerned with whether or not the test items adequately sample the content area: Are they representative and comprehensive? Content validity is based on consensual judgments by subject matter experts.[4] In nursing, the assessment of content validity often has been rather cursory and has historically been reported with a simple statement that a panel of judges agreed that the items possessed content validity.[15] Increasingly, however, content validity is the product of more systematic and elaborate approaches. The contemporary emphasis on concept development and specification in measurement and nursing is stimulating the collection of qualitative data to generate items and enhance content validity. The Mishel Uncertainty in Illness Scale[37] and the Tilden Interpersonal Relationship Inventory[38] were developed in this way. Lynn[36] has described a two-stage process combining qualitative and quantitative activities. In the developmental stage the characteristics of the content domain are identified and items are generated, sampled, and assembled into a useable form. In the judgment-quantification stage, five to ten experts who meet criteria for expertise respond to specific questions about the content relevance of each item, suggest revisions, and identify omissions. An Index of Content Validity showing the proportion of agreement among judges can be calculated for each item and the total scale.

Consistent with contemporary views of validity as a unitary construct, it can readily be seen that content validity is part of construct validity because item content is highly relevant to the eventual meaning of scores. However, because content validity is by definition focused on the test *forms* rather than test *scores*, it also should be obvious that content judgments alone are insufficient for assuming that an instrument is valid, which by definition involves understanding of the meaning and uses of scores.[4] Unfortunately a number of published tool descriptions report content validity as the only form of validity.[5]

Criterion-Related Validity

Criterion-related validity is the correlation between a measure and some outside indicator considered to provide a direct and superior measure of the behavior or characteristic in question. It is most pertinent when a tool will be used for decision making.[15] Two types of criterion-related validity commonly are distinguished, depending on when the criterion data are collected. For concurrent validity, data about the measure and indicator are collected at the same time and indicate the person's present standing on the criterion. For example, a measure of patients' perceived readiness for discharge could be correlated with caregivers' perceptions of their readiness. A high correlation between the scores of the two samples would support concurrent validity.

For predictive validity, data on the criterion variable are collected from the same subjects at a future date. For example, the predictive validity of the Graduate Record Examination for success in graduate study could be evaluated by correlating new students' scores on the test with their final grade point averages.[8] Clinical nursing may be an excellent field for determining predictive validity because of the frequency with which behavioral cycles occur, for example, admission-discharge, crisis, patient teaching, and the availability of multiple respondents. Fox believes that tool users should demand evidence of predictive validity in clinical tools.[21]

In principle, criterion-related validity is a strong form of validity. In practice, there are some important problems. Often, identification of an adequate criterion is not possible,[8] or if a criterion can be identified, reliable measures for it may not be available. Validity coefficients based on a criterion measure with low reliability will underestimate the true strength of the predictor–criterion relationship. Underestimates of validity also will occur if the procedures used to sample the target population do not ensure a representative or random sample or if attrition is high.[15] The validity coefficient may be falsely high if criterion contamination occurs, that is, if raters or judges know how members of the sample performed on the predictor.[21] In addition, a coefficient from a single criterion-related study will tend to inflate the predictor–criterion relationship. Ideally, cross-validation should occur, a procedure in which the predictor–criterion relationship is developed on one sample and tested on a second independent sample from the same population. The cross-validation correlation usually is a lower, more accurate estimate of the true predictor–criterion relationship.[15]

In relating criterion validity to the unitary conceptualization of validity, criterion measures themselves need construct validation. Too often, criterion measures have been chosen because they are available and *apparently* suitable for the task at hand. Evidence should be presented for the theoretical similarity of predictor and criterion measures and the utility of the decisions made with the criterion. Discriminant evidence to rule out the influence of rival constructs that might account for the apparent usefulness of a criterion is particularly needed.[4]

Construct Validity

The focus of construct validity is on the theoretical meanings of measurements, of whether the measurement of one concept is logically related to that of other concepts. As such, it uses the processes of scientific inquiry to link theory with the empirical world and to argue that the relationships found are not attributable to alternative constructs.[4]

There are several approaches to construct validity. In the known-groups approach, the instrument is administered to two groups known to be high and low on the measured concept. If the groups' scores differ significantly in the expected direction, construct validity is supported. In hypotheses testing or the experimental manipulation approach, hypotheses about the behavior of people with varying scores on the measure are proposed and tested experimentally. If the hypotheses are borne out, construct validity is supported.[15]

The use of complex statistical approaches to construct validity is growing rapidly. Although adequate descriptions are beyond the scope of this chapter, tool users should cultivate at least a basic conceptual understanding of them.

The many varieties of factor analysis all aim to reduce a set of variables (the instrument items) to smaller clusters of correlated items called factors. The content of the items within a factor and the mathematical weights of the factors are then used to define the concept or to support prior theorizing about its nature. By identifying items that do not fall into a cluster (do not "load" in factor analysis jargon), factor analysis is useful in refining an instrument. It also sheds light on whether a concept is unidimensional or multidimensional—on whether one or several factors are needed to describe it—and on the issue of whether subscale scores should be calculated. To be credible, factor analysis requires a minimum of five, and preferably ten, subjects per variable (tool item).[39] This guideline is frequently violated in published reports, especially older ones. A newer, more powerful, and much more complex model of factor analysis is the Confirmatory Factor Analysis procedure in LISREL (the analysis of *Li*near *S*tructural *Rel*ations). In conventional (exploratory) factor analysis, the measures may load on any factor and any number of factors may be extracted. With confirmatory factor analysis, the tool developer is required to specify in advance which measures will load on which factors. The analysis tests those exact relationships while (very importantly) taking measurement error into consideration.[40,41]

The multitrait-multimethod approach is based on the principles of convergent and discriminant validity. Convergence is the idea that different measures of the same trait should correlate highly with one another. Discriminant validity means that measures of different constructs should have low intercorrelations. Scores from at least two constructs, each measured in at least two different ways, are entered into a correlation matrix. By reading different diagonals of the matrix, the research can obtain separate correlations for reliability and for convergent, construct, and discriminant validity. The technique is efficient and informative, but it may be burdensome to respondents if the several tools are lengthy. A clear, full description of the procedure is found in Waltz et al.'s *Measurement in Nursing Research*.[15]

Interpretation of Validity Evidence

Because validity evidence often involves the correlation of an instrument with external criteria or indirectly related concepts, validity evidence is harder to interpret than reliability evidence, which essentially involves some correlation of the test with itself. Therefore, validity correlations are usually lower than those for reliability; relationships of r equal to 0.40 to 0.60 may be entirely satisfactory. Unlike reliability coefficients, some validity coefficients will be negative. For example, a measure of happiness should be strongly and negatively correlated with a measure of depression. Tool users should ask: What is being correlated (statistically or logically) with what? How strong can the relationship reasonably be expected to be? Is use of the tool an improvement over use of previous tools or of no measurement at all? How similar is the proposed use to conditions under which the available validity evidence was obtained? What use will be made of the scores?

When correlation coefficients are used as evidence of predictive validity, coefficients in the 0.60 to 0.70 range are usually considered adequate for group prediction purposes. Coefficients in the 0.80s are considered minimal for individual predictions.[7]

Evidence for the construct validity of a tool should be viewed as a cumulative pattern. Each positive study results in greater confidence that a tool is a valid measure of a particular construct. On the other hand, despite many previous successes, one strong negative finding can destroy confidence in the construct as measured. Because validity evidence is specific to an application of the instrument rather than to the instrument itself, users should plan to provide additional evidence of validity from their studies.[15]

Other Desirable Tool Characteristics

Sensitivity is the ability of an instrument to make discriminations of the fineness needed for the study. Often, scales with "Yes" and "No" categories will not allow many subjects to respond accurately. Expanding the scale to five categories ranging from "Strongly Approve" to "Strongly Disapprove" will increase its sensitivity.[42] Sensitivity is especially important when physiologic measurements are being monitored, when measurements will be used to make decisions about an individual rather than a group, and when the experimental and control conditions are not drastically different.[15] These are all common conditions in clinical research. Unnecessary sensitivity may be expensive to achieve and burdensome for either the respondent or the investigator.

Appropriateness is the extent to which subjects can meet the requirements of the instrument. Appropriateness often involves the reading level of a tool and assessment of the fit of the tool to the demographic and cultural backgrounds of the intended subjects. An inappropriate tool will produce invalid responses or refusals to complete it.[42]

Objectivity is the extent to which the data obtained reflect what is being measured rather than some outside influence. Common threats to objectivity are the influence of the race or sex of an interviewer on the subject, instructions that suggest what the answers should be, and observation guides that require the researcher to judge behavior. A tool user should expect the tool developer to spell out the steps taken to protect the objectivity of the data.[21]

The feasibility of an instrument is assessed in terms of the time, cost, and skill needed for the study and in terms of the instrument's acceptability to potential subjects. Cost factors include the time and expense of obtaining subjects, and the purchase price of the tool, printing, photocopying, postage, clerical help, computer time, and consultation. Other things being equal, a short, machine-scorable tool would be more feasible than a longer one that must be hand-scored or interpreted by a specialist.[42] Acceptability involves burden—the time and effort involved for the subject—and the fit between the implicit values or sensitivities of the instrument and the subjects. If subjects consider the items irrelevant or offensive, they may answer casually or not at all.

Psychometric Properties of Biophysiologic Measures

Although data obtained from bioinstrumentation and laboratory procedures are generally accurate, sensitive, and objective, several threats to their reliability and validity (more often referred to as precision and accuracy in physiologic measurement[43]) do exist. Most involve human error (e.g., improper use or calibration of equipment, failure to follow established procedures, or clerical errors in reporting results) or equipment failure. Users of biophysiologic measures often must employ quality-control strategies, such as regular calibrations of equipment and random checks on adherence to procedures. Although biophysical measures are relatively immune to subjects' distortions of readings, the measurement process itself can alter the variable of interest. For example, the presence of a transducer in the bloodstream can reduce the blood flow in the vessel.[15] Other considerations with biophysiologic instruments include direct versus indirect measurement, invasive versus noninvasive measurement, single versus multiple measures, and sensitivity.[44]

Some biophysiologic phenomena (pain, nausea, fatigue) are more subjective than objective and can be assessed by paper-and-pencil instruments. The chief consideration in choosing the instrument is the conceptualization of the phenomenon being studied. If a visual analog scale or short questionnaire captures the variable of interest and adequate psychometric data are available, there is no point in using an expensive, invasive physiologic procedure.[44]

The chapter by DeKeyser and Pugh in this book (Chapter 6) and the texts by Polit and Hungler,[9] Waltz et al.,[15] and Wilson[18] all contain helpful information on choosing and using biophysiologic measures.

Other Helpful Procedures in Instrument Evaluation

Pretesting and Piloting an Instrument

Pretesting (trying out an instrument with a few volunteers) and piloting (trying out the research procedure as a small-scale trial run) can be useful in choosing and using an instrument. The following instrumentation issues can be addressed in a pretest or pilot study:[45]

- Perform reliability and validity checks.
- Reduce random error by assessing subjects' response to the instrument. Are the instructions clear? Do they understand the questions and answer them correctly? Do some questions cause embarrassment or resistance? Is cheating or unwanted collaboration among subjects a problem?
- Obtain accurate estimates of the time required to complete the instrument and of the cost of data collection.
- Determine that the tool will indeed yield the needed data and eliminate the collection of unnecessary data.
- Gain staff experience and confidence in working with the subjects and the tool.
- Standardize rater, interview, and other measurement techniques.

A pilot also can be performed to compare two or more instruments and aid one's final choice. Sometimes piloting should be conducted in phases to allow successive refinements or to address problems in some logical sequence.

Subjects for a pilot study should be as similar as possible to those in the eventual study group but should not serve in both the pilot and data-producing groups. Nurse researchers too often are content to obtain only the views of fellow nurses or graduate students or faculty; although their evaluations may be helpful, they are no substitute for representatives of the study populations. For most trial runs, a sample size of 10 to 20 should suffice. More may be needed if the measurement procedure is complex or if the sample is heterogeneous.[9]

For maximum benefit from a pilot study, the investigator should observe subjects as they complete the tool and then interview them about their reactions. The meaning of subjects' nonverbal responses should be explored. Do frowns, fidgets, and many erasures indicate ambiguity in the tool, resistance to the content or circumstances of administration, or genuine involvement? Because of the small sample size and the relative artificiality of the situation, a pilot study cannot anticipate or solve all problems.[45] Nevertheless, few research procedures are as useful.

Sources of Help with Instrument Evaluation

Several sources of help with instrument selection and use are available if needed. The references at the end of this chapter and the other references in this book can be consulted. As they vary considerably in difficulty, Table 1.1 lists annotated works that are particularly clear and complete.[46-51]

The research faculty of a nearby school of nursing or hospital also may be able to help. One can write to the tool developer or to previous users of a tool. The directories of research and clinical organizations often identify members with expertise in instru-

Table 1.1 Instrument Development Resources

References	Description of Resource
Waltz et al. (15)	Single, most comprehensive treatment of measurement in nursing; covers both norm- and criterion-referenced measurement
	Clearly written, free of jargon, with step-by-step descriptions on how to perform measurement calculations
	Contains outstanding, "user-friendly" chapter on physiologic research (43)
Cox (46)	Excellent description of the conceptualization and early psychometric development of an instrument
	Illustrates item analysis and refinement through item correlations
	Clear example of factor analysis
Foreman (47)	Provides clear illustrations of many aspects of reliability and validity in relation to specific instruments
	Discusses selection of instruments
	Feasibility evaluated
Prescott & Phillips (48) Prescott et al. (49) Castorr et al. (24) Prescott et al. (50) Soeken & Prescott (51)	Provide an unusually clear and complete account of the development of an instrument, from conceptualization through confirmatory factor analysis

Numbers in parentheses correspond to studies used in the References.

mentation and willingness to consult on it. For example, Sigma Theta Tau, the Midwest Nursing Research Society, and the Oncology Nursing Society all publish informative membership directories.

Putting It All Together

These are important questions to consider when evaluating existing instruments:

- *Purpose.* Is the purpose of the tool clearly defined? Is the purpose similar to that of my study?
- *Measurement framework.* Is the measurement framework specified? Is it appropriate for my study?
- *Conceptual base.* Is the conceptual base stated? Implied? Is it at least compatible with my orientation to the problem?
- *Subjects.* Are the intended subjects clearly described? Are they similar to those in my proposed study? If not, how do they differ? Are they more or less heterogeneous than my subjects will be? How many subjects have contributed to the development of this tool?
- *Data-gathering method.* What method is used? Is the method properly used? What are the advantages and disadvantages of this method?
- *Content.* Is the content dated or current? Is a rationale apparent for each item?
- *Administration and scoring.* Are these clearly described? Will the conditions of administration be similar in my study? Will I need help in scoring or interpreting the results?
- *Reliability and validity.* Can the response be faked or distorted easily (a threat to validity)? Are multiple and appropriate forms of reliability and validity reported? Are reliability and validity coefficients appropriately high for the concept being measured?
- *Sensitivity.* Will this instrument make discriminations of the necessary fineness?
- *Appropriateness.* Is the reading level suited to the intended subjects? Do assumptions made about things like standard of living or cultural backgrounds fit the intended subjects?

- *Objectivity.* Has the developer identified steps taken to ensure the objectivity of the data? Are there any unidentified threats to objectivity?
- *Feasibility.* How much time will subjects need to complete this tool? Will subjects be able to do this task under the conditions for my study? Can I afford to use this tool? Will this tool need to be modified before I can use it? Do I have the expertise to make these modifications? If not, can I find help to do this?

Because few instruments have model histories, the evaluation of instruments always is a judgment call. If you answered most questions positively and you generally believe that the tool meets your needs, use it. If there are major doubts, look for another tool or conduct a pilot study. A helpful hint: Saving the written assessment of tools will soon result in a useful tool file.[15] Tools not used for one study may suit another.

Ethical and Legal Aspects of Tools

The ethical and legal use of instruments places obligations on the investigator to the subjects, the developer or publisher of the tool, and the professional and scientific communities. Because obligations to subjects are described in most research texts or can be clarified by research review boards, this discussion will focus on the obligations to the developer and the larger community.

Ethical considerations are inherent in the measurement considerations just discussed. The thoughtful selection of an appropriate instrument and its proper use are themselves ethical acts. Failure to perform them is at best a waste of time and at worst a hindrance to the advancement of nursing knowledge.

Obligations to the Instrument Developer

The user's first obligation to the developer is to obtain his or her written permission to use the tool. Doing so may or may not be simple. Because research literature gives very little guidance about this, the following experiential suggestions are offered.

Ideally, the tool's developer will be at the institution named in the source of the tool. If not, an address may sometimes be obtained from a later publication by the developer, from another user of the tool, or from a publisher. Membership directories of professional organizations, conference brochures, lists of conference participants, and one's own network may also be helpful. For ready reference, this book's Compendium contains sample research tools with their sources.

The letter to the tool's developer should be short and simple. The user should state that he or she wishes to use Instrument X described in Journal Y for Purpose Z. (The name of the tool and the source are important because authors may have published more than one tool in more than one source.) A short abstract or a three- or four-sentence description of the project should be provided. It is permissible to ask authors whether they have more recent information about the tool to share, but they should not be expected to review the literature. The letter should close with an offer to share the findings, an indication of when they may be available, and a statement that a full credit will be given to the developer. If six weeks pass without reply, a courteous second letter may be sent, inquiring whether the previous one was received and requesting a prompt reply.

Although most authors are delighted when people wish to use their instruments, the replies are not always favorable. Some authors do not release their tools until they are highly developed or until they have written a certain article or grant proposal. Others grant permission for use but attach a list of conditions. For example, they may charge for the tool's use, limit the number of copies allowed, stipulate that the instrument may not be altered, request a report of the results, or ask that the responses to the tool be shared for the ongoing validation of the tool. Users are obligated to fulfill those conditions unless they can negotiate otherwise.

The user's second obligation to the tool's developer is to report the results of the tool's use to the developer, whether or not such feedback was requested. Information about difficulties encountered, additional determinations of reliability and validity, and suggestions for modification or future use help the developer to improve the tool and aid the accumulation of knowledge about it.[15]

Obligations to a Test Publisher

Some instruments are available from commercial test publishers. The publisher can be identified in the publication describing the tool, by the author, or by the publisher's catalog. In this case, users purchase the manual and copies and may be asked to document their qualifications for using the instrument properly. Acceptable documentation may consist of a graduate degree in a field that emphasizes measurement, the titles and credit hours of measurement courses, membership in a professional organizations concerned with measurement, and a brief list of one's research activities. Investigators who cannot provide such documentation must order through a qualified individual who consents to supervise the use of the instrument. Improper use could result in the loss of ordering privileges for the supervisor.

Obligations to the Scientific and Professional Communities

Knowledge about tools and their applications cannot accumulate if the research is never published. The most available and enduring form of publication is a journal article.

The goal of a report on tool use is to provide enough information so that a reader can determine that sound measurement principles were observed and reach justified conclusions about the findings. In these reports, full credit must be given to the original developer. Any modifications in tool content, administration, scoring, or interpretation must be clearly described, along with psychometric data about the changes. Information about extraneous or confounding variables that might have influenced subjects' scores should be provided. Reports of problems and failures with a tool are as useful to other investigators as reports of success.[14]

Copyright Considerations

Copyrights involve both legal and ethical aspects of tool use. If an entire instrument is published in a journal, it is considered to be in the public domain and may be used without formal permission unless the author has retained the copyright, which will be indicated by a copyright symbol, ©. An example is found in the article by Hymovich.[52] If the author has the copyright, he or she must be contacted; in either case, it is both wise and courteous to do so because further work may have been done on the tool. The journal retains a copyright on the article regardless of who owns the tool, and proper citation of the published source is mandatory. Permission is needed to adapt items or to alter the tool.

The question, "Can I use a tool if I can't find the author after a reasonable effort to do so?" occasionally arises, usually in reference to a situation in which the author published a tool in full and retained the copyright. The wording of the U.S. copyright law[53] makes this unlikely. Works created on or after January 1, 1978, are protected for the life of the author and for 50 years after the author's death, to be ascertained by mortality records in the Register of Copyrights. An article by Owen[54] presents an excellent explanation of the rights of copyright owners and of the doctrine of fair use that governs copying for personal use. Tool users should be aware that duplicating a copyrighted instrument for use in a research study without permission of the copyright owner is *not* fair use. Questions about reasonable access and use of copyrighted works should be taken to a copyright lawyer. The legal counsel of a hospital or school of nursing also may give advice on these matters.

References

1. American Psychological Association, American Educational Research Association and National Council on Measurement in Education. *Standards for educational and psychological testing.* Washington, DC: American Psychological Association, 1985.
2. Anastasi, A. Evolving concepts of test validation. *Ann Rev Psychol*, 1986, 37:1.
3. Norbeck, J.S. What constitutes a publishable report of instrument development? *Nurs Res*, 1986, 34(6):380.
4. Messick, S. Validity. In R.L. Linn (Ed.), *Educational measurement* (3rd ed.). New York: American Council on Education/Macmillan, 1989, p. 13.
5. Waltz, C.F., & Strickland, O.L. Measurement of nursing outcomes: State of the art as we enter the eighties. In W.E. Field (Ed.), *Measuring outcomes of nursing practice, education, and administration: Proceedings of the First Annual Southern Council on Collegiate Education for Nursing Research Conference.* Atlanta: Southern Regional Education Board, 1982, p. 47.
6. Strickland, O.L., & Waltz, C.F. Measurement of research variables in nursing. In P.L. Chinn (Ed.), *Nursing research methodology: Issues and implementation.* Rockville, MD: Aspen, 1986, p. 79.
7. Gay, L.R. *Educational evaluation and measurement* (2nd ed.). Columbus, OH: Merrill, 1985.
8. Rabkin, J.S., & Struening, C.B. Life events, stress, and illness. *Science*, 1976, 194(3269):1013.
9. Polit, D., & Hungler, B. *Nursing research: Principles and methods* (5th ed.). Philadelphia: Lippincott, 1995.
10. Ellis, R. Characteristics of significant theories. *Nurs Res*, 1968, 17(3):217.
11. Fitzpatrick, J., Whall, A., Johnston, R., & Floyd, J. *Nursing models and their psychiatric mental health applications.* Bowie, MD: Brady, 1982.
12. Jacobson, S.F. Stresses and coping strategies of neonatal intensive care unit nurses. *Res Nurs Health*, 1983, 6(1):33-40.
13. Kearney, B., & Fleischer, B. Development of an instrument to measure exercise of self-care agency. *Res Nurs Health*, 1979, 2(1):25.
14. Walker, L.O., & Avant, K.D. *Strategies for theory construction in nursing.* Norwalk, CT: Appleton-Century-Crofts, 1983.
15. Waltz, C.F., Strickland, O.L, & Lenz, E.R. *Measurement in nursing research* (2nd ed.). Philadelphia: Davis, 1991.
16. Mishel, M.H. Methodological studies: Instrument development. In P.J. Brink & M.J. Wood (Eds.), *Advanced design in nursing research.* Newbury Park, CA: Sage, 1989, p. 238.
17. Kerlinger, F.N. *Foundations of behavioral research* (3rd ed.). New York: Holt, Rinehart, and Winston, 1986.
18. Wilson, H.S. (Ed.) *Research in nursing* (2nd ed.). Redwood City, CA: Addison-Wesley, 1989.
19. Ferketich, S. Aspects of item analysis. *Res Nurs Health*, 1991, 14(2):165-168.
20. Knapp, T.R. Validity, reliability, and neither. *Nurs Res*, 1985, 34(3):189.
21. Fox, D.J. *Fundamentals of research in nursing* (4th ed.). Norwalk, CT: Appleton-Century-Crofts, 1982.
22. Hoskins, C.N. Psychometrics in nursing research: Further development of the interpersonal conflict scale. *Res Nurs Health*, 1983, 6(2):75.
23. Washington, C.C., & Moss, M. Pragmatic aspects of establishing interrater reliability in research. *Nurs Res*, 1988, 37(3):190.
24. Castorr, A.H., Thompson, K.O., Ryan, J.W., et al. The process of rater training for observational instruments: Implications for interrater reliability. *Res Nurs Health*, 1990, 13(5):311.
25. Cohen, J. A coefficient of agreement for nominal scales. *Educ Psychol Meas*, 1960, 20(1):37.
26. Cohen, J. Weighted kappa: Nominal scale agreement with provision for scaled disagreement or partial credit. *Psychol Bull*, 1968, 70(4):213.
27. Topf, M. Three estimates of interrater reliability for nominal data. *Nurs Res*, 1986, 36(4):253-255.
28. Ferketich, S. Internal consistency estimates of reliability. *Res Nurs Health*, 1990, 13(6):437.
29. Zeller, R.P., & Carmines, E.G. *Measurement in the social sciences.* Cambridge, England: Cambridge University Press, 1980.
30. Humenick, S.S. *Analysis of current assessment strategies in the health care of young children and childbearing families.* Norwalk, CT: Appleton-Century-Crofts, 1982.
31. Hartmann, D. Considerations in the choice of interobserver reliability estimates. *J Appl Behav Anal*, 1977, 10(1):103.
32. Landis, J.R., & Koch, G.G. The measurement of observer agreement for categorical data. *Biometrics*, 1977, 33(1):159.
33. Nunnally, J.C., & Bernstein, I.H. *Psychometric theory* (3rd ed). New York: McGraw-Hill, 1994.
34. Feldt, L.S., & Brennan, R.L. Reliability. In R.L. Linn (Ed.), *Educational measurement* (3rd ed.). New York: American Council on Education/Macmillan, 1989, p. 105.
35. Shavelson, R.J., & Webb, N. *Generalizability theory: A primer.* Newbury Park, CA: Sage, 1991.
36. Lynn, M.R. Determination and quantification of content validity. *Nurs Res*, 1986, 35(6):382-385.
37. Mishel, M.H. The measurement of uncertainty in illness. *Nurs Res*, 1981, 30(5):258.
38. Tilden, V.P., Nelson, C.A., & May, B.A. Use of qualitative methods to enhance content validity. *Nurs Res*, 1990, 30(3):172.

39. Bentler, P.M. Factor analysis. In *Research issues 13: Data analysis strategies and designs for substance abuse research.* Report No. 017-024-00562-2. Rockville, MD: National Institute on Drug Abuse, December 1976, p. 139.

40. Boyd, C.J., Frey, M.A., & Aaronson, L.S. Structural equation models and nursing research: Part I. *Nurs Res*, 1988, *37*(4):249.

41. Aaronson, L.S., Frey, M.A., & Boyd, C.J. Structural equation models and nursing research: Part II. *Nurs Res*, 1988, *37*(5):315.

42. Kovacs, A.R. *The research process: Essentials of skill development.* Philadelphia: Davis, 1985.

43. DeKeyser, F.G., & Pugh, L.C. Approaches to physiologic measurement. In C.F. Waltz, O.L. Strickland, & E.R. Lenz (Eds.), *Measurement in nursing research* (2nd ed.). Philadelphia: Davis, 1991, p. 387.

44. Lindsey, A.M., & Stotts, N.A. Collecting data on biophysiologic variables. In H.S. Wilson (Ed.), *Research in nursing* (2nd ed.). Redwood City, CA: Addison-Wesley, 1989, p. 374.

45. Fox, R.N., & Ventura, M. Small scale administration of instruments and procedures. *Nurs Res*, 1983, *32*(2):122.

46. Cox, C.L. The health self-determinism index. *Nurs Res*, 1985, *34*(3):177.

47. Foreman, M.D. Reliability and validity of mental status questionnaires in elderly hospitalized patients. *Nurs Res*, 1987, *36*(4):216.

48. Prescott, P.A., & Phillips, C.Y. Gauging nursing intensity to bring costs to light. *Nurs Health Care*, 1988, *9*(1):17.

49. Prescott, P.A., Soeken, K.L., & Ryan, J.W. Measuring patient intensity: A reliability study. *Eval Health Prof*, 1989, *12*(3):255.

50. Prescott, P.A., Ryan, J.W., Soeken, K.L., et al. The Patient Intensity for Nursing Index: A validity assessment. *Res Nurs Health*, 1991, *14*(3):213.

51. Soeken, K.L., & Prescott, P.A. Patient Intensity for Nursing Index: The measurement model. *Res Nurs Health*, 1991, *14*(4):297.

52. Hymovich, D. The chronicity impact and coping instrument: Parent questionnaire. *Nurs Res*, 1983, *32*(5):275.

53. Farnighetti, R. (Ed.). Copyright law of the United States. In *The world almanac and book of facts.* Mohwah, NJ: Funk and Wagnalls, 1994, p. 270.

54. Owen, S. Copyright law: How it affects your hospital and you. *J Nurs Admin*, 1987, *17*(10):32.

2

Tool Adaptation for Socioeconomically Disadvantaged Populations

Sally P. Weinrich, Marlyn D. Boyd, and Barbara D. Powe

Nearly *one-half* of adult Americans are literacy impaired to the point that they have difficulty holding a job and using everyday written materials such as menus and written directions for taking medications.[1] Similarly, they have difficulty answering questionnaires. Although the number of instruments useful for nursing research are increasing, few are designed specifically for use with socioeconomically disadvantaged (SED) populations. This chapter provides guidelines for the evaluation and adaptation of instruments for use with SED populations.

There is no set definition for SED populations. Definitions usually are based on income and education levels and may include the criterion of Medicaid eligibility. Income qualification may be defined as being at or below the poverty level. Education usually is defined as having little or no formal education, that is, having completed less than the eighth grade. Frequently, SED populations are disproportionately made up of minorities and of persons with limited social experiences. However, minority status should not be the determining criteria in SED classification.[2] For the purposes of this chapter, SED is defined as impaired literacy and/or having an income that is insufficient to meet one's basic needs adequately.

In 1990, over 13% of the population had incomes below the poverty level. Racial percentages for incomes below the poverty level were whites, 11%; African Americans, 32%; and Hispanics, 28%.[3] In 1986, 9 percent of the population was covered by Medicaid.[3] Older persons with their limited income are at risk for being SED. Research often targets SED populations because they, more so than any other group, are less likely to practice prevention measures, are at greater risk for a myriad of conditions and diseases, and have higher mortality rates.

Nearly one-half of all people in the United States read and write so poorly that it is difficult for them to function effectively in a literate society.[1] A high school diploma does not guarantee literacy.[1] Although grade completed of formal schooling and reading ability are not synonymous, there is some correlation. Most studies have found that people tend to read three to five grade levels below the last grade completed.[4-7] If reading is not used in work or leisure activities, skills deteriorate over time.[5-8] SED populations have a disproportionate number of literacy-impaired individuals. It is important for the researcher to remember that impaired literacy does *not* mean that the SED participant has *below-normal intelligence*. Instead, the SED study participant has been undereducated and because of that, has a deficit in the use of written and oral language in a literate society. These limitations can greatly affect test outcomes.

The SED study participant may have difficulty in a number of areas that can affect the validity and reliability of instruments. Impaired language skills including a limited vocabulary can mean that the study participant's viewpoint is limited to his or her own personal experience.[4] Extrapolating to an unknown may be an impossible task for the SED participant. For example, if an SED participant is asked, "What would you do if you started having bad headaches?," the SED participant might answer, "No, I don't ever get bad headaches." The participant may not be able to think abstractly outside of his or her present state.

Another limitation may be that the SED participant may not comprehend the rationale for questions. When asked, "Tell me how you fix your meals," the SED participant may say, "Well you know, just like I always done." The rational for attitude or opinion questions can be especially confusing. For example, in response to questions about fear of cancer, respondents have responded to the authors with "Are you trying to trick me?" Similarly, the rationale for mental status questions can be confusing to older SED populations. The ten mental status questions[9] include questions such as "Who is the current president, and who was the past president?" Noninstitutionalized well elderly participants asked these questions responded with "I'm not crazy," "Don't you think I know what I'm doing?," and even "I'm not going to answer anymore." These authors have reduced the ten mental status questionnaire to two questions dealing with date and location. Experience has shown that these two questions are reliable indicators of mental status in older *noninstitutionalized* SED populations.

Similarly, an SED study participant may have difficulty categorizing data. Asking participants to choose foods low in fat or list several aerobic exercises may result in no response or a jumbled list of several foods and activity items. Literacy-impaired individuals also may have difficulty with abstract concepts, synthesizing data, and problem solving. Asking a cardiac rehabilitation patient to describe how the heart works may net the interviewer a prolonged silence from the participant who cannot conceptualize the heart's physiology.

The literacy-impaired study participant usually has a very limited vocabulary and is not capable of distinguishing between nuances of terms or distinguishing between a spectrum of options. For cxample, asking an SED individual to describe pain in several terms such as burning, stabbing, or radiating may only confuse the respondent. Likewise, some Likert-type scales may be too confusing to respond to with accuracy or reliability. Because reading and/or listening can be difficult, SED study participants may be easily distracted, have short attention spans, refuse to complete a tool, or become irritable or angry.

The high literacy level of patient education materials has been documented in several studies.[7,10-12] Although the reading levels of instruments in the first edition of this book vary considerably, the majority are written on a high school or college level. And the instruments that do have a reading level in the eighth-grade range do so only by using few polysyllabic words. However, unfortunately, these instruments often include single- and two-syllable words that are too sophisticated for the SED reader. Examples of words used in the instruments that the SED persons will probably have trouble understanding include crisis situation, esteem, competency, emotional support, extent, characteristics, attractive, annoyed, and symptoms.

Tools Designed for SED Populations

Few tools exist that were designed specifically for SED population.[13-18] Three of the best tools include the Dartmouth Primary Care Cooperative Information scales (COOP),[16-19] the John Henryism Scale for Active Coping (JHAC-12),[13,20] and the Knowledge of Colorectal Cancer Questionnaire.[14]

Adaptation of Existing Tools

A few studies have adapted instruments for SED populations.[17,21-28] Adaptations have included adjustments for literacy and cultural level and pilot-testing of the instrument. Bill-Harvey et al.'s study with arthritic patients is one of the best studies reported in the literature that has adapted a tool for an SED population.[25]

Existing instruments can and should be adapted when used with an SED population or when used with an SED population that is different from the population for which the instrument was developed.[29] For example, the instrument could have been used with low-income urban persons, and it will now be used for low-income migratory farm workers. Changes in the instrument should include reducing the literacy level, changing individual words, widening the response options, being aware of socially desirable answers, and shortening the instrument. A comprehensive assessment of the SED population is the initial step.

Assessing the SED Population

Population assessment and pilot studies are crucial first steps in the development of a valid and reliable instrument.[30] Data about the population to be studied can be obtained from patient records, regional and local databases, and individuals. Data, such as age, gender, education, ethnicity, and work history, can be obtained from records or databases. A small pilot sample of the study population needs to be interviewed for factors such as instrument readability (if tool is to be self-administered), oral comprehension (if interview format is to be used), and slang or regional terms used by the SED population for concepts that are being measured.

Reducing Literacy Level

The subjects' reading abilities, as well as the literacy level of the instrument, need to be assessed.[4] Every subject's reading level need not be tested; but rather, a random sample of the typical client population should be tested to establish a baseline or profile for the study population. One quick, easy, and accurate method of testing a subject's reading ability is to use the reading subtest of the Wide Range Achievement Test (WRAT). This brief test (five minutes or less) is normed on age versus grade levels and is a good clinical tool for assessing reading ability.[31] It is noteworthy that the authors of this chapter have found major inconsistencies with SED populations in self-reported educational level and actual reading level when using the WRAT.

Measuring the literacy level of the instrument with a readability formula also is important. Readability formulas are mathematical equations that predict the level of reading ability needed to understand a printed piece. Readability formulas measure various grammatical components, such as sentence length, the number of syllables, and word familiarity. The SMOG and Fry's Readability Formula are common readability formulas.[8,32-35] They are accurate to within 1.5 to 2 grade levels.[33] Appendices 2A and 2B provide guidelines for using the SMOG formula. Today, many computer word processing programs have readability assessment programs that can be easily accessed.

Reducing the literacy level of an instrument includes avoiding the use of three- or more syllable words and using short words; short sentences; the active rather than passive voice; boldface type, italic, or underline for emphasis; pictures to illustrate concepts; analogies or examples for abstract terms; and giving simple directions (Exhibit 2.1).[30] For example, consider the differences in wording in the following:

- *College reading level.* With the onset of nausea, diarrhea, or other gastrointestinal disturbances, consult your physician immediately.
- *Twelfth-grade reading level.* If you experience nausea, diarrhea, or other stomach or bowel problems, call your physician immediately.
- *Eighth-grade reading level.* If you start having nausea, loose bowel movements, or other stomach or bowel problems, call your doctor immediately.
- *Fourth-grade reading level.* If you start having an upset stomach, loose bowel movements, or other problems, call your doctor right away.[3]

Exhibit 2.1 Reduction of Literacy Level

- Avoid words with three syllables or more. For example, use "doctor" rather than "physician," and use "cut" instead of "laceration."
- Use shorter words for longer ones. For example, "give" versus "administer" or "wipe clean" versus "thoroughly cleanse."
- Use short sentences of about ten words or less.
- Avoid complex sentence structures.
- Use the active rather than the passive voice.
- Use simple directions.
- Assess your population, and use words that have meaning to your population.
- Use concrete examples rather than abstract ones whenever possible.
- Use boldface type, italicize, or underline words and ideas for emphasis.
- Use pictures to illustrate concepts whenever possible.
- Use analogies or examples for abstract terms.
- Avoid medical abbreviations such as MI, SCAN, or TRP.
- Pilot-test instrument with population.
- Use white space to rest the eyes (double spacing and margins).
- Use uppercase and lowercase letters. ALL CAPS MAKES TEXT HARDER TO READ.
- Use type appropriate for age or vision. For example, 8 to 10 point type should be used for patients with normal vision, and 12 to 14 point type should be used for patients with failing vision and for children:

this is 8 point type
this is 10 point type
this is 12 point type
this is 14 point type

Serif type (letters with horizontal strokes at the bottoms and tops of letters) should be used; it is easier to read than sans-serif.

Adapted from Weinrich, S.P., & Boyd, M. Education in the elderly: Adapting and evaluating teaching tools. *J. Gerontol Nurs,* 1992, *18*(1):15-20.

The effectiveness and reliability of pictures to measure functional status also have been documented. In a study by Larson et al.,[36] no response differences occurred between patients who received functional questions that were depicted with pictures and those who received written text and no pictures.

Wording Changes

Individual words may have different meanings for various populations. Some participants in the authors' study of colorectal cancer[37] thought "stool" meant bar stool and were quite puzzled when asked if they had ever tested their stool for hidden blood. There are no set guidelines for what SED persons will and will not understand. Each instrument must be pilot-tested, and changes made based on target population feedback. Socioeconomically disadvantaged persons often hide the fact that they do not understand. They have had a lifetime of reading incomprehensible material and are not used to an environment where they can feel safe admitting their confusion or lack of understanding. For example, the misinterpretation of stool was identified by another SED person who was hired as a research assistant in the Colorectal Cancer Project.[38] Of special significance was the fact that the researcher failed to detect this misunderstanding in the pilot studies, even though a special effort to check literacy levels and understanding was made.

Medical jargon usually is not understood by the general population, including SED populations. For example, diabetes often is referred to as "sugar," hypertension as "high blood pressure," and anemia as "low blood." Commonly used examples heard by these authors are listed in Table 2.1. Again, the *specific* SED population would need to be interviewed and words that they use identified for each questionnaire.

Socioeconomically disadvantaged persons are primarily concrete thinkers and may have difficulty understanding abstract concepts. For example, an SED participant may have great difficulty understanding the heart's need for oxygen (air), until it is compared to a car engine's need for gas. Testing of the meaning of abstract terms usually takes more time; however, without this step of the process, the instrument may not be valid.

Identifying confusing or misunderstood words in a group setting usually is ineffective as people do not like to admit in public what they do not understand. Pilot-testing

Table 2.1 Laypersons' Terms for Common Medical Conditions

Medical Condition	Laypersons' Terms
Anemia	Low blood, poor blood, tired blood
Arthritis	Stiffness, old joint disease, bursitis, gout, joint misery, old stiffness, rheumatism, Arthur
Cardiovascular disease	Heart trouble, bad heart
Constipation	Stopped up, bowels locked, bowel misery
Diabetes	Sugar, rot, high sugar
Diarrhea	Runs, outhouse trot, runny bowels
Hypertension	High blood pressure, high blood
Migraine headache	Sick headache, period headache
Sickle cell anemia	Blood disease, black curse
Syphilis	Bad blood
Pulmonary disease	The wheeze, breathing disease, bad lungs
Urinary retention	Kidneys won't act, water backed up, can't make water
Impotence	Trouble with my nature
Urinate	Pee, make water, make kidneys act, locked kidneys, piss

should include individual questioning of study participants in a nonthreatening and private setting. To encourage pilot study participants to help to identify confusing words, concepts, or sentences we suggest asking: "We will be asking many people like you these questions. Will you help me find questions that are not clear?" Or "Will you tell me what this means to you?" If the answer is "Yes," the questions should be read one at a time and the goal (identification of confusing words/concepts) repeated often. Also, asking about a specific word is effective. For example, "Many people do not know what 'bran' means. What does it mean to you?"

Changes in Response Options

Many instruments use Likert-type responses that have four- to five-answer options. Some SED persons think in terms of Yes or No rather than variations of Yes and No. The researcher should try to encourage an answer first by saying such things as "Is that a strong Yes or a weak Yes?" if Likert-type responses are more desirable. Results need to be analyzed. If all the responses fall in two categories rather than four, the instrument may need to be changed to Yes and No responses. For example, in developing of the Knowledge of Colorectal Cancer Questionnaire,[14] five response items were originally used: strongly agree, agree, disagree, strongly disagree, and don't know. In the pilot studies, respondents would answer "Yes" or "No." Trying to force a response by asking, "Is that a strong yes or just a Yes?" resulted in confusion and misunderstanding among the participants. From their concrete perspective, they had already answered "Yes" or "No" and did not understand why they were being asked the same question again. Repeating and trying to force an answer to cover all of the questions was a deterrent to the interview process, not an enhancing factor. When the response options were changed to "Yes" or "True" and "No" or "False," the interviewing process ran much more smoothly. The "Yes" or "No" responses were used by most of the respondents. However, a small minority of about 15% would answer "True" or "False." So both options were retained on the questionnaire with the "True, False" option being placed in parentheses under the "Yes, No" option:[14]

Bowel cancer is always a deadly disease.
Yes   No   Don't Know
(True)   (False)

The key point here is to measure what works in *each individually* selected SED population. Research studies are needed to document the effect of changes in response options on the sensitivity and reliability of instruments.

Awareness of Socially Desirable Answers

Socioeconomically disadvantaged persons may have a greater tendency to deny reality[39] or answer in terms of socially desirable answers. For example, questions that measured instrumental activities of daily living (dressing, cooking, shopping, cleaning house, and phone use)[40] were used in a research project that involved older SED people.[37] Most of these people wanted to be independent in their activities of daily living, and data analyses revealed that the majority had answered that they were independent. Experience had taught these authors that the participants were more dependent than the data revealed. Changing the stem from "Can you fix your meals?" to " Tell me what problems you have with fixing your meals." resulted in answers that reflected greater levels of dependence.

Shortening the Instrument

Many SED persons have not had previous or recent experience(s) with questionnaires. It is important to measure the time for administration of the instrument with *your* SED population. Fatigue and/or disinterest can be a factor with lengthy tools. This information is best gathered through a pilot test and observation. The researcher should look for changes in behavior from the beginning to the end of the tool administration. Examples of fatigue and/or disinterest could include looking up frequently, squirming, gazing out a window, and/or failure to complete the questionnaire. In addition, test–retest procedures can be used to check for the effect of test fatigue. For this assessment, the position of items are switched to determine whether items answered at the end of the instrument are answered in a significantly different manner from items answered at the beginning of the instrument. If items are eliminated from an instrument, reliability and validity analyses[41] are critical.

Pilot Studies and Instrument Reliability and Validity

Reliability and validity analyses are mandatory in using instruments with SED populations, including at the pilot study phase (see Chapter 1, "Evaluating Instruments for Use in Clinical Nursing Research). Reliability is affected by the number of items. The shorter the instrument, the lower the reliability. Frequently, short instruments are needed for SED populations. Principal component analyses[42] or Spearman–Brown prophecy formula[43] can be used to obtain improved scores with shorter instruments. Time to revise the instrument and make changes *before* beginning the main research needs to be allocated.

There are no research studies that contrast reliability analyses on SED populations and non-SED populations. It has been the experience of these authors that SED populations tend to have lower questionnaire reliability results than non-SED populations. Additional research is needed in this area.

Administration of Instruments

Different administration procedures are needed with an SED population. These include interviewing, considering environmental conditions, collecting of sensitive data, and wording of informed consent. Socioeconomically disadvantaged persons may not be able to read. If this is the case, the instrument will need to be read to the subject, and responses scored by an interviewer. Uniform procedures for administration of the instrument, as well as interviewer training, are needed. Individual variations in interviewing can have significant effects on responses. Data analyses should include analyses by the interviewer to detect whether trends or consistent differences in responses are occurring. Environmental conditions that reduce noise and provide privacy are important.

Certain data, such as income, are sensitive to collect regardless of the socioeconomic background of the population. If this information is collected in a group setting, identify ways in which the respondents' privacy can be maintained. For example, in the Colorectal Cancer Project, which included reading and scoring of the instrument by an interviewer, the income options were typed in large print on a separate piece of paper. The respondent was asked to point to the monthly income that was most similar to his or her income. The respondent's privacy was maintained, and the income answer was never said out loud by the interviewer.

Informed consents usually accompany instrument administration. Unfortunately, most informed consent forms have a reading level of twelfth grade or college level.[44-46] The discussion about assessing and reducing the literacy level of an instrument to match each SED population applies to the informed consent as well.

References

1. National Center for Education. *Adult literacy in Americans.* Washington, DC: Educational Testing Service, Department of Education, 1993.
2. Krieger, N. Analyzing socioeconomic and racial/ethnic patterns in health and health care. *Am J Public Health*, 1993, *83*(8):1086-1087.
3. U.S. Department of Commerce, Economics and Statistics Administration. *Statistical abstract of the United States, 1992.* Washington, DC: Bureau of the Census, U.S. Government Printing Office, 1992.
4. Doak, C.C., Doak, L.G., & Root, J.H. *Teaching patients with low literacy skills.* Philadelphia, PA: Lippincott, 1985.
5. Boyd, M.D., & Feldman, H.L. Information seeking and reading and comprehension abilities of cardiac rehab patients. *J Cardiac Rehab*, 1984, *4*:343-347.
6. Boyd, M.D., Gallagher, E., & Brunner, C.M. Systemic lupus erythematosus patient education literature: A comparison of reading levels of literature and the reading abilities of patients. *Clin Rheumatol Practice*, 1985, *3*:58-64.
7. Boyd, M.D. Patient education literature: A comparison of reading levels and the reading ability of patients. In J.H. Humphrey (Ed.), *Advances in health education: Current research.* New York: AMS Press, 1988, pp. 101-110.
8. Whitman, N.I., Graham, B.A., Gelit, C.J., & Boyd, M.D. *Teaching in nursing practice: A professional model.* Norwalk, CT: Appleton & Lange, 1992.
9. Kahn, R.L., Goldfarb, A.I., Pollack, M., & Peck, A. Brief objective measure for the determination of mental status in the aged. *Am J Psychiatry*, 1960, *117*:326.
10. Meade, C., Diekman, J., & Thornhill, D. Readability of American Cancer Society patient education literature. *Oncol Nurs Forum*, 1992, *19*(1):51-55.
11. Stephens, S. Patient education materials: Are they readable? *Oncol Nurs Forum*, 1992, *19*(1):83-85.
12. Michielutte, R., Bahnson, J., & Beal, P. Readability of the public education literature on cancer prevention and detection. *J Cancer Educ* 1990, *5*(1):55-61.
13. James, S.A., Hartnett, S.A., & Kalsbeek, W.D. John Henryism and blood pressure differences among black men. *J Behav Med*, 1983, *6*:259-278.
14. Weinrich, S.P., Weinrich, M.C., Boyd, M.D., et al. Knowledge of colorectal cancer among older persons. *Cancer Nurs*, 1992, *15*(5):322-330.
15. Weinrich, S.P., & Weinrich, M.C. Cancer knowledge among elderly individuals. *Cancer Nurs*, 1986, *9*(6):301-307.
16. Nelson, E., Wasson, J., Kirk, J., et al. Assessment of function in routine clinical practice: Description of the Coop chart method and preliminary findings. *J Chron Dis*, 1987, *40*:55S-63S.
17. Nelson, E.C., Landgraf, R.D., Hays, J.W., et al. The COOP function charts: A system to measure patient function in physicians' offices. In WONCA Classification Committee (Eds.), *Functional status measurement in primary care.* New York: Springer-Verlag, 1990, pp. 97-131.
18. WONCA Classification Committee. *Functional status measurement in primary care.* New York: Springer-Verlag, 1990.
19. Nelson, E.C., Landgraf, J.M., Hays, R.D., et al. The functional status of patients: How can it be measured in physicians' offices? *Med Care*, 1990, *28*(12):1111-1126.
20. Weinrich, S.P., Weinrich, M.C., Keil, J.E., et al. The John Henryism and Framingham Type A Scales: Measurement properties in elderly blacks and whites. *Am J Epidemiol*, 1988, *128*(1):165-178.
21. Ammerman, A.S., DeVellis, B.M., Haines, P.S., et al. Nutrition education for cardiovascular disease prevention among low income populations—Description and pilot evaluation of a physician-based model. *Patient Educ Couns*, 1992, *19*:5-18.
22. Reis, J. Medicaid maternal and child health care: Prepaid plans vs. private fee-for-service. *Res Nurs Health*, 1990, *13*:163-171.
23. Flaskerud, J.H., & Nyamathi, A.M. Black and Latina womens' AIDS related knowledge, attitudes, and practices. *Res Nurs Health*, 1989, *12*:339-346.
24. Reis, J., Sherman, S., & Macon, J. Teaching inner-city mothers about family planning and prenatal and pediatric services. *J Pediatr Health Care*, 1989, *3*(5):251-256.
25. Bill-Harvey, D., Rippey, R., Abeles, M., et al. Outcome of an osteoarthritis education program for low-literacy patients taught by indigenous instructors. *Patient Educ Couns*, 1989, *13*:133-142.
26. Brannan, J.E. Accidental poisoning of children: Barriers to resource use in a black, low-income community. *Public Health Nurs*, 1992, *9*(2):81-86.
27. Nelson, E.C., Landgraf, J.M., Hays, et al. The functional status of patients. *Med Care* 1990a, *28*:111-1126.
28. Meyboom-de-Jong, B., Smith, R.J. Studies with the Dartmouth COOP Charts in General Practice: Comparison with the Nottingham Health Profile and the General Health Questionnaire. In WONCA Classification Committee (Eds.), *Functional status measurement in primary care.* New York: Springer-Verlag, 1990, pp. 132-149.
29. U.S. Department of Health and Human Services. Pretesting in health communication methods: Examples and resources for improving health messages and materials. NIH Pub. No. 83-1493. Bethesda, MD: National Cancer Institute, 1982.
30. Weinrich, S.P., & Boyd, M. Education in the elderly: Adapting and evaluating teaching tools. *J Gerontol Nurs*, 1992, *18*(1):15-20.
31. Jastak Associates, Inc. Wide Range Achievement Test. Wilmington, DE: Jastak Associates Inc., 1978.
32. McGraw, H.C. SMOG testing. In C. Doak, L.G. Doak, & J.H. Root (Eds.), *Teaching patients with low literacy skills.* Philadelphia, PA: Lippincott, 1985, pp. 36-37.
33. McLaughlin, G.H. SMOG grading—A new readability formula. *J Reading*, 1969, *12*:639-646.
34. Fry, E. A readability formula that saves time. In International Reading Association *Classroom Strategies for Secondary Reading.* Newark, DE: 1977, pp. 29-35.
35. Fry, E. Fry's Readability Graph: Clarifications, validity, and extension to level 17. *J Reading*, 1977, December:242-252.
36. Larson, C.O., Hays, R.D., & Nelson, E.C. Do the pictures influence scores on the Dartmouth COOP charts? *Qual Life Res*, 1992, *1*:247-249.

37. Weinrich, S.P., Weinrich, M.C., Boyd, M.D., et al. *Effective approaches for increasing compliance with ACS's screening recommendations in socioeconomically disadvantaged populations*. Atlanta: American Cancer Society, 1992, pp. 1-8.

38. Weinrich, S.W., Weinrich, M.C., Stromborg, M., et al. The elderly educator method. *The Gerontologist*, 1993 *33*:7-12.

39. Garrison, C.Z., Schoenbach, V.J., Schluchter, M.D., & Kaplan, B.H. Life events in early adolescence. *J Am Acad Child Adol Psychiatry*, 1987, *26*:865-872.

40. Duke University Center for the Study of Aging and Human Development. *Multidimensional Functional Assessment: The OARS Methodology*. Durham, NC: Duke University Medical Center, 1978.

41. Jacobson, S.F. Evaluating instruments for use in clinical nursing research. In M. Frank-Stromborg (Ed.), *Instruments for Clinical Nursing Research*. Norwalk, CT: Appleton & Lange, 1988, pp. 3-20.

42. Carmines, E.G., & Zeller, R.A. *Reliability and Validity Assessment*. Newbury Park, CA: Sage, 1979.

43. Sax, G. *Principles of educational and psychological measurement and evaluation*. Belmont, CA: Wadsworth, 1980.

44. Berg, A., & Hammilt, K.B. Assessing the psychiatric patient's ability to meet the literacy demands of hospitalization. *Hosp Comm Psychiatry*, 1980, *31*:266-268.

45. Bergler, J.H., Pennington, C., Metcalf, M., & Freis, E.D. Informed consent: How much does the patient understand? *Clin Pharmacol Ther*, 1980, *27*:435-439.

46. O'Connor, R.G. Informed consent: Legal, behavioral, and educational issues. *Patient Couns Health Educ*, 1991, *3*:49-55.

Appendix: SMOG Readability Formula

2A. Samples with at Least Thirty Sentences

1. Select a total of thirty sentences; ten consecutive sentences from the beginning, ten from the middle, and ten from the end of the written piece. A sentence is any string of words punctuated by a period, an exclamation point, or a question mark.

2. Count the words containing *three or more syllables*, including repetitions in the thirty sentences.

   _____ Hyphenated words are *one* word.

   _____ Pronounce numerals aloud, and count the syllables pronounced for each numeral (e.g., for the number 573, five = 1, hundred = 2, seventy = 3, and three = 1, or seven syllables).

   _____ Proper nouns should be counted.

   _____ If a long sentence has a colon, consider each part of it as a separate sentence. However, if possible, avoid selecting that segment of the passage.

   _____ The words for which the abbreviations stand should be read aloud to determine their syllable count (e.g., Oct. = October = 3 syllables).

3. Obtain the nearest perfect square root of the total number of words of three or more syllables and then add a constant of 3 to the square root to obtain the grade level:

   Example: First 10 sentences   = 23 polysyllabic words
   Second 10 sentences   = 22 polysyllabic words
   Third 10 sentences   = 22 polysyllabic words

                         Total 67 polysyllabic words

Obtain square root of 67 = 8.
Add the constant of 3.
8 + 3 = 11th grade.*

You can also use the following conversion method:

SMOG Conversion Table†

Word Count	Grade Level	Word Count	Grade Level
0– 2	4	73– 90	12
3– 6	5	91–110	13
7–12	6	111–132	14
13–20	7	133–156	15
21–30	8	157–182	16
31–42	9	183–210	17
43–56	10	211–240	18
57–72	11		

†Developed by Harold C. McGraw (32), Office of Educational Research, Baltimore County Public Schools, Towson, Maryland.

*McLaughlin, G.H. SMOG Grading—A New Readability Formula, *Journal of Reading*, 1969, 12:639-646.

2B. Samples with Fewer than Thirty Sentences

Number of Sentences	Word Count A (e.g., 6)	Conversion Number B	Reading Level = A × B*
29	6	1.03	7
28	6	1.07	6
27	6	1.1	7
26	6	1.15	6
25	6	1.2	7
24	6	1.25	8
23	6	1.3	8
22	6	1.36	9
21	6	1.43	9
20	6	1.5	9
19	6	1.58	10
18	6	1.67	10
17	6	1.76	11
16	6	1.87	11
15	6	2.0	12
14	6	2.14	12
13	6	2.3	14
12	6	2.5	15
11	6	2.7	16
10	6	3.0	18

*Reading levels rounded to nearest grade level. Developed by Susan Weinrich and Marilyn Boyd (30), University of South Carolina, College of Nursing, Columbia, South Carolina.

3

Measurement Issues with Children and Adolescents

Debra P. Hymovich

This chapter provides an overview of issues involving research and measurement, selection of appropriate instruments, and ethical and legal aspects of research with children and adolescents. Most studies related to children and adolescents involve direct observation, interview, completion of questionnaires or other instruments, or those in which children are studied indirectly through data collected by significant others, such as the child's parents, teachers, or peers. In this chapter, measurement issues are limited to children from birth through 18 years of age who are studied directly. The terms *measure*, *tool*, and *instrument* are used interchangeably.

Considerations in selecting research instruments are: (1) the conceptual or theoretical base and its consistency with the proposed study; (2) appropriateness for the child's age, including available norms for children of the same age and sex in the proposed study; (3) length of time to complete the instrument; (4) whether the instrument is norm-referenced or criterion-referenced; and (5) the validity and reliability of the instrument.

Ethical Issues

Obtaining informed consent for research involving children in numerous research studies and weighing the physical and psychosocial risks and benefits of conducting studies with children are ethical considerations for the researchers.[1]

Informed Consent

Parent Consent

Voluntary and informed consent is one of the most difficult aspects of child research. Parental or guardian consent is required to safeguard the rights of children and adolescents.[2] Traditionally, researchers have relied on proxy consent from parents as a substitute for obtaining informed consent from children. However, proxy consent does not fully meet the requirements for informed consent.

Because parents are legally responsible for all matters pertaining to their children, parental consent to permit their children to participate in a study is mandatory in research ethics codes. Parents may refuse to permit their children to participate in even the most innocent study for a variety of reasons. Parents may distrust scientists in general or a particular researcher; they may not want strangers to talk to their children; or they may be unwilling to endure any inconvenience to themselves.[3]

Child Assent

Although parents have the legal consenting responsibility regarding their children's participation in research, the child who has reached the "age of understanding" has the right to assent.[3] Assent has been referred to as knowledgeable agreement. Children are capable of giving a degree of informed consent, subject to developmental constraints. It is the researcher's responsibility to ensure that the child's rights are respected.

There are limited data regarding children's ability to consent to research. Abramowitz and colleagues[4] describe four studies, using a total of 148 subjects ranging in age from 7 to 12 years, to obtain data on children's ability to consent to psychologic research. Subjects were from suburban, relatively affluent families whose parents were willing to have them participate in the research. Most subjects understood all or most of what they were asked to do in a psychology study, but few younger than 12 years understood or believed that their performance would be confidential. Study results imply that 7- to 12-year-old children have the capacity to assent meaningfully to participation in research, but problems exist in guaranteeing that they make this decision freely. Frame and Strauss[5] investigated the possibility of sample bias resulting from parental consent in 308 grade-school children for whom sociometric and teacher ratings were available prior to requesting parental consent for a research project. Parental consent was lower for socially rejected and neglected students and those who had significantly lower academic performance. Social withdrawal and poor academic performance were the best independent predictors of nonconsent, accounting for 10% of the variance. Teacher ratings of various psychological characteristics failed to differentiate children who gave consent from those who did not.

Recommendations and procedures for obtaining informed consent or assent from children to participate in research generally vary somewhat among institutions. Federal guidelines for research with minors[6] allows institutional review boards (IRBs) to determine the conditions under which parental consent is required. Currently, there is discussion regarding adolescents' rights to consent to participate in research without parental consent or knowledge. The legal–medical model provides a framework for evaluating the conditions under which guardian consent for research might be waived.[7] All states allow adolescents to be treated for venereal disease without guardian consent, and some states allow independent decision making about other treatments as well. As Fisher pointed out, "Decisions regarding whether adolescents should participate in research without parental consent should be based on the potential benefits to the participant rather than the utility needs of the researcher."[2,p8]

It often is a challenge for the researcher to explain the study at the child's level of understanding. Obtaining a child's assent requires time, effort, and respect for the youngster's autonomy. Strategies for obtaining consent are provided by Hughes and Helling,[8] who also highlight the following ethical issues:

- Being sensitive and responsible
- Considering the child's intellectual maturity and comprehension level
- Avoiding taking advantage of subjects' immaturity

- Being sure that children understand that they can refuse or quit at any time (repeat this more than once)
- Realizing that, although the children may enjoy the increased attention, most do not see their role in contributing to a knowledge base
- Determining whether some features of the research can be rewarding to the child
- Giving certificate of acknowledgment to the child for participating
- Offering tangible gifts (pens/pencils, stickers, tape recording) as a "surprise" after the study so that they are not construed as bribes
- Weighing the risks and benefits carefully (physical and psychological harm, social injury against scientific validity of study)
- Ensuring that child is not involved in numerous research studies

Theoretical Model

Investigators need a clear theoretical foundation to conceptualize a study.[9] The majority of nursing studies with children and adolescents have been guided by theories of development. These theories, emerging from the mechanistic and organismic worldviews, include Piaget's cognitive development and Erikson's psychologic development. However, these traditional theories are limited in their ability to inform about the influences of history, culture, and environment on behavioral change.[10] Weekes[10] recommends using the lifespan developmental framework perspective rather than traditional approaches for research with chronically ill adolescents. She believes this permits an understanding of events preceding adolescence. For example, Weekes's study of adolescents with cancer did not support the hypotheses based on Piagetian theory. Similarly, a cross-sequential study of adolescents by Nesselroade and Baltes[11] did not support the age-related developmental changes suggested by Erikson's and Piaget's theories.

The lifespan developmental framework emerges from the dialectic worldview. As Weeks wrote, "The basic aims of the life-span perspective are to describe, explain, and modify developmental change across the lifespan."[10,p42] This theoretical approach may be useful in studying younger children, as well as adolescents. With this approach, the researcher would not only consider children at different stages in their development but also how the developmental, cognitive, and social or emotional changes that occur before and after the study period influence their responses.

Design

The most frequent research designs used for developmental research have been the traditional longitudinal and descriptive designs. Issues in designing a study include the following:

- The need to be efficient and economical without giving a static picture
- Cost (time, money, effort, subject attrition)
- Difficulty in recruiting an adequate number of subjects
- Nonrandom loss of subjects through experimental mortality (refusal, death)
- The need for comparison groups
- Flaws in cross-sectional and longitudinal designs, so that uncontrolled influences (i.e., maturation, new technology) cannot be attributed to random occurrences; viable alternative explanations exist for differences between measurement groups other than age[12]
- The lifespan developmental model, which can be helpful in addressing developmental change in responses to health, illness, and influence of age, time, and cohort on this change[12-14]

- Shaie's redefinition of cohort, time of measurement, and age:[14] *Cohort:* all persons experiencing a particular event at some point in time (age-graded, history-graded, non-normative); *Time of measurement:* time an event has had the opportunity to have an impact on individuals or group (nature of an event rather than time); *Age:* not a threat to validity because maturational effects are considered to be age effects

Longitudinal data usually are essential to investigate directly issues of lifespan development. According to Wohlwill,[15] longitudinal data are necessary (1) to preserve information related to the shape of the function of the developmental response; (2) to provide information on change and the patterning of change; (3) to relate earlier behavior to later behavior; and (4) to relate earlier conditions of life to subsequent behavior.

Weekes[10] suggests that there are sound shortcuts to longitudinal research. Despite its problems, Weekes[10] identifies retrospective data collection as a useful method with adolescents over about 13 years of age. Problems associated with retrospective data collection include inaccurate recall, selective remembering, distortion, projection of the present into the past, and age of child. Another strategy, sequential data collection, involves combining cross-sectional and longitudinal data-collection methods to expedite the collection of developmental data.[16,17] Sequential design strategies can be used to answer questions related to influences of age, cohort, and time of measurement on intraindividual change in behavior. These strategies may be especially useful to researchers who are interested in age and time, or time and cohort influences on developmental change in response to numerous health and illness situations. Problems associated with using sequential designs include the potential for lack of availability of large sample sizes and inability to control for age and time of induction to the study. Certain adjustments may have to be made, such as oversampling certain age groups.

Sampling

Sample size and rigor of sampling methodology are important. Equally important are the developmental level and ethnicity of subjects in considering generalizability.

Beal and Betz[18] evaluated the sample size, study setting, age, and cultural background of subjects of research published in parent–child health nursing journals from 1980 to 1989. In their analysis of 322 articles from 7 journals, 25% had sample sizes of less than 30 subjects, and 66% had sample sizes under 100 subjects. In 5 studies, it was not clear how many subjects were sampled. Nonprobability sampling was the principal technique, with 91% using samples of convenience and only 3% using random sampling. Forty-seven percent of the studies were conducted in the hospital, 12% in the home, and 37% in outpatient clinics and physicians' offices. The remaining studies were conducted in schools ($n = 36$), camps ($n = 3$), and a homeless shelter ($n = 1$). In 3 studies it was unclear where data were collected. In many cases it was difficult to differentiate the age groups of the samples. The majority of studies ($n = 116$, 37%) used parents as samples. Neonates were sampled in 33 studies, and 21 studies sampled toddlers. Overall, Beal and Betz found small samples sizes, accessed through nonprobability sampling techniques, rendering generalizability difficult. Generalizability is further limited when examining ethnicity data. Nonwhite samples were studied in 35% of the 322 studies. In 32 studies, no reference was made to ethnicity. The major focus of the studies was on individual parental response to child behavior, but only 12 studies had a family focus and few studies targeted young children. Beal and Betz[18] suggest that nursing research move into the community to study health promotion issues in high-risk groups. Increasing the sample size and ethnic heterogeneity will further enhance the generalizability and relevance of findings to pediatric practice.

Methodologic Issues

Children may be assessed directly through observation or by having them complete questionnaires and/or answer questions. They can be measured indirectly by asking parents, teachers, or other significant individuals to complete measures about the children. Several studies indicate that parents' perceptions and children's perceptions differ. Research involving children requires an exploration of the child's beliefs, thoughts, feelings, and knowledge rather than just those of the adults. Existing measures of concepts often are completed by parents or other adult observers. Although these instruments may be valid and reliable, they provide information only from the adult's perspective, thus missing the child's perception. Data obtained directly from children and data obtained indirectly from parents are both types of data that might shed light on the issue under study. Whenever possible, researchers should consider collecting data from the perspective of both the children and significant adults.

Instrument Reliability and Validity

Psychometrically sound methods are needed for measuring variables. Because of the wide developmental differences that must be addressed in conducting studies with children and adolescents, the issue of measurement and assessment is complex.[9] Although some measures have been developed for this population, it is still necessary to develop others. Carpenter[9] noted that when different measuring techniques are used with younger and older children, it creates serious problems for interpreting study results. He recommends that instruments be developed that can be applied across the child and adolescent developmental spectrum.

Because reliability estimates vary from sample to sample, instruments reliability should be reestimated for each study. Validity usually is sample invariant; it should be a relatively stable property as long as the technique is used appropriately to derive the type of data for which it was developed. Commonly used measures for assessing validity are correlations with other measures, cluster analyses, and factor analyses. In addition, developmental differences are used as evidence of construct validity, especially to assess instruments devised to evaluate the performance of children.[19]

Developmental Considerations

Although instruments designed for use with adult populations can be used with adolescents, there are very few for use with young children. Tools used with children may have been developed for populations that have little in common with those being studied (sensitivity). Because the items are not sufficiently sensitive, researchers who try to use these instruments may be unable to discriminate important differences between groups or detect changes over time. For example, standardized tests of children's intelligence and academic performance are available and appropriate to study the long-term effects of neurotoxic therapy for childhood leukemia.[20] However, available instruments are not sufficiently sensitive to measure other aspects of cognition, such as memory and attention. In some cases all that is needed may be simply to adapt an existing tool and validate it by obtaining appropriate normative data.

The age and developmental level of the child or adolescent are important considerations in developing or selecting data-collection instruments.[21] The younger the child, the more complex measurement issues become. Cognitive capabilities, psychomotor abilities, and attention span must be considered when selecting and developing instruments for children and adolescents. Appendix 3A highlights developmentally specific measures.[22-32]

Adapting Standardized Instruments

Brown and Haylor identified four areas of development as "most important" when considering how to use standardized tests with young children: (1) psychosocial and emotional development; (2) perceptual-motor development; (3) cognitive development; and (4) linguistic development."[27,p23] Appendix 3B illustrates the steps recommended to adapt standardized tests for preoperational children.

Issues with Special Children

Special children are those children who have conditions, impairments, or disabilities that significantly interfere with normal development and psychologic adaptation. These impairments may be cognitive, sensory, motor, developmental, related to chronic illnesses, and/or learning disabilities. These impairments can interfere with a child's ability to complete many instruments standardized with nonhandicapped children. Several issues require consideration when using psychometric measures with special children.[33] The first issue, of a theoretical nature, has to do with the concept of age equivalence. Although the use of age equivalents makes it easy to summarize and communicate test performance, a direct correspondence of test ages to chronological ages should not be assumed. Two other issues are methodologic in nature. The first concerns the comparability of instruments with similar labels. Identical test ages derived from different tests should not be assumed to be identical conceptually because they may not necessarily measure the same characteristics. Another methodologic issue relates to the concept of standardization and its implications for assessing and interpreting psychometric test results. Most of the tests used with special children have not been standardized with this population. These areas are discussed more fully by Simeonsson.[33]

Measurement Limitations

Characteristics that limit the utility of instruments with special children often are those of reliability and validity. The technical adequacy of instruments is important. Salvia and Ysseldyke[34] have presented tables listing instruments they judge to be inadequate on the basis of reliability and validity as well as those judged inadequate in terms of descriptions and/or construction of norms.

As Simeonsson wrote "The psychometric base for psychological testing of many special children is inadequate."[33,p5] Many tests present stimuli of a visual or auditory nature that cannot be perceived by a child with sensory impairment. Responses requiring speech or manipulation may not be possible for children with hearing or motor impairments. A measurement limitation of a psychomotor nature is the failure to include special children in standardization samples, thus placing restrictions on inferences and generalizations. "A related limitation is truncated normative tables, which do not permit derivation of extreme values," Simeonsson pointed out.[33,p35] The lack of comparability of scores for tests with similar content and purpose is another limiting factor. Ramsey and Fitzhardenge[35] have shown that Bayley Scales of Infant Development and the Griffiths Developmental Scales[36] yielded substantially different scores for 50 high-risk infants. In another study of infants with Down's syndrome,[37] the Bayley Scales and Gessell Developmental Schedules did not yield similar results.

Instrument labels are not always descriptive of the domain they represent. Instruments labeled as intelligence tests, for example, may vary widely in content. Tests with similar labels also may differ dramatically in the nature and comprehensiveness with which a particular domain is assessed. For further discussion of these issues, the reader is referred to Simeonsson.[33]

A final limitation of measurement involves the methodology employed. Diebold, Curtis, and DuBose[38] compared performance of handicapped youngsters using data derived from observation and from testing. In spite of the similarity of the domains being assessed, marked differences were found as a function of methodologies. Performance based on testing was lower than by observation.

Reducing the limitations associated with inappropriate materials can take many forms. The major strategies are to modify, expand, or vary the instruments (such as test stimuli and format) or to modify the testing procedures.[33] Simeonsson[33] advocates using a multivariate approach and recognizing that there are problems in assessing special children that require flexible, rather than rigid, standards of reliability and validity.

Minority Children

Another group of special children are those from minority ethnic, racial, or cultural groups. When planning studies with minority subjects, the researcher needs to consider the client, the instruments, and the evaluator. Few instruments available for children have been normed on these minority groups.

According to Walton and Nuttall, culturally different children "are different from the predominant society," and "this difference is not necessarily a deficit."[39,p281] Most minority parents and children have experienced prejudice, and they bring these previous experiences to the testing situation.

The problem of instrument bias is multifaceted. As Jones noted, instrument bias can exist "at the content level, where decisions are made about what items to include in a test (the perspectives and experiences of minority group children are often thought to be excluded), [and] at the level of standardization, where decisions are made about the population for whom the test is appropriate."[40,p15] Most standardized tests reflect largely white, middle-class values and attitudes. They are biased and unfair to persons from cultural and socioeconomic minorities because they do not reflect the experience and linguistic, cognitive, and other cultural styles and values of minority group persons.[41] The Denver Developmental Screening Test (DDST)[42,43] is an example of an instrument that has been critiqued for its cultural bias. The recent revision, DDST II, was standardized on sample subgroups divided by age, gender, and ethnicity (Anglo, African American, Hispanic), and age-adjusted norms were determined for items in which significant differences exist.[42] In addition, to improve the preparation of screeners, a two-day training course was developed for master trainers. Further documentation is needed to resolve the issue of cultural bias with the revised instrument.

Bias can occur when instruments are administered by researchers who are unfamiliar with the patterns of language, behavior, and customs of the person being examined.[40] When data are collected by persons who do not understand the culture and language of minority group children, they are unable to elicit a level of performance that accurately reflects the child's underlying competence.[40]

Projective techniques frequently used in research with children are detailed in Appendix 3C.[44-48] The most common tests are presented in Appendix 3D.[49-65]

Summary

Much of the research involving child and adolescent subjects is still plagued by sampling bias and design flaws. Most of the nursing research with children and adolescents involves small, nonrepresentative samples; a lack of comparison groups; and the absence of a conceptual framework. Researchers need more valid and reliable instruments; improved designs (qualitative, experimental, multivariate) guided by conceptual or theoretical models; and more representative and larger samples that include minorities, males, and lower-class youth.[66] The content validity, construct validity, and stability of instruments need to be extended and improved for descriptive studies.

References

1. U.S. Department of Health Education and Welfare and National Institutes of Health. Protection of human subjects. *Federal Register*, May 30, 1974.
2. Fisher, C.B. Integrating science and ethics in research with high-risk children and youth. *Soc Pol Rep: Soc Res Child Devel*, 1993, 7(4):1-26.
3. Keith-Spiegel, P. Children's rights as participants in research. In G.P. Koocher (Ed.), *Children's rights and the mental health professions*. New York: Wiley, 1976, pp. 53–81.
4. Abramowitz, R., Freedman, J.L., Thoden, K., & Nikolich, C. Children's capacity to consent to participate in psychological research: Empirical findings. *Child Dev*, 1991, 62(5):1100-1109.
5. Frame, C.L., & Strauss, C.C. Parental informed consent and sample bias in grade-school children. *J Soc Clin Psychol*, 1987, 5(2):227-236.
6. U.S. Department of Health and Human Services. Additional protection for children involved as subjects of research. *Federal Register*, 1983, 48(46):9814-9820.
7. Holder, A.R. Can teenagers participate in research without parental consent? *IRB: Rev Hum Subjects Res*, 1981, 3(2):5-7.
8. Hughes, T., & Hellings, M.K. A case for obtaining informed consent from young children. *Early Childhood Res Q*, 1991, 6(2):225-232.
9. Carpenter, P.J. Scientific inquiry in childhood cancer psychosocial research. *Cancer*, 1991, 67:833-838.
10. Weekes, D.P. Application of the life-span developmental perspective to nursing research with adolescents. *J Pediatr Nurs*, 1991, 6(1):38-48.
11. Nesselroade, J.R., & Baltes, P.B. Adolescent personality development and historical change: 1970-1972. *Monographs of the Society for Research in Child Development*, 1974, 39:1-80.
12. Kosloski, K. Isolating age, period, and cohort effects in development research. *Res Aging*, 1987, 8(4):461-479.
13. Weekes, D.P., & Rankin, S.H. Life-span developmental methods: Application to nursing research. *Nurs Res*, 1988, 37(6):380-383.
14. Schaie, K.W. Beyond calendar definition of age, time, and cohort: The general developmental model revisited. *Developmental Review*, 1986, 6(3):252-277.
15. Wohlwill, J.F. *The study of behavioral development*. San Diego, CA: Academic Press, 1973.
16. Schaie, K.W. A general model for the study of developmental problems. *Psychol Bull*, 1965, 64(2):92-107.
17. Schaie, K.W., & Baltes, P.B. On sequential strategies in developmental research. *Hum Dev*, 1975, 18(5):384-390.
18. Beal, J.A., & Betz, C.L. Sampling issues in parent-child nursing research: Implications for nursing practice. *J Pediatr Nurs*, 1993, 8(4):261-262.
19. Goldman, J., Stein, C.L., & Guerry, S. *Psychological methods of child assessment*. New York: Brunner/Mazel, 1983.
20. Moore, I.M., Kramer, J., & Ablin, A. Late effects of central nervous system prophylactic leukemia therapy on cognitive functioning. *Oncol Nurs Forum*, 1986, 13(4):45-51.
21. Kotzer, A.M. Cognitive strategies for pediatric nursing research: Data collection. *J Pediatric Nurs*, 1990, 5(1):50-53.
22. Moore, I.M., & Ruccione, K. Challenges to conducting research with children with cancer. *Oncol Nurs Forum*, 1989, 16(4):587-589.
23. Keefe, M., Kotzer, A.M., Reuss, J.L., & Sander, L.W. The development of a system of monitoring infant state behavior. *Nurs Res*, 1989, 38(6):344-347.
24. Achenbach, T.M. *Manual for the Youth Self-Report and 1991 Profile*. Burlington, VT: University of Vermont Department of Psychiatry, 1991.
25. Bordens, K.S., & Abbott, B.B. *Research designs and methods: A process approach* (2nd ed.). Mountainview, CA: Mayfield, 1991.
26. Hester, N.K. The preoperational child's reaction to immunization. *Nurs Res*, 1979, 28(4):250-254.
27. Brown, M.S., & Haylor, M. Nursing research with preoperational age children: The use of standardized tests. *J of Pediatric Nurs*, 1989, 4(1):19-25.
28. Hetherington, E.M., & Parke, R.D. *Child psychology: A contemporary viewpoint*. San Francisco: McGraw-Hill, 1986.
29. Romero, I. Individual assessment procedures with preschool children. In E.V. Nuttall, I. Romero, & J. Kalesnik (Eds.). *Assessing and screening preschoolers: Psychological and educational dimensions*. Boston: Allyn and Bacon, 1992, pp. 55-66.
30. Sorensen, E.S. Using children's diaries as a research instrument. *J Pediatric Nurs*, 1989, 4(6):427-431.
31. Savedra, M., & Highly, B. Photography: Is it useful in learning how adolescents cope with hospitalization? *Journal of Adolescent Health Care*, 1988, 9(3):219-224.
32. Hinds, P.S., Weekes, D.P., & Zeltzer, L.K. Identifying threats to data integrity in studies of adolescents with cancer. *Oncology Nursing Forum*, 1988, 15(6):821-824.
33. Simeonsson, R.J. *Psychological and developmental assessment of special children*. Boston: Allyn and Bacon, 1986.
34. Salvia, J., & Ysseldyke, J.E. *Assessment in special and remedial education*. Boston: Houghton Mifflin, 1981.
35. Ramsey, M., & Fitzhardenge, P.M. Comparative study of two developmental scales: The Bayley and the Griffiths. *Early Human Development*, 1977, 1:151-157.
36. Griffiths, R. *The abilities of young children*. Chard, England: Young & Son, 1970.

37. Eippert, D.S., & Azen, S.P. A comparison of two developmental instruments in evaluating children with Down's syndrome. *Physical Ther*, 1978, *58*:1066-1069.

38. Diebold, M.H., Curtis, W.S., & DuBose, R.F. Relationships between psychometric and observational measures of performance in low-functioning children. *AAESPH Review*, 1978, *3*:123-128.

39. Walton, J.R., & Nuttal, E.V. Preschool evaluation of culturally different children. In E.V. Nuttall, I. Romero, & J. Kalesnik (Eds.). *Assessing and screening preschoolers: Psychological and educational dimensions.* Boston: Allyn and Bacon, 1992, pp. 281-299.

40. Jones, R.L. Psychoeducational assessment of minority group children: Issues and perspectives. In R.L. Jones (Ed.), *Psychoeducational assessment of minority group children: A casebook.* Berkeley, CA: Cobb & Henry, 1988, pp. 13-35.

41. Laosa, L.M. Nonbiased assessment of children's abilities: Historical antecedents and current issues. In T. Oakland (Ed.), *Psychological and educational assessment of minority children.* New York: Brunner/Mazel, 1977, pp. 1-20.

42. Frankenburg, W.K., Dodds, J., Archer, P., et al. *Denver II technical manual.* Denver: Denver Developmental Materials, Inc., 1990.

43. Wade, G.H. Update on the Denver II. *J Pediatric Nurs*, 1992, *18*(2):140-141.

44. Krahn, G.L. The use of projective assessment techniques in pediatric settings. *J Pediatric Psychol*, 1985, *10*(2):179-193.

45. Lynn, M.R. Projective technique: A way of getting "hidden" information: Part I. *J Pediatric Nurs*, 1986, *1*(6):407-408.

46. Johnson, B.H. Children's drawings as a projective technique. *J Pediatric Nurs*, 1990, *16*(1):11-17.

47. Poster, E.C. The use of projective assessment techniques in pediatric research. *J Pediatric Nurs*, 1989, *4*(1):26-35.

48. Gardner, E., Rudman, H., Karlsen, B., & Merwin, J. *Stanford Achievement Test* (7th ed.). San Antonio, TX: Psychological Corporation, 1982.

49. Peterson, C., & Schilling, K. Card pull and projective testing. *J Pers Assess*, 1983, *47*:265-275.

50. Waechter, E.H. Children's awareness of fatal illness. *Am J Nurs*, 1971, *71*(6):1168-1172.

51. Bellak, L., & Bellak, S.S. *Children's apperception test* (6th rev. ed.). New York: C.P.S., 1952.

52. Bellak, L., & Bellak, S.S. *Supplement to the children's apperception test.* Larchmont, NY: C.P.S., 1974.

53. Bellak, L., & Bellak, S.S. *The TAT, the CAT and the SAT in clinical use* (3rd ed.). New York: Grune & Stratton, 1975.

54. Myler, B., Rosenkranz, A., & Holmes, G.A. Comparison of the TAT, CAT and CAT-H among second grade girls. *J Personality Assess*, 1972, *36*:440-444.

55. Poster, E., Betz, C.L., McKenna, A., & Mossar, M. Children's attitudes toward the mentally ill as reflected in their human figure drawings and stories. *J Am Acad Child Psychiatry*, 1986, *25*(5):680-686.

56. Scavnicky-Mylant, M. The use of drawings in the assessment and treatment of children of alcoholics. *J Pediatric Nurs*, 1986, *1*(3):178-184.

57. Burgess, A.W. Sexually abused children and their drawings. *Arch Psychiatric Nurs*, 1988, *2*(2):65-73.

58. Engle, P.L., & Suppes, J.S. The relation between human drawing and test anxiety in children. *J Projective Tech*, 1970, *34*:223-231.

59. Rubin, J.A., Schacter, J., & Ragins, N. Intra-individual variability in human figure drawings: A developmental study. *Am J Orthopsychiatry*, 1983, *53*(4):654-657.

60. Blau, T.H. *The psychological examination of the child.* New York: Wiley, 1991.

61. Farel, A.M., Freeman, V.A., Keenan, N.L., & Huber, C.J. Interaction between high-risk infants and their mothers: The NCAST as an assessment tool. *Res Nurs Health*, 1991, *14*:109-118.

62. Coppens, N.M., & Gentry, L.K. Video analysis of playground injury-risk situations. *Res Nurs Health*, 1991, *14*:129-136.

63. Medinnus, G.R. *Child study and observation guide.* New York: Wiley, 1976.

64. Lobo, M.L. Observation: A valuable data collection strategy for research with children. *J Pediatric Nurs*, 1992, *7*(5):320-328.

65. Pellegrini, A.D. *Applied child study: A developmental approach* (2nd ed.). Hillsdale, NJ: Lawrence Erlbaum, 1991.

66. Opie, N.D. Childhood and adolescent bereavement. In J.J. Fitzpatrick, R.L. Taunton, & A.K. Jacox (Eds.), *Annual review of nursing research* (Vol. 10). New York: Springer, 1992, pp. 127-141.

Appendix

3A. Strategies for Measurement across Childhood

Infant (Preverbal)

The following strategies can be used with preverbal children.[22]

Habituation technique. This technique tests discrimination as the infant becomes bored with the repeated presentation of same stimulus; once the infant no longer looks at it, a different stimulus is presented. If the infant looks at the second stimulus, it is inferred that the infant can discriminate.

Preference. The infant is presented with two objects simultaneously, and the length of time the infant looks at each is measured. The infant looks at the preferred object longer.

Discriminant learning. This strategy attempts to have the infant respond differently to different stimuli.

Other measures. Other interventions that can be carried out include assessment of heart rate, cry, sleep–wake patterns before and after an intervention; videotaping or tape recording of behavior or vocalization; noninvasive computerized monitoring.[23]

Preschool-Age Children

Challenge. The lack of adequate instruments and cognitive and social immaturity limit recall and ability to report feelings and behavior,[24] so does the inability to respond to measures designed for older individuals.

Children egocentric. Those aged 4 to 7 years are able to quantify, classify, and relate objects but are unaware of underlying principles.

Strategies.
- Establish and maintain rapport (developmentally appropriate).
- Be sensitive to nonverbal communication.
- Adapt perceptual-motor aspects to developmental level.
- Be flexible and creative (give child maximum opportunity to respond—children will differ in their fatigue and anxiety levels, as well as length of testing time they can tolerate).
- Make measures concrete.[25,26]
- Videotape the child's interaction with environment, recording behavioral and verbal communication.
- Maximum testing time with best time 9:00 A.M. to 11:00 A.M. Worst times are nap time and before and after meals.[27]

School-Age Children

Capacities. School-age children can use instruments requiring concrete or abstract Likert-type responses (e.g., rank-ordering objects),[28] self-administered questionnaires, and qualitative interviews.

Other techniques. A child's drawings of human figures, story telling, using dolls and puppets to elicit information,[21] autobiographical scrapbook,[29] diary or semistructured journal[30] can all be used.

Pilot testing. It is important to pilot questions to ensure understanding and to assure the child that there are no right or wrong answers and that it is okay to say "no."

Adolescence

Capacities. Adolescents can describe feelings and behaviors across situations (self-reports).

Other perspectives. Reports of others who see adolescent in different context should be considered.

Other techniques. Journals, self-recorded interviews, photography[31] can be used.

Reliability and validity. The reliability and validity of adolescent-reported data can be threatened by researcher, adolescent, and nature of research question. For instance, how valid are data gathered when the parent is present?[32]

3B. Adapting Standardized Tests for Preoperational Children

The following adaptations with preoperational children can be considered:[27]

1. Identify and adapt the perceptual-motor appropriateness of the test.
   Use heavy black or colored lines separating every five questions.
   Use cartoons (preferably animals) to illustrate questions.
   Develop alternate forms for Asian and African-American children.
2. Identify and adapt cognitive appropriateness of the test.
   Phrase questions in concrete language.
   Deal with only one variable at a time.
   Avoid words involving time and sequence.
   Use words appropriate for various age groups.
3. Identify and adapt linguistic appropriateness of the test.
   Use simple sentence structure and a sentence length not longer than twelve to fourteen words.
   Avoid double negatives and prepositional and adverbial phrases with more than five words, including exceptions (e.g., "All of the following EXCEPT").
   Use pictures to replace words when needed.
4. Restandardize the measure.
   Assess child's ability to comply.

Individualize the research approach (this may threaten the internal validity of the study, but the responses may be a more accurate reflection of the child's feelings, attitudes, or beliefs and thus may enhance the external validity of the findings).

3C. Projective Testing with Children

Projective Techniques

Projective techniques include the presentation of ambiguous (nonspecific) material or stimuli to enable the child to disclose verbally or nonverbally images or ideas previously undisclosed;[44,45] based on psychoanalytic view of an individual. Useful with child who cannot verbalize.[46]

Categories

A number of categories can be distinguished.[47]

Associative. The child is expected to respond quickly to stimuli word or image (i.e., Rorschach ink-blot technique).

Construction. The child is asked to make up or to create response to stimulus (i.e., Child Apperception Test [CAT]).

Completion. The child completes a partially developed sentence or story (i.e., Gardner's mutual storytelling).[48]

Expressive. The child uses drawings or play.

Tests

- The most commonly used tests are TAT, CAT, Rorschach, and Human Figure Drawings (HFDs).
- Tests require specifically trained individuals to administer and score.
- Overall, there is a lack of reliability and validity data. Many tests are developed to diagnose emotionally disturbed individuals; additional study with comparable "normal" children needs to be done.
- Results "interpreted" based on psychoanalytic theory, so accuracy, quality, and utility of data must be considered.

Techniques for Personality Appraisal

- Structured or unstructured; investigator interprets response in broad psychological terms and behavior dynamics.
- Verbal: word association tests, sentence completion tests, or child asked to tell a story about a picture.
- Nonverbal: expressive or productive, involving children's drawings (i.e., human figures).

3D. Projective Tests Used in Research with Children

Thematic Apperception Test (TAT)

Administration. The child is given ambiguous pictures and asked to make up a story or fantasy including what is happening, what led up to it, and what will happen in the future.[49]

Results. It is assumed that the child will project motives, emotions, and attitudes about self, significant adults, the world, and expectations.

Comments. Requires skillful and sensitive researcher. The TAT has been adapted by Waechter[50] to study death anxiety in children.

Child's Apperception Test (CAT)

Administration. Children aged 3 to 10 years old are given cards with pictures of animals that illustrate themes of sibling rivalry, nighttime loneliness, attitudes toward parents, toileting behavior, aggression, and oral problems.[51-53]

Results. It is assumed that the child will project feelings and attitudes onto animals;[54] various scoring methods can be used (few validity or reliability studies).

Human Figure Drawing (HFD) Tests

Administration. Draw-A-Person (DAP), Kinetic Family Drawing (KFD), and House-Tree-Person (HTP) tests have been used to measure children's perception of mental illness,[55] as well as in measuring children of alcoholics[56] and sexually abused youngsters.[55,57]

Results. Scoring is subjective, depending on the skills, knowledge of child development, and experience of the researcher; many scoring systems exist[58] that provide evidence of interrater reliability. Test–retest reliability and validity are questionable.[59] Difficult to compare study findings because of the differences in subjects, scoring systems, and test environments.[47]

Comments. Complex, so caution should be used with neurologically impaired or developmentally disabled children. Increase reliability and validity by controlled administration, standardize instructions, use together with other measures, obtain at least three drawings from each child, and use concurrent comparison groups.[47] Limit interpretation only to aspects selected for evaluation. Scoring should be done by raters blind to study details and data collection.

Sentence Completion

Administration. Children are asked to complete incomplete sentences, drawing from their own experiences ("my mother . . .").[60]

Results. Considerable face validity, but other psychometric properties are questionable.

Comments. Many differences in stimulus sentences presented to children and adolescents.

Children's Drawings

Administration. Based on psychoanalytic theory. Demonstrates child's usual presentation of self to the world and nature of inner personality.[50]

Results. Interpretation most valid when based on *series* of drawings; should be used in conjunction with other available information about the child; free drawings more physically meaningful than assigned drawings; when drawing, sex of figure child draws first is related to his or her concept of sex role; child adapts own drawing style (psychologically significant); manner that elements are portrayed may be useful indicator of psychological state; drawings may be interspersed as a whole rather than segmentally or analytically.

Comments. Valuable tool in the hands of an expert; ideally child should validate researcher's interpretation.[56]

Observation

Administration. Used for child's interaction with animate or inanimate environment;[61,62] child's behavior is recorded without the use of predetermined categories or arbitrary time intervals (*naturalistic*). It is important not to modify the behavior of the observed child. *Time sampling* can be used to determine the frequency of certain behaviors; the reliability of behaviors is established by observation over time; there is some difficulty in identifying interrelationships among a number of behaviors because the researcher is studying only one behavior.[63] *Event sampling* describes a behavior sequence.

Results. Many rating scales, checklists to quantify observations but these do not provide data about causes or management of the behavior.

Comments. Major concerns[64] include definition; reliability; validity of coding categories; identification of unit of measurement (molar or molecular); method of recording the observation; sampling strategies; observer training; interrater reliability; taxonomy of behaviors (motor or vocal); and instrument and observer reliability. Children's play can be observed in controlled situations where specific materials are provided to elicit specific responses.[65]

Questionnaires and Inventories

Administration. Personality and intellectual ability: observe and record child's behavior and responses when presented with various materials and tasks.

Results. *Tests of ability* are more precise, highly developed, more accurate in predicting behaviors (e.g., school achievement) than personality measures. *Psychometric tests of intelligence* are highly reliable, valid (scores agree with other estimates of intellectual ability and predict school achievement), but they are affected more by the child's motivation, rapport with examiner, physical health, mood, attention, and familiarity with testing situation.

4

Measurement Issues with the Elderly

Joyce H. Rasin

The number of older adults is increasing in this country. In 1992, there were 32.3 million persons 65 years or older representing 12.7% of the population.[1] By 2030, it is projected that there will be approximately 70 million older adults comprising almost 20% of the population. The fastest growing group of elders are those 85 years and older. Their numbers by the year 2030 will be double that of 1990.

In terms of biopsychosocial functioning, elders are very heterogeneous. The majority live in the community, and only 5% were living in nursing homes in 1990. Of those in the community, 10% received help with personal care activities and 22% with home management activities. Although older adults constituted 12% of the population in 1987, they accounted for 36% of the total U.S. personal health-care expenditures and 33% of all hospital stays.

Elders are overrepresented in the health-care system and unless specifically excluded, will be selected as subjects in any study where the population focuses on adults, given that everyone over 18 or 21 years of age is grouped into the category of "adult." There are, however, biopsychosocial factors that make elders different from their younger counterparts. Some of these factors can influence the measurement of study variables in a research project. And, because elders are heterogeneous, the influence of these factors cannot be automatically generalized to all elders. Most elder are healthy and are primarily adapting to changes associated with aging. Some elders are frail because of the interplay of pathologic and age-related changes.

In this chapter, factors that should be considered when developing a measurement plan for elders are discussed. Specifically, concerns about the purpose, conceptualization, and threats to the psychometric properties of instruments are explored. Except for illustrative purposes, instruments to measure specific concepts are not reviewed because the majority of those discussed in this book are applicable to elders. However, the content of this chapter provides information that is foundational for using the instruments presented in the chapters that follow.

Purpose

Congruence between the purpose for which the researcher will use an instrument and the purpose for which the instrument was originally developed is crucial. An instrument is created for a particular population and a particular setting. Many researchers do not consider population specificity when working with elders because of the general propensity to group all adults together. Elders represent a distinct population with specialized requirements. If an instrument is not carefully matched to the population, a ceiling or floor effect may result. With a ceiling effect the scores will cluster in the high range because the questions are too easy. The opposite occurs with a floor effect: The questions are too difficult for the sample and the scores are low. For example, assessing competence in activities of daily living (ADLs) of a cognitively impaired elder in a nursing home with an instrument that was created for healthy community-based elders will produce floor effects. The nursing home residents will be unable to do the same tasks as elders living independently and will have low scores. In this preceding example, the problem occurred because the setting was not considered. Instruments can be designed for use in a particular setting. Assessing the functional status of nursing home residents with an instrumental ADLs scale developed for individuals living in their own home has inappropriate items. For example, ability to do shopping is not relevant to a nursing home resident. Overall, if the setting and the sample of the investigation do not match those for which the instrument was developed, the reliability and validity of the data collected will be compromised.

Conceptualization

The conceptualization of research variables guides the selection of the appropriate measures for operationalization. Conceptualization should consider the complex nature of concepts. The complexity of elder-related concepts is continuously being discovered, and operationalization must reflect this complexity. For example, measures of cognition have been used as indicators of severity of dementia and subsequent ADL and instrumental ADLs function. Reed et al.[2] demonstrated that dementia severity is a complex concept and that the relationship between cognition and ADL function varies by level of cognition. In their study, they found that for subjects with Mini-Mental State Examination (MMSE) scores less than 14.5, there was a significant relationship between MMSE scores and both instrumental and physical ADLs. In the group with greater cognitive functioning (MMSE scores greater than 14.5), MMSE and ADLs scores were independent.

For research that has a direct impact on gerontologic clinical practice, recognizing the complexity of conceptualization is not sufficient; clinical relevance also must reflect the conceptualization. This is a particularly salient issue for researchers interested in measuring elder outcomes. For example, when the improvement of cognitive functioning is the focus, effectiveness should not be limited to the cognitive dimensions of attention and memory because they can be very sensitively measured. Drug (trials) research tells us that additional criteria for success that are related to the impact on everyday life must be added.[3] This focus is particularly relevant to health care providers whose interest is to assist older persons to function at their highest level. A significant change in a memory test is not very important if there is no other change in the level of functioning that can be recognized by the patient, family, or caregiver.

Psychometric Properties

Reliability and validity are fundamental properties of an instrument.[4] *Reliability* is the consistency or stability of measurement. *Validity* refers to the degree to which the instrument actually reflects the concept. There are two different perspectives regarding the definition of validity. According to the revised Standards for Educational and Psychological Testing, validity is a unitary concept, and content, criterion, and construct validity are types of evidence rather than types of validity.[5] Alternatively, Messick, a measurement theorist, argues for the integration of the validity concept and considers content- and criterion-related validity as *evidence* of construct *validity.*[6]

Validity varies from situation to situation and sample to sample. Validity testing validates an instrument with a specific group, not the instrument itself, so any instrument used with elders must be validated with this group. Psychometrically sound measurement instruments are essential for any type of research. Outcomes from a relevant question and a perfectly designed study are useless if the data collected are not accurate and meaningful.

To enhance both reliability and validity, researchers need to minimize both random and systematic measurement error. Random error threatens measurement reliability.[5] Systematic error threatens validity. The following section discusses the potential sources of random and systematic error (1) within the elder respondent; (2) within the measuring device; or (3) related to the instrument administration.

Characteristics of Respondent

Anxiety and primary or secondary physiologic age changes may be sources of error in the measurement process. Primary age changes are those that result from the aging process that all individuals will experience if they live long enough. Secondary age changes are those ensuing from disease processes. Not all older adults experience secondary age changes.

Anxiety

Testing situations can be stressful to elders. Their perception and appraisal of stress depends on personality, health, education, and previous experiences.[7] Many elders were educated in a system that did not use Likert scales, semantic differentials, or multiple-choice questions; they may feel more anxious when confronted with these formats. Increased autonomic arousal can lead to performance deficits. Eisdorfer et al. demonstrated that deficits in verbal learning were associated with heightened autonomic nervous system receptor activity.[8] An experimental group of elders was given an intravenous solution of propranolol, to dampen their autonomic response, while learning a verbal task. The experimental group had significantly higher learning scores than the placebo group, demonstrating that high anxiety impedes the performance of older adults on memory tasks.

Conversely, to determine whether a reduction in anxiety would improve performance, Yesavage taught relaxation techniques to elders before memory training began.[9] Both the experimental and the control groups showed improvements in memory, but improvement was significantly greater in the experimental group receiving relaxation training. Lower anxiety scores at final testing were significantly correlated with recall. These studies indicate the potential effect of anxiety on responses. To obtain reliable data, researchers must create a calm, relaxing atmosphere for test taking.

Primary Age Changes

Primary age changes or age-related changes in vision and hearing can significantly impact the measurement process. Research has demonstrated that visual and hearing function may decrease in old age even when pathology is not found.[10] However, one cannot generalize about the specific changes that might occur because of the intra individual differences in patterns of change and variations in the time of sensory decline. For every physiologic function, some elders will consistently score within the normal range of young adults whereas others will show severe deficits.

Vision. Kosnik et al.[11] conducted a survey of adults 18–100 years to determine the impact of age-related changes on everyday visual performance. They found that five visual dimensions declined with age: visual processing speed, light sensitivity, near vision, dynamic vision, and visual search. The older adults took longer to carry out visual tasks and had more trouble with glare, dim illumination, and near visuals tasks. They also had more difficulty locating a target in a cluttered visual scene. These changes in visual performance are caused by (1) the cornea becoming slightly thicker and more likely to scatter light; (2) the lens becoming denser, more yellow, and less elastic; (3) the pupil becoming smaller, admitting less light; (4) the vitreous gel condensing and collapsing with bits of dense gel appearing as floaters; and (5) a gradual decrease in the number of nerve cells in the retina.[12] Older individuals also have increased difficulty differentiating between blue and green, the short light wavelengths, as opposed to red and yellow that have longer wavelengths.

These age-related visual changes must be considered in instrument development and administration. To enhance near visual tasks the type size is important. Printed materials should be in large type, at least 14 or 16 point.[13] Because low contrast negatively affects acuity, the color of both the paper and the type is important.[10] Black lettering on white paper provides a very high degree of contrast, whereas the contrast of yellow letters on green paper is much lower. Visual acuity is diminished in conditions of low illumination, so the testing environment must be well lit. The type of lighting also may be significant. According to Marmor, "warm" incandescent lighting is often more comfortable than "cold" fluorescent lighting.[12] Although lighting is important, glare also needs to be prevented. Close lighting should be directed onto the reading material, and the elder should not face a window with unfiltered sunlight. Non-gloss paper should be used for the self-report instrument. Vision can be quite good when lighting is optimal and the words are sharply defined.[12] To compensate for the decreased visual processing speed, the research protocol must provide enough time for elders to read self-report instruments.

Hearing. Hearing impairment is more likely to be undetected than visual problems and has been associated with decreased performance on certain cognitive tests.[14,15] Hearing impairment affects up to 23% of persons aged 65 to 74 and over 48% for those over 85.[16] Age-related changes in the anatomy and physiology of the ear result in a change in the quality of hearing—the older person can usually hear but not understand what is being said. Elders have decreasing (1) sensitivity to high-frequency tones (presbycusis); (2) ability to hear rapid speech; and (3) ability to discriminate sounds in the presence of background noise. The researcher should make sure that the subject's attention is obtained before starting to talk. To improve the understanding of speech, stand facing the elder as he or she might be lip-reading. The researcher should not stand so that a bright light is behind him or her as the elder's vision may be diminished. Researchers must also eliminate or minimize background noise and avoid rapid loud speech as volume and speed can distort sounds.

Secondary Age Changes

Chronic illnesses increase with age. The effects of primary aging are complicated by these pathologic processes or secondary aging. The interaction of pathology with age-related changes enhances heterogeneity among elders. The specificity of the health problem will determine the nature of any impairment that may effect the measurement process. For example, a person with arthritis may have difficulty writing or may be uncomfortable sitting for a long time. The elder with a genitourinary problem or who is taking diuretics may need frequent bathroom breaks. Individual physical and mental limitations must be assessed. However, two factors that should be considered with all frail elders are fatigue and the need for proxy respondents.

Fatigue should be considered when working with the frail elderly because it has implications for the item format of a written instrument and/or its administration. Depending on the extent of the fatigue, closed-ended questions that require short answers or just checking off items may be preferable to open-ended questions.[17] If an interview is used, it should be no longer than one to one-and-a-half hours.

Proxy respondents may need to be used when frail elders are involved. Family members most frequently supply information for elders. However, the reliability of these responses also is of concern. There may not be congruency between the elder and the proxy response. Rubenstein and colleagues have reported that, when compared to a professional observer's ratings, elderly individuals tend to overestimate their functional capacity and family members tend to underrate their older relative's capacities.[18] Magaziner and colleagues found similar results.[19] In a study of over 300 elderly and hospitalized patients with hip fractures, proxy respondents tended to underrate the patient's functional independence relative to the patient's ratings. To improve comparability between elder and proxy respondents, researchers recommended that questions refer to explicitly defined behaviors.

Characteristics of a Measuring Device

When developing a measuring device, two questions must be answered: (1) What is the domain to be measured? and (2) How is the domain to be measured? Embedded in the answers to these questions are potential sources of systematic error that can threaten validity.

What Is to Be Measured?

What an instrument measures depends on the definition of the concept. The definition delineates the scope of the content domain. Evidence for content validity is demonstrated when the test items are representative of the content domain.[4] Problems can occur when an instrument created for one age group is used for another. Age-related differences in what comprises the content domain of interest can threaten content validity.[20] A case in point is the measurement of depression.[20,21] Although somatic symptoms are common among the young, they are not sensitive indicators of early depression in elders as many elders without depression have the same somatic complaints. The increased prevalence of somatic complaints by elders on some self-report depression scales results in higher scores, suggesting that depression rates are higher among the elderly.[22] Thus, the items on many depression screening instruments must be carefully examined to ensure that they are valid indicators of depression for elders.

Threats to validity are not limited to domain differences between elders and younger people. Threats to content validity also are present when the same instrument is used among different subgroups of elders. The manifestation of depression may be different for the depressed young-old versus the depressed old-old. Weiss et al.[23] noted that many self-report depression scales do not include the symptoms that are most common for a depressed old-old population. Males and females may differ on instrumental activities of daily living (IADLs). A scale that includes items about cooking, cleaning, and shopping may not be appropriate for this present cohort of married elderly men because they do not usually perform these tasks. The severity of cognitive impairment may affect the validity of some ADL/IADL scales. An ADL Research Project based in Germany evaluated 92 scales that in some way measured ADL/IADL.[24] Preliminary analyses revealed a lack of items for individuals with very mild cognitive decline.

How Is the Domain Measured?

Once the appropriate content domain has been delimited, the specific questions to evaluate that domain have to be developed. Item content, word clarity, readability, and item format can all be potential sources of error that can threaten reliability and validity.

The instrument developer and content experts determine if item content adequately reflects the domain. However, the viewpoint of the elder test taker also is important. Items that are not relevant and that appear childish will not encourage elder participation even if they accurately measure the domain. Elders will not perform tasks that seem trivial or ridiculous.[25] Tasks that are realistic and that seem to be related to real-life activities in daily functioning have face validity.[26] Face validity does not provide evidence for validity[25] or subsequent participation.

Face validity is even more important for the frail elderly. Because it takes physical and/or mental energy to participate, higher levels of motivation are required. Face validity also has been called ecologic validity by some psychologists and psychiatrists.[27] An ecologically valid memory task should appear to relate to the memory tasks faced by elders in their daily lives.[26] Unfortunately, activities such as repeating progressively longer strings of numbers or learning nonsense syllables are frequently taken from neuropsychological test batteries. For example, a method frequently used to assess secondary memory is to ask the person to repeat three words and then later in the interview to ask the person to recall the same three words. If this task seems unimportant, the elderly may not even try to remember the words. Alternatively, the elder may become antagonistic, anxious, and unmotivated. If cooperation diminishes, performance also decreases.

Crook and colleagues[28,29] have developed a number of ecologically valid memory tests. To measure primary memory, instead of being asked to repeat a series of digits, the elder is asked to remember a telephone number or a telephone number with an area code. An ecologically valid test to measure secondary memory is called the Misplaced Object Task.[28] The subject is presented a board showing various rooms of a house. He is given ten objects and asked to place them in various rooms. After 30 minutes, he is asked to indicate where the objects were placed. These types of face-valid tasks should produce less anxiety and higher motivation, resulting in more reliable data.[30]

Lack of *clarity in wording* will threaten validity. Words have different meanings to different groups of people, and the researcher should confirm that there is congruence in meaning between the subject and the researcher and within the subject population itself. In a project to identify cognitive problems with survey questions, using questions from the National Health Interview Survey,[31] it was determined that elders interpreted some words differently. For example, in the question "Do you have any difficulty sitting for two hours?," some elders interpreted sitting as standing for short periods whereas others did not include standing in their definition. Another important feature of this special project was that it identified a method to judge the understandability of questions. Usually an indicator of a problematic survey item is a large number of "I don't know" or "no response" answers. In this project unclear items would not have been detected during a routine instrument administration because elders answered promptly and the responses sounded plausible. Problems were recognized only when probe questions were used to ascertain how questions were answered. Jobe and Mingay[31] recommended that pretesting of new questions be augmented with cognitive interviews.

Low readability of items will influence validity. Although the number of years of formal education of older adults is increasing, there still are a large number of elders of low literacy. Between 1970 and 1990, the percentage who had completed high school rose from 28% to 55%. Among ethnic and racial elderly groups, there are broad differences. In 1993, 37% of whites, 67% of African Americans, and 74% of Hispanics did not have a high school education. Because education levels are still quite variable, it is difficult to develop or select one set of measurement procedures that all elders can use. The researcher cannot automatically assume that if the sample respondents are old and African American or Hispanic that they will not be able to read. It is possible to have a group of high school and college graduates or one with individuals who have only an elementary school education. The researcher must estimate the mean educational level of the elderly population of interest so that measurement procedures are neither too difficult nor too basic. For example, an interview rather than a written format will be needed if the elder has minimal to no literacy skills. When many of the elders have low education levels, evaluating the readability of written material will provide a more objective assessment of difficulty. Several readability formulas are available, but one that has been recommended for patient education materials is the SMOG formula that assesses reading grade level for written text.[3,32] See Chapter 2 for examples of SMOG.

An instrument developer has to make many decisions about *item format*: open-ended versus closed-ended questions and if closed, the specific type. Closed-ended questions with their preset response options may be problematic for some elders because of difficulty categorizing their responses. This was illustrated in Jobe and Mingay's project[31] to evaluate survey questions. When elders were asked how frequently they had attended the senior center during the previous 12 months, many would provide a narrative answer that included frequency information instead of selecting a category (frequently, sometimes, never) as requested. The authors noted that younger respondents did not usually have difficulty selecting categories and attributed this difference to the younger respondents' testing experiences in school. Actually, the older respondent is providing a more accurate response as the categories could be defined differently by each respondent. Because the operationalization of the categories is really the researcher's decision, this type of question could be open-ended rather than fixed choice. Categorization of the response would then be a coding task of the research staff.

Visual analogue scales (VASs) can threaten validity, as many elders have trouble using them. A VAS is used to measure subjective experiences such as dyspnea, mood, anxiety, and pain.[33] In two pain studies, elders had some difficulty with use of the VAS. Kremer et al. obtained intensity estimates from a group of chronic pain patients using a VAS, a numeric scale, and an adjectival scale.[34] The mean age of failures on the VAS was significantly greater (mean 75.3 years) than the mean age of successful patients (mean 54.4 years). It was thought that the failure on the VAS might be related to a deterioration in abstract ability with age. The authors suggested that a numeric scale or an adjectival-numeric scale should be used to measure pain intensity. Similar results were obtained by Jensen et al.[35] Chronic pain patients were asked to rate pain intensity with a visual analog scale, a 101-point numerical rating scale, an 11-point box scale, a 6-point behavioral rating scale, a 4-point verbal rating scale, and a 5-point rating scale. Incorrect responses to the VAS were significantly related to age. There was no significant relationship between age and incorrect responses on the other measures.

Administration

When a lower range of educational levels is expected, the quality of the data may be improved by administering the instruments on a one-to-one or small-group basis. Giving subjects the option either to complete the instruments independently or have the investigator read the instruments to them while they follow along allows those with no or low literacy skills to "save face."[36] It also is less anxiety provoking and allows for immediate detection of misinterpretations by the data gatherer.[37] The disadvantage to this approach is the increased cost in time and money for trained data gatherers. However, the success of a scientific investigation depends on the quality of the data, so these costs need to be considered in the planning stages.

The time allowed to complete instruments is very important. More time is needed for one-on-one than for group administration. Elders should also be allowed to work at their own pace. Kim[38] found that when testing knowledge, when self-paced, elders performed better than those in the experiment-paced response conditions. The time for administration also must take into account the subject's agenda. Their agenda may be different from that of the data collector.[39]

Any interaction with the data collector could be viewed as a time for socialization. When asked a question, the elder may provide much more information than is required and/or may initiate another topic. Data collectors must be skilled interviewers experienced in working with elders. They must know how to maintain flexibility while completing the session in a timely fashion. Response burden also is a concern. Several long instruments can create excessive subject burden. Although longer instruments increase internal consistency,[4] they may not be the best choice for elders who are physically or mentally frail. A demented elder may become unmotivated, uncooperative, or fatigued if the testing sessions are too long. Data-collection sessions should be between one[30] and two hours long.[40] To further ease the burden, either rest periods or two very short data-gathering sessions could be offered to the elders.

Summary

Knowing that an instrument has been used with adults is not an acceptable selection criterion. Because of the interplay of normal age-related changes and pathology, particular attention must be paid to instrument selection and administration. The conceptualization of the study variables, the purpose of the instruments, and any threats to reliability and validity must be considered. Instruments are being developed specifically for elders that consider age-related changes and deal with age-related measurement problems. The Delayed Word Recall Test and the Geriatric Depression Scale[41] are two examples of these instruments. The Delayed Word Recall Test, which measures secondary memory, integrates the concept that healthy elders benefit from encoding enhancement. The subject creates sentences for each of ten words supposed to improve the encoding of these words. After a short time, the subject is asked freely to recall the words. A normal older person is supposed to do very well on this task, whereas one with dementia would not. The Geriatric Depression Scale[41] was developed to deal with domain, item format, and item acceptability issues of preexisting self-report depression scales.

Several instrument resources that have been used with elders: *Assessing the Elderly: A Practical Guide to Measurement* by Robert and Rosalie Kane;[42] the *Sourcebook of Geriatric Assessment*, a two-volume book sponsored by the World Health Organization;[43] and the "Handbook of Geriatric Assessment" by Gallo.[44]

Research is still needed regarding the health needs of elders. However, being cognizant of and attending to the potential measurement problems associated with this population will help to ensure the acquisition of high-quality data.

References

1. Fowles, D.G. *A profile of older Americans.* Washington, DC: American Association of Retired Persons, 1993.
2. Reed, B.R., Jagust, W.J., & Seab, J.P. Mental status as a predictor of daily function in progressive dementia. *Gerontology*, 1989, 29:804-807.
3. Stephens, S.T. Patient education materials: Are they readable? *Oncol Nurs Forum*, 1992, 19:83-85.
4. Waltz, C.F., Strickland, O.L., & Lenz, E.R. *Measurement in nursing research* (2nd ed.). Philadelphia: Davis, 1991.
5. American Educational Research Association. *Standards for educational and psychological testing.* Washington, DC: Author, 1985.
6. Messick, S. Validity. In R.L. Linn (Ed.), *Educational measurement* (3rd ed.). New York: Macmillan, 1989, pp. 13-104.
7. Eisdorfer, C. Stress, disease and cognitive change in the aged. In C. Eisdorfer & R. Friedel (Eds.), *Cognitive and emotional disturbance in the elderly.* Chicago: Year Book Medical, 1977.
8. Eisdorfer, C., Nowlin, J., & Wilkie F. Improvement of learning in the aged by modification of autonomic nervous system activity. *Science*, 1970, 170:1327-1329.
9. Yesavage, J.A. Relaxation and memory training in 39 elderly patients. *Am J of Psychiatry*, 1984, 141:778-781.
10. Owsley, C., & Sloan, M. Vision and aging. In F. Boller & J. Grafman (Eds.), *Handbook of neuropsychology.* New York: Elsevier, 1990, pp. 229–250.
11. Kosnik, W., Winslow, L., Kline, D., et al. Visual changes in daily life throughout adulthood. *J Gerontol*, 1988, 43:63-70.
12. Marmor, M.F. Age-related eye diseases and their effects on visual function. In E.E. Faye & C.S. Stuen, (Eds.), *The aging eye and low vision.* New York: The Lighthouse, 1992, pp. 11-21.
13. Weinrich, S.P., Boyd, M., & Nussbaum, J. Continuing education: Adapting strategies to teach the elderly. *J Gerontol Nurs*, 1989, 15:17-21.
14. Granick, S., Kleban, M.H., & Weiss, A.D. Relationships between hearing loss and cognition in normally hearing aged persons. *J Gerontol*, 1976, 31:434-440.
15. Ohta, R.J., Carlin, M.F., & Harmon, B.M. Auditory acuity and performance on the Mental Status Questionnaire in the elderly. *J Am Geriatr Soc*, 1981, 29:476-478.
16. Havlik, R.J. Aging in the eighties, impaired senses for sound and light in persons age 65 years and over:

Preliminary data from the supplement on aging to the National Health Interview Survey: United States, January-June 1984. *Vital Health Stat NCHS*, 1986, 125:1-8.
17. Sexton, D.L. Some methodological issues in chronic illness research. *Nurs Res*, 1983, 32:378–380.
18. Rubenstein, L.Z., Schairer, C., Wieland, D.S., & Kane, R. Systemic bias in functional status assessment of elderly adults: Effects of different data sources. *J Gerontol*, 1984, 39:686-690.
19. Magaziner, J., Simonsick, E.M., Kashner, T.M., & Hebel, J.R. Patient-proxy response comparability on measures of patient health and functional status. *J Clin Epidem*, 1988, 41:1065-1074.
20. Kasniak, A.W. Psychological assessment of the aging individual. In J.E. Birren & K.E. Schaie (Eds.), *Handbook of psychology of aging* (3rd ed.). Boston: Academic Press, 1990, p. 432.
21. Phillips, L.R. Challenges of nursing research with the frail elderly. *West J Nurs Res*, 1992, 14:721-730.
22. Bolla-Wilson, K., & Bleecker, M.L. Absence of depression in elderly adults. *J Gerontol*, 1989, 2:53-55.
23. Weiss, B.A., Nagel, C.L., & Aronson, M.K. Applicability of depression scales to the old person. *J Am Geriatr Soc*, 1986, 34:215-218.
24. Schmidt-Gollas, N., & Erzigkeit, H. Ways of constructing a therapy sensitive scale for the assessment of ADL aspects in cognitively impaired elderly patients. In M. Bergener, R.H. Belmaker, & M.S. Tropper (Eds.), *Psychopharmacotherapy for the elderly: Research and clinical implications.* New York: Springer, 1993, pp. 119-124.
25. Cunningham, W.R. Psychometric perspectives: Validity and reliability. In L.W. Poon (Ed.), *Clinical memory assessment of older adults.* Washington, DC: American Psychological Association, 1986, pp. 27-31.
26. Ferris, S.H., Reisberg, B., deLeon, M., & Crook, T. Recent developments in the assessment of senile dementia. In J.P. Abrahams & V. Crooks (Eds.), *Geriatric mental health.* New York: Grune & Stratton, 1984.
27. Woods, R.T., & Britton, R.G. *Clinical psychology with the elderly.* Rockville, MD: Aspen, 1985.
28. Crook, T., Ferris, S.H., & McCarthy, M. The misplaced objects test: A brief test for memory dysfunction in the aged. *J Am Geriatr Soc*, 1979, 27:284-287.
29. Crook, T., Ferris, S.H., McCarthy, M., & Rae, D. The

utility of digit recall tasks for assessing memory in the aging. *J Consult Clin Psychol*, 1980, *48*(2):228-233.

30. Ferris, S.H., Crook, T., Flicker, C., Reisberg, B., & Bartus, R.T. Assessing cognitive impairment and evaluating treatment effects: Psychometric performance tests. In L.W. Poon. (Ed.), *Clinical memory assessment of older adults*. Washington, DC: American Psychological Association, 1986, pp. 139-148.

31. Jobe, J.B., & Mingay, D.J. Cognitive laboratory approach to designing questionnaires for surveys of the elderly. *Public Health Rep*, 1990, *105*:518-524.

32. Mclaughlin, G.H. SMOG grading: A new readability formula. *J Reading*, 1969, *12*:639-646.

33. Wewers, M.E., & Lowe, N.K. A critical review of visual analogue scales in the measurement of clinical phenomena. *Res Nurs Health*, 1990, *13*:227-236.

34. Kremer, E., Atkinson, J.H., & Ignelzi, R.J. Measurement of pain: Patient preference does not confound pain measurement. *Pain*, 1981, *10*:241-248.

35. Jensen, M.P., Karoly, P., & Braver, S. The measurement of clinical pain intensity: A comparison of six methods. *Pain*, 1986, *27*:117-126.

36. Rasin, J.H. The relationship between confusion and blood pressure in black, community elders. *Dissertation Abstracts International*, 1989, *50*:2663B.

37. Gueldner, S.H., & Hanner, M.B. Methodological issues related to gerontological nursing research. *Nurs Res*, 1989, *38*:183-185.

38. Kim, K.K. Response time and health care learning of elderly patients. *Res Nurs Health*, 1986, *9*:233-239.

39. Zimmer, A.W., Calkins, E., Hadley, E., et al. Conducting clinical research in geriatric populations. *Ann Int Med*, 1985, *2*:276-283.

40. Applegate, W.B., & Curb, J.D. Designing and executing randomized clinical trials involving elderly persons. *J Am Geriatr Soc*, 1990, *8*:943-950.

41. Yesavage, J.A., & Brink, T.L. Development and validation of a geriatric depression screening scale: A preliminary report. *J Psychiatry Res*, 1983, *17*:37-49.

42. Kane, R.A., & Kane, R.L. *Assessing the elderly*. Lexington, MA: Lexington Books, 1981.

43. Israel, L., Zozaveric, D.S., & Sartorius, N. *Sourcebook of geriatric assessment*. Basel: Karger, 1984.

44. Gallo, J.J., Reichel, W., & Anderson, L. "Handbook of Geriatric Assessment," *Psychopharmacol Bull*, 1988, *24*:1-20.

5

Measurement Issues Concerning Linguistic Translations

Claudette G. Varricchio

The current research climate emphasizes the inclusion in clinical research of representative samples of all ethnic and cultural groups, thereby reflecting the composition of the U.S. population. Many researchers are interested in the cross-cultural aspects of illness and wellness phenomena, symptoms, and other variables. For these reasons, it is important to consider linguistic translations and the cultural appropriateness of research tools. This chapter addresses the issues, controversies, and techniques used for translating and determining the cultural appropriateness of measurement instruments.

Many instruments that assess physical symptoms, functional status, psychologic state, and social interactions, as well as more global constructs, have been developed and validated. If these instruments are considered for cultural adaptation or linguistic translation, a researcher must have operationally defined the concepts. The researcher must then determine whether the concepts exist in the target culture and whether they can be operationalized in the same way. Few existing methods of assessment of health-illness concepts are appropriate for, or have been validated with, subjects from diverse cultural backgrounds. This problem is compounded by the practical difficulties of language barriers, cultural differences, and economic constraints in addition to the cultural and ethnic diversity of the subjects. Thought must be given to the validity of cultural equivalence of meaning when interpreting the scores. Decisions regarding treatment and supportive care or other interventions for persons from special populations often are based on clinical research that includes few participants from these groups.

Language is one of the most obvious barriers to assessment. Simple, direct translation of standardized or new instruments will not solve this problem.[1-5] Psychosocial and other concepts do not necessarily have a one-to-one correspondence between languages, or within a language from dialect to dialect.[6,7] Measures of health-related concepts must be sensitive to these subtle language differences, as well as to cultural differences that influence understanding of the constructs. The development or modification of instruments for people from non-English-derived cultures requires knowledge of the customs, beliefs, and traditions the target subjects practice related to health, illness, independence, and decision making. Methods and instruments must be validated in the target population to ensure that the concepts of interest have the same meaning as in the original language and culture. There is no reason to expect that a reliable and valid research instrument in one language will accurately measure the phenomenon as experienced by people from another culture.[1]

The underlying question is whether the research stimuli are presented in equivalent ways to all of the individuals included in a study, and whether conclusions from a study using a specific set of measures in a primarily white, middle-class U.S. sample can be generalized or compared to conclusions derived from, or applied to, subgroups of Americans or to subjects from other ethnic or cultural groups. The methods of approaching cross-cultural research and the translation, cultural appropriateness, and adaptation of existing instruments are the focus of this chapter.

Instrument Translation

The recommended procedure for translating research instruments is known as back-translation.[1,2] The goal is to ensure the equivalent meaning of items in both languages. This is accomplished by having questions in the source language translated by a bilingual person, preferably from the target culture, into the target language. Another bilingual individual then translates the items from the target language back to the source language. The two source language versions are then compared for equivalence. This process can be repeated until satisfactory equivalence is obtained.

When the original English version is revised to ensure conceptually identical items in the target language and back-translated versions, the result is known as *decentering*. In this process, no one language is the center of attention. Both languages are equally important during the translation procedure. In decentering, both languages contribute to the final set of questions, and both are open to revisions.[8]

Researchers are cautioned not to become overly confident in the outcome of the initial efforts at back-translation. In some instances, seeming equivalence between versions may be the result of factors other than good translations. Brislin[8] suggests that the following factors must be considered when judging the adequacy of a translation: Translators may have a shared set of rules for translating certain nonequivalent words and phrases; some back-translators may be able to make sense out of a poorly written target language version; the bilingual translating from the source to the target may retain many of the grammatical forms of the source. In such situations, the translated document may be worthless for the purpose of asking questions of target language monolinguals because it uses grammar common to the source, not the target group.

A second issue to consider in translation is that of etic versus emic concepts. *Etic* refers to phenomena that are universal or have a common meaning across the cultures of interest. If a concept survives repeated rounds of translation and back-translation, it can be considered etic. An etic concept can be expressed with readily available words and phrases in the languages of the two cultures. *Emic* concepts are group specific or are not readily expressed in the different cultures and do not survive back-translation in a consistent, common interpretation.[1,2] Emic concepts are not readily expressed in one of the languages or do not have a word form with equivalent meaning in both languages.

An ideal translation contains etic concepts and emic concepts added to ensure that the questionnaire is culturally relevant. This process works best when adjustments are made in the wording of the source-language items. Some suggestions for successful translation efforts follow:[1, p144-149]

- Use short simple sentences of less than sixteen words with one dominant idea per sentence.
- Use the active rather than passive voice.
- Repeat nouns rather than using pronouns.
- Avoid metaphors and colloquialisms.
- Avoid the subjunctive: verb forms with could, should, or would.
- Add sentences to provide a context for key ideas.
- Avoid adverbs and prepositions telling "where" or "when." There often are no direct equivalents for these words, and the meaning of the entire item may be changed.
- Avoid possessive forms whenever possible. The concept of ownership may differ in different cultures.
- Use specific rather than general terms.
- Avoid vague terms regarding some event or thing, such as probably, maybe, or perhaps.
- Use words that are familiar to the translator.
- Avoid sentences with two different verbs if the verbs suggest two different actions.

Often a discussion of etic versus emic leads to a philosophical discussion concerning what is the desired outcome—linguistic equivalence or conceptual equivalence. In a linguistically equivalent item, there is a word-for-word translation. If no equivalent word is available in the target language, the item may be dropped or a word is chosen that conveys, as closely as possible, the same idea even if this concept has no meaning to the target group. In a conceptually equivalent translation, an item may use different words, but the intent is to convey an equivalent idea that has meaning and relevance to the target population.

Concept equivalence as a goal may necessitate adaptation of source-language items and changes in an existing instrument. This works best when applied to the translation of new instruments or if the researcher is willing to make changes in the choice of words in an existing instrument and validate both versions of the instrument in the appropriate targeted populations. The intent of the item is maintained, not the exact content. In this situation, the final back-translated version may serve as the source language version in the research setting because it is most likely to be equivalent to the target language version.[1] Some authors of established tools resist any changes in their instruments by others working on translations or cultural adaptations. Some recommendations for the back-translation process can be followed:[8]

- If possible, the translators should be familiar with the content (disease vocabulary, psychosocial concepts, etc.) in the source language and in the target language.
- Use words in the source language that have similar frequency of use in the target language.
- Translators and back-translators should work independently of each other.
- Test the translation on bilinguals. The researcher could use a split half arrangement where one group takes the first half of the test in the source language and the second half in the target language. The process is reversed for group two.
- Refine translations on items where there is ambiguity or discrepancy in responses.
- Discard items where agreement on the wording or meaning cannot be achieved. Modification of the wording of items in the source language may be necessary at this point.
- Test with focus groups or a small pilot group of the target population to ensure that persons representative of the target group understand the items. Administer the items

to bilingual subjects: Some see the source language version, some see the target language version, and some see both. Responses should be similar across groups.

Cultural Appropriateness

Accurate translations can result in linguistic equivalence, but may not elicit accurate responses from subjects using the target language version because appropriate attention was not given to culture-specific aspects in tool development. Cultural or linguistic subgroups may preferentially use different words for an object or an idea. If the word or phrase commonly used by the target population is not used, the translation may be stilted, foreign, or meaningless for those responding.[9] A detailed discussion of this topic can be found in Marin and Marin.[2] A given translation may meet one or many criteria for cross-cultural equivalence. This is one technique for judging the adequacy of the translation. The following five criteria are often used:[10]

1. *Content equivalence.* The content of each item of the instrument is relevant to the phenomena of each culture being studied.
2. *Semantic equivalence.* The meaning of each item is the same in each culture after translation into the language and idiom of each culture.
3. *Technical equivalence.* The method of assessing the concept is comparable in each culture with respect to the data that it yields.
4. *Criterion equivalence.* The interpretation of the findings remains the same when compared with the norm for each culture studied.
5. *Conceptual equivalence.* The instrument is measuring the same theoretical construct in each culture.

An instrument may be cross-culturally equivalent by any of the criteria and not in the others. The goal of true cultural and language equivalence is that an instrument is equivalent in all five of the criteria.[10] This approach to cross-cultural validity is similar in concept to the more familiar types of validity used in research (i.e., face validity, construct validity).

One way to evaluate cultural appropriateness or relevance is to convene a focus group representative of the target population and ask participants to review the proposed items and comment on their meaning, clarity, and currency. Another way is to ask selected individuals in an interview setting, "What does the item mean to you?" and "What ideas are conveyed by this item?" This process is particularly relevant when dealing with translations of standardized instruments that have been normed on English-speaking groups.

The psychometric characteristics of the target language version also must be established. It has been reported that the internal structure of an instrument changes when it is adapted and translated.[2] Different factor structures in a factor analysis may mean that different constructs are being tapped in the two versions.[10] As with the adaptations of all research instruments, any changes in the wording or structure of an instrument requires that validity and reliability be established for the new version.

Acculturation

The culture learning that occurs when immigrants come into contact with a new group, nation, or culture has been labeled *acculturation*.[2,11,12] The degree to which persons from one culture assume the thoughts, behaviors, beliefs, and values of the host culture is a measure of their acculturation. Berry[13] suggested that acculturation involves change in any or all of six areas of psychological functioning: language use, cognitive style, personality, identity, attitudes, and stress.

Measures of acculturation should go beyond demographic information. Self-identity of the subjects, as an outsider or a member of the culture, is an important aspect of this construct. Diversity within cultural or ethnic communities must not be overlooked. Assumptions of homogeneity cannot be made. Varying degrees of acculturation are likely in any given cohort of subjects and are based on the degree of exposure and interaction of the individual or group with the new culture. The researcher must decide to what extent the degree of acculturation is likely to affect the variables of interest in any research study. Excellent discussions of the assessment of acculturation and of existing acculturation scales are available in Marin and Marin.[2,11]

Is it necessary and cost-effective to measure acculturation in the planning phase of the research? Will acculturation be taken into consideration when choosing how to measure the research variables? These questions are increasingly relevant given the current requirement to include women, minorities, and subpopulations in clinical research. The costs of producing appropriate measurement tools must be included in calculating research budgets. The time required for translations and cultural adaptations must be planned into research, and pilot studies for validation of the adapted research tools will be necessary preliminary work until a critical mass of validated and reliable instruments is available.

Additional Resources

Researchers who are considering translating or adapting an existing instrument or creating a new one will find the Additional Readings section at the end of this chapter useful. Translation and cultural sensitivity in research are areas that are developing rapidly and where new information is constantly becoming available. Many of the currently available instruments have had limited validity testing in culturally diverse populations. The researcher is cautioned about the need to establish validity and other parametrics in the target population before making assumptions or interpreting the data. The appendix highlights established research instruments that have been translated or culturally adapted. In some cases the validity of the translated version is still under investigation.

References

1. Brislin, R.W. The wording and translation of research instruments. In W.J. Lonner & J.W. Berry (Eds.), *Field methods in cross-cultural research*. Beverly Hills, CA: Sage, 1986, pp. 137-164.
2. Marin, G., & Marin B.V. *Research with Hispanic populations*. Newbury Park, CA: Sage, 1991.
3. Montero, D. Research among racial and cultural minorities: An overview. *J Soc Issues*, 1977, 33(4):1-10.
4. Hayes-Bautista, D.E., & Chapa, G. Latino terminology: Conceptual bases for standardized terminology. *AJPH*, 1987, 77(1):61-68.
5. Hendricson, W.D., Russel, I.J., Prihoda, T.J., et al. An approach to developing a valid Spanish language translation of a health status questionnaire. *Med Care*, 1989, 27(10):959-966.
6. Schur, C.L., Bernstein, A.B., & Berk, M.L. The importance of distinguishing Hispanic subpopulations in the use of medical care. *Med Care*, 1987, 25(7):627-641.
7. Trevino, F.M. Standardized terminology for Hispanic populations. *JAPH*, 1987, 77(1):69-72.

8. Brislin, R.W. Back-translation for cross-cultural research. *J Cross-Cultural Psychol*, 1970, 1(3):185-216.
9. Bravo, M., Canino, G.J., Rubio-Sitpec, M., & Woodburry-Farina, M. A cross-cultural adaptation of a psychiatric epidemiologic instrument: The diagnostic interview schedule's adaptation in Puerto Rico. *Culture, Med Psychiatry*, 1991, 15(1):1-18.
10. Flaherty, J.A., Gavira, M.F., Pathak, D., et al. Developing instruments for cross-cultural psychiatric research. *J Nerv Mental Dis*, 1988, 176(5):257-263.
11. Marin G., Sabogal, F., Marin, B.V., et al. Development of a short acculturation scale for Hispanics. *Hispanic J Behav Sci*, 1987, 9(2):183-205.
12. Berry, J.W., Trimble, J.E., & Olmedo, E.L. Assessment of acculturation. In W.L. Lonner & J.W. Berry (Eds.), *Field methods in cross-cultural research*. Beverly Hills, CA: Sage, 1986, pp. 291-324.
13. Berry, J. Acculturation as varieties of adaptation. In A.M. Padilla (Ed.), *Acculturation: Theory, models and some new findings*. Boulder, CO: Westview, 1980, pp. 9-25.

Additional Readings

Information on Specific Measurement Tools That Have Been Translated

Bravo, M., Canino, G.J., Rubio-Stipc, M., & Woodbury-Farina, M. A cross-cultural adaptation of a psychiatric epidemiologic instrument: The diagnostic interview schedule's adaptation in Puerto Rico. *Culture, Med Psychiatry*, 1991, 15:1-18.

Bundek, N.I., Marks, G., & Richardson, J.L. Role of health locus of control beliefs in cancer screening of elderly Hispanic women. *Health Psychol*, 1993, 12(3):193-199.

Canino, G.J., Bird, H.R., Shrout, P.E., et al. The Spanish diagnostic interview schedule. Reliability and concordance with clinical diagnoses in Puerto Rico. *Arch Gen Psychiatry*, 1987, 44:720-726.

Cervantes, R.C., Padilla, A.M., & Salgado de Snyder, N. Reliability and validity of the Hispanic stress inventory. *Hispanic J Behav Sci*, 1990, 12(1):76-82.

Deyo, R.A. Pitfalls in measuring the health status of Mexican Americans: Comparative validity of the English and Spanish Sickness Impact Profile. *AJPH*, 1984, 74(6):569-573.

De Beneditis, G., Massei, R., Nobili, R., & Pieri, A. The Italian pain questionnaire. *Pain*, 1988, 33:53-62.

DeVogler-Ebersole, K.L., & Ebersole, P. Meaning in life depth test—"Spanish." In D. Jenerson-Madden, P. Ebersole, A.M. Romero, (Eds.), Personal life meaning of Mexicans. *J Soc Behav Personality*, 1992, 7:151-161.

Erkel, E.A. Conceptions of community health nurses regarding low-income Black, Mexican American, and white families: Part I. *J Comm Health Nurs*, 1985, 2(2):99-107.

Evers, G.C.M., Isengerg, M.A., Philipsen, H., Senten, M., & Btouns, G. Validity testing of the Dutch translation of the appraisal of the self-care agency A.S.A.-Scale. *Int. J Nurs Stud*, 1993, 30(4):331-342.

Flaherty, J.A., Gaviria, F.M., Pathak, D., et al. Developing instruments for cross-cultural psychiatric research. *J Nerv Mental Dis*, 1988, 176(5):257-263.

Franks, F., & Faux, S.A. Depression, stress, mastery, and social resources in four ethnocultural women's groups. *Res Nurs Women's Health*, 1990, 13:283-292.

Garcia, H.B., & Lee, P.C.Y. Knowledge about cancer and use of health care services among Hispanic- and Asian-American older adults. *J Psychosoc Oncol*, 1988, 6(3/4):157-177.

Gaston-Johansson, F., Albert, M., Fagan, E., & Zimmerman, L. Similarities in pain descriptions of four different ethnic-culture groups. *J Pain Symptom Man*, 1990, 5(2):94-100.

Gilson, B.S., Bilson, J.S., Bergner, M., et al. Sickness Impact Profile. In W.D. Hendricson, I.J. Russell, T.J. Prihoda, et al. (Eds.), An approach to developing a valid Spanish language translation of a health status questionnaire. *Med Care*, 1989, 27:959-966.

Gilson, B.S., Erickson, D., Chavez, C.T., et al. A Chicano version of the Sickness Impact Profile (SIP). *Culture, Med Psychiatry*, 1980, 4:137-150.

Gonzales, J.T., & Gonzales, V.M. Initial validation of a scale measuring self-efficacy of breast self-examination among low-income Mexican American women.

Hispanic J Behav Sci, 1990, 12(3):277-291.

Guarnaccia, P.J., Angel, R., & Worobey, J.L. The factor structure of the CES-D in the Hispanic health and nutrition examination survey: The influences of ethnicity, gender and language. *Soc Sci Med*, 1989, 29(1):85-94.

Hendricson, W.D., Russell, I.J., Prihonda, T.J., et al. Sickness Impact Profile—San Antonio format. In W.D. Hendricson, I.J. Russell, T.J. Prihoda et al. (Eds.), An approach to developing a valid Spanish language translation of a health-status questionnaire. *Medical Care*, 1989, 27(10):959-966.

Lobo, A., Perez-Echeverria, M.J., & Artal, J. Validity of the scaled version of the General Health Questionnaire (QHQ-28) in a Spanish population. *Psychol Med*, 1986, 16:135-140.

Lobo, A., Perez-Echeverria, M.J., Jimenez-Aznarez, A., & Sancho, M.A. Emotional disturbances in endocrine patients. Validity of the scaled version of the General Health Questionnaire (GHQ-28). *Brit J Psychiatry*, 1988, 152:807-812.

Lopez-Aqueres, W., Kemp, B., Plopper, M., et al. Health needs of the Hispanic elderly. *J Am Geriat Soc*, 1984, 32(3):191-198.

Lorensen, M., Holter, I.M., Evers, G.C.M., et al. Cross-cultural testing of the "appraisal of self-care agency: ASA scale" in Norway. *Int J Nurs Stud*, 1993, 30(1):15-23.

Madiros, M. A view toward hospitalization: The Mexican American experience. *J Adv Nurs*, 1984, 9:469-478.

Meenan, R.F., Gertman, P.M., & Mason, J.M. Arthritis Impact Measurement Scale. (AIMS). In W.D. Hendricson, I.J. Russell, T.J. Prihoda et al. (Eds.), An approach to developing a valid Spanish language translation of a health-status questionnaire. *Med Care*, 1989, 27:959-966.

Meister, J.S., Warrick, L.H., de Zapien, J.G., & Wood, AH. Using lay health workers: Case study of a community-based prenatal intervention. *J Comm Health*, 1992, 17(1):37-51.

Naughton, M.J., & Wiklund, I. A critical review of dimension-specific measures of health-related quality of life in cross-cultural research. *Qual Life Res*, 1993, 2(6):397-432.

Nielsen, B.B., McMillan, S., & Diaz, E. Instruments that measure beliefs about cancer from a cultural perspective. *Cancer Nurs*, 1992, 15(2):109-115.

Park, K.B., Upshaw, H.S., & Koh, S.D. East Asians: Response to Western health items. *J Cross-Cultural Psychol*, 1988, 19(1):51-63.

Patrick, D.L., Sittamplam, Y., Somesville, S.M., et al. Cross-cultural comparison of health status values. *AJPH*, 1985, 75(12):1402-1407.

Roberts, R.E., Attkisson, C.C., & Mendias, R.M. Assessing the client satisfaction questionnaire in English and Spanish. *Hispanic J Behav Sci*, 6(1):385-396.

Spinetta, J.J. Measurement of family function, communication, and cultural effects. *Cancer*, 1984, 53(10 suppl): 2330-2337.

Vallerand, R.J., & Halliwell, W.R. Vers une méthodologie de validation trans-culturelle de questionnaires psychologiques: Implications pour la psychologie du sport. *Can J Appl Sport Sci*, 1983, *8*(1):9-18.

Walker, S.N., Kerr, M.J., Pender, N.J., & Sechrist, K.R. A Spanish language version of the health-promoting lifestyle profile. *Nurs Res*, 1990, *39*(5):268-273.

Warrick, L.H., Wood, A.H., Meister, J.S., & de Zapien, J.G. Evaluation of a peer health worker prenatal out-

reach and education program for Hispanic farm worker families. *J Comm Health*, 1992, *17*(1):13-26.

Zapka, J.G., Harris, D.R., Hosmer, D., et al. Effect of a community health intervention on breast cancer screening among Hispanic American women. *Health Serv Res*, 1993, *28*(2):223-235.

Cultural Issues

AAN Expert Panel on Culturally Competent Nursing Care. AAN expert panel report: Culturally competent health care. *Nurs Outlook*, 1992, *40*(6):277-283.

Eliason, M.J. Ethics and transcultural nursing care. *Nurs Outlook*, 1993, *41*(5):225-228.

Ell, K.O., Mantell, J.E., & Hamovitch, M.B. Socioculturally sensitive interventions for patients with cancer. *J Psychosocial Oncol*, 1989, *6*(3/4):141-155.

Fong, C.M. Ethnicity and nursing practice. *Topics Clin Nurs*, 1985, *7*(3):1-10.

Frank-Stromborg, M., & Olsen, S.J. *Cancer prevention in minority populations*. St. Louis: Mosby, 1993.

Harwood, A. (Ed.). *Ethnicity and medical care*. Cambridge, MA: Harvard University Press, 1984.

Henderson, G., & Primeaux, M. (Eds.). *Transcultural health care*. Menlo Park, CA: Addison-Wesley, 1981.

Lipson, J.G., & Meleis, A.I. Culturally appropriate care:

The case of immigrants. *Topics Clin Nurs*, 1985, *7*(3): 48-56.

Porter, C.P., & Villarruel, A.M. Nursing research with African American and Hispanic people: Guidelines for action. *Nurs Outlook*, 1993, *41*(2):59-67.

Reinert, B.R. The health care beliefs and values of Mexican-Americans. *Home Healthcare Nurse*, 1986, *4*(5):23-31.

Rogler, L.H. The meaning of culturally sensitive research in mental health. *Am J Psychiatry*, 1989, *146*(3):296-303.

Tripp-Reimer, T. Research in cultural diversity. *Western J Nurs Res*, 1984, *6*(4):457-458.

West, E.A. The cultural bridge model. *Nurs Outlook*, 1993, *41*(4):229-234.

White, E.H. Giving health care to minority patients. *Nurs Clin North Am*, 1977, *12*(1):27-39.

Acculturation

Cuellar, I., Harris, L.C., & Jasso, R. An acculturation scale for Mexican American normal and clinical populations. *Hispanic J Behav Sci*, 1980, *2*(3):199-217.

Mendoza, R.H. An empirical scale to measure type and degree of acculturation in Mexican-American ado-

lescents and adults. *J Cross-Cultural Psychol*, 1989, *20*(4):372-385.

Olmedo, E.L., & Padilla, A.M. Empirical and construct validation of a measure of acculturation for Mexican Americans. *J Soc Psychol*, 1978, *105*:179-187.

Methodological Issues

Aaronson, N.K., Acquadro, C., Alonso, J., et al. International quality of life assessment (IQOLA) project. *Qual Life Res*, 1992, *1*:349-351.

Aday, L.A., Chiu, G.Y., & Andersen, R. Methodological issues in health care surveys of the Spanish heritage population. *AJPH*, 1980, *70*(4):367-374.

Berkanovic, E. The effect of inadequate language translation on Hispanics' responses to health surveys. *AJPH*, 1980, *70*(12):1273-1281.

Berzon, R., Hays, R.D., & Shumaker, S.A. International use, application and performance of health-related quality of life instruments. *Quality of Life Res*, 1993, *2*(6):367-368.

Bullinger, M., Anderson, R., Cella D., & Aaronson, N.K. Developing and evaluating cross-cultural instruments from minimum requirements to optimal models. *Qual Life Res*, 1993, *2*(6):451-459.

Canales, S., Ganz, P.A., & Schag, C.A.C. Translation and validation of a quality of life instrument for Hispanic American cancer patients: Methodological considerations. *Qual Life Res*, 1995, *4*(1):3-11.

Cella, D.F., Wiklund, S.A., & Aaronson, N.K. Integrating health-related quality of life into cross-national clinical trials. *Qual Life Res*, 1993, *2*(6):433-440.

Domino, G., Fragoso, A., & Moreno, H. Cross-cultural investigations of the imagery of cancer in Mexican nationals. *Hispanic J Behav Sci*, 1991, *13*(4):422-435.

Guyatt, G.H. The philosophy of health-related quality of life translation. *Qual Life Res*, 1993, *2*(6):461-465.

Hayes-Bautista, D.E. Identifying "Hispanic" populations: The influence of research methodology upon public health. *AJPH*, 1980, *70*(4):353-356.

Hayes-Bautista, D.E., & Chapa, J. Latino terminology: Conceptual bases for standardized terminology. *AJPH*, 1987, *77*(1):61-68.

Howard, C.A., Samet, J.M., Buechley, R.W., et al. Survey research in New Mexico Hispanics: Some methodological issues. *Am J Epidem*, 1983, *117*(1):27-34.

Kroeger, A. Health interview surveys in developing countries: A review of the methods and results. *Int. J Epidem*, 1983, *12*(4):465-481.

Marin, G., & Marin, B.V. Methodological fallacies when studying Hispanics. *Appl Soc Psychol Ann*, 1982, *3*:99-117.

Marin, G., & Marin, B.V. A comparison of three interviewing approaches for studying sensitive topics with Hispanics. *Hisp J Behav Sci*, 1989, *11*(4):330-340.

Marin, G., Marin, B.V., Perez-Stable, E.J., & Otero-Sabogal, R. Cultural differences in attitudes and expectancies between Hispanic and non-Hispanic white smokers. *Hispanic J Behav Sci*, 1990, *12*(4):422-436.

McArt, E.W., & Brown, J.K. The challenge of research on international populations: Theoretical and methodological issues. *Oncol Nurs Forum*, 1990, *17*(2):283-286.

Montero, D. Research among racial and cultural minorities: An overview. *J Soc Sci*, 1977, *33*(4):1-10.

Munet-Vilaro, F., & Egan, M. Reliability issues of the family environment scale for cross-cultural research. *Nurs Res*, 1990, *39*(4):244-247.

Park, K.B., Upshaw, H.S., & Koh, S.D. East Asians; Responses to western health items. *J Cross-Cultural Psychol*, 1988, *19*(1):51-63.

Schur, C.L., Berstein, A.B., & Berk, M.L. The importance of distinguishing Hispanic subpopulations in the use of medical care. *Medical Care*, 1987, *25*(7):627-641.

Velasquez, R.J., & Callahan, W.J. Psychological testing of Hispanic Americans in clinical settings: Overview and issues. In K.F. Gesinger (Ed.), *Psychological testing of Hispanics*. Washington, DC: American Psychological Association, 1992.

Other Information

Anderson, R. T., Aaronson, N. K., & Wilkin, D. Critical review of the international assessments of health-related quality of life. *Qual Life Res*, 1993, *2*(6):369-395.

Antle, A. Cultural and ethnic dimensions of cancer care. The American Indian. *ONF*, 1987, *14*(3):70-73.

Becker, D.M., Hill, D.R., Jackson, J.S., et al. (Eds.). *Health behavior research in minority populations; access, design, and implementation*. NIH PUB. No. 92-2965. Washington, DC: DHHS, PHS, NIH, The National Heart, Lung and Blood Institute, 1992.

Brisbane, F.L., & Womble, M. *Working with African Americans. The professional's handbook*. Needham, MA: Ginn Press, 1992. Copies are available from HRDI International Press, 222 S. Jefferson St., Suite 200, Chicago, IL, 60611.

Bureau of the Census. *Hispanic Americans Today*. Washington, DC: U.S. Department of Commerce, Economics and Statistics Administration, Bureau of the Census, 1993, pp. 23-183.

COSSMHO. *Delivering preventive health care to Hispanics: A manual for providers*. Washington, DC: Author, 1990. Copies are available from Provider Education Project, 1501 16th St., NW, Washington, DC, 20036.

Guillory, J. Ethnic perspectives of cancer nursing: The Black American. *Oncol Nurs Forum*, 1987, *14*(3):66-69.

Health and psychosocial instruments (HaPI). Behavioral measurement database services. PO Box 110287, Pittsburgh, PA. 15232-0787 Tel.: (412) 687-6850. The HaPI database also is available online through BRS Search Services at your campus/organization library. The Fall 1993 HaPI-CD includes an update of over 3,000 records that describe the following kinds of measurement instruments: questionnaires, rating scales, interview forms, checklists, vignettes/scenarios, indexes, coding schemes/manuals, projective techniques, tests. The database can be queried for instruments in foreign languages. The HaPI database provides information on first published sources of new instruments to access health practices and outcomes. It does not review validity data. The author and address may be provided. The Behavioral Measurements Letter, a companion information source, is available from Linda Perloff, PhD, editor. The Behavioral Measurements Letter, PO Box 110287, Pittsburgh, PA 15232-0787.

Kagawa-Singer, M. Ethnic perspectives of cancer nursing: Hispanics and Japanese-Americans. *Oncol Nurs Forum*, 1987, *14*(3):59-65.

Naughton, M.J., & Wiklund, I. A critical review of dimension-specific measures of health-related quality of life in cross-cultural research. *Qual Life Res*, 1993, *2*(6):397-432.

National Coalition of Hispanic Health and Human Services Organizations. 1501 Sixteenth St., NW, Washington, DC, 20036, tel.: (202) 797-4335. E. Richardson is a source of information about measurement tools that have been translated into Spanish.

Office of Research on Women's Health, National Institutes of Health, 9000 Rockville Pike, Bethesda, MD, 20892, tel.: (301) 402-1770. Coordinates the effort to include women and minorities in clinical research.

Special Populations Studies Branch, National Cancer Institute, Division of Cancer Prevention and Control. George Alexander, MD, Chief. 9000 Rockville Pike, EPN 240, Bethesda, MD 20892, tel.: (301) 496-8589. This branch has special programs and direct interaction with investigators working with African Americans, Hispanics, Native Americans, Hawaiians, Alaskan Native residents, and underserved groups. Specific resources are the National Hispanic Cancer Control Research Network, the Native Hawaiian and American Samoan Cancer Control Research Network, National Outreach Initiatives Project, which includes the National Black Leadership Initiative on Cancer, the National Hispanic Leadership Initiative on Cancer, and the Appalachia Leadership Initiative on Cancer.

Surgeon General's National Hispanic/Latino Health Initiative. *Recommendations to the Surgeon General to Improve Hispanic/Latino Health*. Washington, DC: U.S. Department of Health and Human Services, 1993. Office of the Assistant Secretary for Health, Office of Minority Health. This is a summary of the Executive Planning Committee meeting held on April 22 and 23, 1993, and the implementation strategies identified at the meeting as crucial for prompt action. Office of Minority Health Resource Center. 1-(800)-444-6472. DHHS, PHS, Office of the Assistant Secretary for Health, Office of Minority Health. Health information and education materials and other directories are available for Asian and Pacific Islander Populations, African Americans, Native Americans, and sources of Spanish-language health materials.

The Language Assistants. Software programs to translate English- and foreign-language documents automatically or interactively. Has the capability of bidirectional translation in English, Spanish, French, German, and Italian. Information available by calling 1-(800)-851-2917, or 24-hour FAX 1-(415)-345-5575.

Varricchio, C. Cultural and ethnic dimensions of cancer nursing care: Introduction. *Oncol Nurs Forum*, 1987, *14*(3):57-58.

Appendix: Established Instruments That Have Been Translated

Title and Language	Source
Braden Scale French, Japanese, Italian	**Nancy Bergstrom, PhD, RN, FAAN**, Professor, College of Nursing, University of Nebraska Medical Center, 600 S. 42nd St., Omaha, NE 68198-5330
Brief Pain Inventory Arabic, Mandarin Chinese, French, Hmong, Italian, Norwegian, Polish, Russian, Serbocroatian, Spanish, Tagalog, Thai, Vietnamese	**Charles Cleeland, PhD**, Director of Pain Research Group, MD Anderson Cancer Center, Houston, TX 77030, (713) 790-2824
Cancer Rehabilitation Evaluation System (CARES) Spanish	**Patricia Ganz, MD**, Division of Cancer Control, UCLA, Los Angeles, CA 90024
Functional Assessment of Cancer Therapy (FACT) Spanish, French-Canadian. FACT -B, Spanish; FACT -C, Spanish; FACT -H&N, Spanish; FACT -L, Spanish; FAHI (HIV), Spanish; FACT -P, Spanish; FACT -O, Spanish; FACT -BMT, Spanish	**David Cella, PhD**, The Rush Cancer Institute, Division of Psychosocial Oncology, 1725 West Harrison, Suite 863, Chicago, IL 60612-3824
CES-D China, Taiwan **Breast cancer interview** Egyptian **Activities of daily living** Japanese	**Marjorie Kagawa-Singer, PhD, RN**, 862 Leonard Rd., Los Angeles, CA 90049
EORTC Quality of Life Scale (QOL 30) French-Canadian, Spanish (Texas and California), French	**Alice Kornblith, PhD**, Psychiatry Service, Memorial-Sloan-Kettering Cancer Center, 1275 York Ave., New York, NY 10021
EORTC Quality of Life Scale (QOL 30) Validated for lung cancer patients in 13 countries: Australia, Canada, Finland, United Kingdom, United States, Germany, The Netherlands, Denmark, Norway, Sweden, French-speaking Belgium, France, Italy	**Neil Aaronson**, Head, Division of Psychosocial Research and Epidemiology, The Netherlands Cancer Institute, Antomi van Leeuwenhoik Hospital, Plesmanlaan 121, 1066 CX Amsterdam, The Netherlands
Ferrans and Powers Quality of Life Index (QLI) Mexican Spanish, Mandarin, Arabic, Swedish, Korean, Japanese, Rumanian, Portuguese. Possibly available in versions for Australia, Canada, Chile, India, Japan, Jordan, Korea, Netherlands, New Zealand, Portugal, Rumania, Taiwan, Turkey, Sweden, and United Kingdom	**Carol Estwing Ferrans, PhD**, Assistant Professor, Dept. of Medical Surgical Nursing (M/C 802), College of Nursing, University of Illinois at Chicago, 845 S. Damen Ave., Chicago, IL 60612-7350
Family Environmental Scale, form R (Moos & Moos) Spanish (Puerto Rican), Vietnamese	**Frances Munet-Vilaro, PhD, RN**, Associate Professor, School of Nursing, San Jose State University, Washington Square, San Jose, CA, 95192
Health-Promoting Lifestyle Profile Spanish	**Susan Noble Walker, PhD, RN**, University of Nebraska Medical Center, College of Nursing, 600 S. 42nd St., Omaha, NE 68198-5330
Jaloweic Coping Scale (JCS) Chinese, Greek, Swedish, Tagalog. Possibly available in Dutch, Islandic, Japanese, Korean, Spanish, Taiwanese, Tamil, Thai, and Turkish	**Anne Jaloweic, PhD, RN**, Niehoff School of Nursing, Loyola University Chicago, 2160 S. First Ave., Maywood, IL 60153

Nottingham Health Profile (NHP)
French, Dutch, Spanish, Swedish

Rhodes Index of Nausea and Vomiting (INV)
Spanish, Swedish, Portuguese, Korean, Chinese, and Japanese

Adapted Symptom Distress Scale (ASDS), Form 2
Dutch

Sickness Impact Profile (SIP)
British English, French, Dutch, Norwegian, Swedish, Mexican American Spanish

South West Oncology Group (SWOG) Quality of Life Questionnaire includes a battery of several standardized scales and items from the MOS SF 36, the Symptom Distress Scale, and others. Validation in Spanish for the Southwest USA is under way

Medical Outcomes Study Short Form (MOS SF)
SF-20 (role functioning)
Spanish (Puerto Rico and Southern CA) and French-Canadian

SF-36 (Physical and Social functioning, Mental Health Inventory and single item overall rating of health)
Spanish

International Quality of Life Assessment Project
Translating for 13 countries: French and English Canada, France, Germany, Italy, Japan, Netherlands, U.S. Spanish, the United Kingdom, Australia, Belgium, Spain, Sweden
Mexican American Spanish dialect

Symptom Distress Scale (SDC)
Spanish

LASA Uniscale (Selby and Robertson)
Mexican American Spanish disease/treatment specific items for each protocol, co-morbidity item. These will be translated into Mexican American Spanish in a project under way

The World Health Organization Quality of Life Project (WHOQOL) This is broader in scope than the health-related QOL scales used in most U.S. clinical trials. Currently being translated into versions for Australia, Croatia, France, India, The Netherlands, Panama, Russia, Thailand, the United Kingdom, the United States, and Zimbabwe. Items will be specific to the country or culture and to the group being evaluated.

R.T. Anderson, Dept. of Public Health Sciences, The Bowman Gray School of Medicine, Winston-Salem, NC 27157

Verna Rhodes, EdS, RN, Dept. of Public Health Sciences
University of Missouri-Columbia, School of Nursing, S314 School of Nursing, Columbia, MO

R.T. Anderson, Dept. of Public Health Sciences, The Bowman Gray School of Medicine, Winston-Salem, NC 27157

Carole Moinpour, PhD, SWOG Statistical Center, 1124 Columbia St. MP-557, Seattle, WA 98104-3093

Linda Bertsch, MSN, RN, MOS-SF Burrougs Wellcome, Clinical Research Division, 3030 Cornwallis Rd., Research Triangle Park, NC 27709, (919) 315-3979

Ron Hays, PhD, The Rand Corporation (310) 393-0411

John E Ware, Jr., PhD, New England Medical Center, The Health Institute, Division of Health Improvement, Box 345, 750 Washington St., Boston, MA 02111 (617) 350-8098

Neil K. Aaronson, The Netherlands Cancer Institute Amsterdam, The Netherlands

Carole Moinpour, PhD, SWOG Statistical Center, 1124 Columbia St. MP-557, Seattle, WA 98104-3093

Ruth Mc Corkle, PhD, RN, School of Nursing, University of Pennsylvania, Philadelphia, PA
Carole Moinpour, PhD, SWOG Statistical Center, 1124 Columbia St. MP-557, Seattle, WA 98104-3093
Carol Moinpour, PhD, SWOG Statistical Center, 1124 Columbia St. MP-557, Seattle, WA 98104-3093

John Orley, MD, Mental Health Division of the WHO, 1211 Geneva 27, Switzerland

6

Physiologic Measurement Issues

Freda G. DeKeyser and Linda C. Pugh

Clinical practice involves assessment and intervention in response to both psychologic and physiologic alterations. Those working in clinical practice must be familiar with techniques used to quantify psychologic as well as physiologic parameters. There is also an increasing awareness that education[1] and research[2,3] in the biologic sciences must be enhanced and encouraged within health-related disciplines such as nursing. Therefore knowledge of the principles of measurement related to physiologic variables is needed by clinicians, educators, and researchers.

Sources of Measurement Error

The most common tools used by clinicians to measure physiologic variables are the five senses. For example, we *see* cyanosis, we *hear* crying, and we *smell* infectious exudate. Instruments such as microscopes or stethoscopes aid and directly enhance the performance of the senses. Possibly because many physiologic variables are directly observable and are so commonly performed, they are perceived as "hard data" or as being objective and without error. However, as stated in classical measurement theory, no measurement is without error.

In fact, several sources of potential error have been identified related to physiologic variables.[4] The first source of error is due to biologic variability. When a researcher measures a physiologic parameter at a certain time, it is probable that the value will change seconds later. The researcher does not know whether that change is due to physiologic changes within the individual or to instrument error. There also are differences among individuals. For example, in Western society there is a trend for blood pressure to increase with advancing age. A second source of error is found in specimen collection and handling. For example, the wrong name could be put on a collection tube or a sample could evaporate. Analytical methods also can contribute to error. A technician might not add enough reagent to a step in the analysis or a transducer might not be calibrated correctly. Errors also can be made after the analysis because of mistakes in transcription. Therefore, error variability leads to measurement error and so decreases the reliability and validity of measurements.

Reliability and Validity of Physiologic Measures

Errors associated with physiologic variables may be random or systematic, such as psychosocial variables. The evaluation of these errors also is described using the concepts of reliability and validity. However, the terms *reliability* and *validity* are rarely used in the biometric, medical, and medical technology literature, maybe because of a lack of familiarity with psychometric theory and the parallel development of other terms and methods deemed more appropriate. It is possible to combine aspects of both types of assessments so that practitioners from both backgrounds can evaluate physiologic variables more effectively.

Reliability

Reliability is a measure of the amount of random error of an instrument. Random measurement error refers to one-time, unusual, or chance mistakes made during the measurement process that lead to different scores on the measurement being taken. For example, if a nurse took a patient's blood pressure while the patient was speaking, the blood pressure reading would probably be higher than the patient's true blood pressure.

Within the psychosocial literature, reliability usually is determined by evaluating the internal consistency and the stability of results obtained with a tool. Internal consistency is usually calculated in psychosocial contexts with an alpha coefficient. This coefficient describes the extent to which performance on any one item or question in the instrument is a good indicator of performance on the entire tool.[5] In biomedical research this type of reliability evaluation is not common because the number of items in a measurement technique is usually very small. For some physiologic variables, investigators will take a specified number of readings and report the average or mean. Grip strength has been measured in two selected studies.[6,7] These researchers reported the average of three scores. Price and Fowlow[8] performed at least four cardiac output measures on patients following cardiac surgery. They discarded the first measure and then averaged the next three measures as long as the three were within 10% of each other.

Test–retest, intra- and interrater reliability methods measure the repeatability or stability of psychosocial instruments. *Test–retest reliability* is evaluated by administering an instrument such as a questionnaire at two different times and then determining the correlation between them. This concept is similar to the duplicate measurements taken in clinical laboratories. In this context, the same specimen is divided into several parts, then readings are taken and then correlated.

Precision is a term not often seen in the psychosocial literature, but it often is used in the biometric and medical literature to describe reliability. The standard error is used to describe the variability and precision of measurements in physiologic research. The specimen is divided into several parts, and the standard error is calculated. The higher the standard error, the greater the variability and, therefore, the lower the reliability of the measurement for that sample.

Intrarater reliability can be evaluated by having the same technician analyze separately two halves of specimens and then determining the correlation between the two readings. *Interrater reliability* is performed in a similar manner, except that two people instead of one perform the analyses. Topf and Davis[9] reported interrater reliability in the assessment of sleep stage scoring. Two scorers independently rated one out of every six sleep records in their sample. Sommers, Woods, and Courtade[10] reported that investigators need to attend to interrater reliability and injectate reliability when studying cardiac output.

The Levy–Jennings control chart is a method used by many clinical laboratories to assess precision. A standardized or control sample is divided into at least twenty parts and is then analyzed for a specific metabolite by a specific technique on subsequent days. A chart is made with the day on the x axis and the laboratory value on the y axis. The mean and standard deviations are calculated for all of the days being studied. Lines are drawn through the value of the mean, as well as two standard deviations above and below the mean. It is expected that only one in twenty-two points will be greater than two standard deviations above or below the mean.[11] If more than this number of points are found to be greater than two standard deviations away from the mean, then that method is said to be imprecise or unreliable for that laboratory.

Another method of calculating precision is the coefficient of variation. The coefficient of variation is calculated by dividing the standard deviation by the mean (where coefficient of variation = standard deviation/mean).[11]

Validity

Validity refers to an instrument's ability to measure the true score. Validity can be seen as a measure of the amount of systematic error of a measurement. Calibration is one method commonly used with biomedical instruments to decrease the amount of systematic measurement error. Calibration is the procedure by which an instrument is adjusted to make its readings correspond as closely as possible to the true values of a known substance. For example, Derrico[12] calibrated blood pressure readings from a Dinamap monitor with a mercury gravity manometer before collecting data.

Accuracy, the term used instead of validity in the biomedical literature, is said to reflect the amount of bias or difference between obtained results and the known or assumed truth.[13] Accuracy also can refer to the ability of the instrument to indicate the true value of the variable being measured. Ko[14] has defined accuracy as

$$\text{accuracy} = \frac{\text{True value} - \text{Measured value}}{\text{True value}} \times 100\%$$

Although validity has been defined as accuracy, there are several aspects related to validity that are not included in the concept of accuracy. Validity refers not only to how far empirical measurements are from true values but also whether the instrument is measuring what it is supposed to measure. For example, a researcher who just measured white blood cell counts would only be measuring some of the many aspects of immune functioning. There are many other measures of immune function, and it would be erroneous to conclude that the entire concept was measured by just white blood cell counts.

Accuracy is determined by three parameters: selectivity, sensitivity, and specificity. *Selectivity* refers to the ability of the instrument to identify correctly the signal under study and distinguish it from all other signals.[15] *Sensitivity*, or the true positive rate, is defined as the likelihood that a patient with a given disease will have a positive test result. *Specificity*, or the true negative rate, is the probability that a patient without the disease will have a negative test result (Figure 6.1). No test has 100% specificity and sensitivity. A test that has higher specificity usually has a lower sensitivity. Those deciding which measurement tool to use must decide whether it is more important to have a higher level of true positives or true negatives. For example, Davis[16] compared the sensitivity and specificity of tympanic, oral, and rectal thermometers. She found a 97.1% sensitivity and 75% specificity in comparing tympanic to oral thermometers and a 90.3% sensitivity and 89.3% specificity when comparing tympanic to rectal thermometers.

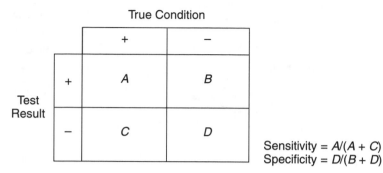

Figure 6.1 Sensitivity and Specificity

Construct Validity

Several approaches to validity can be tested and determined. *Construct validity* provides evidence of the instrument's ability to accurately measure the concept for which it was designed. It can be tested by using contrasted groups or experimental methods. When contrasted groups are used, two groups that are known to be very high and very low on the concept being studied are measured and compared by the instrument. If the groups are found to be significantly different, then the tool has adequately measured the concept. For example, Metheny et al.[17] tried to evaluate whether the pH values of feeding tube aspirates could be used to differentiate between gastric and intestinal tube placement. They hypothesized that aspirates from gastric tubes would have pH readings ranging from 0 to 4 and that intestinal tube aspirates would be greater than 4. They found that aspirates from gastric tubes were significantly more acidic than those from intestinal tubes, thereby supporting their hypothesis. This study lends construct validity to their pH measurement instrument.

If a hypothesis is tested and supported with an instrument, then the instrument is said to possess construct validity via experimental methods. One example of this type of construct validity is a study by McCarthy et al.[18] They hypothesized that meperidine affects temperature regulation. They found that injection of meperidine blocked the onset of fever in rats using a computerized telemetry system for body temperature monitoring. Therefore, their study demonstrated construct validity for their monitoring system.

Criterion Validity

Criterion validity is assessed when one method of analysis is compared to a known definitive method. Specimens are analyzed using this new method and using an older known method that has been shown to be reliable and valid. For example, Finkelstein and coworkers[19] compared a new method of home spirometry to known methods commonly used in hospital clinics, and Derrico[12] compared several methods of direct and indirect blood pressure monitoring in children.

Correlation coefficients are often used to compare the results of known methods with those obtained by newer ones. Bland and Altman[20] discourage this practice. They state that correlation coefficients measure relationships and not agreement between variables. Correlations also are affected by the range of true values in the sample. Tests of significance also are thought to be irrelevant because both instruments are designed to measure the same thing. Therefore, it would be unlikely *not* to find a significant relationship. Bland and Altman prefer the use of the mean absolute difference and the standard deviation of the difference as more appropriate statistics for this type of analysis.

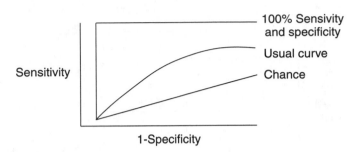

Figure 6.2 Example of ROC Curves

deMonterice and associates[21] report a mean absolute difference between two instruments that measure preterm infant sucking.

Receiver operating characteristic (ROC) curves also are used to compare newer technologies with known standard methods of measurement (Figure 6.2). For each method, the specificity and sensitivity are determined for different test criteria. For example, the blood pressures of known hypertensives were compared to those of normal controls with two types of automatic blood pressure machines. The blood pressures were taken using both machines on each patient. Several criteria for the definition of hypertension were then decided (e.g., systolic blood pressure: >130, >140, >150, >160). The number of true positives and true negatives were then computed for both types of measures, and the values converted into sensitivity and specificity values and plotted on a curve. The curve closest to the "perfect test" curve is the test with the higher validity.

Recovery experiments also are used as a type of criterion validity evaluation. A known amount of substance is added to a sample. The sample with the added substance and the sample without the added substance are then analyzed for that substance in a routine manner. The percentage of the substance found by the analysis is then calculated:[11]

$$\text{Percent recovery} = \frac{\text{Amount recovered}}{\text{Amount added}} \times 100$$

Groups of laboratories analyze the same control material and compare their results, another means of evaluating criterion validity. The results of the analysis by many labs are used to compute a mean and standard deviation. A standard deviation interval (SDI) for each lab can then be calculated as follows:

$$\text{SDI} = \frac{\text{Specific laboratory's value} - \text{Mean of all laboratories using the same method}}{\text{Standard deviation of all laboratories using the same method}}$$

A specific laboratory's results are said to be accurate if the absolute value of the SDI is less than or equal to 1, acceptable if the absolute value is less than 2 but greater than 1, and not acceptable if the absolute value is greater than 2.[11]

Content Validity

Content validity is said to exist when a tool or instrument contains most aspects of the concept being measured and is considered complete when it does not contain extraneous information. This type of validity can be evaluated in psychosocial and physiologic measures in a similar manner. Experts in the field are contacted and asked to evaluate whether the method being used in the analysis is appropriate.

The use of continuous monitoring can be seen as another step at increasing the content validity of monitoring equipment. As technology improves, more physiologic parameters are being measured continuously in more natural settings. For example, 24-hour monitors are now available that can measure activity levels, blood pressure, ECG, and gastric motility. Although problems exist as to what data to actually use in the data analysis, it is thought that information gained from monitoring a person over a longer time in more natural settings has higher validity than a one-time reading taken in a doctor's office or hospital bed.

Biomedical Instrumentation

Many physiologic variables are measured with some form of biomedical instrumentation. These tools may be used in connection with clinical practice and research. They often are electrically powered.[22] Every biomedical instrument is made up of three basic parts: a transducer, signal-conditioning equipment, and a display mode. Transducers convert one form of energy into another. In biomedical instruments, the transducer senses the physiologic event and converts it into an electrical signal usually measured in volts. For example, the voltage in an arterial blood pressure monitor increases as the arterial pressure increases. The transducer usually is separated from the rest of the instrument and often is applied to the body. For example, ECG electrodes are transducers that are placed on the chest.

The signal produced by the transducer is then sent to the signal-conditioning equipment. This component modifies the electrical signal so that it can be understood by other pieces of equipment. For example, the signal might be amplified or extraneous noise might be dampened. Noise or artifacts are unwanted signals that are produced but that are not due to the variable being measured. For example, when a patient moves in bed, noise or artifact often appears on the ECG monitor that is unrelated to electrical conduction in the heart.

The display converts the electrical signals sent by the signal-conditioning equipment into a form that can be understood by practitioners and/or stored in a computer. A strip recorder or an oscilloscope are two types of displays.

Several common properties of biomedical instruments can be used to evaluate their worth as measurement tools. These are the range, sensitivity, stability, and reliability of the instrument. The *range* of an instrument is "the complete set of values over which the instrument is designed to operate properly."[22] For example, Hanneman[23] reports that cardiac output readings are accurate within 5% for values between 0.5 and 1.0 liters/minute. If one expects values to be higher or lower than that range, one should choose another instrument.

Sensitivity, from an instrumentation point of view, refers to the ability of the machine to detect small differences. The higher the sensitivity, the smaller the differences that can be detected. Resolution, one aspect of sensitivity, is the smallest measurable input increment.[14] For example, a thermometer that measures in 0.1^0 differences is less sensitive than one that can detect differences of 0.01^0.[22] Ko[14] defines sensitivity as the ratio of output to input (output–input). Therefore, the larger the level of artifact or noise (or a larger input), the lower the sensitivity of the instrument.

Stability indicates the ability of a machine to maintain accurate values over repeated testings and time. A machine that has unstable readings will be subject to drift. *Drift* is a change in the sensitivity of the machine with time, temperature, or other interfering factors.[14] For example, Hanneman[23] calibrated arterial and pulmonary catheter equipment every 8 hours to control for a drift of 0.3 mm Hg per hour.

Table 6.1   Measurement Techniques Used in Psychosocial versus Physiologic Disciplines

	Psychosocial	Physiologic
Reliability/precision		
a) Internal consistency	Alpha coefficient	If >1 measure taken, average measurements together
b) Stability	Test–retest	Duplicate measurements
	Intrarater	Coefficient of variation
	Interrater	Standard error
Validity/accuracy		
a) Construct	Contrasted groups	Control groups
	Experimental methods	Experimental methods
b) Criterion	Correlations with known tools	Recovery experiments
		Standard deviation interval
		Correlations with known tools
		Receiver operating characteristic curves
c) Content	Content experts	Content experts

Table 6.1 compares the methods used to determine the reliability, precision, and validity or accuracy of measurement tools between the psychosocial and physiologic disciplines. Measures of internal consistency and stability can be replaced with duplicate measurements, coefficient of variation, and standard error measurements to assess the reliability and precision of a physiologic instrument. The accuracy or validity of instruments can be assessed with control groups, experimental methods, and recovery experiments, as well as less well-known methods in the psychosocial disciplines, such as ROC curves and the SDI. The use of these means to evaluate measurement issues should prove useful to those researchers interested in studying complex, multidimensional concepts that include physiologic and psychosocial components.

References

1. Trnobranski, P.H. Biological sciences and the nursing curriculum: A challenge for educationalists. *J Adv Nurs*, 1993, *18*(5):493-499.
2. Sigmon, H. Answering critical care nursing questions by interfacing nursing research training, career development, and research with biologic and molecular science. *Heart Lung*, 1993, *22*(4):285-288.
3. Cowan, M.J., Heinrich, J., Lucas, M., et al. Integration of biological and nursing sciences: A 10-year plan to enhance research and training. *Res Nurs Health*, 1993, *16*(1):3-9.
4. Noe, D. *The logic of laboratory medicine*. Baltimore: Urban & Schwartzenberg, 1985.
5. Waltz, C.S., Strickland, O.L., & Lenz, E.R. *Measurement in nursing research* (2nd ed.). Philadelphia: Davis, 1991.
6. Maloni, J.A., Chance, B., Zhang, C., et al. Physical and psychosocial side effects of antepartum bed rest. *Nursing Research*, 1993, *42*(4):197-203.
7. Pugh, L.C. Childbirth and the measurement of fatigue. *J Nurs Meas*, 1993, *1*(1):57-66.
8. Price, P., & Fowlow, B. Thermodilution cardiac output determinations: A comparison of iced and re-frigerated injectate temperatures in patients after cardiac surgery. *Heart Lung*, 1993, *22*(3):266-274.
9. Topf, M., & Davis, J. Critical care unit noise and rapid eye movement (REM) sleep. *Heart Lung*, 1993, *22*(3):252-258.
10. Sommers, M.S., Woods, S.L., & Courtade, M.A. Issues in methods and measurement of thermodilution cardiac output. *Nurs Res*, 1993, *42*(4):228-233.
11. Williams, G., & Schork, M. Basic statistics for quality control in the clinical laboratory. *CRC Crit Rev Clin Lab Sci*, 1982, *17*(2):171-190.
12. Derrico, D.L. Comparison of blood pressure measurement methods in critically ill children. *Dimensions Crit Care Nurs*, 1993, *12*(1):31-39.
13. Howanitz, P.J., & Howanitz, J.H. *Laboratory quality assurance*. New York: McGraw-Hill, 1987.
14. Ko, W. Biomedical transducers. In J. Kline (Ed.), *Handbook of biomedical engineering*. New York: Academic press, 1988, pp. 3-71.
15. Rubin, S.A. Measurement theory and instrument errors. In S.A. Rubin (Ed.), *The principles of biomedical instrumentation*. Chicago: Yearbook Medical Publishers, 1987, pp. 50-74.

16. Davis, K. The accuracy of tympanic temperature measurement in children. *Ped Nurs*, 1993, *12*(3):267-272.

17. Metheny, N., Reed, L., Wiersema, L., et al. Effectiveness of pH measurements in predicting feeding tube placement: An update. *Nurs Res*, 1993, *42*(6):324-331.

18. McCarthy, D.O., Daun, J.M., & Hutson, P.R. Meperidine attenuates the febrile response to endotoxin and interleukin-1 alpha in rats. *Nurs Res*, 1993, *42*(6):363-367.

19. Finkelstein, S.M., Lindgren, B., Prasad, B., et al. Reliability and validity of spirometry measurements in a paperless home monitoring diary program for lung transplantation. *Heart Lung*, 1993, *22*(6):523-533.

20. Bland, J.M., & Altman, D.G. Statistical methods for assessing agreement between two methods of clinical measurement. *Lancet*, 1986, *1*, 307-310.

21. deMonterice, D., Meier, P.P., Engstrom, J.L., et al. Concurrent validity of a new instrument for measuring nutritive sucking in preterm infants. *Nurs Res*, 1992, *41*(6):342-346.

22. Cromwell, L., Arditti, M., Weibell, F.J., et al. *Medical instrumentation for health care.* Englewood Cliffs, NJ: Prentice-Hall, 1976.

23. Hanneman, S.K.G. Multidimensional predictors of success or failure with early weaning from mechanical ventilation after cardiac surgery. *Nurs Res*, 1994, *43*(1):4-10.

II

Instruments for Assessing Health and Function

7

Measuring Function

Therese Richmond, Ruth McCorkle, Lorraine Tulman, and Jacqueline Fawcett

Function, which has been used as a proxy for health status and as an outcome measure for clinical research, has been receiving increasing attention since the mid-1970s by the members of many health-care disciplines. A major goal of health care is to assist individuals to maintain or regain their pre-illness level of function or to attain the maximal functional level possible given their current health status. The purposes of this chapter are to discuss the significance of measuring function, analyze the concept of function and the methodologic issues in the measurement of function, and review instruments that have been developed or used by health professionals to assess function in seriously ill adults.

Instruments that measure function can assist health professionals in both the research and the clinical arenas. In research, the use of valid and reliable instruments to measure function is critical for the development of an empirically based body of knowledge concerning the outcomes of interventions. Clinically, valid and reliable measures can assist clinicians in assessing baseline function and changes over the course of an illness, as well as in identifying the requirements for care during hospitalization and following discharge to home. The ability to determine baseline function and changes over time provides a mechanism for meaningful assessments of the efficacy of interventions and the quality of care.

The Concept of Function

The concept of function has been defined in various ways both within the discipline of nursing and by other health-care disciplines. The terms *function*, *functioning*, *functional ability*, *functional status*, *physical function*, *impairment*, *disability*, *handicap*, and *health status* are frequently used interchangeably. Lack of clarity concerning the concept of function and its definition has resulted in studies that use the same term with different definitions and different measures, making comparisons across studies and integration of findings difficult, if not impossible. Moreover, different terms used to measure the same concept add to the confusion.

In general, the term *function* refers to "how people perform activities that are relevant to personal expectations and social norms."[1] Nagi[2] explained that the concept of function incorporates both the ability to perform activities or tasks that are important for independent living and the actual performance of activities and tasks crucial to the fulfillment of roles within one's current life circumstances. Although the actual terms are different, the dual approach to the concept, as proposed by Nagi, is used in this chapter. Function is viewed as a concept with two dimensions: functional ability and functional status.

Functional ability refers to the actual or potential capacity to perform the activities and tasks normally expected of an adult.[2] The inability to perform activities within the range considered normal may be temporary or permanent, static or dynamic. Instruments that measure functional ability focus on either basic activities of daily living (BADL),[3] (e.g., bathing, dressing, continence, and feeding), or a combination of BADL and instrumental activities of daily living (IADL),[4] (e.g., housekeeping, food preparation, use of transportation, and shopping).

In contrast, *functional status* refers to individuals' actual performance of activities and tasks associated with their current life roles. Limitations in functional status are said to occur when there is "a discrepancy between individual performance and average expectable role performance."[5] Emphasis is on BADL, IADL, and advanced activities of daily living (AADL), (e.g., working, traveling, engaging in hobbies, or participating in social and religious groups). Instruments designed to measure functional status differ in the breadth of measurement (the number of roles included) and the depth of measurement (the numbers and types of activities included for each role). Furthermore, measurement of functional status *assumes* functional ability. In other words, the assumption is made that the person has the ability to perform the roles and associated activities of interest.

Issues in the Measurement of Function

Several issues surround the selection of an instrument to measure function. Issues to consider include the primary purpose of measurement, the match between the theoretical dimension of function (functional ability, functional status), the focus of the instrument, the unique requirements of the population of interest, and methodologic concerns.

When the primary *purpose* of measuring function is clinical assessment, practical considerations such as the time required to administer the instrument, the ease of use by multiple care providers, the setting in which the measurement is obtained, and the clinical usefulness of the data obtained are particularly important. If the primary purpose of measuring function is research, the time required to administer the instrument continues to be a consideration. Furthermore, when functional assessment is only one of several instruments used, the degree of burden to subjects also must be considered in the choice of the instrument.

The choice of an instrument to measure function in research must be consistent with the *conceptual definition* and scope of function for that particular study. For example, if the purpose is to determine the rate and completeness at which individuals are resuming their job responsibilities following an illness (functional status), then an instrument that yields data on only the extent to which assistance is needed with BADL (functional ability, not including ability to perform job responsibilities) is not appropriate for that study.

The unique aspects of the *population of interest* are an important consideration in choosing a measure of function. In the hospitalized adult, the clinician or researcher may be more interested in the individual's functional ability than functional status. Indeed, measurement of functional status of hospitalized persons usually is not possible because they are in a situation where IADL and AADL cannot be performed. In other situations, such as chronically ill people living in the community, measurement of functional status may be of primary interest.

The needs of the population and the purpose of measuring function may dictate whether functional assessment measures are self-report, based on clinical assessment, or reported by a *proxy*, also known as a *surrogate*. Whenever possible, data should be collected from the patients themselves when they are able and available; otherwise, data may be provided (either totally or partially) by a proxy respondent.

Physicians and other health-care providers often depend on data provided by family members (proxy respondents) in evaluating the health status of elderly and seriously ill patients and deciding on the appropriate treatment. Data provided by proxy respondents are helpful for logistical, economic, and scientific reasons.[6] Proxy respondents usually are asked to provide information when the study subject is unable to respond either because of functional impairments or disabilities, a language barrier, or inability of the interviewer to locate the study subject. The use of proxy-reported data increases sample size, improves representativeness of the study sample, and reduces the need for and the cost of phone or home call-backs. Without proxy data, the rate of nonresponse may be high. Researchers need, however, to weigh the advantages and disadvantages of proxy data. The use of proxy-reported data carries with it the potential for introducing a bias that may result in misclassification of respondents or in misestimated data. Respondents may under- or overestimate the true values of the data provided. Accordingly, the basic methodologic concern associated with using proxy-reported data is related to the extent of agreement between self- and proxy-reported data. When analyzing data that contain both self- and proxy-reported responses, it is important to investigate the role of proxy-reported data as both a potential confounder and an effect modifier.[7]

Floor and ceiling effects must be considered. Specifically, patients may be at the highest level of the measure, resulting in little to no variability. Conversely, if patients have reduced function, they may be at the lowest range of the instrument and have little ability to discriminate between lower levels of function. Examining the original purpose and population for whom the instrument was developed can minimize the risk of floor and ceiling effects. For example, the Barthel Index was designed to assess the progress of patients with chronic diseases during rehabilitation. Instrument developers specifically state that the highest score does *not* imply the ability to live alone, cook, or keep house.[8] Consequently, use of the Barthel Index to assess function in an independent community based sample would predictably result in a ceiling effect.

The degree to which subtle changes in function are of interest to the investigator or clinician should be determined at the outset, as this dimension also influences the choice of an instrument. One reason why changes in function may not be seen is that the rating scale lacks the *sensitivity* to capture differences. Another reason why changes in function may not be detected is that the instrument uses an aggregate score that reflects overall level of function.[9] Use of subscale scores that provide a profile of the patient's level of function in various dimensions (e.g., the subscales of the Sickness Impact Profile) may be more informative.[10]

Another issue is the extent to which the *assumption of existing functional ability* is valid when measuring functional status. For example, illness may compromise one's functional ability. It is, therefore, recommended that both functional ability and functional status be measured. Still another consideration is the selection of an instrument that includes culturally and developmentally relevant roles and associated activities.

Instruments

A plethora of instruments have been developed to measure function. The ones included in Appendix 7A have the following qualities: they (1) were developed, currently used by, or of potential use by health professionals for clinical or research purposes in adult populations; (2) have established validity and reliability; and (3) are consistent with the definitions of function as used in this chapter. Selected instruments and a concise overview of their properties and uses are presented in Appendix 7A. Key properties of the instruments also are provided, and the emphasis is placed on the dimension(s) of function measured, the target population for whom the instrument was developed, the number of items, and methods of administration. Concise descriptions of reliability and validity data also are included. As can be seen, several instruments contain items or discrete subscales that measure functional ability and other items or subscales that measure functional status. Clinicians and investigators who use such instruments are cautioned to be aware of the distinctions, so that appropriate interpretations of data can be made.

Summary

This chapter highlights the significance for health professionals of measuring function. The concept of function is found to consist of the dimensions of functional ability and functional status. Specific issues in the measurement of function, such as the purpose of measurement, the match between the conceptual definition and instrument, the unique requirements of the population of interest, and methodologic considerations, have been explored.

Exemplar Study

McCorkle, R., Benoliel, J.Q., Donaldson, G., Georgiadou, F., Moinpour, C., & Goodell, B. A randomized clinical trial of home nursing care for lung cancer patients. *Cancer*, 1989, 64(6):1375.

This study exemplifies the measurement of function in a prospective clinical trial designed to assess the effects of home nursing care for patients with progressive lung cancer. The three-group experimental design is described in detail, and the methods are rigorous. Several instruments with established validity and reliability are used in this study. The primary measure of function and level of dependency was the Enforced Social Dependency Scale. Significant differences in social dependency were found among the groups, and the results suggest that home nursing care assists in maintaining cancer patients' levels of function longer than for those who do not live in a home with nursing care.

References

1. Granger, C.V. A conceptual model for functional assessment. In C.V. Granger & G.E. Gresham (Eds.), *Functional assessment in rehabilitation medicine.* Baltimore: Williams & Wilkins, 1984, p. 14.
2. Nagi, S. Disability concepts revisited: Implications for prevention. In A.M. Pope & A.R. Tarlov (Eds.), *Disability in America: Toward a national agenda for prevention.* Washington, DC: National Academy Press, 1991, p. 309.
3. Katz, S., Ford, A.S., & Moskowitz, R.W. The index of ADL: A standardized measure of biological and psychosocial function. *JAMA*, 1963, *185*(12):914.
4. Lawton, M.P., & Brody, E.M. Assessment of older people. Self maintaining and instrumental activities of daily living. *Gerontologist*, 1969, 9:17.
5. Moriarty, J.B. Disability concepts: Implications for research. In E.B. Whitten (Ed.), *Pathology, impairment, functional limitations, and disability—Implications for practice, research, program and policy development and service delivery.* Washington, DC: National Rehabilitation Association, 1975, p. 15.
6. Moore, J.C. Self/Proxy response status and survey response quality: A review of the literature. *J Off Stat*, 1988, 4:155.

7. Walker, A.M., Velema, J.P., & Robins, J.M. Analysis of case-control data derived from proxy respondents. *Am J Epidemiol*, 1988, *127*:905.

8. Mahoney, F.I., & Barthel, D. W. Functional evaluation: The Barthel Index. *Rehab Notes*, 1965, *14*(2):61.

9. Feinstein, A.R., Josephy, B.R., & Wells, C.K. Scientific and clinical problems in indexes of functional disability. *Ann Int Med*, 1986, *105*:413.

10. Bergner, M., Bobbitt, R.A., Carter, W.B., & Gilson, B.S. The Sickness Impact Profile: Development and final revision of a health status measure. *Med Care*, 1981, *19*:787.

11. Fredericks, C.M., te Wierik, M., Visser, A., & Sturmans, F. The functional status and utilization of care of elderly people living at home. *J Commun Health*, 1990, *15*:307.

12. Fredericks, C.M., te Wierik, M., Visser, A., & Sturmans, F. A scale for the functional status of the elderly living at home. *J Adv Nurs*, 1991, *16*:287.

13. Fredericks, C.M., te Wierik, M., von Rossum, H., et al. Why do elderly people seek professional home care? Methodologies compared. *J Commun Health*, 1991, *17*:131.

14. Gulick, E.E. Parsimony and model confirmation of the ADL self-care scale for multiple sclerosis persons. *Nurs Res*, 1987, *36*:278.

15. Gulick, E.E. The self-administered ADL scale for persons with multiple sclerosis. In C.F. Waltz & O.L. Strickland (Eds.), *Measurement of nursing outcomes: Measuring client outcomes* (vol. I). New York: Springer, 1988, p. 128.

16. Gulick, E.E. Self-assessment of health and use of health services. *West J Nurs Res*, 1991, *13*:195.

17. Gulick, E.E., & Bugg, A. Holistic health patterning in multiple sclerosis. *Res Nurs Health*, 1992, *15*:175.

18. Hamrin, E.K., & Lindmark, B. The effect of systematic care planning after acute stroke in general hospital medical wards. *J Adv Nurs*, 1990, *15*:1146.

19. Hamrin, E., & Wohlin, A. Evaluation of the functional capacity of stroke patients through an Activity Index. *Scand J Rehab*, 1982, *14*:93.

20. Meenan, R.F., Gertman, P.M., & Mason, J.H. Measuring health status in arthritis: The Arthritis Impact Measurement Scale. *Arthritis Rheumatol*, 1980, *23*:146.

21. Meenan, R.G. The AIMS approach to health status measurement: Conceptual background and measurement properties. *J Rheumatol*, 1982, *9*:785.

22. Meenan, R.F., Anderson, J.J., Kazis, L.E., et al. Outcome assessment in clinical trials: Evidence for the sensitivity of a health status measure. *Arthritis Rheum*, 1984, 27:1344.

23. Meenan, J.H., Anderson, J.J., & Meenan, R.F. A model for health status for rheumatoid arthritis: A factor analysis of the Arthritis Impact Measure. *Arthritis Rheum*, 1988, *31*:714.

24. Brown, J.H., Kazis, L.E., Spitz, P.W., et al. The dimensions of health outcomes: A cross-validated examination of health status measurement. *Am J Pub Health*, 1984, *74*:159.

25. Granger, C.V., Albrecht, G.L., & Hamilton, B.B. Outcome of comprehensive medical rehabilitation: Measurement by PULSES Profile and Barthel Index. *Arch Phys Med Rehab*, 1979, *60*:145.

26. Granger, C., Cotter, A.C., Hamilton, B.B., et al. Functional assessment scales: A study of persons with multiple sclerosis. *Arch Phys Med Rehab*, 1990, *71*:870.

27. Ramiezl, P. CADET, a self-care assessment tool. *Geriatr Nurs*, 1983, *4*:377.

28. Huber, M., & Kennard, A. Functional and mental status outcomes of clients discharged from acute gerontological versus medical/surgical units. *J Gerontol Nurs*, 1991, *17*(7):20.

29. Schag, C.A., Heinrich, R.L., & Aadland, R.L. Assessing problems of cancer patients: Psychometric properties of the Cancer Inventory of Problem Situations. *Health Psychol*, 1990, *9*:83.

30. Schag, C.A., Ganz, P.A., & Heinrich, R.L. Cancer Rehabilitation Evaluation System-Short Form (CARES-SF): A cancer specific rehabilitation and quality of life instrument. *Cancer*, 1991, *68*:406.

31. Benoliel, J.Q., McCorkle, R., & Young, K. The development of a social dependency scale. *Res Nurs Health*, 1980, *3*:3.

32. McCorkle, R., & Benoliel, J.Q. Symptom distress, current concerns, and mood disturbance after diagnosis of life threatening disease. *Soc Sci Med*, 1983, 17:431.

33. Fink, A. Social dependency and self-care agency: A descriptive correlational study of ALS patients. Thesis, University of Washington, Seattle, 1985.

34. Keith, R.A., Granger, C.V., Hamilton, B.B., & Sherwin, F.S. The Functional Independence Measure: A new tool for rehabilitation. In M.G. Eisenberg & R.C. Grzesiak (Eds.), *Advances in clinical rehabilitation*. New York: Springer, 1987, p. 6.

35. Fricke, J., Unsworth, C., & Worrell, D. Reliability of the Functional Independence Measure with occupational therapists. *Austral Occup Ther J*, 1993, *40*:7.

36. Schipper, H., Clinch, J., McMurray, A., & Levitt, M. Measuring the quality of life of cancer patients: The Functional Living Index-Cancer: Development and validation. *J Clin Oncol*, 1984, *2*:472.

37. Monahan, M.L. Quality of life of adults receiving chemotherapy. A comparison of instruments. *Oncol Nurs Forum*, 1988, *15*:795.

38. Jette, A.M. Functional Status Index: Reliability of a chronic disease evaluation instrument. *Arch Phys Med Rehab*, 1980, *61*:395.

39. Jette, A.M., Harris, B.A., Cleary, P.D., & Campion, E.W. Functional recovery after hip fracture. *Arch Phys Med Rehab*, 1987, *68*:735.

40. Calkins, D.R., Rubenstein, L.V., Cleary, P.D., et al. The Functional Status Questionnaire: Initial results of a controlled trial. *Clin Res*, 1985, *33*:244A.

41. Jette, A.M., Davies, A.R., Cleary, P.D., et al. The Functional Status Questionnaire: Reliability and validity when used in primary care. *J Gen Int Med*, 1986, *1*:143.

42. Jette, A.M., & Cleary, P.D. Functional disability assessment. *Phys Ther*, 1987, *12*:1854.

43. Tedesco, C., Manning, S., Lindsay, R., et al. Functional assessment of elderly patients after percutaneous aortic balloon valvuloplasty: New York Heart Association Classification versus Functional Status Questionnaire. *Heart Lung*, 1990, *19*:118.

44. Fries, J.G., Spitz, P., Kraines, R.G., & Holman, H.R. Measurement of patient outcome in arthritis. *Arthritis Rheum*, 1980, *23*:137.

45. Fries, J.F., Spitz, P.W., & Young, D.Y. The dimensions of health outcomes: The Health Assessment Questionnaire, disability and pain scales. *J Rheumatol*, 1982, *9*:789.

46. Tulman, L., Fawcett, J., & McEvoy, M.D. Development of the Inventory of Functional Status-Cancer. *Cancer Nurs*, 1991, *14*:254.

47. Katz, S., Downs, T.D., Cash, H.R., & Grotz, R.C. Progress in development of the Index of ADL. *Gerontologist*, 1970, *10*(1, part I):20.

48. Katz, S., & Akpom, C.A. A measure of primary sociobiological functions. *Int J Health Serv*, 1976, *6*:493.

49. Katz, S. Assessing self-maintenance: Activities of daily living, mobility, and instrumental activities of daily living. *J Am Geriatr Soc*, 1983, *31*:721.

50. Aske, D. The correlation between mini-mental state examination scores and Katz ADL status among dementia patients. *Rehab Nurs*, 1990, *15*:140.

51. Karnofsky D., & Buchenal, J. The clinical evaluation of chemotherapeutic agents in cancer. In C.M. MacLeod (Ed.), *Evaluation of chemotherapeutic agents*. New York: Columbia University Press, 1949, p. 191.

52. Yates, J.W., Chalina, B., & McKegney, F.P. Evaluation of patients with advanced cancer using the Karnofsky Performance Status. *Cancer*, 1980, *45*:2220.

53. Mor, V., Laliberte, L., Morris, J.N., & Wiemann, M. The Karnofsky Performance Status Scale: An examination of its reliability and validity in a research setting. *Cancer*, 1984, *53*:2002.

54. Klein, R.M., & Bell, B. Self-care skills: Behavioral measurement with Klein-Bell ADL Scale. *Arch Phys Med Rehab*, 1982, *63*:335.

55. Venable, S.D. & Mitchell, M.M. Temporal adaptation and performance of daily living activities in persons with Alzheimer's disease. *Phys Occup Ther Geriatr*, 1991, *9*(3/4):31.

56. Longman, A.J., Atwood, J.R., Sherman, J.B., et al. Care needs of home-based cancer patients and their caregivers. *Cancer Nurs*, 1992, *15*:182.

57. Chambers, L.W. The McMaster Health Index Questionnaire. Prepared for the Workshop on Advances in Health Status Assessment, *Proceedings of the First National Meeting of the Association of Health Services Research*, Chicago, IL, June 1984.

58. Chambers, L.W., MacDonald, L.A., Tugwell, P., et al. The McMaster Health Index Questionnaire as a measure of quality of life for patients with rheumatoid disease. *J Rheumatol*, 1982, *9*:750.

59. Fillenbaum, G.G., & Smyer, M.A. The development, validity, and reliability of the OARS multidisciplinary functional assessment questionnaire. *J Gerontol*, 1981, *36*:428.

60. Lawton, M.P., Moss, M., Fulcomer, M., & Kleban, M.H. A research and service-oriented multilevel assessment instrument. *J Gerontol*, 1982, *37*:91.

61. Weaver, T.E., & Narsavage, G.L. Reliability and validity of the Pulmonary Impact Profile Scale. *Am Rev Resp Dis*, 1989, *139*(suppl):A244.

62. Weaver, T.E., & Narsavage, G.L. Physiological and psychological variables related to functional status in chronic obstructive pulmonary disease. *Nurs Res*, 1992, *41*:286.

63. Pollard, W.E., Bobbitt, R.A., Bergner, M., et al. The Sickness Impact Profile: Reliability of a health status measure. *Med Care*, 1976, *14*:146.

64. Gulick, E.E. Reliability and validity of the work assessment scale for persons with multiple sclerosis. *Nurs Res*, 1991, *40*:107.

65. Gulick, E.E. Model for predicting work performance among persons with multiple sclerosis. *Nurs Res*, 1992, *41*:266.

66. Gulick, E.E., Yam, M., & Touw, M.M. Work performance by persons with multiple sclerosis: Conditions that impede or enable the performance of work. *Int J Nurs Studies*, 1989, *26*:301.

Appendix

7A. Instruments Used to Measure Function

Name	Dimensions Measured	Dimensions of Function	Items	Administration	Reliability	Validity
Activities of Daily Living–Household Activities (ADL-HAA) (11-13)	ADL (6 items) Household activities (7 items)	Ability, Status Target: elderly	13	Self or structured interview, takes a few minutes	Test-retest: ADL = 93%, HHA = 43% (81% if 1-point difference allowed) Cohen's kappas 0.49–0.79 Cronbach's alpha = 0.86	Discriminant: higher scores related to increased age and those receiving home care Correlation between ADL and HHA subscales $r = 0.50$
Activities of Daily Living–Multiple Sclerosis (ADL-MS) (14-17)	7 dimensions: lower body, upper body, recreational/social, sensory communication. intimacy, urine elimination, bowel elimination	Ability, Status Target: patients with Multiple Sclerosis	55 (also 15-item short form)	Self-administered	Cronbach's alpha: 0.96 for entire scale, 0.75–0.97 for five of the six factored subscales (0.63 for bowel elimination) Test-retest: 0.73–0.93 (over 2–4 weeks)	Construct: factor analysis yielded 6 factors accounting for 71% of variance (lower body, upper body, intimacy, sensory/communication, recreation/socializing, bowel elimination) Convergent: correlations with Kurtzke Disability Scale and Incapacity Status Scale
Activity Index (18-19)	3 subscales: (1) mental capacity, (2) motor activity, (3) ADL functions	Ability Target: patients with CVA	16	Clinician assessed (must know patient)	Internal consistency: total index 0.94; subscales: (1) 0.83, (2) 0.79, (3) 0.94	Concurrent: high correlation ($r = 0.94$) between Activity Index and Rankin Disability Scale Predictive: predicts scores of 3 and 12 months after stroke; predicts survival during acute hospitalization phase
Arthritis Impact Measure (AIMS) (20-24)	Mobility, physical activity, dexterity, household activities, ADL, social activity, anxiety, depression, pain, general health	Ability, Status Target: patients with rheumatoid arthritis (RA), other chronic illnesses	67	Self, takes 20 minutes	Internal consistency: >0.70 (0.61–0.92) for patients with RA. (0.40–0.92 for other chronic illnesses) Test-retest: 0.84–0.92 (6 months)	Convergent/discriminant: high intercorrelations within and across instruments on physical scales, lower, on psychological scales; discriminates between diabetic and arthritis, and osteoarthritis, and rheumatoid arthritis Concurrent: correlate with functional class and disease activity (overall health) Construct (recent): 5 factors (RA) upper- and lower-extremity function affect, symptoms, social interaction

7A. Instruments Used to Measure Function (*cont.*)

Name	Dimensions Measured	Dimensions of Function	Items	Administration	Reliability	Validity
Barthel Index of ADL Scale (8,25,26)	Physical disability, ADL, mobility 7 subscales: feeding, grooming, bathing, toileting, walking or climbing stairs, propelling a wheelchair, control bowel, bladder	Ability Target: patients with chronic disease	16	Health-care staff familiar with patient; takes 2 minutes	Internal consistency: alpha: 0.943–0.965 Interobserver: $r = 0.99$; correlation between telephone interview and performance assessment >0.97	Predictive: score <60 inversely related to subsequent mortality (CVA) Concurrent: established
CADET (27,28)	Communication, ambulation, ADL, elimination, transfer	Ability Target: geriatric, inpatient settings	5	Person with familiarity with patient	Internal consistency: 0.984 Interrater: 0.936	Not specified
Cancer Rehabilitation Evaluation System (CARES) and CARES-SF (short form) (29,30)	Physical, psychosocial, medical interaction, marital, sexual, miscellaneous subscales	Ability, Status Target: patients with cancer	139 SF-59	Self	Internal consistency: Cronbach's alpha: 0.82–0.94 (CARES); SF: 0.60–0.85 Test-retest: CARES: 84%–86%, SF: 81%–86%	Content: literature, patient, and professional interview Concurrent: correlation between CARES and SF with FLIC, symptom-checklist-90, Karnofsky, Dydadic Adjustment Scale Construct: established by factor analysis
Enforced Social Dependency Scale (31-33)	Personal competence (eating, dressing, walking, traveling, bathing and toileting); Social competence (home, work, recreation)	Ability, Status Target: individuals with cancer; other life-threatening illnesses	10	Semi-structured interview guide (10–20 minutes)	Internal consistency coefficient = 0.82 Test-retest reliability 0.62 (over 30-day elapse)	Content: extensive interviews with patients with life-threatening illnesses Discriminant: demonstrated ability to distinguish between situations in which recovery is likely versus not likely Construct: two factors (personal and social competence) confirmed by factor analysis; correlation with Sickness Impact Profile, $r = 0.89$

Instrument	Dimensions	Type/Target	No. of items	Administration	Reliability	Validity
Functional Independence Measure (FIM) (26,34,35)	Self-care, sphincter control, mobility, locomotion, communication, social adjustment/cooperation, cognition/problem solving	Ability, selected aspects of Status Target: patients with CVA, spinal cord injury	18	Clinician, takes 10 minutes	Interrater: 0.86–0.87 Intraclass correlations: (eating, bathing, dressing, grooming, toilet and tub transfer) 0.88	Predictive: help needed by patients with MS Content: established by interview with expert clinician
Functional Living Index (FLIC) (36,37)	Functional quality of life, 4 factors: physical well-being, psychological state, family/situational interaction, nausea	Status Target: patients with cancer	22	Self, takes <10 minutes	Not published	Construct: established by factor analysis Concurrent: validated against Karnofsky, Katz, ADL, and others
Functional Status Indices (FSI) (38,39)	Basic ADL, Instrumental ADL, Social/role function	Ability, Status Target: rheumatology patients	17	Self or structured interview takes <15 minutes	Internal consistency: Cronbach's alpha: 0.93–0.96	Construct: determined by factor analysis Criterion: agreement for basic and instrumental ADL = 0.71–0.95 when comparing self-report and direct observation
Functional Status Questionnaire (FSQ) (40-43)	7 scales: physical, psychosocial role function, ADL (2), mental health, work performance, social activity, quality of interaction	Ability, Status Target: ambulatory patients	34	Self, takes approximately 15 minutes	Internal consistency: alphas 0.62–0.82; highest (ADL(2), mental health)	Content: established through selection of items from existing instruments Construct: established based on bivariate relationship between each FSQ scale and 7 variables related to function Predictive: early outcome after valvuloplasty
Health Assessment Questionnaire (HAQ) Disability Index (24,44,45)	Disability Scales: dressing/grooming, arising, eating, walking, reaching, personal hygiene, gripping activities	Ability Target: not known	21	Self, takes 5–8 minutes	Test-retest $r = 0.93$–0.95 (1 week); $r = 0.98$ (6 months) Internal consistency: 0.46–0.63 (2 scales, 0.77, 0.87) Interrater: $r = 0.85$, weighted kappa 0.52	Construct: factor analysis (gross motor and fine motor movement) Convergent: high intercorrelations within dimensions and across instruments Discriminant: discriminates between diabetics and arthritics Predictive: greater or lesser disability

Name	Dimensions Measured	Dimensions of Function	Items	Administration	Reliability	Validity
Inventory of Functional Status-Cancer (46)	Personal care, household and family, occupational, social, and community	Status; Target: women with cancer during and after adjuvant phase of treatment	39	Self or interview (<10 minutes)	Subscale item to subscale total scores using Fisher's z transformation: Household and Family Activities: 0.74, Social and Community Activities: 0.82, Personal Care Activities: 0.56, Occupational Activities: 0.72; Subscale to total IFS-CA score correlations range: Household and family activities: 0.92, occupational activities: 0.73; Test-retest: 0.91 (over 4–7 days)	Content: Popham's average congruency established at 98.5%; Construct: subscale correlations from 0.33 to 0.62; Discriminant: total functional status higher for women who completed treatment than for those still in treatment
Katz-Index of Activities of Daily Living (3,47-50)	Bathing, dressing, toileting, transfer, continence, feeding	Ability; Target: patients with hip fracture, chronic illness, and elderly	6	Rater who has health care experience and knowledge of subject, takes a few minutes	Test-retest: 0.95–0.98 (without impairment 0.73)	Predictive: discharge status, function; Construct: correlates highly with Mini-Mental ($r = 0.76$); Guttman characteristics-coefficient of reproducibility of 0.95–0.98
Karnofsky Index of Performance Status (KPS) (51-53)	Ability to do work, perform normal activities, need for assistance	Ability, status; Target: patients with cancer	11	Observer, short time	Interrater: $r = 0.89$, kappa = 0.53; Internal consistency: Cronbach's alpha = 0.97; Test-retest: $r = 0.66$ (1 week, home vs. clinic)	Convergent: significant correlations with cancer inventory of problem situations, Katz ADL scale, and others; Predictive: survival in days
Klein Bell Scale (54)	Dressing, elimination, mobility, bathing/hygiene, eating, emergency, telephone, communication	Ability; Target: long-term care patients	170	Clinician assessed, 15 minutes	Interrater: 0.92	Predictive: ADL scores correlated at discharge with assistance needed ($r = -0.86$)
Lawton Instrumental Activities of Daily Living-Physical Self-Maintenance Scale (IADL-PSMS) (4,55,56)	Instrumental ADL and physical self-maintenance scale	Ability, Status; Target: geriatric	IADL = 8 women, 5 men, PSMS = 6 items	Clinician familiar with subject, takes 10-15 minutes	Internal consistency: IADL: alpha = 0.92, standard alpha = 0.93, PSMS alpha = 0.87, standard alpha = 0.90; Interrater: PSMS 0.87–0.91; IADL: 0.85	Concurrent: significant correlations with physical classification, mental status questionnaire, Adjustment Rating Scale; Construct: significant correlations between severity of Alzheimer's disease and IADL and PSMS; Discriminate: between groups for cancer patient–caregiver dyads

Instrument	Dimensions measured	Ability, Status, Target	N	Administration	Reliability	Validity
McMaster Health Index Questionnaire (MHIQ) (57,58)	Physical, social, emotional	Ability, Status Target: rehabilitation outpatients, patients with chronic disease	59	Interviewer or self takes 20 minutes	Test–retest: physical ($r = 0.53$–0.95), emotional ($r = 0.70$–0.77), social ($r = 0.48$–0.66) (1-week range)	Construct: established (better functioning for younger vs. older adults)
OARS Multidimensional Functional Assessment Questionnaire (OMFAQ) (59-60)	A: OMFAQ (personal functioning) B: Services utilization	Ability, Status Target: community based population	101	Trained interviewer takes 45–75 minutes	Part A Interrater: social (0.823), economic (0.783), mental health (0.803), physical health (0.662) Interclass: correlation coefficients (0.66–0.87)	Part A Construct: Kendell's tau, Spearman's rank-order correlations: economic ($r = 0.68$, tau $= -0.62$), health ($r = 0.67$, tau $= 0.75$), self-care ($r = 0.89$, tau $= 0.83$) Discriminant: excellent vs. totally impaired functioning
Pulmonary Functional Status Scale (PFSS) (61-62)	Daily life, behaviors	Ability, Status Target: patients with chronic pulmonary disease	56	Self, takes 15 minutes	Internal consistency: alpha 0.81–0.83 Test–retest: $r = 0.67$ ($p = 0.002$)	Concurrent: SIP ($r = 0.54$)
Sickness Impact Profile (SIP) (10,63)	Physical, psychosocial, 5 additional subscales	Ability, Status Target: acute and chronic illness	136	Self or structured interview takes 20–30 minutes	Test–retest: $r = 0.88$ (24 hours) Internal consistency: Cronbach's alpha 0.93–0.97	Discriminant: higher correlation between SIP and levels of dysfunction and different groups of patients Convergent: AIMS and SIP ($r = 0.97$)
Work Assessment Scale (WAS) (64-66)	WAS Impediments (WAS-I): mobility, hand function, cognition, body state, pain, environment WAS enhancers (WAS-E); job adjustment, personal attributes, social support, environmental adjustment, health practices	Status Target: patients with MS	52	Self	WAS-I Internal consistency: 0.79–0.91 Test–retest: 0.76–0.91 WAS-E Internal consistency: 0.77–0.89 Test–retest: 0.67–0.81 (2–3 weeks)	Content: content analysis Concurrent: correlates with ADL-MS subscales and MS-symptom-related checklist Construct: factor analysis

Numbers in parentheses correspond to studies cited in the References.

8

Measuring Cognitive Status

Marquis D. Foreman

Cognition is comprised of perception, memory, and thinking—the recognition/registration, storage, and use of information. Cognition can be affected, both positively and negatively, by illness and its treatment. The evaluation of an individual's cognitive status can be instrumental in identifying the presence of specific pathophysiologic states (e.g., delirium, dementia, or depression), a person's readiness to learn, or the effectiveness of a treatment regimen. To evaluate cognitive status, numerous instruments have been developed. These instruments range from comprehensive, full-scale batteries that require a skilled examiner and place intensive pressure on the examinee, to bedside variants that place little demand on the examiner and examinee. The bedside variants will be addressed in this chapter.

The measures of cognitive status reviewed in this chapter are representative of those most frequently used in research and practice and are either considered the "standard" for each aspect of cognition or have been recently developed and show great promise. For each measure of cognition described, the available psychometric information is reviewed, the strengths and limitations presented, and recommendations provided. The content is organized according to: (1) measures of specific areas of cognition; (2) measures of global aspects of cognition; (3) measures for common disorders of cognition; (4) criteria for selecting a measure of cognitive status; and (5) conditions for using a measure of cognition. The two approaches of examination are (1) assessment of *specific* dimensions of cognition; and (2) *global* assessment of cognitive function.[1] Each has advantages and disadvantages:

Testing	Advantages	Disadvantages
Specific dimensions of cognition	Easy to administer to individuals requiring it most (e.g., fatigued, distressed, or with language or sensory limitations)	Not a comprehensive examination and may overlook an important deficit

Acknowledgement: Drs. Sharon K. Inouye and Diane Cronin-Stubbs are gratefully acknowledged for their review and critique of an earlier draft of this chapter.

| Global assessment of cognition | All components of cognition systematically assessed | Time-consuming; may be less sensitive to some aspects of cognition; may overlook important deficits |

Measures of Specific Areas of Cognition

Albert[2] identified five specific, or individual, components of cognition that should be evaluated: attention, visuospatial abilities, language, memory, and conceptualization. Each component, along with its major measures, is presented. The psychometric properties, advantages, and disadvantages of each instrument are detailed in Appendix 8A.

Attention

Attention is the ability to focus on a specific stimulus without being distracted by extraneous environmental stimuli. An individual's ability to sustain attention over time must be established before more complex cognitive functions, such as memory, can be evaluated.[2,3] According to Albert,[2] if the individual has difficulty focusing on a task for 1 to 3 minutes at a time, it will not be possible to assess other areas of cognitive function.

Evaluation of an individual's attentional abilities also is important in determining the nature of the cognitive impairment. Attentional abilities are preserved in some forms of cognitive impairment while deficient in others. For example, attentional ability is preserved in dementia, whereas an attentional deficit is a major feature of acute confusion or delirium.[4-8]

Historically, the attentional abilities of an individual have been assessed using tasks such as serial subtraction; however, these tasks are known to be biased by the individual's premorbid intellectual capability, calculating ability, and socioeconomic status.[3] Hence, in people where these factors could confound the interpretation of results, other tests of attention, such as Digit Span or repetition, the vigilance or "A" test, or trail-making tests, should be substituted. However, these measures are not without limitations. The attentional abilities of individuals who have a significant language disorder, such as aphasia, cannot be assessed validly with the digit span/repetition test or test of vigilance.[3] Similarly, individuals with physical and sensory impairment may not be capable of completing the trail-making tests.[7]

Digit Span

The Digit Span/repetition task consists of a series of numbers that are read to the individual who repeats them in the same sequence. This task is easy to administer and interpret and requires approximately 5 minutes. In administering this task, it is important that the digits not be presented in pairs or sequences, but randomly in a normal tone of voice at the rate of one digit per second. A second attempt by the examinee is permissible; however, if both attempts are failed, the task is terminated. The score on the Digit Span/repetition task is the number of digits correctly repeated by the examinee.

Adequate performance on this task demonstrates that the individual is able to attend to a verbal stimulus and to sustain attention for the period of time required to repeat the digits. Persons of average intelligence can repeat readily five (5) to seven (7) digits without difficulty. According to Strub and Black,[3] repetition of less than five digits by a nonretarded patient without obvious aphasia indicates defective attention.

Test of Vigilance

The test of vigilance, also referred to as the A-test,[3] is a test that is easy to administer and interpret, requiring approximately 2 to 3 minutes. It consists of a series of random letters among which the target letter "a" appears with greater frequency. The examinee is required to indicate whenever the target letter is spoken by the examiner, who reads the list of letters to the examinee at the rate of one letter per second. Normally, an examinee should make no errors; any error is indicative of an attentional deficit. Common are: (1) errors of omission; (2) errors of commission; and (3) perseverative errors. The type of error can assist in determining the nature of the cognitive impairment (e.g., perseverative errors are common with dementia). The score on this test is the absolute number of errors irrespective of their type.

Trail-Making Tests

The Trail-Making Test (TMT) is a standardized timed test to assess visual-motor tracking skills, counting ability, spatial skills, and cognitive flexibility.[6,9] The test has two parts: Part A consists of 25 numbered circles randomly scattered on a sheet of paper. The examinee is instructed to connect these numbered circles in ascending numerical order as rapidly as possible without lifting the pencil from the paper. Part B is approximately 2.5 times more difficult than Part A[10] and consists of 13 numbered circles and 12 lettered circles randomly scattered on a sheet of paper that the examinee is to alternately connect in the proper sequence (e.g., 1-A, 2-B, 3-C, . . . 13). Practice is provided on a brief example. During the task, if a circle is connected out of sequence, the examinee is stopped, corrected, and begun again from that point. Both parts are scored according to the total time in seconds required by the examinee to compete the task. For Part B, times greater than 200 seconds are considered abnormal.[9,11-13]

The TMT has been used with various samples: individuals with organic brain damage,[9] neuropsychiatric patients,[12,14] normal adults,[9] and candidates for liver transplantation.[13,15] Delirious, elderly demented, and chronic schizophrenic patients were found to be severely impaired on the TMT;[12] however, only nine of the 20 patients with delirium could perform the test. Given these characteristics of the TMT shown in Appendix 8A, the TMT may be useful in identifying an attentional deficit, but not in determining the exact nature of the cognitive impairment.[7] Other measures of attention include the Mental Control and the Attention Concentration Index subsections of the Wechsler Memory Scale (discussed later in the memory section), and Digit or Letter Cancellation.[11]

Visuospatial Ability

Because of the prevalence of visual-sensory deficits that accompany aging, the assessment of visuospatial ability is more difficult in the elderly than in the young. Many of the cognitive domains discussed in this chapter can be evaluated either orally or visually. However, this is not possible for visuospatial ability, and alternative means of testing have proven more difficult.

Constructional ability can be evaluated using two methods: figure copying or drawing on command. Albert,[16] however, warns against using drawing on command as a measure of visuospatial ability as it is confounded by conceptual impairments. Figure copying can be assessed simply by asking the examinee to copy a single line drawing, for example the copying of the intersecting pentagons item of Folstein's Mini-Mental State Examination.[17] Figure copying is useful in the diagnosis and localization of cerebral lesion; for example, patients with dementia omit essential features, whereas others oversimplify their drawings.[18] In copying a design, demented individuals also fail to preserve accurate spatial relationships.[18]

In addition to constructional ability, one should assess perceptual capacity. Figure-matching tasks are a good analog for figure copying. They have the added advantage that they can be administered to patients with severe cognitive deficits, patients in whom it is otherwise difficult to meaningfully assess spatial function. However, these measures of perceptual capacity require good visual acuity of the examinee.[1] Single measures of perceptual capacity are not reviewed here, but are found as component elements of the global measures of cognition discussed later in this chapter.

The Clock-Drawing Test

The Clock-Drawing Test is an examination of visuospatial abilities considered useful in screening for global cognitive impairment and dementia.[19-23] There are three components to this test: (1) clock drawing; (2) clock setting; and (3) clock reading. Two different versions exist for the clock-drawing component. In the first, the examinee is instructed to draw a clock on a blank sheet of paper, to number the face of the clock, but to omit placing the hands. In the second version, the examinee is given a sheet of paper with a predrawn circle and is instructed to draw and number the clock face, again omitting the hands on the clock. There are also two versions of the clock-setting component. The examinee is requested to place the hands on the clock depicting one to five specific times in the first version, whereas, in the other version, the examinee is allowed to select the time periods. The last component of the test is clock reading. For this component, the examinee is shown one to five clocks depicting different time periods and is asked to read the times depicted by these clock faces. The method for scoring and interpreting the results of the Clock-Drawing Test also varies.

Language

Language is crucial for assessing most cognitive abilities. Therefore, its integrity must be established early in the evaluation.[3] If deficits in language are identified, subsequent evaluation of higher aspects of cognition are difficult, if not impossible. Assessment of language should include an evaluation of comprehension, repetition, reading, writing, and naming.[4] Several standard batteries are available for this purpose, e.g., the Boston Diagnostic Aphasia Examination,[24] the Western Aphasia Battery,[25] and the Boston Naming Test.[26] Some of these batteries include brief aphasia screening tests that are useful for identifying the existence of a problem without giving a detailed analysis (e.g., the Halstead-Wepman Aphasia Screening Test).[27] Even if aphasia has been ruled out or is not suspected, language abilities should be a part of the assessment of an older individual, because decreases in naming ability occur with age and also are a prominent symptom of a number of disorders among the elderly (e.g., Alzheimer's disease). A variety of these measures of language abilities are presented.

Modified Halstead-Wepman

The Modified Halstead-Wepman[27] is a brief screening test of language and visuographic skills.[1,11] According to Lezak,[11] the Modified Halstead-Wepman is the most widely used of all aphasia tests because it or its variants have been incorporated into many formally organized neuropsychological test batteries, such as the Halstead-Reitan Neuropsychological Test Battery. Various modifications of the Halstead-Wepman exist. As originally devised, this test had 51 items covering all the elements of aphasic disabilities, as well as the most commonly associated communication problems. Reitan[28] pared down the list to 32 items, but still handled the data descriptively in much the same manner as the original. The emphasis of the scoring is on determining the nature of the linguistic problem, once its presence has been established. Errors are coded into a "diagnostic profile" to describe the pattern of the patient's language disabilities. The severity of the language impairment is by breadth (the more errors in more aspects of language abilities, the more severe the impairment) and by depth (the more errors generally, the more severe the impairment). However, no provisions are made to grade test performance or classify patients on the basis of severity.

A second revision contains 37 items, the same as Reitan's with the addition of four easy arithmetic problems and the task of naming a key. A simple error-counting scoring system was established for use with a computerized diagnostic classification system that converts to a six-point rating scale—an attempt to overcome the previous scoring limitations. However, this scoring strategy indicates the severity of an aphasic disorder, but not its nature.

Last, a short version consists of four tasks:[29] (1) copy a square, Greek cross, and triangle without lifting the pencil from the paper; (2) name each copied figure; (3) spell each name; and (4) repeat, "he shouted the warning" and then explain and write it. This version is reputed to aid in discriminating between patients with left- and right-hemisphere lesions, for many of the former can copy the designs but cannot write, whereas the latter have little trouble writing but many cannot reproduce the designs.[11]

Boston Naming Test

The Boston Naming Test[26] examines single-word expressive vocabulary or naming ability by requiring the examinee to name 60 pictured objects ordered in increasing difficulty from "bed" to "abacus." There are various starting points for various groups of examinees: (1) children under ten and aphasic patients start with object 1; (2) older examinees start with item 30 and continue forward unless errors are committed before item 38, if so, they return to item 29 and work backward. The pictures are presented by the examiner to the examinee in order. The examinee is allowed up to 20 seconds to respond, unless the examinee says he does not know the word before the 20 seconds. If the answer is correct, the time in seconds required for the response is noted. For other than correct responses, the verbatim response is recorded. If the examinee is unable to name spontaneously an object, the examiner provides a categorical cue, such as "it's something to eat," that is printed in brackets under the response line for each item. Again, the examinee is allowed up to 20 seconds to name the picture. If the subject still does not recognize the picture after receiving the categorical cue or misnames it, the examiner should note the response and proceed to phonemic cuing. Phonemic cues assist the examinee by providing the opening sound of the target word. It is recommended that a phonemic cue be given after every failure to respond or after any incorrect response. The scoring scheme reflects these administration procedures: (1) object correct without assistance; (2) number of categorical cues given; (3) number of objects correct following categorical cues; (4) number of phonemic cues given; (5) objects correct following phonemic cues. Provisional norms are provided in the manual for children, normal adults, and aphasic adults. However, minimal psychometric information is available.

Western Aphasia Battery

The Western Aphasia Battery[30] (WAB) grew out of efforts to develop an instrument from the Boston Diagnostic Aphasia Examination that would generate diagnostic classifications and be suitable for both clinical and research purposes.[11,30] Seven areas of language abilities are examined: spontaneous speech, auditory comprehension, repetition, naming, reading and writing, praxis, and construction. Some training is required for administration. Shewan and Kertesz[30] report that it takes most aphasics approximately 60 minutes to complete and less time with the more impaired patients. For those individuals unable to withstand such lengthy testing, the WAB can be administered in two parts.

Memory

Memory is an essential component of cognition and is the mental processes for receiving, storing, and retrieving information. It should be evaluated in detail. Memory dysfunction occurs in almost all of the cognitive disorders.[2] To distinguish the type and degree of memory deficit, anatomic localization, the etiologic nature of the pathology, and the impact of the deficit on the individual's ability to function, various aspects of memory should be assessed in some detail.[2,3,10] Albert[2] warns that the assessment of memory in elderly persons is complicated further by the fact that changes in the capacity of memory occur as people age. Therefore, careful testing often is necessary to differentiate normal from pathologic memory performance. In evaluating memory, Strub and Black[3] suggest that the following be considered: (1) the examiner must be able to verify the answers from a source other than the examinee; (2) performance on memory tasks requires sustained attention, therefore, examinees with attentional deficits will not perform optimally; (3) the examinee must be capable of relating to and cooperating with the examiner; and (4) the examinee must have no defect that impairs the comprehension or expression of language. According to Albert,[2] the most common measures of memory in use today are the Wechsler Memory Scale,[7,31] the Benton Visual Retention Test,[32] the Randt Memory Test,[33] and Story Recall. We discuss each.

Wechsler Memory Scale

The Wechsler Memory Scale (WMS)[7] was developed to evaluate rapidly, simply, and practically a rather disparate group of memory functions.[7,34] The objective of the test battery was to create a measure that correlated well with intelligence tests without duplicating them. Seven subtests comprise the WMS and include: (1) personal and current information; (2) orientation; (3) mental control (backward counting, alphabet, and counting by 30); (4) logical memory (two passages read and subject scored on average number of items retained when repeating); (5) digit span (forward and backward); (6) visual reproduction (draw geometric figures from memory); and (7) associate learning (learning 10 pairs in three trials). Performance on the subtests is summed and statistically age corrected to provide a memory quotient (MQ), which in some ways is analogous to a full-scale IQ (mean 100, SD 15). The scoring is most useful on three factors: memory, attention, and concentration. Scoring instructions published by Wechsler[7] and Klonoff and Kennedy[35] show norms for people in their eighties and nineties. For many years, the WMS was the only widely available and standardized objective test of memory for clinical use. Indices of reliability and validity[35-37] are shown in Appendix 8A.

Benton Visual Retention Test

The Benton Visual Retention Test (BVRT)[32] consists of several series of simple and complex line drawings designed to assess short-term or immediate memory. Visual motor construction, visual spatial perception, and visual conceptualization also are reportedly assessed by the BVRT.[3] This series of line drawings is presented to the examinee for varying periods of time (5 to 10 seconds), depending on the administration form, in which the examinee either reproduces the designs directly or after a variable delay (immediate recall or a 15-second delay). The BVRT requires approximately 5 minutes to administer. It is recommended that the BVRT be administered by a trained psychologist, that is, one who knows the test.[38]

The BVRT exists in four alternate forms, C, D, E, and I. Form I was an attempt to remove the motor component of the BVRT to assess a more purely visual skill. In this form the examinee is asked to select the original form from a series of four alternatives.[39,40] In addition, there are three forms of administration, A through C. In Administration A, the subject is shown the stimuli for 10 seconds and then is asked to reproduce them. In Administration B, the subject is shown the stimuli for 10 seconds and is asked to reproduce them after a delay of 5 seconds. In Administration C, the subject is allowed to copy the stimuli directly.

The BVRT has explicit scoring instructions and robust normative data. Performance on the BVRT is positively correlated with IQ and negatively correlated with age. Therefore, the norms are for the expected correct responses and the expected number of errors for each alternate form and administration for six IQ groups crossed with multiple age groups from 8 to 64 years. These norms, created with school children of various IQs and with medically ill adult patients with no history of brain disease, are available in the BVRT manual.[32]

Performance on the BVRT also is influenced by the anatomic location of the neurologic involvement. Individuals with bilateral damage average four to six errors, individuals with right-sided damage 3.5 errors, and persons with left-sided damage one error.[41] Other studies tend to support a right–left differential in defective copying of these designs and find that right-hemisphere patients are two or three times more likely to have difficulties.[42] However, in one study that included aphasic patients in the comparisons between groups with lateralized lesions, no differences were found in the frequency with which constructional impairment was present in the drawings of right- and left-hemisphere–damaged patients.[43] Psychometric indices[44] are shown in Appendix 8A. Form 1 may be solved by a logical strategy unrelated to the visual stimulus and requires a posttesting interview of the subject.[45]

Randt Memory Test

The Randt Memory Test (RMT)[33] is a set of seven subtests specifically designed to quantify mild to moderate memory loss in longitudinal studies of patients with organic brain disease. Five alternate forms were developed for repeated examination of everyday memory. The first and last subtests (General Information and Incidental Learning) are identical in all alternate forms. The other five subtests are reported to be equivalent on the basis of such relevant characteristics as word length, frequency, and imagery levels. The middle five subtests are of recall, digits forward and backward, word pairs, and a paragraph. Recognition of line drawings of common objects also is included.

There is a set order of presentation in which acquisition and retrieval from storage are differentiated by separating immediate recall and recall following fixed tasks (a subsequent subtest serves as the distractor task for each of the four subtests that have delayed recall trials). In addition, the RMT is constructed to use telephone interviews to obtain 24-hour recall data.[11]

Story Recall

Story Recall[3,11] begins with the instructions to the examinee, "I am going to read you a short story. Listen carefully, because when I finish reading, I want you to tell me as much of the story as you can remember." After reading the story, the examinee is instructed, "Now tell me everything that you can remember of that story. Start at the beginning of the story and tell me what happened." The separate items of the story are indicated by slash (/) marks. As the patient retells the story, indicate the number of ideas recalled. When an examinee reports only a few items, the examiner should encourage the examinee to try and recall more. If the examinee still does not produce much, the examiner can provide some structure for the recall through directive questioning such as, "What happened?," "Where did it happen?," "Who was involved?" In this instance, the examiner should note where the directive questioning began to keep track of spontaneous versus directed recall.

Following the first recall, the examiner instructs the examinee, "In a little while, I'm going to ask you to tell me how much of the story you can still remember. I'm going to read the story to you again now so that you'll have it fresh in your memory for the next time." Recall following the second reading follows approximately 20 minutes of testing involving verbal material. Once again, the examiner asks the examinee, "Tell me everything you can remember of that story." Directed questioning should proceed as appropriate. Several versions of Story Recall can be located in Strub and Black[3] and Lezak.[11]

Conceptualization

According to Albert,[16] conceptualization is the most complex and difficult aspect of cognition to assess. Furthermore, an individual's conceptual abilities are easily confounded by general intelligence. As a result, when evaluating conceptualization, general intelligence also must be evaluated. Tasks that examine conceptualization include tests of concept formation, abstraction, set shifting, and set maintenance. These measures are considered to underestimate an individual's practical coping and problem-solving abilities.[1] Therefore, it is recommended that these formal tests be supplemented with observations of an individual's everyday decision making.[1] Other measures of conceptualization include Raven's Progressive, the Similarities subtest of the Wechsler Adult Intelligence Scale-Revised (WAIS-R), and the Verbal-Visual Test.

Proverbs Test

The Proverbs Test[46-48] is a standardized test of proverbs with regard to familiarity and difficulty. There are three alternate forms of the Proverbs Test, each containing 12 proverbs of equivalent difficulty. It is administered as a written test in which the examinee is instructed that the intent of the test is to explain what the proverb means, rather than just telling the examiner more about the proverb. The responses are scored on a five-point rating scale that objectifies the degree of abstraction. One form is a multiple-choice version of 40 items, each with four possible answers (the best answer form). Only one choice is appropriate and abstract, the other three are either concrete interpretations or common misinterpretations.[11]

Modified Card Sorting Test

The Modified Card Sorting Test (MCST)[49] is a widely used test devised to study abstract behavior. The examinee is given a pack of 48 cards on which are printed one to four symbols, triangle, star, cross, or circle, in red, green, yellow, or blue. No two cards are identical; cards do not share more than one attribute with a stimulus card. The examinee is instructed to sort the cards according to a rule or category. Whatever category the examinee chooses first is designated "correct" by the examiner who proceeds to inform the examinee whether each choice is correct or not until the examinee has achieved a run of six correct responses. At that point, the examinee is told that the rule has changed and is instructed to find another rule. This procedure is continued until six categories are achieved or the pack of 48 cards is used up.

Besides a score for the number of categories obtained, Nelson[49] derived a score from the total number of errors and score as perseverative errors only those of the same category as the immediately preceding response. Results obtained from testing with the

MCST readily separate examinees with unilateral neurologic lesions from control examinees. There is a tendency for patients with posterior lesions to perform better than patients whose lesions involved the frontal lobes and for patients with frontal lobe lesions to make more perseverative errors than control patients. Nelson's[49] data also suggest that this method is sensitive to aging effects. Older persons perform more poorly, women outperform men, and persons with higher education perform better.

Judgment: Real-Life Hypothetical Situations

Judgment is not generally evaluated in isolation of other cognitive functions, but rather as component elements in the global measures[50,51] of cognition.

Global Measures of Cognition

Global measures are used to survey multiple aspects of cognition. As a result, global measures are useful screening tools for cognitive impairment. In addition, global measures tend not to be comprehensive measures of cognition but to consist of those elements that increase the sensitivity and specificity for detecting impairment. Diagnosis for other than impairment is problematic using global measures. Psychometric indices, as well as advantages and disadvantages of important measures, are shown in Appendix 8B.

Mental Status Questionnaires

Mini-Mental State Examination

The Mini-Mental State Examination (MMSE),[17] is a simplified, scored form that consists of 11 questions requiring 5 to 10 minutes to complete. Each question is scored as either correct or incorrect; the total score ranges from 0 to 30 and reflects the number of correct responses. A score less than 24 is considered evidence of impaired cognition.[17,52,53] The MMSE is a reliable and valid measure. In a comprehensive review of the information about the MMSE accumulated since the mid-1960s, Tombaugh and McIntyre[54] reported that the MMSE remains psychometrically robust across settings and despite gender, race, ethnicity, and social class. Other studies document this as well.[55-59] The MMSE also is known to discriminate well among normal, depressed, demented, and depressed and demented individuals.[17] In recent reviews of cognitive screening instruments,[53-55] the MMSE was identified as the preferred instrument for use with demented elders and remains the most frequently used bedside test of cognition.

Cognitive Capacity Screening Examination

The Cognitive Capacity Screening Examination (CCSE)[60] was developed to be a sufficiently sensitive and relevant instrument for the detection of a diffuse organic mental syndrome, particularly delirium, in nonpsychiatric patients. The CCSE consists of 30 items requiring 5 to 10 minutes to administer. The test measures a variety of cognitive functions: orientation, digit span, concentration, serial sevens, repetition, verbal concept formation, and short-term verbal recall. According to the researchers, patients who score less than 20 points should be considered cognitively impaired.

Neurobehavioral Cognitive Status Examination

The Neurobehavioral Cognitive Status Examination (NCSE)[50,51] is a relatively newly developed, complete, neurologic mental status screening examination. The NCSE was designed to detect and characterize the nature of cognitive dysfunction in hospitalized adults. The NCSE is reported to provide more detailed and sensitive information about cognitive status while remaining clinically practical, that is, brief, and easy to administer (10 to 20 minutes) and score for the clinician, and not fatiguing to the patient. The NCSE consists of a test and an administration/scoring manual. The instrument assesses the level of consciousness, orientation, and attention, as well as five major ability areas: language, constructions, memory, calculations, and reasoning.[50,51] With the exception of the memory and orientation categories, the other tests begin with a screen item. The screen item is a demanding test of the skill involved, and 10% to 30% of the normal population fail the screen.[50] If the screen is answered correctly, the particular skill is considered intact, and no further testing of that skill is required. If the screen is failed, the metric, a series of test items of increasing complexity, is administered. Within each cognitive ability area, the number of correct responses is totaled and recorded on the front of the test booklet, resulting in independent scores for specific cognitive ability areas rather than a single overall score. Scores below a predetermined criterion are interpreted as reflecting impairment within that particular area of cognitive functioning.[50,51]

The NCSE's clinical utility has been demonstrated in psychiatry and neurology clinics and psychiatry and neurology inpatient services and for neuropsychologic and neurosurgery patients. The NCSE occupies a middle ground between very brief instruments that provide a global estimation of cognitive functioning and exhaustive neuropsychologic test batteries that offer a more thorough assessment.[50,51] It can be administered at the bedside in approximately 15 to 30 minutes.

Measures for Common Disorders of Cognition

Common disorders of cognition to be detected and evaluated relative to their nature and severity include acute confusion, or delirium, dementia, and depression. Instruments for each disorder are presented and discussed. See Appendix 8C for a comparison of clinical features of these disorders.[61]

Acute Confusion/Delirium

Acute confusion, or delirium, is a state of transient, global cognitive impairment (i.e., perception, memory, and thinking) of acute onset. Symptoms of acute confusion that fluctuate diurnally include disturbed consciousness, impaired attention and memory, misperception and misinterpretation of information, disorganized thinking, and variable psychomotor behavior[4] (see Appendix 8C). Various methods have been developed to detect accurately and promptly the presence of acute confusion and to predict its occurrence.[62] Measures, in addition to those discussed, are shown in Appendix 8B.

Clinical Assessment of Confusion-Form A

The Clinical Assessment of Confusion-Form A (CAC-A)[63] was developed to determine the presence, pattern, and severity of confusion as perceived by nurses. The CAC-A is a checklist of 25 psychomotor behaviors, representing five dimensions of confusion: (1) cognition; (2) general behavior; (3) motor activity; (4) orientation; and (5) psychotic/neurotic behaviors. The patient is evaluated on the basis of the presence or absence of each behavior. The score is the total of the weights for each of the observed behaviors. Four or more behaviors, weighted scores greater than 8, indicates the presence of confusion. The CAC-A also implies that the more behaviors observed, the more severe the confusion. Vermeersch[63,64] provides the following recommendations for interpreting test results: 4 to 6 behaviors with a weighted score ranging from 9 to 14 indicates mild confusion; 7 to 9 behaviors with a weighted score ranging from 15 to 24, moderate confusion; more than 9 behaviors and weighted scores greater than 28, severe confusion. Psychometric indices[63-65] are shown in Appendix 8B.

NEECHAM Confusion Scale

The NEECHAM Confusion Scale[66] was designed to evaluate rapidly and nonintrusively a patient's cognitive function and behavioral performance to detect early cues to the development of acute confusion and to monitor recovery. NEECHAM places a minimal response burden on the patient by making maximal use of existing data such as the patient's performance in the environment (self-care, feeding, and use of information) and the patient's physiologic stability (vital signs, oxygen saturation, and urinary incontinence). Ratings can be repeated at frequent intervals to monitor changes in the patient's status.[66] The scale is sensitive to early changes in information processing and documents confused behavior, including delirium.[66]

The instrument consists of nine scaled items divided into three subscales of assessment: responsiveness, performance, and physiologic control. The score ranges from 0 (minimal responsiveness) to 30 (normal function) and is completed by the nurse in a manner similar to other vital function measurements conducted during routine or required nursing assessments. The authors reported that NEECHAM scores lower than 20 were strongly associated with DSM-IV criteria for delirium, whereas scores of 20 to 24 seemed to indicate the patients with borderline confusion.[67]

Delirium Rating Scale

The Delirium Rating Scale (DRS)[12] is a 10-item scale. Each of the 10 items is rated by the clinician using information obtained from an interview and mental status examination of the patient. Information from the patient's hospital record (e.g., medical history, laboratory tests, nursing observations) and family reports are also necessary.[12] The clinician-rater is instructed to complete the DRS using information obtained from at least a 24-hour period of observation of the patient because the fluctuating course of the symptoms of delirium. Operationalizing the DSM-III criteria for delirium, the DRS includes items measuring the temporal onset of symptoms, perceptual disturbances, hallucinations, delusions, psychomotor behavior, cognitive status during formal testing, physical disorder, sleep–wake disturbance, lability of mood, and variability of symptoms. The total score on the DRS is the sum of the items ranging from a minimum of 0 to a maximum of 32 and is intended to reflect the severity of the delirium (the higher the score, the more severe the delirium).

The DRS is considered to represent a significant advance over earlier symptom-rating scales used to detect delirium. The criteria for delirium have been operationalized, thereby providing information on both cognitive and behavioral symptoms.

Confusion Assessment Method

The Confusion Assessment Method (CAM)[5] was developed to assist clinicians who have no formal psychiatric training to identify quickly and accurately patients with delirium. The CAM measures nine dimensions of delirium as defined by the DSM-III-R criteria for delirium. The CAM is suitable at the bedside to identify patients with delirium.

Delirium Symptom Interview

The Delirium Symptom Interview (DSI)[68] was developed in response to previous criticism that the measurement of the symptoms of delirium was too subjective and, therefore, unreliable. Development of the DSI also was predicated on the belief that it was necessary to have structured assessments that could be administered by trained, lay interviewers so that data would be reliably collected and could be replicated by other research groups. To improve reliability and avoid the observation bias introduced by subjective opinions from clinical interviews, the DSI was constructed to structure the assessments of all the symptoms of delirium, and not just the cognitive symptoms, as is typically the case. These structured assessments consist of 17 questions and 45 observations of the examinee. The symptoms assessed by the DSI are the DSM-IV diagnostic criteria for delirium: clouding of consciousness, disorientation, disturbance of sleep, perceptual disturbance, incoherent speech, increased or decreased psychomotor activity, and fluctuating behavior.

The authors report that 10 to 15 minutes are required to complete the DSI. A symptom was identified as having a rapid onset, or as new, if: (1) it was not present at the patient's initial evaluation and developed subsequently in the hospital; or (2) if present when the patient was first seen in the hospital, it had not been observed prior to the patient's hospitalization as documented through a structured interview with a relative or caretaker. Fluctuating behavior is rated, and an etiology is sought, but not required.

Dementia

Dementia is a chronic, insidious, progressive, and permanent form of cognitive impairment. It is an impairment of higher cortical functions, including memory, that is manifested by difficulties in day-to-day functioning, problem solving, and the control of emotions.[69] There are several types of dementia made on the basis of the etiologic agent, such as Primary Degenerative Dementia of the Alzheimer Type, Multi-Infarct Dementia, and AIDS-Related Dementia. A comparison of clinical features of delirium (acute confusion), dementia, and depression is found in Appendix 8A.

Mattis Dementia Rating Scale

The Mattis Dementia Rating Scale (MDRS),[70] examines five areas that are particularly sensitive to behavioral changes that characterize Alzheimer's Dementia: (1) attention; (2) initiation and perseveration; (3) construction; (4) conceptual; and (5) memory.

An interesting feature of the MDRS is that, instead of giving the items in the usual ascending order of difficulty, the most difficult item is given first. Because the most difficult items are within the capacity of most intact older persons, this feature can be a time-saver. An intact patient would only have to have three abstract answers on the first subtest, and the remaining items could be skipped. On the other hand, Mattis reports that the examination of demented patients can take 30 to 45 minutes. A motivation behind the development of the MDRS was to minimize the floor effect frequently observed when testing such persons. Scores range from 0 (poorest performance) to 144 (perfect performance).

Kendrick Cognitive Tests for the Elderly

The Kendrick Cognitive Tests for the Elderly[71-74] were developed to screen and assess the course of dementia and simultaneously differentiate it from depression, as well as to quantify the change in cognitive function over time. Therefore, the Kendrick Battery is recommended for diagnostic, prognostic, and monitoring purposes.[38] The Kendrick Cognitive Tests for the Elderly are considered short, simple, and easy to administer.[71] It consists of: (1) the Kendrick Object Learning Test (KOLT); and (2) the Kendrick Digit Copying Test (KDCT). It is recommended[71] that the battery be administered by either a psychologist, physician (not necessarily a psychiatrist), nurse, social worker, or speech therapist. One half-day training *is* needed; if the test is not used regularly, refresher courses are recommended. Fifteen minutes are required to administer the battery.

The KOLT is a test of recall of everyday objects after viewing for a brief period. There are two alternate forms: A and B, each with four cards of pictures of common objects. The examinee is instructed to look at the objects and memorize as many as is possible in the short time that the card is shown them. When the card is turned over, the examinee is to recall as many of the objects as possible. Card 1, with 10 objects is displayed for 30 seconds; Card 2, with 15 objects, 45 seconds; Card 3, with 20 objects, 60 seconds; and Card 4 with 25 objects, 75 seconds. The examinee is prompted to look at the card for the entire time allotted. When responses are incomplete, the examiner encourages the examinee to try and remember more objects. This is continued until the examinee remembers all objects or indicates that no more can be recalled. It is permissible to confirm responses. For diagnostic purposes, type of errors (e.g., perseverative errors, incorrect, randomly named objects, or similar objects are important). However, the score is the number of *correct* responses only.

The Kendrick Digit Copying Test (KDCT) is a simple test of speed performance. The maximum score is 70. The examinee is given the KDCT form and a pen. The examinee is instructed to copy each number as fast as possible below the line on the form and to continue until the examiner says to stop. Instructions can be repeated, and the examiner can demonstrate the test to the examinee for the task to be understood. In addition, encouragement to continue until the task is completed is permissible. The examinee is allowed two minutes to complete the test. If the examinee completes the test in less than 2 minutes, the score is the amount of time in seconds required to complete the test, otherwise the score is the number of correct responses. Scores are transformed for equivalence and can be converted to an age-scaled score and compared to a table of standardized scores. The Kendrick Battery[71] is not recommended for individuals whose IQ is less than 70 or for diagnostic purposes with institutionalized individuals. However, it is recommended to repeat testing at 6-week intervals to detect changes in cognitive performance.

Consortium to Establish a Registry for Alzheimer's Disease

The Consortium to Establish a Registry for Alzheimer's Disease (CERAD)[75] was organized to establish a brief and accurate method for assessing the presenting clinical manifestations and cognitive alterations in individuals with Alzheimer's Disease (AD).[76] A uniform, reliable, simple, yet accurate, means of evaluation to obtain information about the clinical, neuropsychologic, and neuropathologic aspects of the disease was essential to provide appropriate health services and for research purposes. The CERAD is an extensive, comprehensive composite of other tests separated into two batteries. The first is the Neuropsychological Battery, which consists of tests of: (1) verbal fluency; (2) modified Boston Naming Test; (3) Mini-Mental State Examination; (4) Word List Memory; (5) Constructional Praxis; (6) Word List Recall; and (7) Word List Recognition. The second is a Clinical Battery consisting of (1) demographic information; (2) drug inventory; (3) history of patient by patient and an informant; (4) a physical examination; (5) laboratory studies; and (6) a diagnostic impression.

Depression

Depression is a disturbance of mood, consisting of dysphoria, feelings of sadness, pessimism, hopelessness, and loss of interest or pleasure in most activities.[77] It is a term used to refer to a range of disorders from a subclinical problem—a "blue" mood state and general feelings of hopelessness and demoralization—to a major depressive disorder. Most of these scales were developed to detect the presence of depression and to determine its level of severity.[78] Most scales, however, do not facilitate the identification of the underlying etiologic mechanisms of depression (e.g., endogenous versus non-endogenous depression).

Some problems should be considered with any of the following measures of depression:[12,79] (1) the elderly deny feelings of depression; (2) in the elderly there is a higher prevalence of somatic complaints caused by genuine physical problems and their treatment, thereby making what are generally accepted as common somatic complaints of depression nonspecific in the elderly; and (3) it is difficult to differentiate depression from other cognitive problems, such as dementia and acute confusion. We present some measures in chronological order of development.

Beck's Depression Inventory

Beck's Depression Inventory (BDI) was constructed to screen for the presence and severity of depression in adults[80] and is considered reliable and valid even with the elderly.[81] The BDI contains 21 items, each concerned with a particular aspect of the experience and symptomatology of depression, that are rated on a four-point intensity, rather than frequency, dimension. A rating of three indicates the most severe, and zero indicates an absence of a problem in that area. As a result, the greater the score, the more depressed the individual. The ratings are made by the examinee or by an observer, who is recommended to be either a psychologist or psychiatrist. With brief training, administration takes five minutes.[38] Because the BDI requires a severity rating for each symptom, a finer grained picture of the patient's distress can be obtained with the BDI than with other measures of depression. Furthermore, the BDI contains a suicide item that can be highly relevant in the assessment of older adults. Numerous validation studies[79-81] with psychiatric in- and outpatients have generated indices of reliability and validity shown in Appendix 8B.

Hamilton Depression Rating Scale

The Hamilton Depression Rating Scale (HDRS)[82] was designed to assess the level of depression. As a result of the comprehensive coverage of depressive symptomatology, related psychopathology, and its strong psychometric properties, it has remained the most commonly used rating scale of the level of depression in clinical research settings since the 1960s.[79] The HDRS heavily relies on the skill of the examiner to elicit the information required to make the ratings of depression, and, therefore, it is recommended that the HDRS be administered by a psychiatrist or an adequately trained individual. Training requires background knowledge of psychiatry and experience with about 10 patients.[38] The scale often is administered by two examiners, and the score is the average of both ratings. Comprised of 21 items, 17 of which relate to depression, the HDRS can be completed in about 30 minutes.

Geriatric Depression Scale-Short Form

The Geriatric Depression Scale-Short Form (GDS-SF)[83] was developed for measuring depression in the elderly for whom traditional depression scales may not be appropriate.[84,85] The GDS-SF has proven valid and reliable for measuring depression in the elderly, both those institutionalized[85] and demented.[86] None of its items focuses on the typical somatic complaints, but instead tap psychologic distress (e.g., helplessness, hopelessness, and lack of satisfaction with life).[79] It requires five to seven minutes to administer; all items are answered in a yes or no format for ease of comprehension by even cognitively impaired elders. The brevity and ease of administration of the GDS-SF are important considerations with individuals who are physically frail and among whom depression may coexist with other forms of cognitive impairment (e.g., dementia and acute confusion). Sensitivity and specificity remain acceptable with MMSE scores greater than or equal to 15.

Cornell Depression Scale

The Cornell Depression Scale,[87,88] is a 19-item clinician-administered scale developed to evaluate the full spectrum of depressive symptomatology with both cognitively intact and impaired patients. The examiner rates the individual on each of the 19 items using a four-point grading system: a, unable to evaluate; 0, symptom is absent; 1, symptom is present in mild or intermittent form; 2, symptom is present in severe form. The score is the total of all points assigned and can range from 0 to 38. The higher the score, the more severe the individual's depression. In a recent study by Camus et al.,[89] various parameters of reliability among three measures of depression were compared, and the Cornell Scale was found more reliable than the Sunderland or Hamilton measures.

Using a Measure of Cognition

In using an instrument to measure cognition, the following aspects should be considered:

1. Characteristics of the testing environment
   a. Maximize the comfort and privacy of both examiner and examinee.
   b. Make sure the room is well lit and of a comfortable ambient temperature (prevent glare when using laminated materials with elderly examinees).
   c. Check that area is free from distractions (noise, test material scattered on the examination table, brightly colored or patterned clothing, jewelry; if a timer is needed, keep one that is quiet and out of the examinee's sight, as its presence, visual and auditory, could be a source of distraction).
   d. Avoid testing in the presence of others, and keep the testing emotionally nonthreatening (e.g., older adults are especially sensitive to having any difficulty thinking; therefore, stress the importance of the testing while taking care not to increase the examinee's anxiety about testing so that an environment is created where the examinee is motivated to perform well. The order of presentation of items also can be altered so that the examinee experiences success[11] but with care so as not to alter the psychometric properties).
2. Characteristics of the examinee and examiner
   a. Use 15 to 20 minutes to establish rapport with the examinee and to determine the examinee's capacity to be tested (e.g., establish whether the examinee has any special problems that could influence testing or its interpretation and implement measures to minimize disturbance, e.g., for the elder with hearing impairment, taking a position across from the examinee so that he or she can readily use the examiner's nonverbal language as well as read the examiner's lips).
   b. Be alert for signs of fatigue, observing for physical evidence of being tired, slurring of speech, motor slowing, restlessness,[11] and temporarily terminate testing if necessary; if the examination must be terminated in the middle of a section, it would probably be wise to repeat the entire section when testing is resumed. Dividing of testing should consider the purpose of testing, characteristics of the examinee, and amount and type of information desired.
3. Timing of the measurement. Avoid inappropriate times of the day: immediately upon awakening from sleep; immediately before and after meals; immediately before and after medical diagnostic and therapeutic procedures; or in the presence of discomfort or pain.

Interpreting Results

Interpreting results from cognitive testing is not simple and should consist of more than just the score obtained on testing. The nature and pattern of the examinee's responses to testing; the examinee's behavior during testing; the context of testing; the examinee's health history, physical examination, and results of various laboratory and other tests; educational level; occupation; family history; current living situation; level of social functioning; and presence of sensory and/or motor deficits[11] must be considered when interpreting the results of cognitive testing.

The nature and pattern of the responses to testing can provide valuable information about an individual's cognitive status. Noting the examinee's verbatim responses on testing often is valuable in differential diagnosis. For example, was the examinee not motivated to respond? Did the examinee appear to be capable of performing at a higher level than was attempted? Were "I don't know" responses frequent? If such responses were typical for a given examinee, a likely conclusion would be that the individual is depressed (see Appendix 8C).

Anecdotal notes of the context of testing, the testing environment, and the appearance of the examinee during testing are also important for a better understanding of the performance on testing. Supplementary information from the examinee's health history, physical examination, and laboratory and other tests can provide valuable insight into the individual's performance on testing.

Summary

The available psychometric information, the strengths and limitations of global measures of cognition, measures of specific aspects of cognition, and measures for common disorders of cognition were reviewed in this chapter. Points to consider in selecting and using a measure of cognition and interpretations of test results were discussed. Clearly, the determination of an individual's cognitive status is important in the process and outcomes of illness and its treatment. However, additional testing and refinement of these measures of cognitive status is warranted.

Exemplar Studies

Vermeersch, P.E.H., & Henly, S.J. The theoretical structure of the "Clinical Assessment of Confusion-A." Unpublished Manuscript, University of North Dakota, Grand Falls, ND, 1993.

This study exemplifies the need to continue debate of the theoretical properties of the concept of confusion and the accompanying measurement issues. This is a replication study to further evaluate the structure of confusion as measured by the Clinical Assessment of Confusion-A (CAC-A). In the development study, dimensions of confusion were identified: cognition, general behavior, motor activity, orientation, psychotic/neurotic behavior, and two uninterpretable factors. In this study, data from 556 nurses were analyzed to evaluate and compare three completing models of confusion: a single factor unidimensional model, an orthogonal six factor model, and an oblique six factor model similar to the structure suggested in the development study. The oblique six factor model provided the best fit in the predictive sense, and was the most satisfactory from a theoretical sense. Implications for the clinical use of these data were discussed.

Pompei, P., Foreman, M.D., Cassel, C.K., Alessi, C.A., & Cox, D. Detecting delirium among hospitalized older patients. *Arch Int Med*, 1995, 155:301.

This study exemplifies many of the inherent dilemmas in the measurement of delirium in older hospitalized patients. The study was a prospective cohort design of 432 elderly patients to examine the diagnostic characteristics of four instruments commonly used clinically to detect delirium: Digit Span, Vigilance "A" test, the Clinical Assessment of Confusion-A (CAC-A), and the Confusion Assessment Method (CAM). The analysis of the diagnostic characteristics of the tests was novel. Diagnostic properties were examined for each instrument, for worst, best, and median scores on each instrument, and for various combinations of the four instruments. In addition to determining sensitivity and specificity, positive and negative likelihood ratios were examined—information clinically useful for determining a specific individual's probability, or likelihood, of being delirious given their performance on the test(s). Results consistently indicated the CAC-A to possess the best diagnostic characteristics.

References

1. La Rue, A. *Aging and neuropsychological assessment.* New York: Plenum, 1992.
2. Albert, M.S. Assessment of cognitive dysfunction. In M.S. Albert & M.B. Moss (Eds.), *Geriatric neuropsychology.* New York: Guilford, 1988, pp. 57-81.
3. Strub, R.L., & Black, F.W. *The mental status examination in neurology* (2nd ed.). Philadelphia: Davis, 1985.
4. Foreman, M.D. Acute confusion in the elderly. *Ann Rev Nurs Res*, 1993, *11*:1.
5. Inouye, S.K., van Dyke, C.H., Alessi, C.A., et al. Clarifying confusion: The Confusion Assessment Method. A new method for detection of delirium. *Ann Intern Med*, 1990, *113*(12):941.
6. Levkoff, S., Liptzin, B., Cleary, P., et al. Review of research instruments and techniques used to detect delirium. *Int Psychogeriatr*, 1991, *3*(2):253.
7. Wechsler, D. A standardized memory scale for clinical use. *J Psychol*, 1945, *19*:87.
8. Pompei, P., Foreman, M.D., Cassel, C.K., et al. Detecting delirium among hospitalized older patients. *Arch Int Med*, 1995, *155*:301.
9. Reitan, R.M. Validity of the Trail Making Test as an indicator of organic brain damage. *Percept Motor Skill*, 1958, *8*(4):271.
10. Khan, A.U. *Clinical disorders of memory.* NY: Plenum, 1986.
11. Lezak, M.D. *Neuropsychological assessment* (2nd ed.). New York: Oxford University Press, 1983.
12. Trzepacz, P.T., Baker, R.W., & Greenhouse, J. A symptom rating scale for delirium. *Psychiatr Res*, 1988, *23*(1):89.
13. Trzepacz, P.T., Brenner, R.P., Coffman, G., & van Thiel, D.H. Delirium in liver transplantation candidates: Discriminant analysis of multiple test variables. *Biol Psychiatr*, 1988, *24*(1):3.
14. Smith, T.E., & Boyce, E.M. The relationship of the Trail Making Test to psychiatric symptomatology. *J Clin Psychol*, 1962, *18*(4):450.
15. Trzepacz, P.T., Maue, F.R., Coffman, G., & van Thiel, D.H. Neuropsychiatric assessment of liver transplantation candidates: Delirium and other psychiatric disorders. *Int J Psychiatr Med*, 1986–1987, *16*(2):101.
16. Albert, M.S. Assessment of cognitive function in the elderly. *Psychosomatics*, 1984, *25*(4):310.
17. Folstein, M., Folstein, S., & McHugh, P. Mini-Mental State Examination: A practical guide for grading the cognitive state of patients for clinicians. *J Psychiatr Res*, 1975, *12*(3):189.
18. Moore, V., & Wyke, M. Drawing disability in patients with senile dementia. *Psychol Med*, 1984, *14*(1):97.
19. Ainslie, N.K., & Murden, R.A. Effect of education on the Clock-Drawing Dementia Screen in nondemented elderly persons. *J Am Geriatr Soc*, 1993, *41*(3):249.
20. Mendez, M.F., Ala, T., & Underwood, K.L. Development of scoring criteria for the Clock Drawing Task in Alzheimer's Disease. *J Am Geriatr Soc*, 1992, *40*(11):1095.
21. Sunderland, T., Hill, J.L., Mellow, A.M., et. al. Clock Drawing in Alzheimer's Disease: A novel measure of dementia severity. *J Am Geriatr Soc*, 1989, *37*(8):725.
22. Tuokko, H., Hadjistavropoulos, T., Miller, J.A., & Beattie, B.L. The Clock test: A sensitivity measure to differentiate normal elderly from those with Alzheimer Disease. *J Am Geriatr Soc*, 1992, *40*(6):579.
23. Watson, Y.I., Arfken, C.L., & Birge, S.J. Clock completion: An objective screening test for dementia. *J Am Geriatr Soc*, 1993, *41*(11):1235.
24. Goodglass, H., & Kaplan, E. *The assessment of aphasia and related disorders.* Philadelphia: Lea & Febiger, 1972.
25. Kertesz, A. *The Western Aphasia Battery.* New York: Grune & Stratton, 1982.
26. Kaplan, E., Goodglass, H., & Weintraub, S. (Eds.) *Boston Naming Test.* Philadelphia: Lea & Febiger, 1983.
27. Halstead, W.C., & Wepman, J.M. The Halstead-Wepman Aphasia Screening Test. *J Speech Hear Dis*, 1949, *14*(1):9.
28. Reitan, R., & Davison, L.A. *Clinical neuropsychology: Current status and applications.* New York: Hemisphere, 1974.
29. Heimburger, R.F., & Reitan, R.M. Easily administered written test for lateralizing brain lesions. *J Neurosurg*, 1961, *18*(3):301.
30. Shewan, C.M., & Kertesz, A. Reliability and validity characteristics of the Western Aphasia Battery (WAB). *J Speech Hear Dis*, 1980, *45*(3):308.
31. Horner, J., Dawson, D.V., Heyman, A., & Fish, A.M. The usefulness of the Western Aphasia Battery for differential diagnosis of Alzheimer's dementia and focal stroke syndromes: preliminary evidence. *Brain Lang*, 1992, *42*(1):77.
32. Benton, A.L. *The Revised Visual Retention Test.* Iowa City: University of Iowa Press, 1955.
33. Randt, C.T., Brown, E.R., & Osborne, D.P., Jr. A memory test for longitudinal measurement of mild to moderate deficits. *Clin Neuropsychol*, 1980, *2*(4):184.
34. Kane, R.A., & Kane, R.L. *Assessing the elderly: A practical guide to measurement.* Lexington, MA: Lexington Books, 1984.
35. Klonoff, H., & Kennedy, M. Memory and perceptual functioning in octogenarians and nonoctogenarians in the community. *J Gerontol*, 1965, *20*(3):328.
36. Baker, E.L., Feldman, R.G., White, R.F., et al. Monitoring neurotoxins in industry: Development of a neurobehavioral test battery. *J Occup Med*, 1983, *25*(2):125.

37. Erickson, R.C., & Howieson, D. The clinician's perspective: Measuring change and treatment effectiveness. In L.W. Poon (Ed.), *Handbook for clinical memory assessment of older adults.* Hyattsville, MD: American Psychological Association, 1986, pp. 69-80.

38. Israel, L., Kozarevic, D., Sartorius, N. *Source book of geriatric assessment* (vol. 1). Geneva: World Health Organization, 1984.

39. Benton, A.L. A multiple choice type of visual retention test. *Arch Neurol*, 1950, *64*:699.

40. Benton, A.L., Hamsher, K. de S., & Stone, F.B. *Visual retention test: Multiple choice I.* Iowa City, IA: University of Iowa Hospital and Clinics, 1977.

41. Benton, A.L. Differential behavioral effects in frontal lobe disease. *Neuropsychologia*, 1968, *6*(1):53.

42. Benton, A.L. *Contributions to clinical neuropsychology.* New York: Aldine, 1969.

43. Arena, R., & Gainotti, G. Constructional apraxia and visuopractic disabilities in relation to laterality of cerebral lesions. *Cortex*, 1978, *14*(4):463.

44. Crookes, T.G., & McDonald, K.G. Benton's Visual Retention Test in the differentiation of depression and early dementia. *Br J Soc Clin Psychol*, 1972, *11*(1):66.

45. Blanton, P.D., & Gouvier, W.D. A systematic solution to the Benton Visual Retention Test: A caveat to examiners. *Int J Clin Neuropsychol*, 1985, *7*(2):95.

46. Gorham, D.R. A proverbs test for clinical and experimental use. *Psychol Rep*, 1956, 2 (monograph suppl. 1):1.

47. Fogel, M.L. The Proverbs Test in appraisal of cerebral disease. *J Gen Psychol*, 1965, *72*(2):269.

48. Bromley, D.B. Some effects of age on the quality of intellectual output. *J Gerontol*, 1957, *12*(3):318.

49. Nelson, H.E. A modified card sorting test sensitive to frontal lobe defects. *Cortex*, 1976, *12*(4):313.

50. Kiernan, R.L., Mueller, J., Langston, J.W., & Van Dyke, C. The Neurobehavioral Cognitive Screening Examination: A brief but differentiated approach to cognitive assessment. *Ann Intern Med*, 1987, *107*(4): 481.

51. Schwamm, L.H., Van Dyke, C., Kiernan, R.J., et al. The Neurobehavioral Cognitive Status Examination: Comparison with the Cognitive Capacity Screening Examination and the Mini-Mental State Examination in a neurological population. *Ann Intern Med*, 1987, *107*(4):486.

52. Anthony, J.C., LeResche, L., Niaz, U., et al. Limits of the "Mini-Mental State" as a screening test for dementia and delirium among hospital patients. *Psychol Med*, 1982, *12*(2):397.

53. Kaufman, D.M., Weinberger, M., Strain, J.J., & Jacobs, J.W. Detection of cognitive deficits by a brief mental status examination: The Cognitive Capacity Screening Examination, a reappraisal and a review. *Gen Hosp Psychiatr*, 1979, *1*(3):247.

54. Tombaugh, T.N., & McIntyre, N.J. The Mini-Mental State Examination: A comprehensive review. *J Am Geriatr Soc*, 1992, *40*(9):922.

55. Omer, H., Foldes, J., Toby, M., & Menczel, J. Screening for cognitive deficits in a sample of hospitalized geriatric patients: A re-evaluation of a brief mental status questionnaire. *J Am Geriatr Soc*, 1983, *31*(5):266.

56. Bird, H.R., Canino, G., Stipec, M.R., & Shrout, P. Use of the Mini-Mental State Examination in a probability sample of a Hispanic population. *J Nerv Ment Dis*, 1987, *175*(12):731.

57. Bleecker, M.L., Bolla-Wilson, K., Kawas, C., & Agnew, J. Age-specific norms for the Mini-Mental State Exam. *Neurology*, 1988, *38*(10):1565.

58. Escobar, J.I., Burnam, A., Karno, M., et al. Use of the Mini-Mental State Examination (MMSE) in a community population of mixed ethnicity: Cultural and linguistic artifacts. *J Nerv Ment Dis*, 1986, *174*(10):607.

59. Magaziner, J., Bassett, S.S., & Hebel, J.R. Predicting performance on the Mini-Mental State Examination: Use of age- and education-specific equations. *J Am Geriatr Soc*, 1987, *35*(11):996.

60. Jacobs, J.W., Bernard, M.R., Delgado, A., & Strain, J.J. Screening for organic mental syndromes in the medically ill. *Ann Intern Med*, 1977, *86*(1):40.

61. Marcantonio, E.R., Goldman, L., Mangione, C.M., et al. A clinical prediction rule for delirium after elective noncardiac surgery. *JAMA*, 1994, *271*(2):134.

62. Foreman, M.D. Acute confusion in the hospitalized elderly: A research dilemma. *Nurs Res*, 1986, *35*(1):34.

63. Vermeersch, P.E.H. The Clinical Assessment of Confusion-A. *Appl Nurs Res*, 1990, *3*(3):128.

64. Vermeersch, P.E.H., & Henly, S.J. Structure of the Clinical Assessment of Confusion-A. Unpublished manuscript, University of North Dakota, Grand Forks, ND, 1993.

65. Mion, L.C., & Nagley, S.J. Clinical Assessment of Confusion in Long-Term Care. *Appl Nurs Res*, 1992, *5*(2):100.

66. Neelon, V.J., Champagne, M.T., McConnell, E., et al. Use of the NEECHAM Confusion Scale to assess acute confusional states of hospitalized older patients. In S.G. Funk, E.M. Tournquist, M.T. Champagne, & R.A. Wiese (Eds.), *Key aspects of elder care: Managing falls, incontinence, and cognitive impairment.* New York: Springer, 1992, pp. 278-289.

67. Neelon, V.J., Funk, S.G., Carlson, J.R., & Champagne, M.T. The NEECHAM Confusion Scale: Relationship to clinical indicators of acute confusion in hospitalized elders. *Gerontologist*, 1989, *29*(special issue):65A.

68. Albert, M.S., Levkoff, S.E., Reilly, C., et al. The Delirium Symptom Interview: An interview for the detection of delirium symptoms in hospitalized patients. *J Geriatr Psychiatr Neurol*, 1992, *5*(1):14.

69. Bondareff, W. Biomedical perspective of Alzheimer's disease and dementia in the elderly. In M.L.M. Gilhooly, S.H. Zarit, & J.E. Birren (Eds.), *The dementias: Policy and management.* Englewood Cliffs, NJ: Prentice-Hall, 1986, pp. 13-37.

70. Mattis, S. Mental status examination for organic mental syndrome in the elderly patient. In L. Bellak, & T.B. Karasu (Eds.), *Geriatric psychiatry: A handbook for psychiatrists and primary care physicians.* New York: Grune & Stratton, 1976, pp. 77-121.

71. Kendrick, D.C. *Kendrick Cognitive Tests for the Elderly.* Windsor, England: NFER-Nelson, 1985.

72. Kendrick, D.C. Administrative and interpretive problems with the Kendrick Battery for the Detection of Dementia of the Elderly. *Br J Clin Psychol*, 1982, *21*(2):149.

73. Knight, R.G., & Moroney, B.M. An investigation of the validity of the Kendrick Battery for the detection of dementia in the elderly. *Int J Clin Neuropsychol*, 1985, VII(3):147.

74. Rabbitt, P. How to assess the aged? An experimental psychologist's view. Some comments on Dr. Kendrick's paper. *Br J Clin Psychol*, 1982, 2(1)1:55.

75. Morris, J., LaBarge, E., Clark, C., et al. CERAD clinical and neuropsychological assessment of Alzheimer's disease: A preliminary report of standardized procedures and reliability [abstract]. *Neurology*, 1988, *38*(suppl 1):287.

76. Welsh, K., Butters, N., Hughes, J., Mohs, R., & Heyman, A. Detection of abnormal memory decline in mild cases of Alzheimer's disease using CERAD neuropsychological measures. *Arch Neurol*, 1991, *48*(3):278.

77. Stabb, A., & Lyles, M. *Manual of geriatric nursing.* Glenview, IL: Scott-Foresman, 1990, pp. 528-529.

78. Thompson, L.W., Futterman, A., & Gallagher, D. Assessment of late-life depression. *Psychopharmacol Bull*, 1988, *24*(4):577.

79. Thompson, L.W., Gong, V., Haskins, E., & Gallagher, D. Assessment of depression and dementia during the late years. *Ann Rev Gerontol Geriatr*, 1987, 7:295.

80. Beck, A.T., Ward, C.H., Mendelson, M., et al. An inventory for measuring depression. *Arch Gen Psychiatr*, 1961, 4(6):561.

81. Gallagher, D., Breckenridge, J., Steinmetz, J., & Thompson, L. The Beck Depression Inventory and Research Diagnostic Criteria: Congruence in an older population. *J Consult Clin Psychol*, 1983, 51(6):945.

82. Hamilton, M. Development of a rating scale for primary depressive illness. *Br J Soc Clin Psychol*, 1967, 6(4):278.

83. Brink, T.L., Yesavage, J.A., Lum, O., et al. Screening tests for geriatric depression. *Clin Gerontol*, 1982, 1(1):37.

84. Burke, W.J., Nitcher, R.L., Roccaforte, W.H., & Wengel, S.P. A prospective evaluation of the Geriatric Depression Scale in an outpatient geriatric assessment center. *J am Geriatr Soc*, 40(12):1227.

85. Parmalee, P.A., Lawton, M.P., & Katz, I.R. Psychometric properties of the Geriatric Depression Scale among the institutionalized aged. *J Consult Clin Psychol*, 1989, 57(1):92.

86. Yesavage, J.A., Brink, T.L., Rose, T.L., & Adey, M. The Geriatric Depression Rating Scale: Comparison with other self-report and psychiatric rating scales. In T. Crook, S. Ferris, & R. Bartus (Eds.), *Assessment in geriatric psychopharmacology.* New Canaan, CT: Mark Powley, 1983, pp. 153-167.

87. Alexopoulos, G.S., Abrams, R.C., Young, R.C., & Shamoian, C.A. Use of the Cornell Scale in nondemented patients. *J Am Geriatr Soc*, 1988, 36(3):230.

88. Alexopoulos, G.S., Abrams, R.C., Young, R.C., & Shamoian, C.A. Cornell Scale for depression in dementia. *Biol Psychiatr*, 1988, 23(3):271.

89. Camus, V., Schmitt, L., Ousset, P.J., et. al., A comparative study of Hamilton, Cornell, and Sunderland depression rating scales [abstract]. *J Am Geriatr Soc*, 1993, 41:SA42.

Appendices

8A. Advantages and Disadvantages of Specific Measures

Dimension Tested	Psychometric Properties	Advantages	Disadvantages
Attention			
Digit Span	Sensitivity 0.34 (8) Specificity 0.90 (8)	Brief norms available (7)	Insensitive to mild inattentiveness; confounds attention with primary memory
Test of vigilance (A-test)	Sensitivity 0.722 (7) Specificity 0.564 (7) (when used with moderately demented elderly examinees)	Can test nonverbal patients with predetermined method (eye blink); does not have educational, intellectual or socioeconomic bias	Cannot be used with hearing-impaired persons
Trail-making test (TMT)	Sensitivity: Part A: 0.75; Part B: 0.917 Specificity: Part A: 0.821; Part B: 0.731	Useful in identifying attentional deficit but not in determining exact nature of impairment	Reliability altered by variability in examiner's reaction time and time for patient to make correction (11) High false-positive rates Practice effects; age bias; poor tolerance by older hospitalized patients (8)
Visuospatial ability			
Clock-drawing test	Internal consistency: 0.95 (20) Test–retest reliability 0.70 (20,22) Interrater reliability 0.48–0.95 Concurrent validity varies (Folstein Mini-Mental 0.4; Rey Complex Figure 0.66) (17,19) Criterion-related validity (dementia): sensitivity 0.478–0.901, specificity 0.418–1.00 Clock setting has greatest sensitivity (87%), specificity (82%), test–retest reliability 0.82, Kappa 0.63 and interrater reliability 0.90–0.93		Lack of standardized performance instructions between versions preventing direct comparisons Variable methods of scoring and interpreting results Biased against poorly educated persons May measure more complex and higher aspects cognition (abstraction, reasoning)
Language			
Halstead-Wepman	Not available	Brief (<30 minutes) Covers essential language abilities Discriminates among various types of aphasia	No guidelines for clinical applications so must be used by experienced examiners; no standardized scoring procedure

105

8A. Advantages and Disadvantages of Specific Measures (*cont.*)

Dimension Tested	Psychometric Properties	Advantages	Disadvantages
Boston-Naming Test	Sensitive (1) Internal consistency reliability 0.68–0.96 (26)	Relieves examinee's frustration of failure by providing possibility of success Differentiates among types of aphasic individuals Provides evidence that a word is in examinee's potential vocabulary	
Western Aphasia Battery	Cronbach's alpha 0.905 Bentler's coefficient theta 0.975 Correlations among subtests >0.60 Test–retest reliability >0.88 Overall interrater reliability >0.90 Construct validity Face and content validity	Discriminates aphasia from other brain damage language problems	Least able to classify patients with hemisphere strokes (31)
Memory			
Wechsler Memory Scale (WMS)	Validity questioned as to whether test measures motivation, cooperation, willingness to memorize material of little value (27) Test–retest for subscales: 0.41–0.60 (recall), 0.75–0.89 (total score) Cronbach's alpha 0.686 (figural; 0.44; digit 0.88 Construct validity (3 factors) (7,35-37)	Easy to use, short (15–30 minutes) Allowance made for memory variances with age Memory quotient directly comparable to other intellectual functions Useful in the detection of special memory defects with specific brain injuries	Highly verbal test Overemphasis on very basic processes Combining widely variable tests to make "memory quotient" Age correction may invalidate data (3) Reliance on mental quotient when memory is multidimensional
Benton Visual Retention Test	Difficult to interpret as may use alternate form and administration Test–retest reliability (Adm A): 0.85 (41); Form C 0.58–0.60 with interrater reliability 0.95 (11) Discriminant validity for depression and dementia (standard admin, A) (44)	Three alternative forms allow use of one for a copy trial (11)	Alternative forms may not be equivalent (11,32)

Rand Memory Test	Validity of incidental learning questioned (1) Traditional indices not reported	Short (20 minutes) Accuracy in evaluating conditions associated with aging and diffuse brain diseases (11)	Highly verbal so penalizes patients with language disorders Insensitive to memory impairments involving nonverbal material (11) Requires skilled examiner so patient not questioned to point of discomfort but can push when low-level responses occur
Story Recall	Sensitive for short-term verbal recall (3,11) Traditional indices of reliability and validity not reported Equivalence among versions not done		
Conceptualization Proverb Test	Not reported	Objective scores of abstractness and concreteness and can be compared with norms Decreased variation in administration and scoring (decreased bias) (11) Marginal discrimination	Scores vary by level of individual's education Concrete responses increase with age
Modified Card Sorting Test	Not reported		No scoring norms but may be rarely needed

Numbers in parentheses correspond to studies cited in the References.

8B. Advantages and Disadvantages of Global Measures

Testing Dimension	Psychometric Properties	Advantages	Disadvantages
Mental Status			
Mini-Mental State Exam	Reliable and valid Test-retest reliability 0.82–0.98 Interrater reliability 0.88 (52) Internal consistency 0.96 Criterion-related validity (confusion), Spearman's rho = 0.76 Discriminant validity (depression), $r = 0.38$ Concurrent validity (confusion), c, $r = 0.80$; vas-c, $r = 0.83$	Robust measurement across settings Discriminates among normal, depressed, demented, and demented depressed individuals	Total scores do not reveal precise neuropsychiatric diagnosis May be ecologically invalid
Neurobehavioral Cognitive Status Exam	More sensitive for detecting cognitive impairment than MMSE, CCSE (51) because it scores each cognitive area separately, uses graded series of test items, and assesses a larger number of areas of cognitive function	Brief (10–20 minutes) Easy to administer Provides differential profile of patient's cognitive status	
Cognitive Capacity Screening Exam	Validation studies (77,75,83–88) Interrater reliability 100% Sensitivity 0.71–0.79; specificity 0.45 (55) Internal consistency reliability 0.97 Concurrent validity (MMSE) is 0.78, (SPMSQ) is 0.71	Brief (5–10 minutes)	Performance influenced by age, education level, ethnicity, language (17,56-59) Cannot distinguish between acute and chronic impairment All aspects of cognition not assessed Verbal, so cannot be used with nonverbal persons
Delirium			
Clinical Assessment of Confusion-Form-A	In hospitalized adults (63): interrater reliability 0.98; concurrent validity with SPMSQ 0.71, VAS-C 0.81 Test-retest 0.85	Checklist of 25 psychomotor behaviors Easy scoring	Recent studies show different psychometric indices (65) Nurses in acute care may perceive confused behavior differently from nurses in intermediate care (63)

Scale	Reliability/Validity	Advantages	Disadvantages
NEECHAM Confusion Scale	Internal consistency 0.80 Cohen's kappa 0.70 (in hospitalized elders 0.75) Statistically significant correlation with Folstein's MMSE $r = 0.80$ (25) and VAS-C, $r = 0.82$ Hospitalized and institutionalized elders (66) Interrater reliability 0.96 Test-retest reliability 0.98 Internal consistency (Cronbach's alpha = 0.86) Correlations to MMSE 0.76–0.81 Sensitivity (67): NEECHAM Score $\leq 24 = 0.95$ Specificity 0.78	Reflects clinical reality	Subjective Immature scale
Confusion Assessment Method (CAM)	Face and content validity Sensitivity 0.94–1.0 Specificity 0.90–0.95 Positive predictive accuracy 0.91–0.94; negative predictive accuracy 0.90–1.0 Convergent validity: (MMSE) $k = 0.64$, (story recall) $k = 0.59$, (VAS-C) $k = 0.82$, (Digit Scan) $k = 0.66$ Item analysis: inattention and disorganization of thought most diagnostic for delirium Interobserver reliability: high Cohen's kappa 0.81–1.0	Suitable for use at bedside to assist in identifying patients with delirium (8)	
Delirium Rating Scale	Correlations (15) with MMSE (–0.43), and TMT-B (0.66) Interrater reliability 0,97 ($k = 0.90$) (62)	Differentiates delirious patients from normal and from those with schizophrenia and dementia Superior over earlier symptom rating scales	Scoring relies on subjective clinical judgements from unstructured clinical assessments Expensive

8B. Advantages and Disadvantages of Global Measures (*cont.*)

Testing Dimension	Psychometric Properties	Advantages	Disadvantages
Delirium Symptom Interview (DSI)	(Sample: 50 elders in acute care) Sensitivity 0.90 Specificity 0.80 Positive predictive value 0.87 Negative predictive value 0.84 Interrater reliability–Cohen's kappa 0.90 Interrater agreement on symptom domains 0.46 (fluctuating behavior) to 1.0 (disorientation, sleep disturbance) Internal consistency reliability: Cronbach's alpha, disturbance of consciousness 0.80; disorientation 0.75; incoherent speech 0.61; psychomotor behavior 0.56; sleep disturbance 0.45	Can be used with any population (i.e., sensory, communication deficits, very ill) Lay individuals can reliably use the DSI Less subjective rating of symptoms All domains evaluated DSI can be administered daily without burden or a learning effect	Constructed in outdated diagnostic criteria (DSM-III vs. DSM-IV) Indices of internal consistency are marginally acceptable DSI has not been used by other teams
Dementia			
Mattis Dementia Rating Scale (MDRS)	High test–retest reliability (1 week interval correlation was >0.90) Internal consistency reliability 0.90 Concurrent validation with other similar measures >0.67 (70)	Correlation of scores with cerebral blood flow >0.80 while scores <100 associated with death (105)	Can take 30–45 minutes
Kendrick Cognitive Tests for Elderly	Validation with variety of elders Testing (no coefficients) for external validity, construct validity, discriminant validity, predictive validity, test–retest, standardization (38) KOLT: test–retest form-A, 0.92; Form-B, 0.91 Interest correlation: 0.91 (71) Percent agreement between psychiatric diagnosis and test performance = 0.83 and 0.86 on retest 6 weeks later to 0.96	Discriminates between demented and nondemented patients (72) Ecologically valid so may more accurately reflect true levels of residual capacity and ability to function in daily living Repeat testing every 6 weeks to detect changes in cognitive performance	Considerable overlap in scores between depressed and normal patients No norms for individuals younger than 55 years First testing of patients: hospitalized >3 weeks is confounded (71); anxiolytic, antidepressant, or antipsychotic medications reduce test performance Not recommended if IQ <70

Consortium to Establish a Registry for Alzheimer's Disease (CERAD)	(Sample: 354 patients with AD, 278 nondemented subjects) Interrater agreement: 0.092 (constructional praxis) to 1.0 (word list recall) Test–retest reliability: 0.44–0.90 (1-month interval) Discriminant validity = distinguishes AD from nondemented individual Construct validity: factor analysis: 3 factors accounting for 73% variance	More recent testing of sensitivity (76) (Sample 549 with AD and 390 controls): 0.86–0.96 Classification ability 0.91	Classification ability decreases to 0.84 when attempting to discriminate mildly from moderately impaired individuals
Depression			
Beck's Depression Inventory (BDI)	Split half reliability: 0.86–0.93 Test–retest reliability 0.74 (3-month interval); with elderly, depressed subjects, 0.090 Internal consistency 0.91 Excellent congruence with Research Diagnostic Criteria Specificity 0.82 (cutpoint 10), vs. 0.96 (cutpoint 17) Sensitivity 0.89 (cutpoint 10), 0.57 (cutpoint 17) DSM-II criteria for depression (cutpoint 10): sensitivity 0.89, specificity 0.82; (cutpoint 17): sensitivity 0.50, specificity 0.92 Predictive validity 0.85, 0.88–0.91 Correct classification of patients, interrater reliability 0.73	Can identify major > minor depressive disorders (81)	Self-rating nature of scale so susceptible to manipulation or socially desirable answers
Hamilton Depression Rating Scale (HDRS)	Sensitive to change in elderly depressives Psychometric problems, but most laboratories report high reliability (118) Interrater reliability: 0.80–0.90 (78)	Provides common denominator for communicating information about level of depression across samples	Weighting shifts from frequency to intensity factor depending upon dimension tested Heavily weighted toward somatic symptomatology so in elderly may result in false positives

8B. Advantages and Disadvantages of Global Measures (*cont.*)

Testing Dimension	Psychometric Properties	Advantages	Disadvantages
	Construct validity-factor analysis up to 3 factors: (1) general factor of depression, (2) anxious depression factor, (3) index of instability	Reasonable reliability with young subjects	High number of false-positives in older adults
Zung's Self-Rating Depression Scale Geriatric Depression Short-Scale Form GDS-SF	Various studies but coefficients not reported (38) (Cutpoint 10): sensitivity: 0.84–0.89; specificity: 0.73–0.095 (compared to RDC and DSM-II criteria) Discriminant validity with clinical diagnosis: 0.84 Concurrent validity with HDRS and SDS	Simple yes/no response format for symptom evaluation so may be more appropriate with cognitively impaired elders or low educational level Sensitivity and specificity acceptable when MMSE scores > 15	
Cornell Depression Scale	High correlation with RDC definition of depression High sensitivity, correlates significantly with RDC diagnoses Concurrent validation with independent psychiatric diagnoses if depression R(s) = 0.81 Interrater reliability: 0.82–0.93, Cohen's kappa = 0.74 Internal consistency = 0.98	Equally sensitive in cognitively intact and impaired individuals Easy to administer and score Cornell scale most reliable compared to Hamilton and Sutherland (89)	

Numbers in parentheses correspond to studies cited in the References.

8C. Comparison of the Clinical Features of Delirium, Dementia, and Depression

Feature	Delirium	Dementia	Depression
Onset	Acute/subacute; depends on cause	Chronic, generally insidious; depends on cause	Coincides with life changes; often abrupt
Course	Short, diurnal fluctuations in symptoms; worse at night, in the dark, and upon awakening	Long, no diurnal effects; symptoms progressive yet relatively stable over time	Diurnal effects; typically worse in morning; situational fluctuations, but less than with delirium
Progression	Abrupt	Slow but even	Variable, rapid-slow but uneven
Duration	Hours to less than 1 month, seldom longer	Months to years	At least 2 weeks, but can be several months to years
Awareness	Reduced	Clear	Clear
Alertness	Fluctuates, lethargic, or hypervigilant	Generally normal	Normal
Attention	Impaired, fluctuates	Generally normal	Minimal impairment, distractibility
Orientation	Fluctuates in severity, generally impaired	May be impaired	Selective disorientation
Memory	Recent and immediate impaired	Recent and remote impaired	Selective or patchy impairment; "islands" of intact memory
Thinking	Disorganized, distorted, fragmented, slow, or accelerated incoherent speech	Difficulty with abstraction; thoughts impoverished; judgment impaired; words difficult to find	Intact but with themes of hopelessness, helplessness, or self-deprecation
Perception	Distorted, illusions, delusions, and hallucinations; difficulty distinguishing between reality and misperceptions	Misperceptions often absent	Intact; delusions and hallucinations absent, except in severe cases
Psychomotor behavior	Variable, hypokinetic, hyperkinetic, or mixed cycle reversed	Normal, may have apraxia	Variable; psychomotor disturbed; often early morning awakening
Associated features	Variable affective changes; symptoms of autonomic hyperarousal; exaggeration of personality type; associated with physical illness	Affect tends to be superficial, inappropriate, and labile; attempts to conceal deficits in intellect, personality changes, aphasia, agnosia may be present; lacks insight	Affect depressed; dysphoric mood; exaggerated and detailed complaints; preoccupied with personal thoughts; insight present; verbal elaboration
Mental status testing	Distracted from task	Failings highlighted by family; frequent "near-miss" answers; struggles with test; great effort to find an appropriate reply	Failings highlighted by the examinee; frequent "don't know" answers; little effort; frequently gives up, indifferent; does not care or attempt to find an answer

Adapted from Foreman, M.D. Acute confusion in the hospitalized elderly: A research dilemma. *Nurs Res*, 1986, *35*(1):34.

9

Single Instruments for Measuring Quality of Life

Geraldine V. Padilla and Marilyn Frank-Stromborg

The proliferation of Health Related Quality of Life (HQOL) instruments since the mid-1970s makes it necessary to narrow this chapter's focus to general measures of HQOL, many of which have been adapted for use with specific diseases, such as cancer, heart, or arthritis. Also included are instruments specifically designed for persons with cancer or HIV. Some cancer-related quality-of-life (QOL) measures have several versions for different types of cancers or treatments.

Definitions of Quality of Life

Two definitions of quality of life reflect current notions of the meaning of this construct. An international group of investigators led by Drs. Orley, Kuyken, and Sartorius and working under the auspices of the Division of Mental Health of the World Health Organization defined quality of life as "an individual's perception of their position in life in the context of the culture and value systems in which they live and in relation to their goals, expectations, standards and concerns." These investigators define six broad domains of quality of life: physical health, psychologic state, levels of independence, social relationships, environmental features, and spiritual concerns, including personal beliefs. This definition reflects the view that quality of life refers to a subjective evaluation, which is embedded in a cultural, social, and environmental context. As such, quality of life cannot be equated simply with the terms *health status*, *lifestyle*, *life satisfaction*, *mental state*, or *well-being*. Rather, it is a multidimensional concept incorporating the "individual's perception of these and other aspects of life."[1,p1]

At a U.S.P.H.S. National Institutes of Health Workshop on Quality of Life Assessment led by Drs. Furberg and Schuttinga, a group of scientists agreed that a concise, clearly stated, operational definition of HQOL was preferable to a global definition.[1] Workshop participants adopted this working definition, "Health-related quality of life is the value assigned to duration of life as modified by the impairments, functional states, perceptions and social opportunities influenced by disease, injury, treatment or policy."[2]

The World Health Organization definition emphasizes the subjective nature of QOL evaluations, the importance of the cultural and value context in which judgments are made, and the relevance of goals, expectations, and standards.[1] The NIH QOL Workshop definition reflects the scientific need for specificity and objectivity.[2] Quality is based on a value that may be assigned to the duration of life by the patient, family, health care provider, policymaker, or other person. QOL is limited to those aspects of life that are important to the evaluator in the context of health and illness. This chapter does not adhere to a specific conceptual or operational definition of QOL except to focus on HQOL measures.

Definitional differences summarized by Bard in 1984 are true today. He stated that the term *quality of life* is too broad and inclusive to be meaningful. It is operationally defined in very different ways by different investigators leading to measures of different things.[3] Representative HQOL conceptual frameworks are offered in Appendix 9A. Strickland points out that some QOL conceptualizations have included not only dimensions of the concept but also covariates.[4] For example, Strickland questions the inclusion of coping ability or self-esteem in QOL definitions because these variables may be covariates, not dimensions.

The division between subjective and objective QOL measures may be artificial, because objective and subjective dimensions found in the literature do not seem congruent. For instance, Evans et al.'s study of QOL in patients with end-stage renal disease found that "patients on dialysis were clearly not functioning like people who were well, despite the fact that they were enjoying life."[5,p557] Because the definitions of HQOL and approaches to measurement vary considerably from study to study, meaningful comparisons between studies are difficult to make.

Examples illustrating this criticism are found in the work of Palmer et al.[6] and Cookfair and Cummings.[7] Palmer's QOL measurement consists of asking women with primary breast cancer receiving adjuvant chemotherapy, "How much did the full course of treatment interfere with your life?"[6] Cookfair's QOL assessment was based on the measurement of three variables (employment, functional status, and nursing needs) in 1,902 cancer patients with varying diagnoses and demographic characteristics.[7] Obviously, there can be no QOL comparison between these two studies.

Wellisch emphasizes that the optimal measurement approach to QOL is the prospective design in which the same group of patients is interviewed sequentially.[8] Evans et al. believe that subjective QOL (i.e., the individual's attitudes) is a state rather than a trait and is thus subject to variation over time.[5] If measurement takes place at only one point in the patient's experience, the true QOL picture may not emerge. Wellisch's recommended methodologic strategies for quality of life research are shown in Appendices 9B and 9C.[8]

Guyatt et al. have recognized the value of both cross-sectional and longitudinal studies.[9] The former allows comparisons between persons at one point in time and the latter evaluations of QOL changes in a person. The authors state that HQOL measures should be interpretable in a clinical sense. Differences in scores should represent the range of clinical changes from trivial or small to moderate or large.

Health as a Dimension of Quality of Life

Regardless of the approach, research has indicated clearly the importance of health in determining life satisfaction and overall HQOL.[3,5-8,10,11] Health indices have been developed to define QOL as it applies to the state of wellness of the individual. Earlier health indices tended to concentrate on the physical functions of patients and to rely on a cross-sectional (one-time) analysis of the health status of persons. The literature indicates that this narrow functional definition of health status is changing. For instance, Ware advocates the use of a multidimensional conceptual model to measure health status, mental status, social status, general status (i.e., self-ratings of health, physical symptoms, psychosomatic symptoms), and diagnostic indicators (i.e., blood pressure).[12] Patrick and Bergner discuss health status measurement issues that are relevant for the 1990s.[13]

The Centers for Disease Control and Prevention's Behavioral Risk Factor Surveillance System (BRFSS), added four questions about HQOL to its 1993 survey.[14] These questions asked about subjective perceptions of general health, physical health, mental health, and impact of poor physical or mental health on usual activities (self-care, work, recreation). The BRFSS is a continuous, state-based random-digit–dialed telephone survey conducted by states. Survey information for 1993 was available on 44,978 persons over 18. The survey found that good health days were more likely to be enjoyed by college graduates, Asian/Pacific Islanders, and those with incomes over $50,000. Poorest good health day scores were found among persons over age 75, who smoked 20 or more cigarettes a day, were told they had high blood pressure or diabetes, were unemployed, were separated from their spouse, had less than a high school education, and had annual incomes under $10,000.

What emerges from a review of the literature about health indices for determining QOL is the general consensus that attributes of mind, body, and spirit all need to be included in any comprehensive approach. This approach is recommended because numerous domains of social and physiologic function may be substantially affected by changes in health status. For instance, Berg et al. constructed a values scale that included cognitive, emotional, social, and physical functions. Berg's results indicate that any attempt to define health operationally, as it relates to quality of life, must include more than just physical functions.[10]

Other Dimensions of Quality of Life

Although health is a major QOL component, other dimensions are equally important. An early attempt to define the dimensions that constitute QOL was made by Flanagan, who studied 3,000 Americans of varying ages and health statuses in terms of their perceptions of what constitutes QOL.[11] Using the critical incident technique, he identified those factors a healthy population would consider important for quality of life.[11] A sample question is "Think of the last time you did something very important to you or had an experience that was especially satisfying to you. What did you do or what happened that was so satisfying to you?[11,p57]

Flanagan asked two critical incident questions and obtained 6,500 critical incidents. Categorization by independent judges resulted in 15 factors that included all of the 6,500 critical incidents. A sample of 3,000 people (ages 30 to 70 years) was then asked one question about each of these 15 factors: "At this time in your life, how important is _____?" Flanagan found that six dimensions were extremely important to overall QOL: health, having and raising children, material comforts, work, close relationship with a spouse, and understanding oneself. The conceptual frameworks in Appendix 9A show that investigators have espoused a multidimensional model of HQOL consisting of physical and functional well-being that include symptom distress and nutritional status; environmental and economic well-being; social functioning and well-being; psychological, emotional, and spiritual well-being; and subjective health perceptions. A review of the HQOL measurement literature in cancer provided five additional lessons: Observers are poor judges of how patients feel about their QOL; high compliance with self-reports of HQOL is possible; HQOL can be improved with aggressive therapy; symptoms are associated with disruptions in HQOL; and pre-treatment HQOL scores can predict QOL outcomes during treatment as well as survival.[15]

Selecting a Quality-of-Life Instrument

The assessment of an HQOL is an evolving area of clinical research. The researcher desiring to measure this construct must consider multiple issues and choose from various instruments. Numerous measurement review articles by Cella and Tulsky,[16] Anderson and colleagues,[17] Naughton and Wiklund,[18] books by Spilker,[19] McDowell and Newell,[20] Wenger et al.,[21] Walker,[22] and Bowling[23] are available to assist the researcher in making this selection. Of particular help in identifying instruments is the bibliography authored by Spilker et al.,[24] which indexes QOL measures by author, instrument, and therapeutic categories.

Multiple versus Single Instruments

The following must be considered when selecting QOL instruments:

1. Can a concept be measured by a single instrument, or does it require multiple instruments? Multiple tests: consider the feasibility, design, costs, variety of staff needed, and patient's ability to tolerate lengthy administration.
2. Qualitative versus quantitative data: subscale scores
    a. Qualitative instruments: subscale scores capture multiple dimensions of the construct.
    b. Quantitative instruments: descriptive and may focus on facets of life affected by illness that have changed overall QOL.
3. Objective versus subjective instruments
    a. Objective: observable data.
    b. Subjective: patient evaluates own quality of life, not the health professional's perception of patient's QOL.[25,26]
4. Objective versus subjective QOL dimensions
    a. Focus on measuring objective dimensions: housing, work, education, environment, socioeconomic status.
    b. Focus on measuring subjective dimensions: psychosocial, spiritual well-being.
    c. Combination of objective and subjective dimensions.[5,27]
5. Conceptual or linguistic translation
    a. Conceptual congruity or merely linguistically accurate when translated?
    b. Diversity within minority groups so that direct translation may not be conceptually accurate.
    c. Ideal is interactive translation to achieve both conceptual and linguistic equivalence.[28]

In summary, the choice of instrument will depend on research and pragmatic considerations (e.g., resources available to do content analysis of qualitative data, computer availability, stamina of the sample that may influence the length of the instrument desired). Sugarbaker et al.'s study is a comprehensive approach to the measurement of QOL.[29] This cooperative, multidisciplinary effort uses multiple QOL assessment methodologies such as objective and subjective dimensions, an interview, and self-reports. This all-inclusive approach may not always be possible or practical (see Appendix 9C). Thus, single HQOL instruments represent a realistic option for the researcher.

Objective Scales Yielding Quantitative Data

Karnofsky Performance Index

Early attempts to measure QOL in patients focused on one dimension of the patient's life, the ability to perform activities of daily living (ADL). Karnofsky and colleagues developed a scale that rates physical activity from 0 (dead) to 100 (a person able to carry on normal activities) in increments of 10.[30] Although the Karnofsky scale is designed as an objective QOL measure, one researcher used it as a subjective tool by having patients evaluate their own physical status.[31] Examples of Karnofsky ratings are:

100   Normal, no complaints, no evidence of disease.
 60   Requires occasional assistance, but is able to care for most needs.
 20   Very sick, hospitalization necessary, active supportive treatment necessary.
  0   Dead.

Grieco and Long reevaluated the Karnofsky scale and reported that:

> Tests of inter-rater reliability, concurrent validity, and discriminant validity indicate that, with standardized observational procedures based on a mental status exam, the Karnofsky scale is acceptably reliable and valid as a global measure, but it does not adequately capture the conceptual domain of quality of life.[25,p129]

Zubrod Scale

The Zubrod Scale, a 0-to-4 scale in increments of 1, evaluates the patient's ability to remain ambulatory and to perform ADL.[32] Both the Karnofsky and Zubrod scales have been used extensively by cooperative cancer research groups because they show a correlation with tumor response to treatment and survival.

QL-Index

An objective scale that has been used primarily by physicians, but has a broader orientation than the Zubrod or Karnofsky scales, was developed by Spitzer et al.[33] The QL-Index is a brief measure (1 minute) of health, family support, activity, daily living, and outlook completed by a health professional. The range of scores is 0 to 10. An example from one category on the QL-Index is: "During the last week the patient: has been appearing to feel well or reporting feeling 'great' most of the time (+2); has been lacking energy or not feeling entirely up to par more than just occasionally (+1); has been feeling very ill or 'lousy,' seeming weak and washed out most of the time or was unconscious (0)."

Spitzer reports that the instrument has discriminant construct validity, content validity, high internal consistency (Cronbach's coefficient alpha 0.775), and statistically significant interrater Spearman rank correlation ($r = 0.81$, $p < 0.001$). The QL-Index was piloted by more than 150 physicians who rated 879 patients. It was standardized on cancer patients with several levels of seriousness of diagnosis as well as on people with several other chronic diseases as controls. Cella and Tulsky report that the QL-Index is the most widely used observer-rated QOL scale.[16] However, the ability of the instrument to stand alone is questionable because correlations between observer and patient ratings are modest. Grieco and Long state that the QL-Index has the advantage of brevity, but, like the Karnofsky scale, lacks standardized observational procedures.[25] In other words, there are no standardized instructions for how observers should score these two instruments. Additional instruments are described in Appendix 9D.[34-38]

Subjective Scales Yielding Quantitative Data

Quality of Life Scale for Cancer (QOL-CA), Bone Marrow Transplant (BMT), and Pain

The multidimensional Quality of Life Scale for Cancer (QOL-CA) was originally known as the Quality of Life Index (QLI) when it was published in 1983.[39] However, since Ferrans and Powers published their QLI in 1985[40] and Spitzer et al. published the QL-Index in 1981,[33] Padilla and colleagues changed the name of the instrument to avoid confusion. The name was first changed to the MQOLS-CA and then to the QOL-CA. The QLI/MQOLS-CA/QOL-CA has been revised a number of times and is available in several versions with instructions.

Based on an earlier instrument by Presant et al.,[41] Padilla developed a 14-item linear analog scale.[39,42,43] The scale includes three general areas: (1) psychologic well-being (general quality of life, fun, satisfaction, usefulness, sleep); (2) physical well-being (strength, appetite, work, eating, sex); and (3) symptom control (pain, nausea, vomiting). Each item is anchored by a word or phrase that describes an extreme response to the item stem. For example, to the question, "How good is your quality of life?" The person would mark an "x" somewhere along the 100-mm line to best reflect his or her quality of life. One end of the line is anchored by the phrase "extremely poor quality of life," and the other end is anchored with "excellent quality of life." All items are scored from 0 (poorest quality of life) to 100 (excellent quality of life). Some items have the 0 on the left end of the line and some on the right end of the line. Total and subscale scores are obtained by adding the scores for each item in a scale and dividing by the number of items. Thus, the range of scores possible for any scale is 0 (poorest quality of life) to 100 (best quality of life). Scoring of the subscales is recommended.

The original QLI was tested with five subject groups: (1) oncology outpatients receiving chemotherapy ($n = 43$) or (2) radiation therapy ($n = 39$); (3) oncology inpatients receiving chemotherapy ($n = 48$); (4) nonpatient volunteers ($n = 48$); and (5) diabetic females ($n = 77$).[42] Test–retest reliability coefficients were satisfactory ($r = 0.60$, $p < 0.01$), and internal consistency was good at 0.88 ($p < 0.01$). Validity was supported by factor analysis, by significant differences between mean scores of groups expected to be higher and lower in quality of life, and by significant correlations between MD ratings of the patient's QOL and the patients' own score on the psychologic well-being subscale.

Ryan used the QLI/QOL scale in her study of 422 veterans with lung or colon cancer from 11 Veterans Administration medical centers.[44] She reported internal consistency as significant ($r = 0.93$, $p < 0.01$). In test-retest, the percentage of retest responses within 1 cm on the original linear analog scale response was 72% in a group of veterans before treatment.[44]

The 14-item QLI version has been revised several times. Additional QOL versions were developed for persons with colostomies;[42,43] patients receiving radiation for cancer of the pelvic[42,45] and head and neck areas;[42,45] cancer patients with pain;[46,47] persons with gynecologic cancer;[42,48] survivors of bone marrow transplants;[49] and family caregivers of persons with cancer pain.[50-52]

For each of these versions, satisfactory reliability and validity were reported. For example, the QLI-Pain version was used on a sample of 150 cancer patients with pain.[47] The study yielded significant content validity (> 0.90). Internal consistency was supported by alpha coefficients superior or equal to 0.65 for all scales. Construct validity also was demonstrated by the fact that patients with pain had significantly poorer QOL scores than patients without pain or without cancer (analysis of variance, $p < 0.05$). Concurrent criterion validity was expressed in the significant correlations between the QLI-Pain scale and the Karnofsky Performance Scale ($r = 0.59$) and the pain assessment tool ($r = 0.54$).

The QOL-BMT was used with a sample of 205 bone marrow transplant (BMT) survivors who returned the mailed questionnaire.[49] This version of the QOL scale used a 10-point linear analog scale instead of the 100-mm scale. Initial psychometric testing yielded a test–retest reliability coefficient of 0.71 and an overall alpha coefficient of internal consistency of 0.85. Satisfactory content validity was established, as well as construct validity. The results of the factor analysis confirmed three of the QOL dimensions (psychologic well-being, physical well-being, and social concerns) described in the multidimensional model proposed by the authors.

A 30-item version of the QOL-CA was used in a study of a heterogeneous group of 227 cancer patients discharged to home care. Psychometric data for this recent generic version is presented here. Items 1, 2, 5–7, 9, 12–14, 16, 17, 18, 20–23, 28, and 29 are scored from left (0) to right (100). Items 3, 4, 8, 10, 11, 15, 19, 24–27, and 30 are scored from right (0) to left (100). An alternative scheme is to score all items from left (0) to right (100) and then subtract the score from 100 for items 3, 4, 8, 10, 11, 15, 19, 24–27, and 30. In comparing the factor analysis results of these data with previous studies, the following subscales emerge.[42] Psychosocial existential well-being (items 1, 2, 6–11, 16, 17, and 20); physical functional well-being (items 5, 12–15, 18, 28, and 29), symptom distress—nutrition (items 21, 23, and 25–27), symptom distress—pain, bowel patterns (items 4, 19, and 22), and attitude of worry (items 3, 24, 30). The two symptom distress subscales can be further combined into one. The resulting subscales support the predicted multidimensional structure of the instrument. The worry scale lacks conceptual clarity. Correlations with scales on the OARS Multidimensional Functional Assessment Questionnaire from the Duke Center for the Study of Aging and Human Development[102] yielded significant coefficients ($p \leq 0.05$) between the QOL-CA scores and OARS scores. These were: QOL-CA psychosocial score and OARS perceived mental/emotional health (0.47), and OARS social resources for care (0.32); QOL-CA physical function and OARS perceived physical health (0.49), and OARS activities of daily living (0.33); QOL-CA symptom distress and OARS functional impairments (–0.26), and OARS perceived physical health (–0.34). Internal consistency alpha coefficients for the total scale and subscales ranged from 0.68 to 0.91, with the exception of the three-item worry scale (0.52).

Ferrans and Powers's Quality of Life Index (QLI)

Ferrans and Powers's Quality of Life Index (QLI) was developed to measure the QOL of healthy people, as well as those who are experiencing an illness.[40] The original generic version of the QLI consisted of 32 items to which subjects provided self-ratings on two six-point scales from "very dissatisfied" to "very satisfied" and from "very unimportant" to "very important." Reliability was supported with data from 69 graduate students (test–retest reliability = 0.87, internal consistency alpha coefficient = 0.93). Criterion-related validity was established by comparing the QLI with a question on overall satisfaction with life. Subjects were asked to rate their overall satisfaction with life on a six-point rating scale, which ranged from "very dissatisfied" to "very satisfied." The correlation between scores from the QLI and the life satisfaction question for graduate students was 0.75.[40]

The current generic version of the QLI, like the original, includes two sections: Section 1 measures satisfaction with various life domains; section 2 measures the importance of each domain to the respondent.[40] This approach to QOL measurement is unusual among the HQOL instruments. The revised generic version includes 34 items that assess the satisfaction with and importance of four QOL domains: health and functioning, socioeconomic, psychologic/spiritual, and family domains. Responses are the same as in the original. Scores are adjusted to reflect how satisfied one is with each domain, as well as how much one values each domain. The scoring procedure requires that satisfaction scores be first recoded to center the scale to zero by subtracting 3.5 from the satisfaction response for each item. Second, satisfaction scores are adjusted by multiplying the recoded satisfaction score by the importance score. Third, the overall adjusted score is obtained by summing all adjusted scores and dividing by the number of items answered (to account for any missing items). To eliminate negative scores, 15 is added to every score. Scores can range from 0 to 30 with a score of 30 indicating the best quality of life. Dr. Ferrans developed a computer program (available upon request) that performs the calculations.

Different versions of the QLI address QOL issues for patients with different diagnoses or undergoing different procedures. Satisfactory reliability and validity data are published for the hemodialysis version,[53] the cancer version,[54] the cardiac version,[55] and the liver transplant version.[56] Other forms of the QLI for diagnostic groups such as arthritis, diabetes, and chronic fatigue syndrome also are available. The QLI has been translated into Mexican-Spanish, Arabic, Mandarin Chinese, Korean, Japanese, Swedish, and Romanian. Reliability and validity data on the Mexican-Spanish and Mandarin Chinese[57] versions, as well as an extensive bibliography of the QLI, are available from Dr. Carol Ferrans. The most requested versions of the QLI are the generic, cancer, and cardiac versions (Ferrans, personal communication, January 7, 1994). An instruction manual is available.

Quality of Life Questionnaire (QLQ)

In their pilot study of QOL in people with melanoma, Young and Longman developed a short Quality of Life Questionnaire (QLQ) and correlated this scale with several other instruments (i.e., social dependency scale, symptom distress scale, behavior-morale scale).[58] Their instrument uses a Likert-type scale, and subjects are instructed to rate their current quality of life from 1 (poor) to 6 (excellent). In another question, subjects are asked to rate, on a scale from 1 (not at all satisfied) to 10 (very satisfied), their feelings of satisfaction with their current quality of life. These two questions were found to be strongly associated (0.81) and statistically significant ($p < 0.0001$).[59] The QLQ correlated positively with behavior-morale and negatively with symptom distress and social dependency. As quality of life was ranked higher, symptom distress and social dependency were ranked lower.

Sickness Impact Profile (SIP)

The Sickness Impact Profile (SIP) has been used by researchers to measure QOL. An instruction manual is available. The SIP was initially developed by Bergner et al. in 1972 and, after pilot-testing on a sample of 278 subjects and revisions, resulted in a measure that contains 136 items grouped into 12 categories of life activities.[60] The categories are physical dimension (body movement, mobility, ambulation); psychosocial dimension (intellectual function, social interaction, emotional behavior, communication); sleep and rest; taking nutrition; usual daily work; household management; leisure; and recreation. Typical statements on the SIP are: (1) "I laugh or cry suddenly" or (2) "I just pick or nibble at my food." The instrument takes between 20 and 30 minutes to administer, and "scores that range from zero to one hundred percent disruption can be calculated for each scale category, for each dimension of the scale, or categories can be disregarded and one total disruption score calculated."[61,p37] Investigators report that the SIP scores discriminate among subsamples, and correlations between criterion measures and SIP scores provide evidence for the validity of the instrument. The SIP has been used with patients with coronary artery disease, pulmonary disease, and hyperthyroidism as an outcome measure in evaluating treatments.[62-64] Johnson et al. used the SIP with radiation oncology patients and believe that this instrument is an acceptable QOL measure.[61] The criticism has been made that, because the SIP assesses a fairly broad functional state, it may not discriminate among more subtle changes produced by the disease state or treatment.[65] The lack of ability to detect change becomes important in studies attempting to show "before" and "after" QOL changes. Additional instruments are found in Appendix 9E.[66-85]

Cancer Rehabilitation Evaluation System (CARES) and Short Form (CARES-SF)

The Cancer Rehabilitation Evaluation System (CARES) is a cancer-specific, self-administered rehabilitation and treatment planning questionnaire that assesses HQOL.[82] The CARES was originally called the CIPS.[82]

The CARES long form consists of 139 potential problems experienced by persons with cancer. The first 88 items pertain to all patients. The next 51 are different for each person depending on the course of treatment. The minimum number of items completed is 93, and the maximum is 132. Each item is answered on a five-point scale from not at all (0 no problem) to very much (4 severe problem). If used for clinical purposes, a form is available wherein patients indicate whether they want help with the problem (Yes) or not (No). The CARES consists of a global HQOL scale, five summary scales (physical, psychosocial, marital, medical interaction, and sexual), and 31 subscales measuring everyday functioning (ambulation, weight loss, pain, difficulty working, body image, sexual and psychosocial distress, etc.). The scoring procedure is: (1) Add individual item scores for all items rated 1 to 4 for a severity score; (2) add the number of potential problems that can apply to a particular person; (3) add the number of endorsed problems, problems scored from 1 to 4. These three scores are then used to obtain the average severity rating (severity score divided by number of endorsed problems), and the global score (severity score divided by number of potential problems). Raw scores can be converted to T scores to provide a profile of the individual patient that can be compared to normative data. Norms exist for six groups of cancer patients: (1) prostate; (2) breast; (3) female non-breast; (4) male non-prostate; (5) male (prostate and other); and (6) female (breast and other). These are published in the manual.[83]

The CARES-SF (short form) contains 59 items, and patients complete a minimum of 38 and a maximum of 57.[84] The ratings are the same as for the long form. If used for research purposes only the 0-to-4 scales are used to rate each problem. If used for clinical purposes, then a clinical form also allows the patient to indicate which problems require help. Scoring is similar to the CARES long form. Norms exist for the CARES-SF and also are provided in the manual.[83]

Psychometric information for the CARES long form supports the reliability and validity of the instrument.[82] Test–retest reliability correlations are all above 0.82 for a sample of 120. Test–retest percent agreement for whether a problem existed ranged from 84% to 88%. Test–retest agreement of the exact same rating showed that 77% of ratings were exactly the same, and of the disagreements, 70% were off by only one rating value.

This means that 93% of the time the retest rating was exactly the same or one rating different from the first test. Alpha coefficients for three samples of 479, 1,047, and 114 cancer patients ranged from 0.82 to 0.94.[84]

Validity information is provided by Schag et al.[82] Construct validity of the five major scales was supported by factor analysis. Convergent and discriminant validity was supported by the patterns of correlations with other measures. Correlations with the Karnofsky Performance Scale measure of physical function and the CIPS/CARES were at 0.46 for the global score, at 0.64 for the physical factor, and under 0.42 for all other higher-order factors. Correlations between the SCL-90 measure of symptoms were at 0.76 for the global score, 0.61 for the physical and 0.74 for the psychosocial factors, and under 0.49 for all the other higher-order factors. Correlations with a visual analog scale of current functioning were at 0.54 for the global score, 0.55 for the physical factor, 0.50 for the psychosocial factor, and under 0.27 for all other factors. Correlations between the CIPS/CARES global and higher-order scores and the visual analog scale for the time prior to cancer were low. These findings were expected and support the validity of the instrument. The authors comment that validation of the CIPS/CARES is difficult because it does not measure one clearly definable construct.

Psychometric information for the CARES-SF (short form) is provided by Schag et al.[84] The integrity of the short form is supported by correlations with the long form that range from 0.98 to 0.90 for the global and higher-order scores with samples of 1,047 heterogeneous cancer patients, and 114 homogeneous, newly diagnosed breast cancer patients in a rehabilitation evaluation trial. Alpha coefficients for the five higher-order factor scales ranged from 0.60 to 0.85 for a sample of 479 heterogenous cancer patients and the two samples above. Percent agreement of ratings between test and retest for presence or absence of a problem ranged from 81% to 86%.

Convergent and discriminant validity for the CARES-SF was supported by the pattern of correlations between the CARES-SF global and higher-order scores and other instruments.[84] The pattern of correlations was similar to the pattern described for the CARES. Factor analysis further supported the construct validity of the higher-order factors. The CARES-SF was also found to be sensitive to change. The global CARES-SF improved over time, as expected. Additional instruments are shown in Appendix 9E.

Subjective Scales Yielding Qualitative Data

Cain and Henke Survey

One of the first qualitative nursing studies to investigate QOL in cancer patients was conducted by Cain and Henke in 1978.[86] They developed a survey that assessed primarily the nonmedical needs of 50 ambulatory cancer patients. The survey, which took approximately 20 minutes to complete, asked about pain, nausea and vomiting, work, leisure activity, dependency needs, future concerns, religious beliefs, and overall QOL. This survey served to identify specific areas that had changed the QOL of the patients with cancer.

The rest of the qualitative instruments discussed in this chapter are all similar in that they result in a description of the changes that have occurred in the person's life (rather than a single score) and thus indirectly assess overall QOL. Most of the qualitative instruments are a result of a desire by clinicians to have a tool that systematically assesses the impact of cancer on the lives of patients and targets the specific areas that have changed, thus enabling them to develop appropriate, focused interventions.

Freidenbergs et al. Questionnaire

One such tool yielding descriptive data was developed by Freidenbergs et al. to measure the psychosocial problems of cancer patients and thus indirectly assess QOL.[87] Their tool is a structured problem-oriented interview that assesses 122 potential cancer-related problems grouped into 13 areas of life functioning: physical discomfort; medical treatment; hospital service; mobility; housework; vocational; financial; family; social; worry; affect; body image; and communication. Patients were asked to report the severity of each acknowledged problem on a 10-point scale (1 mild, 10 severe). The instrument takes one-half to one hour to administer. Two typical questions on this instrument are: (1) "Are there any changes in activities with friends? If so, how severe is the change?"; and (2) "Are there any changes in family role? If so, how severe is the change?"

Health Survey

Stromborg and Wright's Health Survey instrument includes both qualitative and quantitative measures.[88] It differs from other qualitative instruments in that it not only identifies the specific areas altered by the diagnosis of cancer but also obtains patients' perceptions of the severity of the change and their attitude toward the alteration in lifestyle.[88] Ratings on the severity of the change were obtained from seven options on a Likert-type scale ranging from "extremely negative" to "extremely positive." The Health Survey employs both open-ended and closed-ended questions and consists of the following sections: (1) demographic data (18 items); (2) physical impact data (18 items, such as taste, weight, activity); (3) psychosocial impact data (12 items, such as sex, finances, self-image); and (4) patient/health professional relationship data (5 items, such as who they communicate with, how often, and why). Content validity for the Health Survey was pilot-tested on 340 ambulatory cancer patients.

Summary

Early QOL measures (e.g., Karnofsky)[30] focused on one dimension, functional status. Instruments developed later are based on a multidimensional conceptualization of QOL and a broader definition of health within the QOL construct. Health includes physical and mental health and function; health perception; physical and psychosomatic symptoms and side effects of disease and treatment; and diagnostic indicators. As the definition of QOL is broadening, investigators are insisting on more precise definitions and recommend that QOL be considered in relation to health concerns. Thus, the HQOL conceptual frameworks espouse a multidimensional model consisting of physical and functional well-being, including symptom distress and nutritional status; environmental and economic well-being; social functioning and well-being; psychologic, emotional, and spiritual well-being; and subjective health perceptions. Whether these dimensions hold true over time, disease state, and across cultures awaits further research.

Exemplar Study

Stewart, A.L., & Ware, J.E. *Measuring functioning and well-being: The medical outcomes study approach.* Durham, NC: Duke University Press, 1992.

This study exemplifies current efforts to measure HQOL with a single, multidimensional, brief, self-rating scale. The Medical Outcomes Study (MOS) is a landmark, observational study of 20,000 English-speaking adult patients from Boston, Chicago, and Los Angeles, 523 physicians, as well as clinical psychologists and social workers. The chronic diseases of interest were hypertension, Type II diabetes, advanced coronary artery disease, and depression. Persons over 60 were overrepresented in the sample. In each city, patients and physicians were sampled from five practice settings that differed in structural characteristics. Cross-section and longitudinal data (over 4 years) were collected. The Rand 36-item Health Survey, Version 1.0 (i.e., the SF-36 Health Survey) is one of several versions of the larger Rand MOS Functioning and Well-Being Profile Questionnaires. The popular 36-item scale reflects physical, mental, and social functioning and well-being as well as health perceptions. The study supported the theoretical basis, reliability, and validity of the 36-item version.

References

1. World Health Organization. *WHOQOL Study Protocol: The development of the World Health Organization Quality of Life assessment instrument.* Publication MNH/PSF/93.9. Geneva, Switzerland: Division of Mental Health, World Health Organization, 1993.
2. Patrick, D.L., & Erickson, P. *Health status and health policy: Quality of life in health care evaluation and resource allocation.* New York: Oxford University Press, 1993.
3. Bard, M. Summary of the informal discussion of functional states: Quality of life. *Cancer* 1984; 53(10): 2327.
4. Strickland, O. Measures and instruments. *Patient outcomes research: Examining the effectiveness of nursing practice.* Proceedings of the state of the science conference sponsored by the National Center for Nursing Research, September 1991. NIH Publication No. 93-3411, 1992.
5. Evans, R., Manninen, D.L., Garrison, L.P., Jr., et al. The Quality of life with end-stage renal disease. *N Engl J Med*, 1985; 312(9):553-559.
6. Palmer, B., Walsh, G., McKinna, J., & Greening, W. Adjuvant chemotherapy for breast cancer: Side effects and quality of life. *Br Med J*, 1980, 281(6253): 1594-1597.
7. Cookfair, D., & Cummings, K. Quality of life among cancer patients. In: *Advances in cancer control: Research and development.* New York: Liss, 1983, p. 445.
8. Wellisch D. Work, social, recreation, family, and physical status. *Cancer* 1984, 53(10):2290-2302.
9. Guyatt, G.H., Feeny, D.H., & Patrick, D.L. Measuring health-related quality of life. *Ann Int Med*, 1993, 118(8):622-629.
10. Berg, R., Hallauer, D., & Berk, S. Neglected aspects of the quality of life. *Health Serv Res*, 1976, 11(4):391.
11. Flanagan, J. Measurement of quality of life: Current state of the art. *Arch Phys Med Rehabil*, 1982, 63(2):56-59.
12. Ware, J. Conceptualizing disease impact and treatment outcomes. *Cancer*, 1984, 53(10):2316-2326.
13. Patrick, D.L., Bergner, M. Measurement of health status in the 1990s. *Ann Rev Pub Health*, 1990, 11:165-183.
14. Centers for Disease Control and Prevention. Current Trends: Quality of life as a new public health measure-Behavioral risk factor surveillance system, 1993. *MMWR*, 1994, 43(20):375-380.
15. Osoba, D. Lessons learned from measuring health-related quality of life in oncology. *J Clin Oncol*, 1994, 12(3):608-616.
16. Cella, D.F., & Tulsky, D.S. Measuring quality of life today: Methodological aspects. *Oncology*, 1990, 4(5): 29-38.

17. Anderson, R.T., Aaronson, N.K., & Wilkin, D. Critical review of international assessments of health-related quality of life. *Qual Life Res*, 1993, 2(6):369-395.
18. Naughton, M.J., & Wiklund, I. A critical review of dimension-specific measures of health-related quality of life in cross-cultural research. *Qual Life Res*, 1993, 2(6):397-432.
19. Spliker, B. *Qualify of life and pharmacoeconomics in clinical trials* (2nd ed.). Philadelphia: Lippincot-Raven, 1996, pp. 301-308.
20. McDowell, I., & Newell, C. *Measuring health: A guide to rating scales and questionnaires.* New York: Oxford University Press, 1987.
21. Wenger, N.K., Mattson, M.E., Furberg, C.D., & Elinson, J. (Eds.). *Assessment of quality of life in clinical trials of cardiovascular therapies.* New York: LeJacq Publishing, 1984.
22. Walker, S.R. *Quality of life assessment: Key issues in the 1990's.* CMR Workshops Series. Boston: Kluwer, 1992.
23. Bowling, A. *Measuring health: A review of quality of life measurement scales.* Chicago: Taylor and Francis, 1991.
24. Spilker, B., Molinek, F.R., Johnson, K.A., et al. Quality of life bibliography and indexes. *Med Care*, 1990, 28(suppl 12):DS1-DS77.
25. Grieco, A., & Long, C.J. Investigation of the Karnofsky Performance Status as a measure of quality of life. *Health Psychol*, 1984, 3(2):129-142.
26. Danoff, B., Kramer, S., Irwin, P., & Gottlieb, A. Assessment of the quality of life in long-term survivors after definitive radiotherapy. *Am J Clin Oncol (CCT)*, 1983, 6(3):339-345.
27. U.S. Department of Commerce Bureau of the Census. *Social indicators.* Washington, DC: U.S. Government Printing Office, 1976.
28. Guyatt, G.H. The philosophy of health-related quality of life translation. *Qual Life Res*, 1993, 2(6):461-465.
29. Sugarbaker, P., Barofsky, I., Rosenberg, S., & Gianola, F. Quality of life assessment of patients in extremity sarcoma clinical trials. *Surgery*, 1982, 91(1): 17-23.
30. Karnofsky, D., & Burchenal, J. *The clinical evaluation of chemotherapeutic agents in cancer.* New York: Columbia University Press, 1949.
31. Waterhouse, J., & Metcalfe, M. A tool for measuring sexual adjustment in postoperative cancer patients. Proceedings of the Oncology Nursing Society, 9th Annual Congress, Toronto, Canada, 1984.
32. Zubrod, C.G., Schneiderman, M., Frei, E., et al. Appraisal of methods for the study of chemotherapy of cancer in man: Comparative therapeutic trial of nitrogen mustard and triethylene thiophosphoramide. *J Chron Dis*, 1960, 11(1):7-33.

33. Spitzer, W.O., Dobson, A.J., Hall, J., et al. Measuring the quality of life of cancer patients: A concise QL-Index for use by physicians. *J Chron Dis*, 1981, *34*(12): 585.

34. Nelson, E.C., Landgraf, J.M., Hays, R.D., et al. The functional status of patients: How can it be measured in physicians' offices? *Med Care*, 1990, *28*(12):1111-1126.

35. Nelson, E.C., Landgraf, J.M., Hays, R.D., et al. The Coop function charts: A system to measure patient function in physician's offices. In M. Lipkin, Jr. (Ed.), *Functional status measurement in primary care*. New York: Springer-Verlag, 1990, pp. 97-131.

36. van Weel, C., & Scholten, J.H.G. Report of an international workshop of the WONCA Research and Classification Committee. In J.H.G. Scholten (Ed.), *Functional status assessment in family practice*. Meditekst: Lelystad, 1992, pp. 5-51.

37. Kaplan, R.M., & Anderson, J.P. The general health policy model: An integrated approach. In B. Spilker (Ed.), *Quality of life and pharmacoeconomics in clinical trials* (2nd ed.). Philadelphia: Lippincott-Raven, 1996, pp. 309-322.

38. Holzmer, W.L., Bakken, H.S., Stewart, A., & Janson-Bjerklie, S. The HIV quality audit marker (HIV-QAM): An outcome measure for hospitalized AIDS patients. *Qual Life Res*, 1993, *2*(2):99-107.

39. Padilla, G.V., Presant, C., Grant, M.M., et al. Quality of life index for patients with cancer. *Res Nurs Health*, 1983, *6*(3):117-126.

40. Ferrans, C.E., & Powers, M.J. Quality of life index: Development and psychometric properties. *ANS*, 1985, *8*(1):15-24.

41. Presant, C.A., Klahr, C., & Hogan, L. Evaluating quality-of-life in oncology patients: Pilot observations. *Oncol Nurs Forum*, 1981, *8*(3):26-30.

42. Padilla, G.V., Grant, M.M. Lipsett, J. et al. Health quality of life and colorectal cancer. *Cancer*, 1992, *70* (5 suppl): 1450-1456.

43. Padilla, G.V., & Grant, M.M. Quality of life as a cancer nursing outcome variable. *Adv Nur Sci*, 1985, *8*(1):45-60.

44. Ryan, L. Quality of life and lung or colon cancer: A prospective study to determine the impact of an experimental treatment. Paper presented at the Tenth Annual Oncology Nursing Society Congress, 1985.

45. Padilla, G.V., Grant, M.M., Lipsett, J. et al. Health quality of life and colorectal cancer. *Cancer*, 1992, *70*(5 suppl):1450-1456.

46. Ferrell, B.R., Wisdom, C., Wenzl, C., & Brown, J. Controlled release vs. short acting analgesia: Effects on pain and quality of life. *Oncol Nurs Forum*, 1989, *26*(4):521-526.

47. Ferrell, B.R., Wisdom, C., & Wenzl, C. Quality of life as an outcome variable in the management of cancer pain. *Cancer*, 1989, *63*(11 suppl):2321-2327.

48. Padilla, G.V., Mishel, M.H., & Grant, M.M. Uncertainty, appraisal and quality of life. *Qual Life Res*, 1992, *1*(3):155-165.

49. Grant, M., Ferrell, B., Schmidt, G.M., et al. Measurement of quality of life in bone marrow transplant survivors. *Qual Life Res*, 1992, *1*(6):375-384.

50. Ferrell, B.R., Ferrell, B.A., Rhiner, M., & Grant, M. Family factors influencing cancer pain. *Post Grad Med J*, 1991, *67*(suppl 2):S64-S69.

51. Ferrell, B.R., Rhiner, M., Cohen, M., & Grant, M. Pain as a metaphor for illness. Part I: Impact of cancer pain on family caregivers. *Oncol Nurs Forum*, 1991, *18*(8):1303-1309.

52. Ferrell, B.R., Cohen, M., Rhiner, M., & Rozak, A. Pain as a metaphor for illness. Part II: Family caregivers' management of pain. *Oncol Nurs Forum*, 1991, *18*(8):1315-1321.

53. Ferrans, C., & Powers, M. Psychometric assessment of the quality of life index. *Res Nurs Health*, 1992, *15*(1):29-38.

54. Ferrans, C.E. Development of a quality of life index for patients with cancer. *Oncol Nurs Forum*, 1990, *17*(3) suppl:15-19.

55. Bliley, A.V., & Ferrans, C. Quality of life index after angioplasty. *Heart Lung*, 1993, *22*(3):193-199.

56. Hicks, F., Larson, J., & Ferrans, C. Quality of life after liver transplant. *Res Nurs Health*, 1992, *15*(2):111-119.

57. Hsueh-Erh, L. Factors related to the quality of life of Chinese caregivers. Thesis in partial fulfillment of the Doctor of Philosophy in Nursing Science, University of Illinois at Chicago, 1991.

58. Young, K.J., & Longman, A.J. Quality of life in persons with melanoma: A pilot study. *Cancer Nurs*, 1983, *6*(3):219-225.

59. Longman, A. Personal communication on quality of life questionnaire tool development (Phase 1), May 9, 1984.

60. Bergner, M., Bobbitt, R., Pollard, W., et al. The Sickness impact profile: Validation of a health status measure. *Med Care*, 1976, *14*(1):57-67.

61. Johnson, J.E., King, K.B., & Murray, R.A. Measuring the impact of sickness on usual functions of radiation therapy patients. *Oncol Nurs Forum*, 1983, *10*(4):36-39.

62. Ott, C.R., Sivarajan, E.S., Newton, K.M., et al. A controlled randomized study of early cardiac rehabilitation: The sickness impact profile as an assessment tool. *Heart Lung*, 1983, *12*(2):162-170.

63. Nocturnal Oxygen Therapy Trial Group. Continuous or nocturnal oxygen therapy in hypoxemic chronic obstructive lung disease. *Ann Intern Med*, 1980, *93*(3):391-398.

64. Rockey, P., & Griep, R. Behavioral dysfunction in hyperthyroidism. *Arch Intern Med*, 1980, *140*(9):1194-1197.

65. Deyo, R. Measuring functional outcomes in therapeutic trials in chronic disease. *Cont Clin Trials*, 1984, *5*(3):223-240.

66. Cantril, H. The pattern of human concerns. New Brunswick, NJ: Rutgers University Press, 1965.

67. Coates, A., Gebski, V., Bishop, J.F., et al. Improving quality of life during chemotherapy for advanced breast cancer. *N Engl J Med*, 1987, *317*(24): 1490-1495.

68. Selby, P.J., Chapman, J.A.W., Etazadi-Amoli, J., et al. The development of a method for assessing the quality of life of cancer patients. *Br J Cancer*, 1984, *50*(1):13-22.

69. Llewellyn-Thomas, H.A., Sutherland, H.J., Hogg, S.A., et al. Linear analogue self-assessment of voice quality in laryngeal cancer. *J Chron Dis*, 1984, *37*(12):917-924.

70. Baum, M., Priestman, T., West, R.R., & Jones, E.M. A comparison of subjective responses in a trial com-

paring endocrine with cytotoxic treatment in advanced carcinoma of the breast. *Eur J Cancer*, 1980, 16(suppl 1):223-226.

71. Cotanch, P. Measuring nausea and vomiting in clinical nursing research. *Oncol Nurs Forum*, 1984, 11(3):92-94.

72. Schipper, H., Clinch, J., McMurray, A., & Levitt, M. Measuring the quality of life on cancer patients: The functional living index-Cancer: Development and validation. *J Clin Oncol*, 1984, 2(5):472-483.

73. Morrow, G.R., Lindke, J., & Black, P. Measurement of quality of life in patients: Psychometric analysis of the Functional Living Index-Cancer (FLIC). *Qual Life Res*, 1992, 1(5):287-296.

74. Romsaas, E., Juliani, L., Briggs, A., et al. A method for assessing the rehabilitation needs of oncology outpatients. *Oncol Nurs Forum*, 1983, 10(3):17-21.

75. RAND. *RAND 36-item Health Survey 1.0: RAND Health Sciences Program (Scoring manual)*. Santa Monica, CA: RAND, 1992.

76. Hays, R.D., Sherbourne, C.D., & Mazel, R.M. The RAND 36-items health survey 1.0. *Health Econ*, 1993, 2(3):217-227.

77. Stewart, A.L., & Ware, J.E. *Measuring functioning and well-being: The medical outcomes study approach*. Durham, NC: Duke University Press, 1992.

78. McHorney, C.A., Ware, J.E., Jr., & Raczek, A.E. the MOS 36-item short health survey (SF-36):II. Psychometric and clinical tests of validity in measuring physical and mental health constructs. *Med Care*, 1993, 31(3):247-263.

79. Kurtin, P.S., Davies, A.R., Meyer, K.B., et al. Patient-based health status measurements in outpatient dialysis: Early experiences in developing an outcomes assessment program. *Med Care*, 1992, 30(suppl 5):MS136-MS149.

80. Aaronson, N.K., Acquadro, C., Alonso, J., et al. International quality of life assessment (IQOLA) project. *Qual Life Res*, 1992, 1(5):349-351.

81. Cella, D.F., Tulsky, D.S., Gray, G., et al. The functional assessment of cancer therapy scale: Development and validation of the general measure. *J Clin Oncol*, 1993, 11(3):570-579.

82. Schag, C.A., Heinrich, R.L., Aadland, R., & Ganz, P.A. Assessing problems of cancer patients: Psychometric properties of the Cancer Inventory of Problem Situations. *Health Psychol*, 1990, 9(1):83-102.

83. Schag, C.A.C., & Heinrich, R.L. *Cancer Rehabilitation Evaluation System CARES Manual*. Santa Monica, CA: CARES Consultants, 1988.

84. Schag, C.A.C., Ganz, P.A., & Heinrich, R.L. Cancer Rehabilitation Evaluation System—Short Form (CARES-SF). *Cancer*, 1991, 68(6):1406-1413.

85. Ganz, P.A., Schag, C.A.C., Kahn, B., et al. Describing the health-related quality of life impact of HIV infection: Findings from a study using the HIV Overview of Problems-Evaluation System (HOPES). *Qual Life Res*, 1993, 2(2):109-119.

86. Cain, M., & Henke, C. Living with cancer: A random sample of 50 patients in a hematology-oncology clinic. *Oncol Nurs Forum*, 1978, 5(3):4-5.

87. Freidenbergs, I., Gordon, W., Hubbard, M., & Diller, L. Assessment and treatment of psychosocial problems of the cancer patient: A case study. *Cancer Nurs*, 1980, 3(2):111-119.

88. Stromborg, M., & Wright, P. Ambulatory cancer patients' perceptions of the physical and psychosocial changes in their lives since the diagnosis of cancer. *Cancer Nurs*, 1984, 7(2):117.

89. Cella, D.F. *Manual: Functional Assessment of Cancer Therapy (FACT) scales and the Functional Assessment of HIV Infection (FAHI) scale*. Unpublished manual. Chicago: Rush-Presbyterian-St. Luke's Medical Center, 1993.

90. Bergner, M., Bobbitt, R.A., Carter, W.B., & Gilson, B.S. The sickness impact profile: Development and final revision of a health status measure. *Med Care*, 1981, 19(8):787-805.

91. Bergner, M. Measurements of health status. *Med Care*, 1985, 23(5):696-704.

92. Stewart, A.L. The medical outcomes study framework of health indicators. In A.L. Stewart & J.E.J. Ware (Eds.), *Measuring functioning and well-being: The medical outcomes study approach*. Durham, NC: Duke University Press, 1992, pp. 12-26.

93. Ware, J.E., & Sherbourne, C.D. The MOS 36-item short-form health survey (SF-36): I. Conceptual framework and item selection. *Med Care*, 1992, 30(6):473-483.

94. Padilla, G.V., Ferrell, B.R., Grant, M.M., & Rhiner, M. Defining the content domain of quality of life for cancer patients with pain. *Cancer Nurs*, 1990, 13(2):108-115.

95. Andrews, F., & Withey, S. *Social indicators of well-being*. New York: Plenum, 1976.

96. Campbell, A. *The sense of well-being in America*. New York: McGraw-Hill, 1981.

97. Campbell, A. Subjective measures of well-being. *Am Psychol*, 1976, 31(2):117-124.

98. Campbell, A., Converse, R., & Rogers, W. *The quality of American life*. New York: Russell Sage Foundation, 1976.

99. Kilpatrick, F., & Cantril, H. Self-anchoring scaling: A measure of individual's unique reality worlds. *J Individ Psychol* 1960, 16:158.

100. Levy, N., & Wynbrandt, G. The quality of life on maintenance hemodialysis. *Lancet*, 1975, 1(7920):1328.

101. Study protocol for the World Health Organization project to develop a quality of life assessment instrument (WHOQOL). *Qual Life Res*, 1993, 2(2):153-159.

102. Center for the Study of Aging and Human Development. *Multidimensional functional assessment: The OARS methodology* (2nd ed.). Durham, NC: Duke University Press, 1978.

103. Penckofer, S., & Holm, K. Early appraisal of coronary revascularization on quality of life. *Nurs Res*, 1984, 33(2):60-63.

104. Laborde, J., & Powers, M. Satisfaction with life for patients undergoing hemodialysis and patients suffering from osteoarthritis. *Res Nurs Health*, 1980, 3(1):19-24.

Appendices

9A. HQOL Conceptual Frameworks

	Cella et al. (81); Cella (89)	Bergner et al. (90); Bergner (91)	Stewart (92); Ware and Sherbourne (93)	Ferrans (54); Ferrans and Powers (53)	Grant, Ferrell et al. (49)	Strickland (4)	Padilla et al. (94)
Physical dimension	Physical well-being: energy, unwellness, distress from side effects (i.e., nausea, pain), meeting family needs, cancer/HIV disease and treatment-specific concerns Functional well-being: able to work, accept illness, sleeping well, enjoy life, enjoy leisure, enjoy quality of life	Physical dimension: ambulation, mobility, body care and movement, eating, home management, work, sleep and rest, recreation and pastimes	Physical functioning and well-being: physical functioning, energy/fatigue, pain, psychophysiologic symptoms, sleep problems	Satisfaction and importance of health and functioning domain: usefulness, physical independence, responsibilities, health, stress, sex life, health care, and treatment, leisure activities, retirement, travel, long life	Physical well-being and symptoms: strength and stamina, functional activities, disease-specific symptoms (e.g., visual disturbance), coping with chronic symptoms (e.g., GVHD), nutrition	Physical function: activity level or mobility, fitness or exercise tolerance, energy or stamina, nutritional balance, sexual activity, physical symptoms, impairments, disease, tissue alterations, biochemical alterations, sleep/rest, somatic comfort	Physical well-being: general functioning, disease- and treatment-specific attributes
Interpersonal dimension	Social/family well-being: support or communication from friends, family, and neighbors, sexual intimacy Relationship with doctor: confidence, communication	Psychosocial function (focus on social): social interaction	Social functioning and well-being: social activity limitations from health, role limitations from physical health, role limitations from emotional problems	Satisfaction and importance of family domain: family's happiness, children, relationship with spouse/significant other, family's health	Social well-being: appearance, roles and relationships, affection/sexual function, caregiver burden, leisure activities, return to work, financial burden	Social function: limitations in social roles/role fulfillment, interpersonal relationships or well-being, ability to communicate usefulness to others, recreational participation Family: relationship with partner and children, family health and happiness	Interpersonal well-being: social support, social/role functioning

Economic/environmental dimension

Emotional well-being: feeling sad, nervous, hopeless, worry about dying, coping with illness		Satisfaction and importance of socio-economic domain: standard of living, financial independence, home, job, neighborhood, overall USA conditions, friends, emotional support, education		Satisfaction with economic status: financial status/income, standard of living, employment/work, neighborhood, housing, education	

Psychologic/spiritual dimension

Psychosocial function (focus on psychologic): communication, alertness behavior, emotional behavior	Mental functioning and well-being: cognitive functioning, psychologic distress, psychologic well-being	Satisfaction and importance of psychologic/spiritual domain: satisfaction with life, happiness, satisfaction with self, achievement of goals, peace of mind, personal appearance, faith in God	Psychologic well-being: anxiety, fear of recurrence, depression, changed priorities, cognition/attention, normalcy, second chance, coping with survival Spiritual well-being: strengthened belief, hope, despair, religiosity, inner strength	Psychologic function: affect or mood, cognitive ability, stress, anxiety, worries, contentment, satisfaction with life, enthusiasm for life, control over life, achievement of life goals, adjustment to illness	Psychologic well-being: affective and cognitive responses, coping ability, meaning of pain and cancer, feeling of accomplishment

Health perception dimension

Health perceptions: current health perceptions, health outlook				Health status/perceptions: health indicators, satisfaction with health, general health perceptions, acceptability of treatment, satisfaction with treatment and health care, self-care ability	

Numbers in parentheses correspond to studies in the References.

9B. Methodologic Approaches to Quality-of-Life Research

	General Strategy of Approach	When Data Collected	Benefits	Limitations
Most optimal	Prospective	Several times in course of treatment, usually from diagnosis through posttreatment period	Offers true process evaluation of same group of patients. Offers baseline to follow-up comparisons and higher reliability estimate of quality of life	Expensive; data takes long time to obtain; patient attrition
	Single data collection per patient, same time posttreatment	At same time posttreatment for each patient	Offers uniformity of posttreatment patient evaluation	Limited view of quality of life; possible low reliability
	Cross-sectional/ separate groups	At different phases of illness or treatment with patients with same illness, e.g., three groups of patients with breast cancer, at diagnosis, recurrence, and near death	Offers some view of flow of quality of life in relation to illness with less expense than prospective design; possibly increases reliability	Patients may not be well matched other than on disease variable, therefore, true phase comparisons risky
Least optimal	Single data collection/patients at variable times posttreatment	At variable times after treatment, e.g., patients range 1–10 years postmastectomy	Offers ability to assess maximal number of patients; least expensive method of data collection	Severe limit to comparability of patient responses due to history, effects, variability of time since diagnosis, and treatment

Based on Wellish D. Work, social, recreation, family, and physical status. *Cancer*, 1984, *53*(10):2292.

9C. Strategies and Technologies for Quality-of-Life Research

	Tools	Administrator	Advantages	Disadvantages
Most optimal	Combination structured interviewing; analog scales; behavioral functioning/ activities	Some self-administered; some administered by project staff (not treating physician)	Very comprehensive; can be both general and tailored to specific illness/ treatment; better content and construct validity	Expensive to design; can be lengthy to administer; convergent validity (between measures) can suffer
Least optimal	Unstructured clinical interview	Treating physician	Low cost, easy, and plentiful patient access	Physician bias severe; patient often skews response set to please doctor; no objective measures; low reliability
	Semistructured interview	Usually treating physician	Low cost, easy, and plentiful patient access	Less biased than unstructured interview, but physician and patient bias still problem; low validity; questionable reliability
	Analog rating scales	Can be physicians	Very brief; can be closely tailored to specific tumor types, sites, and regimens	Overly restrictive view of patient life; validity problems
	Psychologic tests	Self-administered	In-depth look at emotional status of patient	Often are very poorly standardized for cancer patients; confounded with preillness issues; only covers emotional issues

Based on Wellish D. Work, social, recreation, family, and physical status. *Cancer*, 1984, *53*(10):2293.

9D. Objective Instruments That Yield Quantitative Data

Name/Description	Psychometric Testing	Comments
Dartmouth Cooperative (COOP) Word-picture assessment charts to measure patient function in busy clinical practices. Measure: social/role functioning; pain and emotional condition; perceptions of changes in health, overall health, quality of life; social support. Simple drawing of picture to illustrate word scale	2,000 points, 4 settings (34,35) Test–retest: 0.78–0.98 elderly, 1 hour apart: 0.73–0.98 low-income After 2 weeks: 0.42–0.88 Validity: correlations between scores on RAND scales of same dimension to acceptable convergent validity (0.62); average discriminant validity correlation 0.39 at one site; significant correlations between symptoms and chart scores for overall health (0.51)	Useful measures of function in busy practices: World Organization of General Practitioners/Family Physicians (WONKA) used COOP in international feasibility study, revised charts (36). Instrument may "detect moderate effects in physical and emotional functioning secondary to changes in health status." (17) Weaknesses: physical condition chart omits disability and does not measure major daily activities; some charts not criterion-based; needs further testing (physical fitness tool in elderly, cross-cultural usefulness, interpretation of daily and social activities)
Quality of Well-Being (QWB) Scale (37) Utility/preference measure of HQOL outcomes. Summarizes HQOL by well years (WY) = quality adjusted life years (QALY) Scores: 0 (death) to 1.0 (optimal function) by combining preference weighted measures of symptoms and functions at a specific point in time Challenge: selection of values that determine the weights Available in Spanish, French, German, Mandarin, Taiwanese, other languages	Validity supported in a number of studies	Applies utility analyses to treatment and policy decision Function scales: mobility, physical activity, social activity Advantages: can compare very different treatment programs and disease outcomes; sensitive to changes in health outcomes; reflects relative importance of HQOL dimensions
HIV Quality Audit Method (HIV-QAM) Measures nursing care–related changes in hospitalized AIDS patients (38) Nurse completes instrument based on judgments made from observations, interviews, reports/records 10 items: 9 scaled 1 (total dependence/severe stress) to 4 (full self-care/no distress); 1 scaled 0 (bedridden) to 4 (asymptomatic) Higher score, better QOL Used in non-HIV populations as well Available in Spanish, Japanese	Content validity secondary to item selection from preexisting scales Construct validity: confirmatory factor analysis and multitrait scaling analysis led to 3 factors: self-care, ambulation, psychologic distress Internal consistency alpha reliability for subscales: 0.89, 0.88, 0.84, respectively Concurrent and predictive validity supported	Useful disease-specific, objective, quantitative scale Focus on nursing care Brief, easy to use

Numbers in parentheses correspond to studies cited in the References.

9E. Additional Subjective Instruments That Yield Quantitative Data

Name/Description	Psychometric Testing	Comments
Self-Anchoring Life Satisfaction Scale (66,99) Measures general sense of well-being Subjective scale: subject identifies best (rung 10) and worst (rung 1) possible life on a ladder image Subject then selects placement 5 years ago, present, and 5 years in future	Content and face validity and reliability established	Similar procedure for health status Used successfully in patients undergoing treatment (i.e., dialysis or coronary revascularization, as well as patients with severe osteoarthritis) (103,104)
Linear Analog Self-Assessment (LASA) Numerous scales (67-70) May evaluate life areas such as feeling of well-being, activity, pain, nausea, appetite	Reliability and validity data inadequate (70) LASA correlates well with patient's clinical status (70,71)	10-cm line is drawn for each tested area, with descriptive words of extremes of that area on each end of the line Patient marks the line at point representing feelings at that moment The distance (in cm) gives the score out of 10
Danoff et al. questionnaire 4 sections: descriptive, demographic items, medical data, perceptual QOL, health status Subject rates feelings on 41 perceptual QOL questions on a 7-point scale ranging from "delighted (1)" to "terrible (7)"	Demographic, perceptual, health status data have been compared to national database Standardized instrument allowing data replication and comparison with baseline and future studies (26)	Quality of life defined objectively (education, income, housing, employment) and in terms of subjective (psychosocial) criteria
Functional Living Index-Cancer (FLIC) (72,73) 22-item questionnaire Likert format (1–7 range) FLIC measures a composite of distinct factors contributing to overall functional living (physical well-being, psychologic state, family situational interaction, social ability, somatic sensation)	Validity and reliability supported by two studies, one on 837 patients over 3 years (72), and another on 530 cancer patients (73). A similar 5-factor structure was described in both studies (72,73) Concurrent validity tested against classic instruments: physical function and ability factor correlates well with those measuring physical attributes/consequences but not with psychosocial measures. Emotional function factor correlates stongly with measures of depression and anxiety but weakly with physical ability measures. (72) Convergent and discriminant validity supported (measures of symptoms and anxiety) (73) Internal consistency supported (73): physical functioning (0.83), psychologic functioning (0.87), gastrointestinal symptoms (0.83), but modest for current well-being (0.64), social functioning (0.65)	Designed for easy, repeated patient self-administration Popular measure of quality of life in studies of persons with cancer Instructions available from Dr. Schipper

9E. Additional Subjective Instruments That Yield Quantitative Data (*cont.*)

Name/Description	Psychometric Testing	Comments
Romsaas et al. Questionnaire (74) Checklist of 15 categories (information, fatigue, pain, nutrition, speech/language, respiration, bowel/bladder, transportation, mobility, self/home care, vocation/ education, interests/activities, emotion, family, interpersonal relationships)	Primarily checklist but some open-ended questions inviting concerns not on checklist Data from tool is used to develop interventions designed to improve quality of life	Chief function of tool is to identify rehabilitation and continuing care needs of ambulatory cancer patients
RAND 36-item (version 1.0), and SF-36 Health Survey (75-79) Self-rating scale of HQOL 36 items measuring 8 scales: physical functioning, bodily pain, role limitations, emotional well-being, social functioning, energy/fatigue, general health perceptions, perceived change in health Scored in 2-step procedure: (1) recoding with resulting scores 0 to 100 (0, poorest health; 100, best health); (2) subscale score determined by averaging items within each of 8 scales	Internal consistency alpha coefficients for 8 scales: 0.78 to 0.93 (75) Construct validity established (77) Bodily pain score has weak convergent validity in relation to severity of medical illness (78) SF-36: floor effects (role functioning scales) (79) and potential ceiling effects (17)	Medical outcomes study: landmark 4 year observational study of 20,000 adult patients from 3 U.S. cities and 523 physicians from 5 practice settings Revised version 1.1 under development RAND and SF-36 essentially same items; SF-36 has different, more complicated scoring (76) International Quality of Life Assessment Project: translating/validating SF-36 in 13 countries (80) Instruction manuals available: RAND Corp. Santa Monica, CA; and Dr. Ware (The Health Institute, New England Medical Center, Boston, MA)
Functional Assessment of Cancer Therapy (FACT) Scales Self-report by persons with cancer or HIV infection (81) 10 scales: FACT-G (general) and tumor-specific or HIV-specific FACT-G has 28 items in 5 subscales	Internal consistency alpha 0.65– 0.82 for subscales, 0.89 for total instrument (630 patients) Concurrent validity with mood state measure Factor analysis: 6 factors, supporting subscale structure Test–retest reliability: 0.82–0.92 (60 patients)	5 subscales of FACT-G: well-being, physical, social/family, emotional, functional; relationship with doctor; item at end of each subscale queries effect on quality of life (QOL) Specific scoring guidelines: the higher the score, the better the QOL Detailed instruction manual available (Dr. Cella)
HIV Overview of Problems-Evaluation Systems (HOPES) (82-85) Self-administered questionnaire Derived from CARES questionnaire 165 items, but not all items applicable to all respondents	Mean alpha coefficient 0.82 across summary scores (good internal consistency) Significant correlations between HOPES and other HQOL measures (criterion-related validity) Construct validity supported by differences between asymptomatic and symptomatic persons' scores	Overall HQOL scale, 5 summary scales (physical, psychosocial, significant other, medical interaction, sexual) plus 35 subscales measuring everyday functioning Specific scoring guidelines Instruction manual available from Dr. Schag

Numbers in parentheses correspond to studies cited in the References.

10

Multiple Instruments for Measuring Quality of Life

Hannah Dean

Health-care reform and managed competition are the buzz words for the 1990s. The drive to offer cost-effective, quality care accessible to all demands efficient and appropriate use of resources. Allocating or rationing of resources is a current and future reality. Quality of life is proposed as a goal of health care,[1,2] as an endpoint,[3-6] as an outcome of treatment,[7,8] and as a means of rank-ordering treatments for allocating resources.[9,10] Kaplan and Coons[11,p30] assert that "health care concerns can be reduced to just two categories: life duration and quality of life." Callahan[1,2] advocates redirecting the goals of health care from extending life to favoring interventions and therapies that improve quality of life.

Padilla et al.[12] identified five purposes for examining quality of life in research. Researchers use quality of life to describe patient responses to disease, patient responses to symptom management, patient and family responses to cancer treatment, patient responses to rehabilitation efforts, and distress trajectories in the course of patients' disease experiences.

The proposed uses for quality-of-life measurements demand that policymakers, researchers and clinicians be rigorous in their approach to choosing instruments and measurement schemes. The inclusion of two chapters on quality of life in this book reflects a recognition of this need for rigor. This chapter proposes using multiple instruments for measuring quality of life. Investigators will find relevant instruments in several other chapters of this book including: functional status, mental status, social support, coping, hope, spirituality, sexuality, anxiety, depression, loneliness, pain, and dyspnea.

Importance of Measuring Quality of Life

The conceptualization and measurement of quality of life are vital to health policy, evaluation research, and clinical decision making. References to the importance of health-related quality of life for health policy and evaluation research abound.[10,13-16] They indicate the need for a means to compare the outcomes across different interventions, disease groups, and populations. Some advocate a means of rank-ordering interventions by their cost-effectiveness with quality of life as one of the factors in making the determinations.[9-10,17]

Working groups at a National Cancer Institute (NCI)–sponsored workshop recommend quality-of-life assessment as an endpoint measure in Phase III clinical trial protocols, along with tumor response, survival, and toxicities of therapy.[6] Hayden et al.[3] emphasize the Southwest Oncology Group's[3] recommendation of commitment to gathering quality-of-life data because sometimes quality of life is *the* endpoint of interest when comparing one intervention against another. Caution must be exercised when using quality of life as an outcome measure. For example, in the early 1980s, two evaluation studies startled the hospice community when their results failed to indicate significant differences in the quality of life for persons dying in hospice versus nonhospice settings.[18,19] Souquet et al.[20] published a metaanalysis of clinical trials comparing polychemotherapy and supportive care in patients with nonresectable lung cancer. Although two of the studies they reviewed were unsuccessful in assessing quality of life because the subjects were too ill, other studies were able to demonstrate that polychemotherapy helped to reduce pain, coughing, and dyspnea. Some interventions might prove to extend life at the cost of quality of life. Vaisrub alludes to the importance of quality of life as a measure of the usefulness of cardiac revascularization when he says, "The attained 'quality of life' [after cardiac revascularization] is apt to be void of social usefulness."[21,p236] Research findings, if considered valid and replicable, could lead to limitations in funding for programs. Researchers must ensure that measures of quality of life used are valid and sufficiently sensitive to detect differences in quality of life.

Practitioners are admonished to incorporate assessment of quality of life into their clinical practices.[11,22-24] Schipper et al.[25] suggest that patients should be informed about quality of life and survival statistics as part of informed consent regarding the management of their cancers. Lynch[26] moderated grand rounds in critical care in which Engelhardt discussed the "quality of life" versus the "quality of morbidity." Engelhardt makes a strong case for the importance of providing patients with a clear picture of the impact of treatment. Informed consent requires that patients have information from which to decide whether increased lifespan is worth the morbidity associated with their conditions or their treatment or both. For example, Sugarbaker et al.[27] report evidence that suggests that amputation for sarcoma is less disruptive to quality of life than is a limb-sparing procedure involving surgery and radiation.

Clinical decision making also requires attention to factors that influence compliance. An extensive study of the effects of antihypertensive therapy on the quality of life compared three antihypertensive agents. Croog et al.[28] report this excellent quality-of-life study using multiple instruments and a comparative design. The resulting data provide health-care professionals with information that will assist them in choosing medications to improve compliance with the medical regimen for hypertension.

Issues to Consider in Measuring Quality of Life

Significant health policy and clinical decisions may depend on the perceived effect on quality of life of various approaches to providing care. The data on which such decisions are made must be replicable, valid, and sufficiently sensitive to yield meaningful results. Several significant problems have been raised by quality-of-life scholars. Yancik and Yates[29] express concern about the indiscriminate and superficial use of quality of life in clinical trials. They identify as a problem the use of a single instrument to discern differences in quality of life in patients across cancer diagnoses. In a related argument, Braden et al.[30] point to the difficulty of using quality of life as an outcome measure because the factors that affect it are so complex. They suggest that specific components of quality of life be measured that are consistent with the theoretical framework of the study and the specific expected effects or outcomes of the disease, treatment, or intervention.

Kagawa-Singer[31] questions the validity of Euro-American quality-of-life instruments applied to non-Euro-American populations. She asserts that the Japanese, for example, hold values opposite to those of Euro-Americans. According to Kagawa-Singer, in Japanese culture life is not sacred, the individual is not autonomous, suffering is a part of life, and verbal language is viewed as a negative quality. She warns that measurements of items that have no conceptual equivalency in another culture are invalid. Kagawa-Singer recommends a framework including security, integrity, and belonging as basic needs essential to quality of life, the means of achieving which vary depending on culturally based values.

Rosser[32] advocates a single instrument and a unitary index for ease of use for planning purposes; however, he points out that the conceptualization of quality of life has shifted, making it difficult to compare data over time. Stewart[33,p13] indicates that variations in conceptualizations also occur depending on the frame of reference of the observer. She says that "only one category, functioning or behavior is included in all schemes."

Approaches to Measuring Quality of Life

Multiple instruments to measure the multidimensional concept of quality of life are advocated because of the need for reliable, comparable, valid, and sensitive measurements. Gotay et al.[5,p576] urge researchers to choose instruments based on a careful definition of quality of life; they say, "in a particular study, there may not be a single instrument available to carry out such a collection [of both functional and satisfaction data]." Use of multiple instruments allows flexibility in the conceptualization of quality of life while permitting comparability of specific dimensions across studies. Employing increasingly sensitive measures for specific domains may be more feasible with the use of multiple instruments. Such an approach permits the investigator to avoid either a ceiling or a floor effect.[16] Jalowiec[34] concludes that, after a thorough examination, the advantages of the multiple-instrument approach outweigh the disadvantages. In another article, Jalowiec[35] recommends methods to overcome the practical, measurement, data quality, and data analysis issues in a multidimensional assessment of quality of life.

Three general approaches to the use of multiple measures have emerged in the quality-of-life literature in the past several years: a core instrument and specific modules to be used for particular situations or conditions,[36,37] a battery of instruments, and composite instruments constructed using parts of existing instruments. The core and module approach stems from work in Europe. The instruments are under development and will be capable of being tailored to fit cultural, disease, respondent, and setting characteristics.[36]

The studies cited later in this chapter are examples of the battery approach to measuring the multiple dimensions of quality of life. In the early 1980s, Ware[38] suggested the wisdom of selecting a battery of health status measures because of the lack of consensus about the dimensions of the concept. In the early 1990s, Stewart[39] reiterated the breadth of the concept and indicated that there continues to be fairly wide diversity depending on the frame of reference of the researcher. Moinpour et al.[4] recommend separate measures of physical functioning, emotional functioning, symptoms, and global quality of life; they further recommend including measures of social functioning and other "protocol-specific" variables when appropriate. Schumaker et al.[40,p97] and Guyatt and Jaeschke[41] identify a range of problems with using a battery approach, including difficulty analyzing across time and interpreting the results of the multiple measure when they point in different directions, the complexity of study design, and the burden on the patient and staff. Nevertheless, Schumaker et al.[40] advocate a battery approach with instruments that "correspond to the dimensions of quality of life most likely to be either positively or negatively affected by treatment, and to use the best instruments to assess each of these dimensions." Spilker,[42] Spilker et al.,[43] and McDowell and Newell[44] provide valuable resources for identifying measures to be included in a battery. Many discussions and examples of the battery approach are reflected in the literature.[6,7,45-52]

The third approach to using multiple measures involves constructing composite instruments from existing measures. Cleary et al.[53] developed an instrument for examining health-related quality of life in persons with AIDS by combining specific subscales from several instruments, including the Functional Status Questionnaire, a fatigue scale from the Medical Outcomes Study short form, several questions from the Health Interview Survey, and two questions from the Memory Assessment Clinic Self-Rating Scale. DeLeo et al.[54] constructed a 31-item instrument to assess quality of life in the elderly by selecting items from eight other scales. Other examples of this approach can be found in works by Lubeck and Fries,[55] Sherbourne et al.,[56] Tuchler et al.,[57] and Wiklund et al.[58] Such an approach carries the same potential problems found in the use of a battery, with the added question of reliability and validity when previously validated instruments are cannibalized and reconstructed in new forms.

Frank-Stromborg[59] reports on selecting a single instrument to measure quality of life. She emphasizes four decisions a researcher must make in choosing an instrument: qualitative versus quantitative measures, subjective versus objective reporters of data, subjective versus objective dimensions, and single versus multiple instruments. Other choices emerge from the literature, such as global versus domain-specific measures, societal versus individual perspectives, cognitive versus affective evaluations, global versus disease-specific measures, and population specific measures. As Spitzer et al. point out:

> Global measures of quality of life include those that seek responses, such as the following: Please mark with an X the appropriate place within the bar to indicate your rating of this person's quality of life during the past week. (100 mm bar with "lowest quality" on the left and "highest quality" on the right).[60,p589]

This approach assumes that the respondent can provide a valid overall assessment of quality of life. A global approach implies unidimensionality. Domain-specific approaches seek assessments of variables related to a multidimensional concept. Domain-specific data may be achieved by either single or multiple instruments. The choice depends on whether one defines quality of life as a unidimensional or multidimensional concept.

Societal versus individual perspectives of the quality of life may vary considerably. The researcher should clarify which approach is being used. Conclusions should reflect limitations to generalizations based on the approach used. Campbell[61] alludes to this distinction when he argues that the individual's experience of quality of life may not relate directly to societal indicators, such as education, mortality, and employment.

George[62] distinguishes between cognitive and affective evaluations of life quality. Cognitive evaluations are those based on the facts of a person's circumstances. Affective evaluations reflect how respondents feel about their quality of life irrespective of the objective facts. Both approaches have value in measuring quality of life.

Increasingly investigators recognize the need to examine quality of life from a disease-specific perspective. The specific effects of one disease compared to another can be expected to have consequences for quality of life in different dimensions. Quality of life has been investigated in patients with rheumatoid arthritis,[46] acquired immune deficiency syndrome[5] and HIV infection,[55] stroke,[47] cardiovascular disease,[58,63] chronic lung disease,[64] hypertension,[11,28] physical disabilities,[65,66] coronary artery surgery,[67,68] heart transplants,[51] depression,[50] and cognitive impairments.[69] In addition, the range of specific cancer diagnoses and treatments addressed in the quality-of-life literature is broad, including breast cancer,[3,30] bone marrow transplant patients,[70,71] head and neck cancer,[72] endometrial cancer,[73] and non-small-cell lung cancer.[20]

Gotay and Moore[72] illustrate the issue of choosing population-specific methods of measuring quality of life in their examination of studies of quality of life in head and neck cancer patients. The problem goes beyond disease-specific to population-specific issues with this patient population for whom the comorbidities of alcohol and nicotine abuse complicate quality-of-life assessment. Other population specific considerations include culture,[16,31,74] age,[22,52,54,55,69,75] and gender.

Conceptualizing Quality of Life

In spite of frequent references to quality of life in health-care issues in the professional and public press, the definition of the concept remains elusive. A review of the literature reveals a variety of terms equated with quality of life, such as life satisfaction,[65,76-78] self-esteem,[79] well-being,[69,75,80-83] health status,[15,22,23,27,38,84,85] happiness,[86] adjustment,[87] value of life,[88] meaning of life,[89,90] and functional status.[64,91,92]

In addition, the dimensions of the concept of quality of life vary from study to study. Hutchinson et al.[93] identify physical, social, and emotional dimensions. Flanagan[94] describes 15 aspects in five categories, including physical and material well-being; relations with other people; social, community, and civic activities; personal development and fulfillment; and recreation. McSweeney et al.[95] define quality of life as emotional functioning, social role functioning, and participation in activities of daily living (ADL) and recreational pastimes. Linn and Linn[96] operationalize quality of life as scores on scales of depression, self-esteem, life satisfaction, alienation, and locus of control. Levy and Wynbrandt[97] report on quality of life in terms of income, sexual activity, and lifestyle. Aaronson et al.[74,p842] point out that "research on single dimensions of quality of life, such as pain, nausea and vomiting, insomnia and psychologic distress, have lead to improvements in symptom control." Guyatt et al.[64] specified dyspnea as a measure of quality of life in patients with chronic airflow limitations. City of Hope researchers expanded their quality-of-life framework to include spiritual well-being, based on extensive research with bone marrow transplant survivors.[70,71]

Acceptance of the premise that quality of life is a multidimensional concept demands a conceptual framework identifying the elements of which it is comprised. Three authors present specific frameworks that may prove useful in clinical nursing research.

The Ware Framework

Ware[98] proposes five elements to be used as guides in selecting instruments to measure quality of life: (1) disease; (2) personal functioning; (3) psychologic distress, or well-being; (4) general health perceptions; and (5) social or role functioning. Disease is central because it is the focus of our interest, the reason we are interested in a particular population for study. Ware recommends disease-specific measures because of the heterogeneity of the concept. Personal functioning is defined as the performance of or capacity to perform ADL, such as self-care, mobility, and physical activities.

Ware insists that the third element, psychologic distress and well-being, be measured using specific measures of psychologic status. General health perceptions refers to self-rated measures of general health and well-being. Finally, role functioning is distinguished from personal functioning and refers to the performance of or capacity to perform activities associated with an individual's usual role, such as father, mother, companion, helpmate.

The George and Bearon Framework

George and Bearon[99] selected four dimensions to define quality of life, including both subjective evaluations and objective conditions. Their subjective evaluations include life satisfaction and self-esteem; their objective conditions include general health/functional status and socioeconomic status. They present detailed accounts of 21 instruments for and methods of measuring the proposed dimensions, with descriptions, measurement properties, and recommendations for use of each.

The Cella Framework

Based on a review of factor analytic and aggregate index studies, Cella[100] presents four dimensions of health-related quality of life: physical, functional, emotional, and social. Cella's model is particularly apt for the purpose of this chapter because of subordinate domains linked the larger dimensions and additional areas for which the linkages are less well established. The physical dimension includes symptoms and side effects; the functional dimension, role performance and ADL; the emotional dimension, distress and well-being; and the social dimension, sociability and intimacy. Additional areas for consideration are work, sexuality, leisure, spirituality, family functioning, and treatment satisfaction.

Instruments Used to Measure Quality-of-Life Elements

Frank-Stromborg[59] describes 13 methods of measuring quality of life with a single instrument. Some of the instruments she describes might also be suitable in a multiple-instrument approach. For example, the Sickness Impact Profile (SIP), the Karnovsky Performance Status Scale, and Cantril's Self-Anchoring Striving Scale can serve as measures of elements within a conceptual framework.

The instruments described in this section are organized according to major studies in which they were used as measures of quality of life. This arrangement illustrates conceptual frameworks and multiple instruments in quality-of-life research.

Burckhardt Study

Burckhardt[101] studied the impact of physical, psychologic, and social factors on the perception of quality of life among 94 people with arthritis in a community. She created a quality-of-life index using a single question rating the subject's overall quality of life, the Life Satisfaction Index (LSI-Z), and the Domain Satisfaction Scale.

Life Satisfaction Index (LSI-Z)

Wood et al.[102] developed the LSI-Z as a short form of the Life Satisfaction Rating (LSR). The LSI-Z consists of 13 items to which the subject is asked to respond with "agree," "disagree," or "?" An example of an item is: "This is the dreariest time of my life."

"Agree" answers score 2 points, and "?" answers score 1 point. All items must be answered. The validity and reliability coefficients between the original LSR and the LSI-Z were 0.57 and 0.79, respectively.

Domain Satisfaction Scale

Burckhardt describes the Domain Satisfaction Scale as developed from empirical data by Flanagan[94] using a 7-point rating scale developed by Andrews and Withey.[103] She refers to Campbell et al.[104] when describing the reliability and validity of the tool.

Index of Domain Satisfactions

The Index of Domain Satisfactions was developed by Campbell et al.[104] Respondents rate their satisfaction with each domain on the seven-point rating scale ranging from "completely satisfied" to "completely dissatisfied." The domains explored include marriage, family life, health, neighborhood, friendships, housework, job, life in the United States, city or county, nonwork, housing, usefulness of education, standard of living, amount of education, and savings. The nonwork item follows several questions about leisure time and are scored as: 1, completely satisfied to 7, completely dissatisfied. An example of an item is: "Overall, how satisfied are you with the ways you spend your spare time?" Results are reported with overall distribution of responses on each scale and average score values. Campbell et al. report stability correlations ranging from 0.42 to 0.67 for the individual domains and 0.76 for the sum of the 14 domain satisfactions.[104] Validity is not addressed explicitly. However, the domains selected relate to everyday life and are similar to those identified by Flanagan[94] and Andrews and Withey.[103]

The Evans et al. Study

Evans et al.[105] report a study of quality of life of 859 patients with end-stage renal disease. Objective measures of functional ability were obtained using the Karnovsky Index and the patient's response to the question: "Are you *now able* to work for pay full time, part time, or not at all?" Subjective indicators were drawn from the work of Campbell et al.,[104] including the Index of Psychological Affect, the Index of Overall Life Satisfaction, and the Index of Well-Being.

Index of Psychological Affect

The Index of Psychological Affect (called the Index of General Affect by Campbell et al.[104]) consists of eight semantic differential items: (1) boring/interesting; (2) miserable/enjoyable; (3) useless/worthwhile; (4) lonely/friendly; (5) empty/full; (6) discouraging/hopeful; (7) rewarding/disappointing; and (8) brings out the best in me/doesn't give me much of a chance.[105] Respondents place an X in one of seven boxes between the bipolar items indicating their feelings about their present lives. Campbell et al. report a reliability coefficient of 0.89 on the Index of General Affect.[104] Correlations with the overall life satisfaction item ($r = 0.55$) and the happiness item ($r = 0.52$) provide indications of validity.

Index of Overall Life Satisfaction

Evans et al. are unclear about their use of the Index of Overall Life Satisfaction.[105] Campbell et al.[104] measure the Index of Domain Satisfactions, and they include an overall life satisfaction item:

> "We have talked about various parts of your life, now I want to ask you about your life as a whole. How satisfied are you with your life as a whole these days? Which number on the card comes the closest to how satisfied or dissatisfied you are with your life as a whole?" (1 completely satisfied; 7 completely dissatisfied.)

In a repeat interview with 285 subjects 8 months after the initial data collection, the stability correlation for the Index of Overall Life Satisfaction was 0.43.[104] Campbell et al. do not address validity explicitly.

Index of Well-Being

The Index of Well-Being[104] is a composite of the Index of Overall Life Satisfaction and the Index of General Affect. The estimated reliability coefficient is reported to be 0.89. Validity is not addressed.

The Lewis Study

Lewis's study of late-stage cancer patients is the third major study from which instrument examples are drawn.[106] Lewis chose the Rosenberg Self-Esteem Scale, the Crumbaugh Purpose-in-Life Test, and the Lewis et al. Anxiety Scale as indicators of the psychosocial aspects of quality of life.

Rosenberg Self-Esteem Scale

The Rosenberg Self-Esteem Scale[107] purports to measure a basic feeling of self-worth. It consists of 10 items to which the subject responds on a four-point scale from "strongly agree" to "strongly disagree." Lewis reports reliability coefficients from 0.85 to 0.92 and validity correlations ranging from 0.56 to 0.83 with similar measures.

Crumbaugh Purpose-in-Life Test (PIL)

The Crumbaugh Purpose-in-Life Test[108] is a 20-item instrument to which subjects respond on a seven-point scale. A sample item is: "In life I have no goals or aims at all" (1) to "very clear goals and aims" (7) or "I am a very irresponsible person" (1), to "a very responsible person" (7). The Purpose-in-Life Test is designed to measure the degree to which the subject experiences a sense of meaning and purpose in life. Split-half correlations are reported to be 0.85 in a sample of church parishioners. PIL Scores correlated with therapist ratings (0.38, $n = 50$) and minister ratings (0.47, $n = 120$).

Lewis et al. Anxiety Scale

The Lewis et al. Anxiety Scale[109] was developed for cancer patients. Subjects respond to nine items on a five-point scale (1 none of the time; 5 all of the time). An example is "I feel more nervous than usual." Lewis[106] reports stability reliability at 0.90 and split-half reliability at 0.79. According to Lewis, validity was established by its inverse relations with an attitude scale measuring perceived functional effectiveness.

The King et al. Study

King et al.[67] examined patient perceptions of quality of life after coronary artery surgery in a sample of 155 men and women 1 year post coronary artery bypass grafting. Their conceptual framework for quality of life encompassed life satisfaction, affect, functional disruption, and relief of angina. Data for the four elements of quality of life were collected by means of a self-administered instrument that included the measures chosen: the Satisfaction with Life Scale, the Bi-polar Profile of Mood States, the Sickness Impact Profile, and an Angina Severity Index they developed.[67] The Angina Severity Index is not included in this chapter because King et al. fail to report validity or reliability for it.

Satisfaction with Life Scale

The Satisfaction with Life Scale is a five-item scale with a response set of 1 to 7 (higher score indicates greater satisfaction). The items include: "In most ways my life is close to my ideal; the conditions of my life are excellent; I am satisfied with my life; so far I have gotten the important things I want in life; if I could live my live over, I would change almost nothing."[110] In the original report of the study, Diener et al.[110,p72] report correlations from 0.58 to 0.75 with eight measures of subjective well-being. King et al.[67] report pre- and postoperative reliability coefficients of 0.82 and 0.87.

Bi-polar Profile of Mood States

The Bi-polar Profile of Mood States[111] is a 72-item instrument on which subjects indicate how they have been feeling during the past week with a response set of 0 to 4. A response of 0 indicates not at all, a response of 4 indicates extremely. Half of the items represent six positive mood states (six items for each of six positive mood states: composed, elated, agreeable, energetic, clear-headed, confident), the other half represent six negative mood states (six items for each of six negative mood states: anxious, depressed, hostile, tired, confused, unsure). High scores indicate more of the mood state, whether positive or negative. Subscale score for positive and negative mood states are calculated separately. The publisher indicates that only college norms are available for the Bi-polar Profile of Mood States.

Sickness Impact Profile (SIP)

King et al.[67] used only six of the 12 SIP scales: sleep and rest, home management, ambulation, social interaction, intellectual function, and recreation and pastimes. Other scales in the SIP include mobility, body care and movement, communications, alertness behaviors, emotional behavior, eating, and work.[112] Subjects identify which items in each scale apply to them. A sample item is:[112] "I sit during much of the day." Weighted scores for each item are identified by the subject and summed, divided by the total possible score, and multiplied by 100. The result is a percentage disruption score. The widely used SIP is sometimes referred to at the "gold standard."[113] King et al.[67] report an alpha coefficient of 0.86 for the combination of the six scales in their study.

The Kinney and Coyle Study

Kinney and Coyle[65] analyzed data from structured interviews of 344 adults with physical disabilities. This study illustrates the need to design studies based on a conceptual framework appropriate to the study population. The instruments chosen afford the opportunity to examine results across populations. The interviews included four instruments aimed at measuring quality of life: the Center for Epidemiological Studies Depression Scale, Rosenberg's Self-esteem Scale, the Life 3 Scale, and 35 related life domain items from Andrews and Withey[38] and Campbell et al.[104] The authors offer clear descriptions of the first three instruments, the fourth is unclear and, therefore, omitted from our discussion.

The Center for Epidemiological Studies
Depression Scale (CES-D)

The CES-D is a 20-item instrument devised using items from five sources, all previously validated depression scales. A sample item is:[114] "I was bothered by things that usually don't bother me." The response set for each symptom indicates how often in the past week the subject has experienced the symptom: not at all to 1 day in the week; 1 to 2 days in the week; 3 to 4 days in the week; or 5 to 7 days in the week. Scores range from 0 (not at all to 1 day in the week for all 20 symptoms) to 60 (5 to 7 days in the week for all 20 symptoms). Kinney and Coyle[65] report a Cronbach alpha value of 0.83 on this scale for their study. They indicate previous validity and reliability studies resulted in Cronbach alphas of 0.84 to 0.90.

Rosenberg Self-Esteem Scale

This scale was described previously in this chapter among the instruments used in the Lewis et al. study. Kinney and Coyle[65] report a Cronbach alpha of 0.83 for their study. This instrument consistently produces highly reliable values.

Life 3 Scale

Kinney and Coyle[65] use the Life 3 Scale as a criterion variable of life satisfaction, a subjective assessment of quality of life. They interjected the question "How do you feel about your life in general?" into their interviews at two separate points. Subjects were offered a response set from 1 (terrible) to 7 (delighted). The two responses were averaged for the Life 3 Scale score. Kinney and Coyle[65] report a test–retest correlation of 0.44 at 6 months. Kinney and Coyle cite Andrews and Withey[103] and Diener[115] in their discussion of the validity of the Life 3 Scale, claiming convergent validity with other measures of life satisfaction of 0.39 to 0.73.

Summary

The use of multiple instruments has the potential for solving problems of comparability and sensitivity. The researcher must, however, consider the problems that may result from this strategy such as administration, time requirements, and directions. Administration of instruments varies; instruments may require completion by the researcher, a health-care professional, the subject, or a significant other. When choosing multiple instruments to measure quality-of-life elements, the research must attend to variations in administration. The time required of respondents affects willingness to participate in research.[29,34] The cumulative time required to complete multiple instruments is a prime consideration. Flanagan[116] cautions about ensuring that directions to respondents are clear. The use of multiple instruments may increase the possibility of confusion.

Choosing multiple instruments for measuring quality of life has the advantage of allowing flexibility in the conceptualization of quality of life. As the concept is refined and clarified, researchers using multiple instruments can compare specific dimensions. As more sensitive instruments are developed, substitutions may be made without having to change all instruments in a battery.

Exemplar Studies

de Haan, R., Aaronson, N., Limburg, M., Hewer, R.L., & van Crevel, H. Measuring quality of life in stroke. *Stroke*, 1993, 24(2):320-327.

This study examines quality of life conceptually, outlines methodologic problems in measuring quality of life, reviews quality-of-life instruments, identifies criteria for selecting instruments, and proposes future directions for quality-of-life studies in stroke patients. The authors review 10 quality-of-life instruments to report their length, time needed for administration, content, scoring, and psychometric evaluation. They point out that choice of instruments depends on the specific questions addressed and on the characteristics of the patients studied. Patient and staff burden affect the feasibility of using long, comprehensive instruments; shorter instruments targeted at the specific questions of the research and compatible with patient characteristics are likely to result in a higher yield of data. The authors strongly recommend refining existing instruments rather than generating new instruments.

Bendtsen, P., & Hörnquist, J.O. Change and status in quality of life in patients with rheumatoid arthritis. *Qual Life Res*, 1992, *1*(5), 297-305.

This study exemplifies an assessment package approach to measuring quality of life. The mailed package included measures of six life domains: somatic, psychologic, social, behavioral/activity, structural, and material. Subjects were asked to rate their quality of life in the various domains, statically (current performance) and dynamically (change in status related to the disease). In addition, significant others were asked to rate the patients' lives in shortened versions of the assessment package. This study is one in a series of studies published by a Swedish team anchored by J.O. Hörnquist since 1982. The team has addressed quality of life in diabetes mellitus, alcohol abuse, cancer, and rheumatoid arthritis.

References

1. Callahan, D. *Setting limits: Medical goals in an aging society.* New York: Simon & Schuster, 1987.
2. Callahan, D. *What kind of life: The limits of medical progress.* New York: Simon & Schuster, 1990.
3. Hayden, L.A., Moinpour, C.M., Metch, B., et al. Pitfalls in quality of life assessment: Lessons from a Southwest Oncology Group breast cancer clinical trial. *Oncol Nurs Forum*, 1993, *20*(9):415-419.
4. Moinpour, C.M., Feigl, P., Metch, B., et al. Quality of life end points in cancer clinical trials: Review and recommendations. *J Nat Cancer Inst*, 1989, *81*(7):485-495.
5. Gotay, C.C., Korn, E.L., McCabe, M.S., et al. Quality of life assessment in cancer treatment protocols: Research issues in protocol development. *J Nat Cancer Inst*, 1992, *84*(8):575-579.
6. Nayfield., S.G., Ganz, P.A., Moinpour, C.M., et al. Report from a National Cancer Institute (USA) workshop on quality of life assessment in cancer clinical trials. *Qual Life Res*, 1992, *1*(3):203-210.
7. Schron, E.B., & Shumaker, S.A. The integration of health quality of life in clinical research: Experiences from cardiovascular clinical trials. *Progr Cardiovasc Nurs*, 1992, *7*(2):21-36.
8. Morreim, E.H. Medical ethics and the future of quality of life research. *Progr Cardiovasc Nurs*, 1992, *7*(2):12-17.
9. Menzel, P.T. Oregon's denial: Disabilities and quality of life. *Hastings Center Report*, 1992, *22*(6):21-25.
10. Capron, A.M. Oregons disability: Principle or politics? *Hastings Center Report*, 1992, *22*(6):18-20.
11. Kaplan, R.M., & Coons, S.J. Relative importance of dimension in the assessment of health-related quality of life for patients with hypertension. *Progr Cardiovasc Nurs*, 1992, *7*(2):29-36.
12. Padilla, G.V., Grant, M.M., & Ferrell, B. Nursing research into quality of life. *Qual Life Res*, 1992, *1*(5):341-348.
13. Kaplan, R., & Bush, J. Health-related quality of life measurement for evaluation research and policy analysis. *Health Psychol*, 1981, *1*(1):61.
14. Faden, R., & Leplege, A. Assessing quality of life. *Med Care*, 1992, *30*(5) suppl:MS166-175.
15. Goldberg, H.I., Pantell, R.H., & Weber, J.R. Final panel. Reactions, reflections and predictions. *Med Care*, 1992, *30*(5) suppl:MS283-293.
16. Guyatt, G.H., Feeny, D.H., & Patrick, D.L. Measuring health-related quality of life. *Ann Int Med*, 1993, *118*(8):622-629.

17. Williams, A. The importance of quality of life in policy decisions. In S.R. Walker & R.M. Rosser (Eds.), *Quality of life: Assessment and application.* Boston: MTP Press, 1988, pp. 279-296.
18. Wales, J., Kane, R., Robbins, S., et al. UCLA hospice evaluation study. *Med Care*, 1983, *21*(7):734.
19. Greer, D., & Mor, V. *A preliminary report of the National Hospice Study.* Washington, DC: Department of Health and Human Services, 1984.
20. Souquet, P.J., Chauvin, F., Boissel, J.P., et al. Polychemotherapy in advanced non small cell lung cancer: A meta-analysis. *Lancet*, 1993, *342*(8862):19-21.
21. Vaisrub, S. Quality of life manqué. *JAMA*, 1976, *236*(4):387.
22. Rubenstein, L.V., Calkins, D.R., Greenfield, S., et al. Health status assessment for elderly patients: Report of the Society of General Internal Medicine Task Force on Health Assessment. *J Am Geriatr Soc*, 1989, *37*(6):562-569.
23. Lohr, K.N. Applications of health status assessment in clinical practice: Overview of the third conference on advances in health status assessment. *Med Care*, 1992, *30*(5) suppl MS1-14.
24. Hopwood, P. Progress, problems, and priorities in quality of life research. *Eur J Cancer*, 1992, *28A*(10):1748-1752.
25. Schipper, H., Clinch, J., McMurray, A., & Leavitt, M. Measuring the quality of life of cancer patients: The Functional Living Index—Cancer: Development and validation. *J Clin Oncol*, 1984, *2*(5):472.
26. Lynch, E. To treat or not to treat—The dilemma. *Heart Lung*, 1978, *7*(3):499.
27. Sugarbaker, P.H., Barofsky, I., Rosenberg, S.A., & Gianola, F.J. Quality of life assessment of patient in extremity sarcoma clinical trials. *Surgery*, 1982, *9*(1):17.
28. Croog, S.H., Levine, S., Testa, M.A., et al. The effects of antihypertensive therapy on the quality of life. *N Engl J Med*, 1986, *314*(26):1657.
29. Yancik, R., & Yates, J.W. Quality of life assessment of cancer patients: Conceptual and methodologic challenges and constraints. *Cancer Bull*, 1986, *38*(5):217-222.
30. Braden, C.J., Mishel, M.H., Longman, A., et al. Symposium: Quality of life in treatment for breast cancer. Presented at the 1993 Scientific Session of the American Nurses Association Council of Nurse Researchers, Washington, DC, November 1993.

31. Kagawa-Singer, M. Quality of life: Cross-cultural differences. Draft manuscript from the author, 1994.

32. Rosser, R. Quality of life: Consensus, controversy and concern. In S.R. Walker & R.M. Rosser (Eds.), *Quality of life: Assessment and application.* Boston: MTP Press, 1988, pp. 297-304.

33. Stewart, A.L. The medical outcomes study framework of health indicators. In A.L. Stewart & J.E. Ware, Jr. (Eds.), *Measuring functioning and well-being: The medical outcomes study.* Durham, NC: Duke University Press, 1992, pp. 12-24.

34. Jalowiec, A. Issues in using multiple measures of quality of life. *Sem Oncol Nurs,* 1990, 6(4):271-277.

35. Jalowiec, A. Multidimensional assessment of quality of life in clinical studies. *Progr Cardiovasc Nurs,* 1992, 7(2):7-12.

36. Orley, J. News from World Health Organization. *Qual Life Res,* 1992, 1(4):277.

37. Aaronson, N.K. Quality of life research in cancer clinical trials: A need for common rules and language. *Oncology,* 1990, 4(5):59-66.

38. Ware, J.E., Jr. Methodological considerations in the selection of health status measures. In N.K. Wenger, M.E. Mattson, C.D. Furberg, & J. Elinson (Eds.), *Assessment of quality of life in clinical trials.* New York: LeJaq, 1984, pp. 87-117.

39. Stewart, A.L. Conceptual and methodologic issues in defining quality of life: State of the art. *Progr Cardiovasc Nurs,* 1992, 7(1):3-11.

40. Schumaker, S.A., Anderson, R.T., & Czajkowski, S.M. Psychological tests and scales. In B. Spilker (Ed.), *Quality of life assessments in clinical trials.* New York: Raven, 1990, p. 95.

41. Guyatt, G.H., & Jaeschke, R. Measurements in clinical trials: Choosing the appropriate approach. In B. Spilker (Ed.), *Quality of life assessments in clinical trials.* New York: Raven, 1990, pp. 37-46.

42. Spilker, B. (Ed.). *Quality of life assessments in clinical trials.* New York: Raven, 1990.

43. Spilker, B., Molinek, F.R., Jr., Johnston, K.A., et al. Quality of life bibliography and indexes. *Med Care,* 1990. 28(12) suppl.

44. McDowell, I., & Newell, C. *Measuring health: A guide to rating scales and questionnaires.* New York: Oxford University Press, 1987.

45. Hyland, M.E. A reformulation of quality of life for medical science. *Qual Life Res,* 1992, 1(4):267-272.

46. Bendtsen, P., & Hornquist, J.O. Change and status in quality of life patients with rheumatoid arthritis. *Qual Life Res,* 1992, 1(5):297-305.

47. deHaan, R., Aaronson, N., Limburg, M., et al., Measuring quality of life in stroke. *Stroke,* 1993, 24(2):320-327.

48. Ferrans, C.E. Conceptualizations of quality of life in cardiovascular research. *Progr Cardiovasc Nurs,* 1992, 7(2):2-7.

49. Hornquist, J.O., Hansson, B., Akerlind, I., & Larsson, J. Severity of disease and quality of life: A comparison in patients with cancer and benign disease. *Qual Life Res,* 1992, 1(2):135-141.

50. Revicki, D.A., Turner, R., Brown, R., & Martindale, J.J. Reliability and validity of a health-related quality of life battery for evaluating outpatient antidepressant treatment. *Qual Life Res,* 1992, 1(4):257-266.

51. Strauss, B., Thormann, T., Strenge, H., et al., Psychosocial, neuropsychological and neurological status in a sample of heart transplant recipients. *Qual Life Res,* 1992, 1(2):119-128.

52. Wray, J., Radley-Smith, R., & Yacoub, M. Effect of cardiac or heart-lung transplantation on the quality of life of the paediatric patient. *Qual Life Res,* 1992, 1(1):41-46.

53. Cleary, P.D., Fowler, F.J., Weissman, J., et al. Health-related quality of life in persons with acquired immune deficiency syndrome. *Med Care,* 1993, 31(7):569-580.

54. DeLeo, D., Rozzini, R., Bernardini, M., et al. Assessment of quality of life in the elderly assisted at home through a Tele-Check service. *Qual Life Res,* 1992, 1(6):367-374.

55. Lubeck, D.P., & Fries, J.F. Changes in quality of life among persons with HIV infection. *Qual Life Res,* 1992, 1(6):359-366.

56. Sherbourne, C.D., Meredith, L.S., Rogers, W., & Ware, J.E., Jr. Social support and stressful life events: Age differences in their effects on health-related quality of life among the chronically ill. *Qual Life Res,* 1992, 1(4):235-246.

57. Tuchler, H., Hofmann, S., Bernhart, M., et al. A short multilingual quality of life questionnaire—practicability, reliability and interlingual homogeneity. *Qual Life Res,* 1992, 1(2):107-117.

58. Wicklund, I., Gorkin, L., Pawitan, Y., et al., for the CAST Investigators. Methods for assessing quality of life in the Cardiac Arrhythmia Suppression Trial (CAST). *Qual Life Res,* 1992, 1(3):187-201.

59. Frank-Stromborg, M. Selecting an instrument to measure quality of life. *Oncol Nurs Forum,* 1984, 11(5):88.

60. Spitzer, W., Dobson, A., Hall, J., et al. Measuring the quality of life of cancer patients. *J Chronic Dis,* 1981, 34(12):585.

61. Campbell, A. Subjective measures of well-being. *Am Psychologist,* 1976, 31(2):117.

62. George, L. Subjective well-being. Conceptual and methodological issues. In C. Eisdorfer (Ed.), *Annual review of gerontology and geriatrics* (vol. 2). New York: Springer, 1981, p. 345.

63. Fletcher, A.E., Hunt, B.M., & Bulpitt, C.J. Evaluation of quality of life in clinical trials of cardiovascular disease. *J Chron Dis,* 1987, 40(6):557-566.

64. Guyatt, G.H., Townsend, M., Keller, J., et al. Measuring functional status in chronic lung disease: Conclusions from a randomized control trial. *Resp Med,* 1991, 85 (suppl B):17-21.

65. Kinney, W.B., & Coyle, C.P. Predicting life satisfaction among adults with physical disabilities. *Arch Phys Med Rehabil,* 1992, 73(9):863-869.

66. Evans, R.L., Dingus, C.M., & Haselkorn, J.K. Living with a disability: A synthesis and critique of the literature on quality of life, 1985–1989. *Psychol Rep,* 1993, 72(3, part 1):771-777.

67. King, K.B., Porter, L.A., Norsen, L.H., & Reis, H.T. Patient perceptions of quality of life after coronary artery surgery: Was it worth it? *Res Nurs Health,* 1992, 15(5):327-334.

68. Prevost, S., & Deshotels, A. Quality of life after cardiac surgery. *AACN Clin Issues Crit Care Nurs,* 1993,

4(2):320-328.

69. Burgener, S.C., & Chiverton, P. Conceptualizing psychological well-being in cognitively-impaired older persons. *Image*, 1992, 24(3):209-213.

70. Ferrell, B., Grant, M., Schmidt, G.M., et al. The meaning of quality of life for bone marrow transplant survivors. Part 2. Improving quality of life for bone marrow transplant survivors. *Cancer Nurs*, 1992, 15(4):247-253.

71. Grant, M., Ferrell, B., Schmidt, G.M., et al. Measurement of quality of life in bone marrow transplantation survivors. *Qual Life Res*, 1992, 1(6):375-384.

72. Gotay, C.C., & Moore, T.D. Assessing quality of life in head and neck cancer. *Qual Life Res*, 1992, 1(1):5-17.

73. Lamb, M.A. The influence of endometrial cancer on intimate relationships. Part II. *Qual Life Nurs Chall*, 1993, 2(2):32-38.

74. Aaronson, N.K, Meyerowitz, B.E., Bard, M., et al. Quality of life research in oncology: Past achievements and future priorities. *Cancer*, 1992, 67(3) suppl:839-843.

75. Stearns, D.M., & Whedon, M. Social well-being and quality of life: Analysis of a journey of cancer survivorship. *Qual Life Nurs Chall*, 1993, 2(2):23-31.

76. Brown, J., Rawlinson, M., & Hilles, N. Life satisfaction and chronic disease: Exploration of a theoretical model. *Med Care*, 1981, 19(11):1136.

77. Laborde, J., & Powers, M. Satisfaction with life for patients undergoing hemodialysis and patients suffering from osteoarthritis. *Res Nurs Health*, 1980, 3(1):19.

78. Ferrans, C.E., & Powers, M.J. Quality of life index: Development and psychometric properties. *Adv Nurs Sci*, 1985, 8(1):15.

79. Ziller, R. Self-other orientations and quality of life. *Social Indic Res*, 1974, 1:301.

80. Fletcher, A., & Bulpitt, C. The treatment of hypertension and quality of life. *Qual Life Cardiovasc Care*, 1985, 1(3):140.

81. House, P., Livingston, R., & Swinburn, C. Monitoring mankind: The search for quality. *Behav Sci*, 1975, 20:57.

82. Carstensen, L., & Cone, J. Social desirability and the measurement of psychological well-being in elderly persons. *J Gerontol*, 1983, 38(6):713.

83. Dow, K.H. Introduction: Social well-being and quality of life: Part II. *Qual Life Nurs Chall*, 2(2), 21-22.

84. Bergner, M., Bobbitt, R., Pollard, W., et al. The Sickness Impact Profile: Validation of a health status measure. *Med Care*, 1976, 14(1):57.

85. Lerner, M. Conceptualization of health and social well-being. *Health Serv Res*, 1973, 8(1):6.

86. Shinn, D., & Johnson, D. Avowed happiness as an overall assessment of quality of life. *Soc Indic Res*, 1978, 5:475.

87. Crewe, N. Quality of life: The ultimate goal in rehabilitation. *Minn Med*, 1980, August:586.

88. Bayles, M. The value of life—By what standard? *Am J Nurs*, 1980, 80(12):2226.

89. Berg, R., Hallauer, D., & Berk, S. Neglected aspects of quality of life. *Health Serv Res*, 1976, 11(4):391.

90. Mount, B., & Scott, J. Whither hospice evaluation? *J Chronic Dis*, 1983, 36(11), 731.

91. Hochberg, F., Linggood, R., Wolfson, L., et al. Quality and duration of survival in glioblastoma multiforme. *JAMA*, 1979, 24(10):1016.

92. Gilbert, H., Kagan, A., Nussbaum, H., et al. Evaluation of radiation therapy for bone metastases: Pain relief and quality of life. *Am J Roentgenol*, 1977, 129(6):1095.

93. Hutchinson, A., Farndon, J., & Wilson, R. Quality of survival of patients following mastectomy. *Clin Oncol*, 1979, 5:391.

94. Flanagan, J. A research approach to improving our quality of life. *Am Psychologist*, 1978, 33(2):138.

95. McSweeney, A., Grant, I., Heaton, R., et al. Life quality of patients with chronic obstructive pulmonary disease. *Arch Intern Med*, 1982, 142(3):473.

96. Linn, B., & Linn, M. Late stage cancer patients: Age differences in their psychophysical status and response to counseling. *J Gerontol*, 1981, 36(6):689.

97. Levy, N., & Wynbrandt, G. The quality of life on maintenance hemodialysis. *Lancet*, 1975, 1(7920): 1328.

98. Ware, J. Conceptualizing disease impact and treatment outcomes. *Cancer*, 1984, 53(10):2316.

99. George, L., & Bearon, L. *Quality of life in older persons: Meaning and measurement*. New York: Human Sciences Press, 1980.

100. Cella, D.F. Functional status and quality of life: Current views on measurement and intervention. In *Functional status and quality of life in persons with cancer*. Atlanta, GA: American Cancer Society, 1991, pp. 1-12.

101. Burckhardt, C. The impact of arthritis on quality of life. *Nurs Res*, 1985, 34(1):11.

102. Wood, V., Wylie, M., & Sheafor, B. An analysis of a short self-report measure of life satisfaction: Correlation with rater judgments. *J Gerontol*, 1969, 24(4):465.

103. Andrews, F., & Withey, S. *Social indicators of well-being: Americans' perceptions of life quality*. New York: Plenum, 1976.

104. Campbell, A., Converse, P., & Rodgers, W. *The quality of American life: Perceptions, evaluations, and satisfactions*. New York: Russell Sage, 1976.

105. Evans, R., Manninen, D., Garrison, L., et al. The quality of life of patients with end stage renal disease. *N Engl J Med*, 1985, 312(9):553.

106. Lewis, F. Experienced personal control and quality of life in late-stage cancer patients. *Nurs Res*, 1982, 31(2):113.

107. Rosenberg, M. *Society and the adolescent self image*. Princeton, NJ: Princeton University Press, 1965.

108. Crumbaugh, J. Cross validation of purpose-in-life test based on Frankl's concepts. *J Individ Psychol*, 1968, 24(1):74.

109. Lewis, F., Firisch, S., & Parsell, S. Clinical tool development for adult chemotherapy patients: Process and content. *Cancer Nurs*, 1979, 2(2):99.

110. Diener, E., Emmons, R.A., Larsen, R.J., & Griffin, S. The satisfaction with life scale. *J Pers Assess*, 1985, 49(1):71-75.

111. Lorr, M., & McNair, D. *Profile of mood states: Bi-polar form (POMS-BI)*. San Diego, CA: Educational and Industrial Testing Service, 1982.

112. Bergner, M. The sickness impact profile. In N.K.

Wenger, M.E. Mattson, C.D. Furburg, & J. Elinson (Eds.), *Assessment of quality of life in clinical trials of cardiovascular therapies.* New York: LeJaq, 1984, pp. 152-159.

113. Cella, D.F., & Tulsky, D.S. Measuring quality of life today: Methodological aspects. *Oncology,* 1990, *4*(5):29-38.

114. Radloff, L.S. The CES-D scale: A self report depression scale for research in the general population. *Applied Psychol Meas,* 1977, *1*(3):385-401.

115. Diener, E. Subjective well-being. *Psychol Bulletin,* 1984, *95*(3):542-575.

116. Flanagan, J. Measurement of quality of life: Current state of the art. *Arch Phys Med Rehab,* 1982, *63*(2):56.

11

Social Support
Conceptualization and Measurement Instruments

Ada M. Lindsey

Some people at risk for illness become ill, whereas others with similar risk do not, and people diagnosed with the same condition experience considerable variation in recovery patterns and in adaptation or adjustment to living with the condition. These observations have led clinicians and investigators to consider the possible contribution of other variables in influencing the onset of and the responses to illness. Social support is one variable that has received increased attention as a possible contributing factor to the observed variances in health outcomes.

There is now considerable literature to illustrate this burgeoning interest. There are reviews of social support,[1-10] descriptions of the properties of social support,[1,2,6,10,11] studies including social support as a variable,[12-23] and reports of instrument development to measure social support.[24-63]

Current theories suggest that social support may have a protective function, serve a stress-buffering or moderating role in health maintenance, and/or be related to positive health outcomes.[64-68] The quality and availability of social support may have an important role in preventing illness or in recovery after illness. Loss or lack of social support has been linked with a variety of conditions and illnesses.[13,69-71]

Cassel,[72] one of the few investigators who has proposed a mechanism for the role of social environment in disease etiology, suggests that social environmental stressors alter the neuroendocrine balance and thus increase susceptibility to disease. People deprived of meaningful social contact do not receive adequate information or feedback. Cassel speculates that this is a key property of those with inadequate social environments. In contrast, people with adequate social support are helped in coping with crisis and adapting to change.

Socially competent individuals are likely to have well-developed social networks and, as a result, may be more resistant to stressors.[73] Persons considered to be well inte-

Acknowledgment: I want to recognize the contributions of Jenny Cashman, research assistant, in obtaining the references and of Marla Crow, administrative assistant, in the preparation of this chapter.

grated and who function well receive more assistance from others.[74] Cobb[75] suggests there is evidence that high levels of social support influence recovery from illness, and this facilitation may occur through increased compliance with the prescribed medical regimen. Caplan[76] proposed that having social support implies that the person has an enduring pattern of relationships over time. A social support network provides "psychosocial supplies" for the individual, and these "supplies" provide for the maintenance of health of the individual. "A common impression of social support is that it provides armor to individuals who need it, can find it and use it."[5,p158]

The quality and availability of social support may have an important role in an individual's recovery from or adaptation to an illness or surgery or in preventing illness. For example, social support perceived to be adequate may facilitate the ability to cope with stressful life events or a major crisis, to maintain health, or to adapt to changes.

Conceptualizations of Social Support

Further study is necessary to determine how social support influences health, what types of support are more important under what specific circumstances, and the mechanisms by which social support exerts an influence. Because of the heightened interest in social support as a moderator variable, definitions, conceptualizations, identification of distinguishing characteristics, and the creation of instruments to measure social support have evolved. The major conceptualizations of social support are reviewed in detail elsewhere.[1-11] They are briefly summarized here to provide a context for the selection of an instrument to measure social support.

Definitions and Relationships

Cobb[64] defines social support as the provision of information that leads people to believe they are cared for, loved, esteemed, valued, and a member of a network of communication and mutual obligation. Caplan[77] recognizes that support comes from continuing, enduring relationships. Significant others help to mobilize psychologic resources and master emotional burdens; they are a refuge or sanctuary for stability and comfort. They share tasks and provide material supplies, skills, and cognitive guidance to improve the individual's ability to handle situations.

The perception of having a confidant or at least one close, confiding relationship is a strong indicator of social support.[78] Weiss[79] expressed social relationships as the major construct and identified six multiple functions: (1) social integration; (2) reliable alliance; (3) guidance; (4) opportunity for nurturance; (5) reassurance of worth; and (6) attachment/intimacy. Social integration is provided through a network of relationships in which participants share concerns, information, and ideas. A sense of reliable alliance is provided primarily through relationships with kin in which the person is assured of continuing assistance. Obtaining guidance occurs during stressful situations when the individual seeks emotional support and cognitive guidance from a trusted and authoritative figure. Opportunity for nurturance refers to an adult taking responsibility for the well-being of another. Reassurance of worth occurs through recognition of a person's competence in a social role. Attachment or intimacy refers to gaining a sense of security and place.

Transactions

The conceptualization of social support proposed by House[80] has four supportive behavior categories: emotional, instrumental, informational, and appraisal. These reflect four types of support. *Emotional support* behaviors provide empathy and demonstration of love, trust, and caring. *Instrumental support* behaviors directly help in time of need. *In-*

formational support behaviors provide information that can be used in coping with personal and environmental problems. *Appraisal support* behaviors transmit information relevant to self-evaluation. Kahn[81] conceptualized social support as interpersonal transactions that express positive affect of one person toward another, affirm another's behaviors, perceptions, or expressed views, and provide symbolic or material aid to another person. The term *convoy* denotes the set of significant people through whom support is given or received. The characteristic of reciprocity is included in the conceptualization of social support by both Kahn[81] and Caplan.[77]

Lindsey et al.[4] note that the social support system is a composite of interpersonal relationships that satisfy specific personal social needs. Social support is a component of human relationships. These relationships are the formal and informal social support systems.

Bloom[3] presents a conceptual overview of social support systems and cancer and addresses well the problem of differences and imprecisions in definitions of the multidimensional construct of social support. In Bloom's review, five components of social support were identified: (1) feedback to the individual about himself or herself; (2) the expression of acceptance and affection; (3) tangible material support; (4) information; and (5) affiliative aspects.

Two studies conducted in elderly persons provide examples of differences in conceptualization of social support. Rundall and Evashwick[12] make a distinction between social network and support network in their study of social network and help-seeking among 883 elderly persons. A typology of four categories was developed: engaged, abandoned, trapped, and disengaged. The typology includes the level of interaction with the network and the satisfaction with the level of interaction. The use of health and social services was found to vary with the behavior category (e.g., engaged versus abandoned). Blazer[14] measured the adequacy of social support in 33 older adults (≥65 years) living in a community. Social support was conceptualized as three parameters: (1) roles and available attachments; (2) perceived support; and (3) frequency of social interaction. In this study, all three components of social support predicted mortality.

An individual's social support system is comprised of multiple networks. These include the kinship network (spouse or partner, family members, and other relatives), social and role networks (friends, neighbors, and work associates), professional networks (health-care providers and other professionals), and community networks (church and community groups and agencies).[4]

Family and Support Network

Social support also has been examined in the context of family functioning. Caplan[82] acknowledges that support system functions depend on stability, intactness, and integration of the family. Eight family support system functions of the contemporary U.S. family were identified; examples of these functions are family as collector and disseminator of information, as source of practical service and concrete aid, as source and validation of identity, and as haven for rest and recuperation.[77]

There are distinctions between the support network and perceived or actual social supportive behaviors. A network is the group of people with whom the person has social connections; these formal or informal relationships are described by size, density, and complexity. The network serves such functions as the provision of information and aid. The perceived impact that these network functions have on the person is social support.[28] The extent to which a person believes or feels that the supportive behaviors provided by the network meet his or her needs is the perceived level of social support.

Quantitative descriptions of the social network and network analysis are beyond the scope of this chapter and are available elsewhere.[83]

Some authors suggest that the functional aspects of social support are stronger predictors of health-related outcomes than are the structural aspects, such as network size.[2,34] They make a case for the importance of focusing on the measurement of functional properties of social support particularly in relationship to health outcomes.

The perception of support and the actual support provided may be incongruent. Individual traits, attitudes, and moods can influence both the perceived and the actual support available and provided. In stressful circumstances, a person may include available social support in the appraisal process, and the subsequent seeking of support may be a response to obtain information or other support to deal with the stressful event.[28] The social support available may thus influence the individual's subsequent coping or adaptation to the circumstance.

Demographic Effects

Social support has both qualitative and quantitative dimensions and includes both subjective and objective perceptions. Social support varies according to age and life situation.[71] Social support varies with availability of sources of support, accessibility to those sources, nature and intensity of the relationship, and changes in level of functioning. Thus, measuring social support at one point in time will not reflect this variability. Past experiences, perceived need, and other demands may influence provision and perception of social support available.

Social support is derived from people, places, and activities. Factors influencing the giving or receiving of social support include interpersonal, cultural, environmental, and physical; for example, the geographic proximity of support network members may facilitate or constrain the provision of supportive behaviors. The ability to generate support for oneself also influences the perceived adequacy of social support available. Measurement instruments must be sufficiently sensitive to capture these subtle differences.

Norbeck[11] developed a model that includes elements of social support and nursing practice and proposed relationships between the two that need to be studied. Properties of the individual and of the situation and the influences of these on the need for social support and on the availability of support are described.

Nonsupportive Dimensions

Much of the research and the conceptualization underlying the development of social support measures have emphasized the positive aspects of social support; a few instruments have included the negative dimensions of social support. Tilden and Galyen[32] describe a "darker side" of social support. Others[30,34,80] have noted there may be a "cost" in social relationships; for example, the need for reciprocal exchanges, interpersonal interchanges that are not benevolent, and the stresses of maintaining relationships. Malone[84] suggests that a continuum exists between social support and social dissupport. Much research focuses on the stress-buffering effects of social support and many instruments focus on the supportive dimensions of relationships, but it may be more appropriate to use instruments that tap not only the support aspects but also the "cost" or conflict aspects involved in the perceptions of social support and their effects on health outcomes, as these negative aspects of supportive relationships may have adverse effects.

Gaps and Further Work

There is a need to examine the cost or conflict dimensions of supportive relationships. There is a need to determine levels of social support in healthy people to use as normative data for comparison with levels of social support in people who are ill. There is a need to study the reciprocity of social support, not just the receiving aspect. Some unresolved questions include: identification of the critical supportive behaviors, and how they differ in relation to different stressful life events and in relation to specific health outcomes. What types and sources of support are most important in which circumstances? What are the most important structural properties of social support networks that allow the individual to evaluate the support as being adequate? What is the nature of the support relationships that leads to improved coping or that facilitates adjustment? Are the same elements of social support perceived to be important in all cultures? Bloom[85] challenges researchers to determine how social support contributes to health. It is apparent that many very important questions about social support remain unanswered.

If, in fact, social support is a moderator variable influencing health maintenance and health outcomes, determining the level of perceived social support, the availability of support, the "costs" of support, and the changes in support over time become important clinical considerations. Enhancing or facilitating the quality or quantity of support may be a crucial intervention strategy. If this is the case, there is a need for a measure of social support to document baseline support in health as well as at the time of diagnosis and throughout the illness and treatment trajectory.[86]

Instruments to Measure Social Support

Social support is a multidimensional construct. As yet, there is no universally accepted definition or conceptualization of social support. Efforts to create instruments to measure social support also reflect this range of diversity. For example, Vaux[8] categorized social support instruments into several categories: measures of support network resources; measures of supportive behavior; measures of support appraisals; help-seeking and support mobilization; support incidents; and support participation. Several instruments are included in more than one category, indicating that they tap more than one dimension of support.

Murawski et al.[10] suggest that measurement of social support should determine the individual's interpersonal support system, characteristics of his or her social roles in the primary support group, beliefs about sources of support that would be available during an illness, patterns of social affiliation, and need for social affiliation. The authors perceive these aspects to be critical elements of social support.

A variety of approaches to measure social support have been used. For example, questions were embedded in studies to assess social support resources, such as marital status; frequency of contacts with parents, children, friends; living arrangements; and other indicators of social ties. Other measurement approaches included assessment of the respondent's perceptions of the supportive aspects of their social environments,[87] of receiving supportive behaviors,[27] of satisfaction with support available,[26] and of the potential availability of affect, affirmation, and aid.[24,25]

As recently as 1977, Dean and Lin[66] were unable to locate any social support instruments with known or acceptable reliability or validity data. In 1985, Tardy[88] reviewed seven instruments designed to measure social support. He published brief descriptions and the reported validity and reliability estimates. He suggested that lack of measurement precision in the field precluded theory development and the application of findings to practice. Wood[89] reviewed 11 social support instruments in 1985 and reported similar constraints.

Orth-Gomer and Unden[90] reviewed 16 social support instruments for use in population surveys. They categorized them into two groups: those that measured social network and interaction and those that measured the functional aspects and adequacy of social support. In tabular form they described psychometric data, if reported, for these instruments and the characteristics of the groups used for testing. For those that had available information, they also summarized the predictive capacity of each instrument (e.g., mortality, smoking reduction, and psychologic distress).

Stewart[23,91] reviewed studies conducted by nurse researchers and identified 21 instruments developed by nurses to measure social support. She examined these instruments according to eight dimensions she considered important in the social support literature: type (positive/negative); direction (received/given); disposition (available/enacted); description/evaluation; content (e.g., emotional, instrumental, appraisal); network/source (e.g., family, friends); duration of relationship; and level of support (e.g., satisfaction with, perceived amount of, frequency of interaction). Stewart concluded that the emphasis of most of the nurse-developed measures was emotional (available and enacted) and instrumental support from family and friends. Validity and reliability testing was reported for 7 of the 21 instruments; only six instruments had been used in more than one study. These results are comparable to Norbeck's[92] earlier finding that only 28% of the 40 social support studies used instruments with established validity and reliability.

O'Reilly[93] examined 24 measures of social support on several dimensions; one was the conceptual dimension used for the development of the instrument. Only 14 of the 24 measures were based on some conceptual definition. Problems with operational definitions of social support also were identified. Examples of issues addressed included: whether the support measure was to be used with a general or a specific population; whether the support measure focused on everyday support or support at critical times; and whether the questions addressed who provided the support or what support was provided. Only 11 investigators reported validity and reliability data, and several reported one or the other. O'Reilly also examined nine social network measures. Like others, he clearly distinguishes between measurement of social support and social networks.

Comparing the list of 21 nurse researcher–developed social support instruments[91] with the 24 instruments reviewed by O'Reilly,[93] only one nurse-developed instrument, the Norbeck Social Support Questionnaire,[24,25] was included in the latter list. This suggests that nurse researcher–developed instruments are not being accessed by researchers in disciplines other than nursing.

Rock and colleagues[94] examined the psychometric properties of the social support and social network scales reported in 29 behavioral science studies accessed between 1967 and 1982. They did not distinguish between the two types of measures (support and network), but only six scales also were reviewed by O'Reilly.[93] Only two of the social support measures developed by nurse researchers[16,24,25] were cited by Rock. Originally Rock and colleagues[94] identified 12 criteria to evaluate the psychometric properties of the scales, but found that 8 criteria were not available in the published works. Only three studies included 10 of the 12 criteria; thus, Rock et al. reduced their criteria to four. Only a third of the studies reported reliability estimates.

The reviews cited suggest that there are a number of investigator-developed instruments that purport to measure social support. However, many of these instruments need considerable conceptual and operational development as well as psychometric testing. Others[9,92,95] also have addressed conceptual and methodologic issues in the measurement of social support.

The instruments included in this chapter purport to measure social support or some aspect of it, and represent the instruments for which there is more evidence of validity and reliability estimates. Appendix 11A alphabetically highlights important points as well as psychometric indices of each instrument.

Arizona Social Support Interview Schedule (ASSIS)

The Arizona Social Support Interview Schedule (ASSIS)[27] uses Likert-type scales to determine perceived available social support, perceived need for support, and degree of satisfaction with the support received for the supportive activities specified in seven separate categories: (1) intimate interaction; (2) material aid; (3) advice; (4) physical assistance; (5) positive feedback; (6) social participation; and (7) negative interaction. The inclusion of sources of negative support is a dimension not frequently assessed by social support instruments.

Respondents indicate the persons who are perceived to be available to provide the type of support specified and which persons actually provided that specific support during the past month.[27] The ASSIS can be used to assess the size of the network perceived to be available to provide specific types of support as well as the size of the network that provided actual specific types of support in the past 30 days.

Close Persons Questionnaire (CPQ)

The Close Persons Questionnaire (CPQ) was developed to asses both social network and quality and types of social support (emotional, instrumental, and negative aspects of support) for up to four close persons identified by the respondent.[31] The support questions included assessment of the type of support needed, whether it was received in the last 12 months, and whether more support was desired.

Cost and Reciprocity of Social Support Scale (CARSSS)

A self-report instrument, the Cost and Reciprocity of Social Support Scale (CARSSS), was created to measure the potentially stressful dimensions of supportive relationships.[32] This instrument is unique in this focus. Theories of social exchange and equity were used in conceptualizing this measure. The CARSSS has six subscales: (1) size of network; (2) sources of support; (3) cost; (4) conflict; (5) reciprocity; and (6) equity. The cost subscale, for example, includes items that address time and effort, services, and tangible aid. The conflict subscale has items that address stress, worry, and trouble (reflecting contention or discord). The respondent lists up to 20 individuals perceived to be supportive and indicates their relationship. Twenty-five questions on the cost, conflict, reciprocity, and equity subscales are all rated on a four-point scale from 0 (not at all) to 4 (a great deal) only for the first five persons listed in the network. The authors state that the instrument has undergone repeated revisions based on use with small samples. Although further testing is necessary, this instrument is included in this review because it taps the nonbenevolent components of social support. This dimension is largely excluded from other social support measures.

Duke Social Support and Stress Scale (DSSSS)

The Duke Social Support and Stress Scale (DSSSS) measures family and nonfamily social support and stress.[33] It is a self-report, 24-item questionnaire. Six categories of family are used (spouse or significant other, children/grandchildren, parents/grandparents, brothers/sisters, other blood relatives, and relatives by marriage); four categories of nonfamily members are included (neighbors, coworkers, church members, and other friends). Each support source category is rated as providing no support, some support, or a lot of support. Separate scores are derived for total family support and total nonfamily support. This instrument is somewhat unique in that it assesses social support from the family separate from support provided by nonfamily members. This is a strength if separation of social support from family and nonfamily is of interest.

Duke-UNC Functional Social Support Questionnaire (D-UNC FSSQ)

The Duke-UNC Functional Social Support Questionnaire (D-UNC FSSQ) is a two-scale, eight-item instrument designed for self-administration.[34] Five items assess confidant support, and three items assess affective support. The confidant support items reflect a relationship in which important life matters are discussed and shared; affective support items reflect emotional or caring support. Responses are rated on a five-point Likert scale ranging from "as much as I would like" to "much less than I would like." An example of an item is: "I get . . . love and affection." The authors describe the development and evaluation of the D-UNC FSSQ. However, this instrument measures only two dimensions of social support (confidant support and affective support).

Family Stress and Support Inventory (FSSI)

The Family Stress and Support Inventory (FSSI) is a self-report instrument designed to assess intrafamilial stress and support provided by each family member as perceived by the respondent.[35] For each family member, the respondent rates the amount of stress and the amount of support they feel they receive on a continuum of 1 to 10. The scores can be tabulated by generation (e.g., by grandparent, parent, or children generation), for the whole family, for individual family members, or some other grouping of family members. Arithmetic means of stress and support for each grouping can be determined, and a ratio of stress to support also can be calculated. Development and testing of this instrument with a sample of 382 people are described.

Interpersonal Support Evaluation List (ISEL)

The Interpersonal Support Evaluation List (ISEL)[36,37] measures perceived availability of support for four dimensions of support: tangible, appraisal (informational), belonging (emotional), and self-esteem. There are two forms of the ISEL: one is designed for college students, and the other for use with a general population. However, most of the testing of the general population form has also been done with college student samples (one exception is use with a smoking cessation community sample). The student version of the instrument has 48 statements related to perceived availability of potential social resources, and the general population version has 40 items. Each of the four subscales has 12 and 10 items, respectively. Respondents are asked to indicate whether each statement is probably true or probably false for them. Half of the statements reflect a positive direction, and half are negatively stated. Items for the college student version are based on the elements of social relationships expected for college students. Examples of items for this version are: "I know someone who would loan me $100 to help pay my tuition" or "I hang out in my friend's room or apartment a lot." Examples of items from the general population form are: "If I needed a quick emergency loan of $100, there is someone I could get it from" and "I feel that I'm on the fringe in my circle of friends."

The authors make the case that they designed the ISEL to be different from other measures. They suggest that different types of support are received from the same network persons. The authors also examined the buffering effects of social support on stress using the ISEL. Descriptions of instrument development and testing are well reported.[36,37]

Interview Schedule for Social Interaction (ISSI)

The Interview Schedule for Social Interaction (ISSI) assesses via four subscales the perceived availability and adequacy of social relationships.[38-40] One subscale assesses the availability of confiding and emotionally intimate relationships, a second subscale assesses the availability of more diffuse relationships (e.g., friends, work associates, neighbors), and the other two subscales assess the adequacy and satisfaction with each of the two types of relationships (intimate or more diffuse). The authors describe pilot development of the instrument with various groups of subjects. The final 52-item measure was tested in a general population survey of 151 individuals and also in other samples.

The instrument is designed to be administered as an interview. Four scores are derived: (1) the Availability of Attachment; (2) the Perceived Adequacy of Attachment; (3) the Availability of Social Integration; and (4) the Adequacy of Social Integration. Scoring variations are provided in the report.

The instrument has been found useful to tap the dimensions of social support that reflect interest in specific clinical populations, such as poststroke hospitalized patients.[20] In addition, Unden and Orth-Gomer[41] shortened and adapted the ISSI for use in population surveys. They tested the original and the shortened versions in middle-aged Swedish men and demonstrated the reliability (internal consistency and split-half) and validity of the shorter version. They concluded that the shortened version had no major disadvantages.

IPR Inventory (IPRI)

The IPR Inventory (IPRI) is a 39-item instrument developed to measure interpersonal relationships; it extends the measurement of social support to include reciprocity and conflict.[42] Based on evidence that conflict does occur in social relationships and that it may be deleterious to health, this instrument, by including assessment of conflict, extends beyond the more support-focused aspects of social support measures. Instrument development was based on social exchange and equity theories; thus consideration was given to the cost–benefit ratios of relationships and of reciprocation in relationships. The IPR Inventory was refined from a previous version of a 74-item Interpersonal Relationship Index.[43] The current IPR Inventory has three subscales: (1) social support (13 items); (2) reciprocity (13 items); and (3) conflict (13 items). Stems of the items are provided; examples include: "Someone I could go to . . ." and "Takes advantage of me."

About half the items ($n = 22$) measure perceived sentiment on a five-point Likert-type scale (strongly agree to strongly disagree), and the remaining items ($n = 17$) measure perceived frequency on a five-point continuum (very often to never). Three additional items assess the structural aspects of the support network. Respondents list their network members, indicate household size, and provide information on the proximity of their relatives. The brief descriptions of the underlying theory for conceptualization and construction of this instrument, the type of testing, and the completeness of descriptions of this testing make this a particularly useful reference for instrument development in general, as well as providing data on the reliability and validity of the IPRI.

Inventory of Socially Supportive Behaviors (ISSB)

Barrera et al.[27] developed a 40-item instrument that measures the frequency with which respondents were the recipients of supportive actions. The inventory assesses help received from natural support systems. Scores on the ISSB were significantly correlated with the size of the network and perceived support of the family. The subjects for the initial testing were college students. Social support was conceptualized to include both tangible and intangible forms of assistance, such as provision of goods and services as well as guidance. Each of the 40 items is rated by the respondent on a five-point scale according to the frequency (ranging from 1, not at all, to 5, about every day) with which they occurred during the preceding month. Examples of items are: "Was right there with you (physically) in a stressful situation" and "Helped you understand why you didn't do something well." An important feature of the ISSB is that it can be used to assess the respondents' perceptions of the helping transactions actually received within a specified time. However, the ISSB does not measure the socializing dimension well.[96]

MOS Social Support Survey (MOS SSS)

A good example of instrument development and evaluation is provided for the MOS Social Support Survey (MOS SSS).[44] This instrument was tested on almost 3,000 adult patients in three different geographic locations. It was developed for chronically ill patients in a medical outcomes study. The MOS SSS is a 19-item self-administered questionnaire comprised of four subscales to assess functional dimensions of social support. The subscales are emotional/informational; affectionate; tangible; and positive social interaction. Subscale scores or the total index score can be used. Emphasis is on the perceived availability of support if needed. This instrument assesses the types of support, but not the sources of support. Respondents are asked to indicate on a Likert-type scale from 1 (none of the time) to 5 (all of the time) how often the type of support is available if needed. Examples of items are: "Someone you can count on to listen to you when you need to talk" and "Someone to help with daily chores if you were sick." The instrument also includes one item to measure the structural support dimension, that is, the number of close friends and relatives. Psychometric testing supports the view that social support is multidimensional.

Multidimensional Scale of Perceived Social Support (MSPSS)

The Multidimensional Scale of Perceived Social Support (MSPSS) is a 12-item self-report measure that assesses perceived social support from family, friends, and a significant other.[45-47] Respondents rate the 12 items on a seven-point Likert-type scale ranging from very strongly agree to very strongly disagree. An example of an item is "There is a special person with whom I can share my joys and sorrows." As the psychometric testing has been conducted primarily with college student samples, it is important to test its use with samples that are different.

My Family and Friends (MFF)

My Family and Friends (MFF) is a three-part instrument developed to assess the perceptions of social support of children (6–12 years old).[48] The instrument uses 12 dialogs and props to engage children and obtain information about the availability of individuals to provide social support and the child's level of satisfaction with the type of support received. In developing and testing the instrument, the authors provide evidence that children understand and can differentiate among types of support, e.g., informational, emotional, companionship, and instrumental. They also claim that the instrument is sensitive to variations in perceived social support by the children when there is "family upheaval." Development of the instrument was based on cognitive developmental theory and on the social support work that has been done with adults to differentiate types of social support (emotional, instrumental, affiliative, informational, and conflictual). The addition of a dialog that indicates conflict recognizes there may be some negative interactions in supportive relationships.

The instrument has three parts. The first orients the child and the child identifies support network members. Props are included in the orientation and consist of the following: (1) cards with the names of the people in the child's network (they also may be drawings or pictures of these network members); (2) a board to insert the cards in a ranked order; and (3) a large barometer with a movable indicator with points at intervals of 10 ranging from 0 to 50. The second part engages the child in the 12 dialogs.

There are five dialogs for emotional support, two each for informational, instrumental, and companionship support, and one that focuses on conflict. For each dialog, using the cards and the board, the child ranks the network members in the order in which the child goes to the individual for the type of support indicated in the dialog. After all network members are ranked, using the barometer movable indicator, the child is then asked how satisfied she or he is with the support provided by the individual. The authors recommend administering the 12 dialogs in two 12- to 15-minute sessions to keep the child engaged. The third part is designed to determine other persons who are important to the child (i.e., an inventory of other important people). In testing and using this instrument, the examiners were carefully selected and trained to conduct the interviews with the children. The training was structured and fairly extensive; it occurred in four 3-hour sessions. An example of the dialog stem for emotional support is: "When you want to share your feelings (like feeling happy, sad, or mad). . . ." For each item, the child is asked which person they go to most often. Then, if that person is not available, whom they go to next. For the level of satisfaction for the dialog stem, the questions are: (1) "When you talk to (name of person ranked) about your feelings, how much better do you feel?" and (2) "How good does (name of person ranked) make you feel about yourself or about being you?"

An example of a dialog stem for instrumental support is: "When you need help doing something around the house, such as making or fixing something, finding something you lost, or moving something, who do you go to most often?" The satisfaction level with the instrumental support provided is assessed by the answer to the question "When you go to (name of person ranked) for help, how helpful is she/he?"

The authors note that it is possible to add other dialogs to the instrument, if there are specific areas for which information is desired. For example, constructing dialog about social support during illness or a specific clinical situation may be of interest.

The MFF scale represents significant work in the development of an instrument to measure the perceptions of types of social support in children 6 to 12 years of age and to assess their level of satisfaction with the type of support received. It also allows the addition of dialogs that can be created to be specific for a given situation.

Norbeck Social Support Questionnaire (NSSQ)

The Norbeck Social Support Questionnaire (NSSQ)[24,25] is another instrument that has been developed by nurse researchers to measure the multidimensional construct of social support. It is a short, self-administered questionnaire that taps three major components: functional aspects, network, and loss. Affect, affirmation, and aid are the functional aspects assessed, and number in the network, duration of relationships, and frequency of contact are the network properties measured. Total loss includes the number of "source of support" categories in which a loss occurred and the perceived amount of support lost.

Conceptual definitions of social support proposed by Kahn[81] were used as the theoretical basis for the NSSQ. Social support is defined as "interpersonal transactions that include one or more of the following: the expression of positive affect of one person toward another; the affirmation or endorsement of another person's behaviors, perceptions, or expressed views; the giving of symbolic or material aid to another."[81,p85] The term *convoy* was suggested by Kahn as representing the vehicle for provision of social support: "An individual's convoy at any point in time thus consists of the set of persons on whom he or she relies for support and those who rely on him or her for support."[81,p84] The NSSQ includes items to tap the three supportive transaction components (affect, affirmation, and aid) and to assess representative convoy or network properties (number in network, frequency of contact, and duration of relationships).

The first item on the NSSQ asks the respondent to list each significant person in their life, considering "all the persons who provide personal support for you or who are important to you." For the next set of six questions, the respondent is asked to identify the extent of support provided by each of the individuals listed in the network. For example, one of the questions used for affect is: "How much does this person make you feel liked or loved?" An item used to tap affirmation is: "How much does this person agree with or support your actions or thoughts?" To assess long-term aid, the question used is: "If you were confined to bed for several weeks, how much could this person help you?" The rating scale ranges from 0 (not at all) to 4 (a great deal).

Other items are included to determine the duration of individual relationships (ranging from less than 6 months to more than 5 years), the frequency of contact (ranging from daily, weekly, to once a year or less), and loss (number of persons no longer available to the individual and the amount of support lost). The NSSQ has been used in various populations, such as the elderly,[97] cancer patients [15,18,19] or chronically ill women.[98]

Perceived Social Support from Friends (PSS-Fr) and from Family (PSS-Fa)

Procidano and Heller[28] developed measures of Perceived Social Support from Friends (PSS-Fr) and from Family (PSS-Fa). The authors report that these were separate valid constructs distinct from network. These represent two different source of support categories and tap different dimensions of social relationships. Each of the measures has 20 items; a "yes," "no," or "don't know" response is given for each item. The items include receiving of supportive behaviors and a few that tap the notion of reciprocity, that is, the individual provides support to network members. An example of an item from the PSS-Fr is: "Most other people are closer to their friends than I am." An example of an item from the PSS-Fa is: "I get good ideas about how to do things or make things from my family."

Personal Resource Questionnaire (PRQ) (PRQ85)

Brandt and Weinert[26] developed the Personal Resource Questionnaire (PRQ) as a measure of the multidimensional characteristics of social support. The instrument has two parts. Information about the person's resources and satisfaction with these resources is obtained from part one. Information about the existence of a confidant is obtained from one item in part one. Part two is based on the social relationship dimensions described by Weiss.[79] There is a 25-item Likert scale and a five-item self-help ideology scale included as part two of the PRQ.

Eight life situations were created for part one of the PRQ. The situations include circumstances in which the person may need assistance, and the respondent is asked to whom or what they could turn to for help (e.g., no one, spouse, child, relative, friend, spiritual advisor, professional person, agency, books, or prayer). Following identification of the sources of support, the individual is asked whether he or she has actually experienced the situation recently and, if so, what was the extent of satisfaction felt with the assistance obtained.

Part two has five items for each of Weiss's five social relationship dimensions[79] (intimacy, social integration, nurturance, worth, and assistance). A seven-point Likert scale is used for the respondent to rate each of 25 items from "strongly agree" to "strongly disagree." A sample item is: "Sometimes I can't count on my relatives and friends to help me with important problems." The last five items of part two of the PRQ estimated the respondents' ideologic stance toward self-help. These items were used to determine whether the PRQ was measuring the constructs of social support.[26] Development of the PRQ is reported as part of a study in which the PRQ was used as a measure of social support; the stress of long-term illness (multiple sclerosis) on the well spouses and family functioning was investigated.

Quality of Relationships Inventory (QRI)

The Quality of Relationships Inventory (QRI) assesses relationship-based perceptions of social support and conflict.[53] This instrument is unique in that it provides for examination of relationship-specific perceptions on three subscales (support, conflict, and depth of relationship) rather than generalized perception of social support. Respondents complete the 29-item instrument for mother, father, and up to four other relationships they consider important, such as a friend. Examples of items include: "To what extent can you turn to this person for advice about problems?" and "How often does this person make you feel angry?" Results from their instrument development testing support the underlying hypothesis that perceptions of relationship-specific support are distinct from the perceptions of general support.

Social Support Appraisals Scale (SSAS)

The 23-item Social Support Appraisals Scale (SSAS) examines the extent to which a person feels loved, respected, and involved with family, friends, or others.[54,55] The instrument development was based on Cobb's[64] conceptualization of social support. The scale can be scored as a total measure, or scores can be determined for family (8 items) and for friends (7 items). The respondents rate the items on a four-point scale from 1 (strongly agree) to 4 (strongly disagree). Examples of items are: "My friends respect me" and "Members of my family don't rely on me." Descriptions of the testing of this instrument are quite helpful for those interested in instrument development.

Social Support Behaviors (SSB)

The Social Support Behaviors (SSB) is a 45-item instrument developed to assess five types of support: emotional, assistance, financial, guidance, and socializing.[56] Respondents indicate how likely a family member or a friend would be to provide the type of supportive behavior characterized in the items if needed. Perceptions of the supportive behaviors of family members and of friends are assessed separately. Examples of items are: "Visited with me or invited me over" and "Gave me a ride where I needed it."

Social Support Questionnaire (SSQ)

Another measure of social support, the Social Support Questionnaire (SSQ), has been developed and tested by Sarason et al.[29] Scores for the perceived number of social supports and satisfaction with the social support available are obtained using the SSQ. The SSQ consists of 27 items, each of which asks the respondent to list the people on whom they can rely for the set of circumstances described and to indicate the degree of satisfaction they have with the support provided. An example of an item is: "Whom do you really count on to be dependable when you need help?" One of the options allows the respondent to answer "no one," but then the degree of satisfaction with the support is still rated (ranging 1 to 6 points from "very satisfied" to "very dissatisfied").

Social Support Questionnaire (SSQ)

Schaefer et al.[30] developed and used another instrument, the Social Support Questionnaire. It is a two-part questionnaire. Nine situations are presented in part one as a measure of tangible support; in part two, the respondent lists network members by specific categories, such as spouse, friends, work or school associates, and so forth, and then is asked to rate the people listed for one question about informational support and for four questions about emotional support. An example of an item from part one is: "Often people rely on the judgment of someone they know in making important decisions about their lives. Is there anyone whose opinion you consider seriously in making important decisions about your family?" Respondents list the individual(s) by initials and check the appropriate relational category. The informational question in part two is: "How much did this person give you information, suggestions and guidance over the last month that you found helpful?" One of the emotional items is: "How much does this person boost your spirits when you feel low?"

For part two questions, the ratings range from 1, not at all, 2, slightly, to 5, extremely. The conceptualization and health-related functions of social support are described by Schaefer et al.[30] The SSQ and the Brandt and Weinert[26] PRQ have been administered concurrently with the NSSQ, and the findings are reported.[24,25]

Social Support Rating Scale (SSRS)

The Social Support Rating Scale (SSRS) developed by Cauce and colleagues[57,58] is one of the few instruments created for use with children and adolescents. Respondents indicate on a five-point Likert scale the extent to which persons provide emotional support and caring, help, and guidance and the extent to which the person may have upset them. On a seven-point Likert scale they indicate the extent of their satisfaction with the emotional support and help provided and the extent to which they are the type of person who seeks help. The instrument also allows the examination of separate sources of support.

Social Support Scale (SSS)

Funch and colleagues[59] describe the development and use of a short scale to measure social support that can be modified for specific situations, such as support when goal is weight loss/dieting. This is a somewhat unique approach in terms of examining the specificity of social support relative to some particular desired health outcome. An example of an item they used with subjects in a health maintenance organization who were involved in a weight loss program is: "When people try to diet, the people around them can sometimes help and sometimes make things harder, even if they don't realize it." The respondent is asked to indicate on a Likert-type scale, ranging from 1 (not at all helpful) to 5 (completely helpful), how helpful each person (spouse, children, other relatives, friends, coworkers) is relative to the specific situation described. More work is required in establishing the psychometric properties of the SSS, but the idea of measuring social support specifically in relationship to an identified health outcome is very important.

Social Support Instruments for Special Populations

A few social support instruments have been designed to be used with specific populations. Investigators are devoting effort to developing measures that are more sensitive to the particular social support needs of specific groups, such as mothers and stroke survivors. Specific situation examination of social support may be more helpful in some cases than is a global assessment. Selected instruments are presented. Their psychometric properties are highlighted in Appendix 11B.

Hughes Breastfeeding Support Scale (HBSS)

An example of beginning development of an instrument for a specific population is the Hughes Breastfeeding Support Scale (HBSS).[60] The 30-item instrument is designed to assess emotional (10 items), instrumental (10 items), and informational (10 items) support as perceived by breastfeeding mothers. It is a self-administered questionnaire using a 1-to-4 Likert-type scale format. Although the HBSS is designed to measure support in a specific population, some of the 30 items also tap the global dimensions of social support. Examples of specific and more global items are: "Answered my questions about breastfeeding" and "Showed concern when I felt blue." This instrument, like many others, needs further testing to establish acceptable psychometric properties, but it is included here because it is an example of a measure of support in a specific situation.

Maternal Social Support Index (MSSI)

The Maternal Social Support Index (MSSI) was developed to assess a mother's perception of the amount of social support (emotional and tangible) and her satisfaction with the support provided.[61] It is a 21-question tool that can be self-administered and obtains information in seven areas: (1) help with daily tasks; (2) satisfaction with visits from kin; (3) help with crises; (4) emergency child care; (5) satisfaction with communication from male partner (6) from another support person; and (7) community involvement. An example of one of the 10 questions related to help with daily tasks is: "Who does the grocery shopping?"

Whether the social support measured by this instrument specific to mothers would be similar to that measured by the more global measures of social support remains unknown. However, it may be useful to think of social support in more specific contexts, such as in relationship to the role of a mother. This specific examination of social support may be more helpful in some cases than a global assessment.

Support Behaviors Inventory (SBI)

The Support Behaviors Inventory (SBI) was developed to use with expectant couples.[62] It is a 45-item instrument where half of the items specifically reference pregnancy and the other half are generally applicable. The items were developed from the generation of a list of supportive behaviors identified in interviews with expectant parents. The author used House's[80] typology as the basis for the four categories of support: emotional, material, informational, and appraisal. On a six-point scale, respondents are asked to indicate the degree of satisfaction (1 very dissatisfied to 6 very satisfied) they experience for each supportive behavior, first for their partner relationship and then their satisfaction of support from other people. Two scores are derived: one is satisfaction with partner support score, and the other is satisfaction with other people support. Conceptually, most instruments have been developed on the theory that social support is multidimensional; however, discriminant validity and factor analytic testing of the SBI suggest a broad, single dimension. Obviously, further study of this issue is required. Other studies with other instruments do support the multidimensionality of social support.

Social Support in Chronic Illness Inventory (SSCII)

Development of the Social Support in Chronic Illness Inventory (SSCII)[99] was based on Kahn's[81] concept of convoy and a model of stress, coping, and health. It is designed for use with people with chronic illnesses, such as diabetes, hypertension, end-stage renal disease, or cardiac disease. The instrument can be completed by the chronically ill individual or the provider of support. Respondents are asked to indicate the degree of satisfaction with the specified supportive behaviors. It is designed to examine perceived satisfaction with each supportive behavior relative to a specific situation, chronic illness, and the analysis is a dyadic or group relationship rather than from a support network perspective.

The SSCII is a 38-item measure (9 are chronic illness specific) using a six-point Likert scale that ranges from 1 (dissatisfied) to 6 (very satisfied). It has four subscales: (1) intimate interaction; (2) guidance/feedback; (3) tangible assistance; and (4) positive social interaction. The respondents rate each item for one individual they identify as being the most important to them at the present time. Examples of these items are: "Provided transportation for me" and "Helped me understand about my disease."

Social Support Inventory for Stroke Survivors (SSISS)

The Social Support Inventory for Stroke Survivors (SSISS) is a self-report inventory to be used in a structured interview format; it taps eight aspects of social support.[63] The sources of social support are personal, friend, and community and professional groups; support is measured by the three dimensions of quality, quantity, and satisfaction. Some inventory items are specific to stroke (e.g., change in available support since the stroke). The inventory is scored by the three dimensions for each of the five sources of support and by each of the dimensions across all five support sources, resulting in eight scores. Preliminary estimates suggest that the inventory has merit with a stroke-specific population, but additional testing is required to establish acceptable psychometric properties.

Examples of Instruments Related to Social Support

A variety of other instruments purport to measure some aspects or concepts relevant to social support, but they do not measure social support specifically. A full description of these instruments is beyond the confines of this chapter, but several are included as illustrations.

Family Environment Scale (FES)

A related measure is the Family Environment Scale (FES) consisting of 10 subscales (90 true–false statements) designed to obtain subjective assessments of the respondent's family social environment.[87,100,101] However, social environment, although possibly contributing to or influencing, is conceptually different from social support. This tool, however, may capture some aspects of the context necessary for social support.

Interview Measure of Social Relationships (IMSR)

The Interview Measure of Social Relationships (IMSR) measures the size and density of the primary network group, the contacts and acquaintances of others, the supportiveness of relationships, adequacy of interactions, and crisis support.[102]

Self-Evaluation and Social Support Schedule (SESSS)

The Self-Evaluation and Social Support Schedule (SESSS) was created as an interview-based instrument to provide a comprehensive description of an individual's social milieu.[103] It is lengthy and complex and examines women's beliefs and attitudes about relationships and activities; it includes an assessment of actual behavior. Thus, although it is related to the measurement of social support, the dimensions assessed by this instrument are more inclusive.

Selection of a Measure of Social Support

With the current surge of interest in social support, additional measures will be created and existing instruments will be revised and refined. Some social support measures include both general social support items as well as situation-specific support items. Some instruments are very short and others are lengthy; some have been designed to be completed in a reasonable time for clinically ill people. Many measures, however, were tested with college-age students and thus will require testing with other populations, particularly if they are to be used with clinical samples.

Whether selecting an instrument for purposes of clinical assessment or to measure a variable for research, similar criteria need to be used in the selection process. There are some major considerations. The primary question is, does the instrument purport to measure the phenomenon or variable of interest and does it tap the major dimensions of interest to you? Are the clinical, theoretical, and empirical premises/bases from which the conceptualizations of the instrument items were derived explicit and congruent with your clinical or research focus? If it is of interest to measure a variable, such as social support, over time, it is important to determine whether the instrument is a sufficiently sensitive measure for changes to be detected.

Space limitations in a book chapter place constraints on providing a full description of every social support measure, the theoretical basis (when available) for the construction of the instrument, a full description and critique of the validity and reliability and other psychometric testing, and descriptions of samples used in the instrument development phases. In all cases, when selecting an instrument, it is necessary to review the original information given about the conceptual basis used to develop the measure, the samples for which it was designed, and the psychometric properties. As indicated throughout this chapter, although there are many choices of instruments designed to measure social support or some dimensions of it, not all are at the same level of development. For additional information about selecting an instrument, refer to Chapter 1.

Summary

Social support is one component of the human context of the individual's social environment. Early work has suggested that social support plays a role in mediating the effects of stressful life events, in protecting health, and in buffering against stressful circumstances or crises. Conceptualizations and measurement of social support remain varied, and several instruments designed to measure one or more dimension of social support are available and have published validity and reliability data. Many instruments require further psychometric testing. The final selection of an instrument must be based on the congruency between what variable(s) you want to measure and what dimension(s) an instrument has been designed to assess.

As reflected in the diverse dimensions of social support assessed by the various instruments, there is as yet no universally accepted definition of social support. Although most authors have viewed social support as multidimensional, and most instruments have been developed to tap one or more dimensions of social support, a few investigators have found that the subscales of the instruments they have used are very highly intercorrelated and that factor analytic techniques yield one dominant factor, suggesting that social support be viewed as one major construct. Many other investigators have found some dimensions/subscales to be separate, lending support to the contention that social support is a multidimensional construct. Obviously, much more work is required.

Beyond instrument development and selection, the future emphasis must be to determine more specifically how social support, or how various social support functions, affects situation- and population-specific health outcomes.

Exemplar Study: Measuring Social Support

McNett, S.C. Social Support, Threat, and Coping Responses and Effectiveness in the Functionally Disabled. *Nurs Res*, 1987 *36*(2):98-103.

Social support and coping were studied in a sample of 50 functionally disabled, wheelchair-bound adults discharged from rehabilitation facilities. Perceived availability of social support was significantly positively related to coping effectiveness, but not use of social support. The strengths of the study include use of theoretical bases, hypothesized causal model, some standardized instruments, and discussion of analysis and findings relevant to theoretical contentions.

This study was selected for several reasons as an example of research that has incorporated social support as a variable. The reasons for selection include: the discussion of the theoretical underpinnings of the selection of variables to be studied; the development and graphic depiction of a hypothesized causal model; the use of some standardized instruments and some investigator-developed items; the selection of a clinical population as subjects; and the discussion of findings based on the model and the evidence for the support or lack thereof for the theoretical bases. McNett[104] studied perceived availability, effectiveness, and use of social support in 50 functionally disabled, wheelchair-bound individuals. She created and tested a causal model to determine the effects of social support variables, threat appraisal, and coping responses on coping effectiveness.

She adapted the Interpersonal Support Evaluation List (ISEL) to measure the availability of support (tangible, informational, and belonging). The self-esteem subscale of this instrument was not used because it was viewed as being a potentially confounding variable for another measure selected to measure coping effectiveness. McNett reported the adapted ISEL internal consistency reliability for her study sample as 0.96; she found the three subscales to have high intercorrelations and thus combined them for a total social support score for the analysis. Investigator-developed items were used to determine perceived effectiveness of social support and perceived personal constraints. Other instruments were used to measure the other variables. There is ample description of the analyses used. From the path analysis using a LISREL computer program, the indices suggested the model fit the data. For additional reference, see another example of path analysis in the social support field.[105]

McNett found, that for this group of wheelchair-bound functionally disabled individuals, the perceived availability of social support was significantly (1) positively related to coping effectiveness via mediating variables (emotion and problem-focused coping); (2) positively related to the use of social support; and (3) related to reduced threat appraisal. In contrast, use of social support was not significantly related to coping effectiveness, but use of social support was positively related to perceived effectiveness of social support. The discussion section considers these and other findings in relation to the theoretical contentions that guided the study.

Many of the instrument development reports also include studies. Those interested in additional examples are referred to those reports[24,63] and to other studies referenced in this chapter.[12-23]

References

1. Wortman, C.B. Social support and the cancer patient. Conceptual and methodological issues. *Cancer,* 1984, *53*(suppl.):2339.
2. House, J.S., & Kahn, R.L. Measures and concepts of social support. In S. Cohen & L. Syme (Eds.), *Social support and health.* New York: Academic, 1985, p. 83.
3. Bloom, J.R. Social support systems and cancer: A conceptual view. In J. Cohen, J.W. Culler, & L.R. Martin (Eds.), *Psychosocial aspects of cancer.* New York: Raven, 1982, p. 129.
4. Lindsey, A.M., Norbeck, J.S., Carrieri, V.L., & Perry, E. Social support and health outcomes in postmastectomy women: A review. *Cancer Nurs,* 1981, *4*(5):377.
5. Bruhn, J.G., & Philips, B.U. Measuring social support: A synthesis of current approaches. *J Behav Med,* 1994, *7*(2):151.
6. Barrera, N., & Ainlay, S.L. The structure of social support: A conceptual and empirical analysis. *J Comm Psychol,* 1983, *11*(April):133-143.
7. Stewart, M.J. Social support: Diverse theoretical perspectives. *Soc Sci Med,* 1989, *28*(12):1275-1282.
8. Vaux, A. *Social Support Theory, Research and Intervention.* New York: Praeger, 1988.
9. Tilden, V.P. Issues of conceptualization and measurement of social support in the construction of nursing theory. *Res Nurs Health,* 1985, *8*(2):199-206.
10. Murawski, B.J., Penman, D., & Schmitt, M. Social support in health and illness: The concept and its measurement. *Cancer Nurs,* 1978, *1*(5):365.
11. Norbeck, J.S. Social support: A model for clinical research and application. *Adv Nurs Sci,* 1981, *3*(4):43.
12. Rundall, T.G., & Evashwick, C. Social networks and help-seeking among the elderly. *Res Aging,* 1982, *4*(2):205.
13. Berkman, L.F., & Syme, S.L. Social networks, host resistance and mortality: A year follow-up study of Alameda County residents. *Am J Epidemiol,* 1979, *109*(2):186.
14. Blazer, D.G. Social support and mortality in an elderly community population. *Am J Epidemiol,* 1982, *115*(5):684.
15. Lindsey, A.M., Ahmed, N., & Dodd, M. Social support network and quality as perceived by Egyptian cancer patients. *Cancer Nurs,* 1985, *8*(1):37.
16. Dimond, M. Social support and adaptation to chronic illness: The case of maintenance hemodialysis. *Res Nurs Health,* 1979, *2*(3):101.
17. Fitzpatrick, R., Newman, S., Archer, R., & Shipley, M. Social support, disability, and depression: A longitudinal study of rheumatoid arthritis. *Soc Sci Med,* 1991, *33*(5):605-611.
18. Larson, P.J., Lindsey, A.M., Dodd, M.J., et al. Influence of age on problems experienced by patients with lung cancer undergoing radiation therapy. *Oncol Nurs Forum,* 1993, *20*(3):473-480.
19. Lindsey, A.M., Larson, P., Dodd, M., et al., Co-morbidity, nutritional intake, social support, weight, and functional status over time in older cancer patients receiving radiation therapy. *Cancer Nurs,* 1994, *17*(2):113-124.
20. Morris, P.L.P., Robinson, R.G., Raphael, B., & Bishop, D. The relationship between the perception of social support and post-stroke depression in hospitalized patients. *Psychiatry,* 1991, *54*(August):306-315.
21. Norbeck, J.S., & Anderson, N.J. Life stress, social support, and anxiety in mid- and late-pregnancy among low income women. *Res Nurs Health,* 1989, *12*(5):281-287.
22. Norbeck, J.S., & Anderson, N.J. Psychosocial predictors of pregnancy outcomes in low-income black, Hispanic and white women. *Nurs Res,* 1989, *38*(4):204-209.
23. Stewart, M.J. Social support intervention studies: A review and prospectus of nursing contributions. *Int J Nurs Stud,* 1989, *26*(2):93-114.
24. Norbeck, J.S., Lindsey, A.M., & Carrieri, V.L. The development of an instrument to measure social support. *Nurs Res,* 1981, *30*(5):264.
25. Norbeck, J.S., Lindsey, A.M., & Carrieri, V.L. Further development of the Norbeck social support questionnaire: Normative data and validity testing. *Nurs Res,* 1983, *32*(1):4.
26. Brandt, P.A., & Weinert, C. The PRQ-A social support measure. *Nurs Res,* 1981, *30*(5):277.
27. Barrera, N., Sandler, I.N., & Ramsay, T.B. Preliminary development of a scale of social support: Studies on college students. *Am J Comm Psychol,* 1981, *9*(4):435.
28. Procidano, M.E., & Heller, K. Measures of perceived social support from friends and from family: Three validations studies. *Am J Community Psychol,* 1983, *11*(1):1.
29. Sarason, I.G., Levine, H.M., Basham, R.B., & Sarason, R. Assessing social support: The social support questionnaire. *J Pers Soc Psychol,* 1983, *44*(1):127.
30. Schaefer, C., Coyne, J.C., & Lazarus, R. The health-related functions of social support. *J Behav Med,* 1981, *4*(4):381.
31. Stansfeld, S., & Marmot, M. Deriving a survey measure of social support: The reliability and validity of the Close Persons Questionnaire. *Soc Sci Med,* 1992, *35*(8):1027-1035.
32. Tilden, V.P., & Galyen, R.D. Cost and conflict. The darker side of social support. *West J Nurs Res,* 1987, *9*(1):9-18.
33. Parkerson, G.R., Nichener, J.L., Wu, L.R., et al., Associations among family support, family stress, and personal functional health status. *J Clin Epidemiol,* 1989, *2*(3):217-229.
34. Broadhead, W.E., Gehlbach, S.H., deGruy, E.V., & Kaplan, B.H. The Duke-UNC Functional Social Support Questionnaire: A measurement of social support in family medicine patients. *Med Care,* 1988, *26*(7):709-723.
35. Halvorsen, J.G. The Family Stress and Support Inventory. *Fam Prac Res,* 1991, *11*(3):255-277.
36. Cohen, S., & Hoberman, H. Positive events and social supports as buffers of life change stress. *J App Soc Psychol,* 1983, *13*(2):99-125.
37. Cohen, S.C., Mermelstein, R., Kamarck, T., & Hoberman, H. Measuring the functional components on social support. In I. Sarason and B. Sarason (Eds.), *Social Support: Theory, Research, and Application.* The Hague, Holland: Martin Niijhoff, 1985, pp. 73-94.

38. Henderson, S., Duncan-Jones, P., Byrne, D., & Scott, R. Measuring social relationships: The Interview Schedule for Social Interaction. *Psychol Med*, 1980, 10(4):723-734.

39. Duncan-Jones, P. (1981). The structure of social relationships: Analysis of a survey instrument, Part I. *Soc Psychiatry*, 1981, 16(2):55-61.

40. Duncan-Jones, P. The structure of social relationships: Analysis of a survey instrument, Part II. *Soc Psychiatry*, 1981, 16(3):143-149.

41. Unden, A-L, & Orth-Gomer, K. Development of a social support instrument for use in population surveys. *Soc Sci Med*, 1989, 29(12):1387-1392.

42. Tilden, V.P., Nelson, C.A., & May, B.A. The IPR Inventory: Development and psychometric characteristics. *Nurs Res*, 1990, 39(6):337-343.

43. Tilden, V.P., Nelson, C.A., & May, B.A. Using qualitative methods to enhance the content validity of a measure. *Nurs Res*, 1990, 39(3):172-175.

44. Sherbourne, C.D., & Stewart, A.L. The MOS Social Support Survey. *Soc Sci Med*, 1991, 32(6):705-714.

45. Zimet, G.D., Dahlem, N.W., Zimet, S.G., & Farley, G.K. The Multidimensional Scale of Perceived Social Support. *J Pers Assess*, 1988, 52(1):30-41.

46. Zimet, G.D., Powell, S.S., Farley, G.K., et al. Psychometric characteristics of the Multidimensional Scale of Perceived Social Support. *J Pers Assess*, 1990, 55(3-4), 610-617.

47. Dahlem, N.W., Zimet, G.D., & Walker, R.R. The Multidimensional Scale of Perceived Social Support: A confirmation study. *J Clin Psychol*, 1991, 47(6):756-761.

48. Reid, N., Landesman, S., Treder, R., & Jaccard, J. "My Family and Friends": Six- to twelve-year-old children's perceptions of social support. *Child Dev*, 1989, 60(4):896-910.

49. Weinert, C., & Brandt, P.A. Measuring social support with the Personal Resource Questionnaire. *West J Nurs Res*, 1987, 9(4):589-602.

50. Weinert, C. Measuring social support: Revision and further development of the Personal Resource Questionnaire. In C.F. Waltz & O.L. Strickland (Eds.) *Measurement of nursing outcomes. Vol. 1. Measuring client outcomes*. New York: Springer, 1988, pp. 309-320.

51. Weinert, C., & Tilden, V.P. Measures of social support: Assessment of validity. *Nurs Res*, 1990, 39(4):212-216.

52. Yarcheski, A., Mahon, N.E., & Yarcheski, T.J. Validation of the PRQ85 social support measure for adolescents. *Nurs Res*, 1992, 41(6):332-337.

53. Pierce, G.R., Sarason, I.G., & Sarason, B.R. General and relationship-based perceptions of social support: Are two constructs better than one? *J Pers Soc Psychol*, 1991, 61(6):1028-1039.

54. Vaux, A., Phillips, J., Holly, L., et al. The Social Support Appraisals (SS-A) Scale: Studies of reliability and validity. *Am J Commun Psychol*, 1986, 14(2):195-219.

55. Vaux, A. Appraisals of social support: Love, respect, and involvement. *J Commun Psychol*, 1987, 15(October):493-502.

56. Vaux, A., Riedel, S., & Stewart, D. Models of social support: The Social Support Behaviors (SS-B) Scale. *Am J Commun Psychol*, 1987, 15(2):209-237.

57. Cauce, A., Felner, R., & Primavera, J. Social support in high risk adolescents: Structural components and adaptive impact. *Am J Commun Psychol*, 1982, 10(4):417-428.

58. Cauce, A. Social networks and social competence: Exploring the effects of early adolescent friendships. *Am J Commun Psychol*, 1986, 14(6):607-628.

59. Funch, D.P., Marshall, J.R., & Gebhardt, G.P. Assessment of a short scale to measure social support. *Soc Sci Med*, 1986, 23(3):337-344.

60. Hughes, R.B. The development of an instrument to measure perceived emotional, instrumental, and informational support in breastfeeding mothers. *Issues Comp Pediatr Nurs*, 1984, 7(6):357-362.

61. Pascoe, J.M., Ialongo, N.S., Horn, W.F., et al. The reliability and validity of the Maternal Social Support Index. *Fam Med*, 1988, 20(4):271-276.

62. Brown, M.A. Social support during pregnancy: A unidimensional or multidimensional construct? *Nurs Res*, 1986, 35(1):4-9.

63. Friedland, J., & McColl, M.A. Social support and psychosocial dysfunction after stroke: Buffering effects in a community sample. *Arch Phys Med Rehab*, 1987, 68(8):475-480.

64. Cobb, S. Social support as a moderator of life stress. *Psychosom Med*, 1976, 38(5):300.

65. Kaplan, B.H., Cassel, J.C., & Gore, S. Social support and health. *Med Care*, 1977, 15(suppl 5):47.

66. Dean, A., & Lin, N. The stress buffering role of social support. *J Nerv Ment Dis*, 1977, 165(6):403.

67. Kahn, R., & Antonucci, T. Convoys over the life course: Attachment, roles and social support. In P.B. Baltes & O. Brim (Eds.), *Life-span development and behavior* (vol. 3). New York: Academic, 1981, p. 253.

68. Broadhead, W.E., Kaplan, B.H., James, S.A., et al. The epidemiologic evidence for a relationship between social support and health. *Am J Epidemiol*, 1983, 117(5):521.

69. Nuckolls, J.B., Cassel, J., & Kaplan, B.H. Psychosocial assets, life crisis and the prognosis of pregnancy. *Am J Epidemiol*, 1972, 95(5):431.

70. Lin, N., Simeone, R., Ensel, W., & Kuo, W. Social support, stressful life events and illness: A model and an empirical test. *J Health Soc Behav*, 1979, 20(2):108.

71. Pilisuk, M., & Froland, C. Kinship, social networks, social support and health. *Soc Sci Med*, 1978, 12(B):273.

72. Cassel, J. The contribution of the social environment to host resistance. *Am J Epidemiol*, 1976, 104(2):107.

73. Heller, K. The effects of social support: Prevention and treatment implications. In A.P. Goldstein & F.H. Kanfer (Eds.), *Maximizing treatment gains: Transfer enhancement in psychotherapy*. New York: Academic, 1979, p. 353.

74. Croog, S.H., Lipson, A., & Levine, S. Help patterns in severe illness: The roles of kin network, non-family resources and institutions. *J Marriage Fam*, 1972, 34:32.

75. Cobb, S. Social support and health through the life course. In H.I. McCubbin, A.E. Cauble, & J.M. Patterson (Eds.), *Family stress, coping and social support*. Springfield, IL: Charles C. Thomas, 1982, p. 189.

76. Caplan, G. *Support systems and community mental health*. New York: Behavioral Publications, 1974.

77. Caplan, G. The family as a support system. In G. Caplan & M. Killilea (Eds.), *Support systems and mutual help: Multidisciplinary explorations.* New York: Grune & Stratton, 1976, p. 19.

78. Conner, K.A., Powers, E.A., & Bultera, G.L. Social interaction and life satisfaction: An empirical assessment of late-life patterns. *J Gerontol,* 1979, *34*(1):116.

79. Weiss, R. The provision of social relationships. In Z. Rubin (Ed.), *Doing unto others.* Englewood Cliffs, NJ: Prentice-Hall, 1974, p. 17.

80. House, J.S. *Work stress and social support.* Reading, MA: Addison-Wesley, 1981.

81. Kahn, R.L. Aging and social support. In M.W. Riley (Ed.), *Aging from birth to death: Interdisciplinary perspectives.* Boulder, CO: Westview Press for American Association for the Advancement of Science, 1979, p. 77.

82. Caplan, G. The family as a support system. In H.I. McCubbin, A.E. Cauble, & J.M. Patterson (Eds.), *Family stress, coping and social support.* Springfield, IL: Charles C. Thomas, 1982, p. 200.

83. Mitchell, R.E., & Trickett, E.J. Social networks as mediators of social support: An analysis of the effects and determinants of social networks. *Comm Ment Health J,* 1980, *16*(1):27.

84. Malone, J. The social support dissupport continuum. *J Psychosoc Nurs,* 1988, *26*(12), 18-22.

85. Bloom, J.R. The relationship of social support and health. *Soc Sci Med,* 1990, *30*(5):635-637.

86. Lindsey, A.M. Social support: Selection of a measurement instrument. *Oncol Nurs Forum,* 1984, *11*(2):88.

87. Moos, R.H. *Evaluating educational environments: Procedures, measures, findings, and policy implications.* San Francisco: Jossey-Bass, 1979.

88. Tardy, C.H. Social support measurement. *Am J Comm Psychol,* 1985, *13*(2):187-202.

89. Wood, Y.R. Social support and social networks: Nature and measurement. In P. McReynolds & G.J. Chelune (Eds.), *Advances in Psychological Assessment.* San Francisco: Jossey-Bass, 1985, pp. 312-353.

90. Orth-Gomer, K., & Uden, A.L. The measurement of social support in population surveys. *Soc Sci Med,* 1987, *24*(1):83-94.

91. Stewart, M.J. Social support instruments created by nurse investigators. *Nurs Res,* 1989, *38*(5):268-275.

92. Norbeck, J.S. Social support. *Ann Rev Nurs Res,* 1988, *6*:85-109.

93. O'Reilly, P. Methodological issues in social support and social network research. *Soc Sci Med,* 1988, *26*(8):863-873.

94. Rock, D.L., Green, K.E., Wise, B.K., & Rock, R.D. Social support and social network scales: A psychometric review. *Res Nurs Health,* 1984, *7*(4):325-332.

95. Depner, C.E., Wethington, E., & Ingersoll-Dayton, B. Social support: Methodological issues in design and measurement. *J Soc Issues,* 1984, *40*(4):37-54.

96. Stokes, J.P., & Wilson, D.G. The inventory of socially supportive behaviors: Dimensionality, prediction and gender differences. *Am J Commun Psychol,* 1984, *12*(1):53-69.

97. Nelson, P.B. Social support, self-esteem, and depression in the institutionalized elderly. *Issues Ment Health Nurs,* 1989, *10*(1):55-68.

98. Primomo, J., Yates, B.C., & Woods, N.F. Social support for women during chronic illness: The relationship among sources and types to adjustment. *Res Nurs Health,* 1990, *13*(3):153-161.

99. Hilbert, G. Measuring social support in chronic illness. In O. Strickland & C. Waltz (Eds.), *Measurement of nursing outcomes. Vol. 4. Measuring clients self care and coping skills.* New York: Springer, 1990, pp. 79-91.

100. Moos, R., & Moos, B. *Family Environment Scale Manual* (2nd ed.). Palo Alto, CA: Consulting Psychologists Press, 1986.

101. Roosa, N.W., & Beals, J. Measurement issues in family assessment: The case of the Family Environment Scale. *Family Process,* 1990, *29*(2):191-208.

102. Brugha, T.S., Stuart, E., MacCarthy, B., et al. The Interview Measure of Social Relationships: The description and evaluation of a survey instrument for assessing personal social resources. *Soc Psychiatr,* 22(2):123-138.

103. Brown, G.W., Bifulco, A., Veiel, H.O.F., & Andrews, B., Self-esteem and depression. II. Social correlates of self-esteem. *Soc Psychiatr Epidemiol,* 1990, *25*(5):225-234.

104. McNett, S.C. Social support, threat, and coping responses and effectiveness in the functionally disabled. *Nurs Res,* 1987, *36*(2):98-103.

105. Vaux, A., & Wood, J. Social support resources, behavior, and appraisals: A path analysis. *Soc Behav Pers,* 1987, *15*(1):105-109.

Appendices

11A. Measures of Social Support

Instrument	Description	Psychometric Indices
Arizona Social Support Interview Schedule (ASSIS) (27)	Uses Likert-type scale to determine: perceived available social support, perceived need for support, degree of satisfaction with the support received; 7 categories: intimate interaction, material aid, advice, physical assistance, positive feedback, social participation, negative interaction) Respondents indicate persons perceived to be available to provide type of support specified, and which persons actually provided the support during the past month Useful in assessing size of perceived and actual support networks Assesses dimension of sources of negative support	Frequency of socially supportive interactions measured by Inventory of Socially Supportive Behaviors (ISSB) correlated moderately yet significantly with ASSIS social support network size of those available and those actually providing support (27)
Close Persons Questionnaire (CPQ) (31)	Assesses both social network and quality and types of social support (emotional, instrumental, negative aspects) of up to 4 persons close to respondent	Beginning psychometric testing reported May have utility for large population/epidemiologic surveys
Cost and Reciprocity of Social Support Scale (CARSSS) (32)	Self-report measure of potentially stressful dimensions of supportive relationships; unique in this regard Combines theories of social exchange and equity Taps nonbenevolent components of social support 6 subscales (size of network, sources of support, cost, conflict, reciprocity, equity) Conflict subscale: items addressing stress, worry, trouble Cost subscale: items addressing time, effort, services, tangible aid Cost, conflict, reciprocity, equity subscales: 25 questions, rated on a 4-point scale for top 5 listed persons	Internal consistency (Cronbach's alpha): 0.69–0.76 (normal subjects) 0.50–0.87 (cancer sample) Strong positive correlation between the giving and receiving dimensions of reciprocity; no association between cost and conflict Further testing warranted
Duke Social Support and Stress Scale (DSSSS) (33)	Self-report measure of family and nonfamily social support and stress 24-item questionnaire 6 categories of family (spouse/significant other, children/grandchildren, parents/grandparents, brothers/sisters, other blood relatives, relatives by marriage) 4 categories of nonfamily (neighbors, coworkers, church members, other friends)	Pearson correlation for test–retest (range 7- to 39-day interval): 0.76 (family support), 0.67 (nonfamily support)

Instrument	Description	Reliability/Validity
Duke-UNC Functional Social Support Questionnaire (D-UNC-FSSQ) (34)	Each support category rated as to degree of support provided (none to a lot) Separate total scores for family and nonfamily support 2-scale, 8-item self-administered measure of 2 dimensions of social support 5 items assess *confidant* support (reflect relationship in which important life matters discussed and shared) 3 items assess *affective* support (reflect emotional or caring support) Responses rated on 5-point Likert scale ranging from "as much as I would like" to "much less than I would like"	Test-retest reliability: 0.66 (1- to 4-week interval, for 22 of 40 married, young females in a primary care clinic) Construct and concurrent validity reported with significant correlations with other measures Further testing in other populations necessary
Family Stress and Support Inventory (FSSI) (35)	Self-report measure of intrafamilial stress and support provided by each family member as perceived by the respondent For each family member, respondent rates amounts of stress and support received on 1-to-10 continuum Scores can be tabulated by generation, whole family, or individual family members Arithmetic means of stress and support for each grouping determined; ratio of stress to support can be calculated	Test-retest reliability: 0.78 (support), 0.68 (stress). Concurrent validity determined in a predominantly white, married female sample with mean age of 41.7 years Halvorsen (35) used Marlowe-Crown Social Desirability Scale to determine whether respondents had a social desirability bias in their responses or based responses on true perception of support or stress
Interpersonal Support Evaluation List (ISEL) (36,37)	Measures perceived availability of support for 4 dimensions of support: tangible, appraisal (informational), belonging (emotional), self-esteem 2 forms: one for college students (48 statements, 12 items per subscale), one for general population (40 items, 10 items per subscale) Respondents asked to indicate whether statement is probably true or false for them 50% of items positively worded, 50% negatively worded	Internal reliabilities (alpha coefficients): *total* student (0.77–0.86), *total* general (0.88–0.90), *subscales* Student General Appraisal (0.77–0.92) 0.70–0.82 Tangible (0.71–0.74) 0.73–0.81 Belonging (0.75–0.78) 0.73–0.78 Self-esteem (0.62–0.73) 0.62–0.73 Test-retest (total student, 4-week interval): 0.87, subscales: 0.80–0.87 Test-retest (general): (2-day interval) 0.87, (6-week interval) 0.70; (subscales): (2 day) 0.67–0.84, (6-week interval) 0.63–0.69 Validity testing reported Additional testing warranted for use with other samples
Interview Schedule for Social Interaction (ISSI) (38–40)	Measure of perceived availability and adequacy of social relationships	Cronbach's alpha: coefficients 0.79–0.90 Test-retest reliability (Pearson product moment correlations): 0.63–0.80

11A. Measures of Social Support (*cont.*)

Instrument	Description	Psychometric Indices
	4 subscales (availability of intimate relationships, more diffuse relationships; adequacy and satisfaction with each of those 2 subscales) 52 items, administered as an interview 4 scores (availability of attachment, perceived adequacy of attachment, availability of social integration, adequacy of social integration)	Convergent and divergent validity studied Has been modified for use with poststroke hospitalized patients (20) Has been shortened and adapted without loss of reliability or validity (41)
IPR Inventory (IPRI) (42)	39-item measure of interpersonal relationships (includes reciprocity and conflict) Based on theories of social exchange and equity, and refined from a previous 74-item Interpersonal Relationship Index (43) 3 subscales: social support (13 items), reciprocity (13), conflict (13) Items either measure perceived sentiment on 5-point Likert-type scale (agree to disagree) or measure perceived frequency on a 5-point continuum (very often to never) 3 additional items assess structural aspects of support network	Internal consistency reliability coefficients: (Cronbach's alpha), 0.92 (support), 0.83 (reciprocity), 0.91 (conflict) Factor analysis determined (detailed description) Criterion-related validity determined for support and conflict Normative scores developed for 3 subscales is an important contribution
Inventory of Socially Supportive Behavior (ISSB) (27)	40-item measure of the frequency with which respondents receive support from natural support systems Scores significantly correlate with size of network and perceived family support Items rated on 5-point scale as to frequency during preceding month (1, "not at all," to 5, "about every day")	Test–retest reliability: 0.88 Internal consistency (coefficient alphas): 0.93, 0.94 Principal components factor analysis: Appropriate to use ISSB total score as global measure of social support (96) ISSB does not measure socializing dimension well (96)
MOS Social Support Survey (MOS SSS) (44)	Developed for use with chronically ill patients in a medical outcomes study 19-item, self-administered questionnaire measuring functional dimensions of social support 4 subscales (emotional/informational, affectionate, tangible, positive social interaction) Can use subscale scores (recommended) or total index score Assesses types of support but not sources Respondents indicate how often the type of support is available if needed on Likert-type scale (1, "none of the time," to 5, "all of the time")	Tested on approximately 3,000 adult patients in 3 sites Internal consistency reliability (Cronbach's alpha): all above 0.91 (each subscale, total scale) Validity tested with multitrait scaling test to high convergent and discriminant validity Findings support view that social support is multidimensional

Instrument	Description	Psychometric properties
Multidimensional Scale of Perceived Social Support (MSPSS) (45–47)	Self-report measure of 3 subscales: perceived social support from family, friends, and a significant other; 12 items rated on a 7-point Likert-type scale (very strongly agree to very strongly disagree); 1 item measures structural support dimension; Good example of instrument development and evaluation	Testing performed on college students; Internal reliabilities (Cronbach's alpha) for subscales and total score: 0.81–0.95; Factor analysis showed factors loading on each of subscales; significant low to moderate correlation
My Family and Friends (MFF) (48)	3-part measure of perceptions of social support of children aged 6–12 years old; 12 dialogs (5, emotional support; 2 each, informational, instrumental, and companionship support; 1, conflict), and props used to engage children and gather data about availability of individuals to provide social support and child's level of satisfaction with type of support received; Based on cognitive developmental theory and social support work; Significant contribution and allows the addition of dialogs created for specific situations	Sensitive to variations in perceived social support during "family upheaval"; Test-retest reliability: 0.68 (network member rankings), 0.69 (satisfaction with support); Overall internal consistency (Cronbach's alpha): dialogs: 0.72, emotional support: >0.75, instrumental support: teacher 0.28, sibling 0.83 (range attributed to stems: 1 focused on help with schoolwork, other on help around the house)
Norbeck Social Support Questionnaire (NSSQ) (24,25)	Developed by nurse researchers to measure multidimensional construct of social support; Short, self-administered questionnaire tapping 3 areas: functional aspects (affect, affirmation, aid); network (number in network, duration of relationships, frequency of contact); loss (number of support categories in which loss occurred and perceived amount of support lost); Theoretical bases are Kahn's conceptual definitions of social support (81); Rating scale ranges from 0 (not at all) to 4 (a great deal); Has been used in diverse populations (low-income pregnant women (21,22); elderly (97); patients with cancer (15,18,19); chronically ill women (98)	Test–retest reliability: functional and network property items: 0.85–0.92; Internal consistency (each of 3 functional aspects of social support): 0.89 or higher; Correlations: among 3 network property items (0.88–0.96), 3 loss items (0.54–0.68); Concurrent validity with Social Support Questionnaire: moderate (0.31–0.56 for subscales); Construct validity demonstrated; Normative database (working adults) reported (25)
Perceived Social Support from Friends (PSS-Fr) and from Family (PSS-Fa) (28)	Measure of valid constructs distinct from network; 20-item, "yes, no, or don't know" response for each instrument (friends, family); Items include receiving supportive behaviors and reciprocity (providing support to network members); Scores on PSS-Pr more related to social competence than those on PSS-Fa (those with high PSS-Fr had significantly lower scores on trait anxiety than those with low PSS-Fr scores)	Internal consistency (Cronbach's alpha): PSS-Fr (0.88); PSS-Fa (0.90); Factor analysis: single factor for each scale; Undergraduate college students used in validity and reliability testing; Scores on PSS-Fr related more closely to social competence than on PSS-Fa; Subjects with high PSS-Fr scores had significantly lower scores on trait anxiety

11A. Measures of Social Support (*cont.*)

Instrument	Description	Psychometric Indices
Personal Resource Questionnaire (PRQ) (PRQ85) (26,50)	Measure of multidimensional characteristics of social support 2 parts: (I) subject's resources and satisfaction with them (e.g., existence of a confidant) measured by 8 life situations; (II) social relationship dimensions (5 subscales) measured on a 25-item 7-point Likert scale, and a 5-item self-help ideology scale Used in studies of healthy adults and adolescents Part II revised to eliminate age references and expand its usefulness; renamed PRQ-85-Part II (50)	High internal consistency reliability coefficient for part II (a = 0.89); Moderate intercorrelations for intimacy, social integration, worth, assistance (some overlap) Nurturance subscale independent Established reliability and validity (49-52)
Quality of Relationships Inventory (QRI) (53)	Measure of relationship-based perceptions of social support and conflict, using 3 subscales (support, conflict, depth of relationship), not generalized perception 29-item questionnaire completed for mother, father, and up to 4 other important relationships Testing in populations beyond undergraduate students is warranted	Alpha coefficients: support subscale for (M) mother (0.83), (F) father (0.88), (Fr) friend (0.85); conflict subscale M (0.88), F (0.88), Fr (0.91); depth subscale M (0.83), F (0.86), Fr (0.84) Moderate to strong associations of 3 subscales for each relationship category
Social Support Appraisals Scale (SSAS) (54,55)	23-item measure of extent to which person feels loved, respected, and involved with friends, family, others Based on Cobb's conceptualization of social support (64) Scale scored as total measure or subscales (family, 8 items; friend, 7 items) Items rated on a 4-point scale (1, strongly agree, to 4, strongly disagree) Instrument testing helpful to researchers interested in instrument development	Convergent and divergent validity studied using 5 college and 5 community samples Internal consistency (Cronbach's alpha): 3 scales (0.80–0.90) Attempts to derive subscales to tap love, respect, and involvement resulted in 3 factors, but difficulty with third factor (55)
Social Support Behaviors (SSB) (56)	45-item measure of 5 types of support: emotional, assistance, financial, guidance, socializing Respondents indicate how likely a family member or friend would provide identified support	High internal consistency reliabilities reported for subscales Subscale validity, content validity, and subscale sensitivity demonstrated
Social Support Questionnaire (SSQ) (29)	27-item measure of perceived number of social supports, and satisfaction with them Respondent asked to list people on whom they can rely for the set of circumstances described in each item and degree of satisfaction with support	Correlations of SSQ with personality, adjustment, life change measures reported Correlations of items with total score (0.48–0.72); satisfaction of items scores (coefficient alpha) was 0.94 Test–retest (4-week interval) correlations for satisfaction (0.83), and for the number listed (0.90) Stability and high internal consistency among items reported

Social Support Questionnaire (SSQ) (30)	2-part questionnaire: (1) measure of tangible support (9 situations); (2) network members listed by specific categories and rated for 1 item about informational support and 4 items about emotional support Has been used in combination with other measures (24,25)	Test–retest (9-month interval) reliability: tangible support (0.56); emotional support (0.68) Internal consistency: information, emotional support (0.81); tangible support (0.31)
Social Support Rating Scale (SSRS) (57,58)	One of few instruments developed for use with children, adolescents Uses 5-point Likert scale to measure extent to which persons provide emotional support and caring, help, guidance, and the extent to which the person may have upset them Uses 7-point Likert scale to measure their satisfaction with emotional support, help, and extent to which they seek help Allows examination of separate sources of support	Internal consistency reliability estimates >0.75
Social Support Scale (SSS) (59)	Short scale used to measure social support; unique in that tool can be modified for use with specific situations (desired health outcome, e.g., weight loss) Likert-type scale used to measure how helpful each person is relative to specific situation (1, "not at all helpful," to 5, "completely helpful")	Requires more work in establishing psychometric properties of scale

Numbers in parentheses correspond to studies listed in the References.

11B. Social Support Instruments for Special Populations

Instrument	Description	Psychometric Indices
Hughes Breast feeding Support Scale (HBSS) (60)	30-item measure of support: emotional (10 items), instrumental (10 items), and informational (10 items) as perceived by breastfeeding mothers Self-administered questionnaire using 1-4 Likert-scale format Measures specific and global dimensions	Corrected split-half reliability scores for 3 subscales 0.85–0.89 Internal consistency alpha coefficients: 0.84–0.88 Warrants further testing
Maternal Social Support Index (MSSI) (61)	Measure of mother's perception of amount of social support (emotional and tangible) and her satisfaction with provided support 21-item, self-administered measure directed to 7 areas: help with daily tasks, satisfaction with visits from kin, help with crises, emergency child care, satisfaction with communication from male partner, other support person, community involvement	Test-retest reliability: 0.72 (6-8 week interval), correlations for individual items 0.58–0.81 Internal consistency (coefficient alphas): 0.60–0.63, If clustered child care and non-child care items into 2 groups, was 0.72 (child care) and 0.78 (non-child care) Warrants further study
Support Behaviors Inventory (SBI) (62)	Developed for use with expectant couples 45-item instrument with 50% of items specific to pregnancy, remainder generally applicable House's typology basis for 4 categories (subscales) of support: emotional, material, informational, appraisal (80) Uses 6-point scale to assess degree of satisfaction for each supportive behavior, first for partner relationship, then satisfaction of support from other people 2 satisfaction scores derived: partner support, other people support	Internal reliability (Cronbach's alpha): scores (1) partner support (0.97), (2) other people support (0.98); subscales (4) 0.83–0.96; subscales very highly intercorrelated Discriminant validity and factor analytic techniques support broad single dimension not 4 separate dimensions Warrants further study
Social Support in Chronic Illness Inventory (SSCII) (99)	38-item measure of perceived satisfaction with specified supportive behaviors, relative to a specific situation (chronic illness) Can be completed by provider of support or chronically ill individual Based on Kahn's (81) concept of convoy, and a model of stress, coping, health Designed for use with persons with chronic illness, e.g., diabetes, hypertension, end-stage renal, cardiac disease Uses 6-point Likert scale (1, "dissatisfied" to 6, "very satisfied") 4 subscales: intimate interaction, guidance/feedback, tangible assistance, positive social interaction	Internal consistency (alpha coefficients): total scale (0.98), subscales (0.84–0.94) Test-retest reliability (2-week interval): 0.48 Factor analysis did not confirm 4 separate subscales but one main factor (intimate interaction) Further refinement may be necessary
Social Support Inventory for Stroke Survivors (SSISS) (63)	Self-report inventory of 8 aspects of social support, administered in a structured interview format Source of social support: personal, friend, community, groups, profession Support measured by 3 dimensions (quality, quantity, satisfaction) Inventory items specific to stroke 8 scores, scored by 3 dimensions for (1) each of 5 sources of support; and by (2) each of dimensions across all 5 support sources	Test-retest reliability (2-week interval): 0.76 Internal consistency (Cronbach's alpha): 0.84 Warrants further testing

Numbers in parentheses correspond to studies listed in the References.

12

Measuring Coping

Jo Ann Wegmann

Coping as a concept has received much attention in the literature and has been investigated by various disciplines and avenues of study. Early work concerning coping as a stress response includes empirical studies by Angell,[1] Koos,[2] and Hill.[3] Interest in family stress has continued to develop systematically. As a result of this systematic research, there are currently available examples of research strategies, methods, and reliable and valid instruments to study coping.[4]

Multiple, often overlapping, definitions of coping exist. In this chapter, coping is defined as the cognitive and behavioral strategies used to master conditions of harm, threat, or challenge when a normal or routine response is not available.[1,5] As such, coping involves two separate frameworks,[5] psychologic and sociologic. According to Lazarus,[5] the psychologic taxonomy of coping includes direct action and palliative modes. Direct actions are associated with (related to) physiologic responses to stress and become evident with threats of change in one's social or physical environment. Palliative coping encompasses thoughts or actions designed to relieve the emotional impact of stress. Unlike direct actions, palliative coping does not alter threatening or damaging events but serves to make the person feel better.

Sociologic coping behaviors rely on the resources of individuals or groups, such as families. Early research into families recognized the importance of family resources, such as cohesion and adaptability, to maintain family organization and functioning during stressful events.[3] Such coping tendencies are closely related to aspects of social support discussed elsewhere in this book (e.g., Chapter 11).

Research into coping evolved from research on responses and the effects of stress. Lyon and Werner[6] identified four theoretical approaches to stress research. They viewed stress as (1) a stimulus; (2) a response; (3) a transaction; and (4) a theoretical approach. In relation to stress, coping has been considered an important concept, within a diverse scope of theoretical orientations.[7]

Instruments to Measure Coping

A comprehensive list of data-collection techniques or instruments used to measure coping would be extensive, and there would be much duplication among tools. The purpose of this chapter is to identify instruments used for research into coping. Resources include family sociology, psychology, psychiatry, and nursing. All the instruments described are designed to measure the effect of adequate coping behaviors on some outcome and appear to be suitable for clinical studies.

Typically, coping processes have been investigated for two reasons: validation or confirmation of a particular theory and evaluation of a patient with a diagnostic clinical instrument.[8] It also is valuable to investigate individual and family coping strategies to identify inappropriate or inadequate coping patterns that can impact health outcomes.

When beginning to identify instruments for the study of coping, it is valuable first to explore broader issues of research into this phenomenon. Because coping represents responses to stressors, the astute investigator must be aware of the sensitive nature of such research, as well as the ethical issues inherent in such exploration. Brailey[9] identifies three research issues in the study of coping strategies: (1) obtaining an accurate picture of routine personal coping strategies; (2) delineating the functions of coping, to determine the effectiveness of coping; and (3) determining appropriate measurements of coping efficacy. Brailey describes four methods of data collection or types of instrumentation used in the study of coping:[9] (1) direct observation during normal events; (2) use of vignettes to elicit personal responses to stressful events; (3) use of structured instrumentation to obtain usual responses to general sources of stress; and (4) personal accounts of coping responses to actual stressful events.[9]

Direct observation of the subject while he or she is coping with normal events is the first method described by Brailey. This strategy typically involves a longitudinal study, with the risk for observer effect on responses. Another means of data collection involves the use of vignettes of stressful situations, from which subject responses are obtained. This may provide information about coping strategies, but Brailey cautions that vignettes may not represent realistic situations.

A third data-collection technique seeks responses to how subjects usually cope with general stressors. Structured instruments typically provide a list of coping responses, rated by the subject on a Likert-type scale. Many instruments that measure coping are designed in this format, yet Brailey cautions that discrepancies may exist between what subjects say they do and what they actually do in specific situations.

The fourth data-collection method involves the use of real events from subjects' own lives and asks them to describe the coping strategies they used. Although this use of real-life events appears advantageous, a potential problem with self-report is selective distortion; this method of data collection is used infrequently.

Singer[8] elaborates somewhat on Brailey's descriptions. This psychologist identifies two types of coping studies. One strategy assumes a theoretical position on how people function. From such a position, the researcher identifies categories or descriptors for coping behaviors. Scales and other measurement instruments can then be developed based on the identified categories. Examples of studies that arise from a theoretical position include comparisons of the relative successes of people employing one category of coping style with those in another.

The second type of coping study described by Singer examines the particular stress or stresses, such as illness or bereavement. Examples include inferential studies about patterns of reactions and functional adaptation to common stressors.

The instruments designed to measure coping described here are organized into two broad categories: those related to family sociology research and those derived from studies of health-care outcomes. In discussing specific instruments, attempts are made to address the methods of data collection described by Brailey,[9] as well as the two types of coping studies identified by Singer.[8] Issues of reliability and validity also are addressed for each instrument. The specific instruments discussed are summarized in Appendix 12A.

Family Inventories

Early attempts at defining and measuring coping arose from research into families and family stress management. Much of the recent literature on coping is grounded in sociology. McCubbin et al.[10] explore recent investigations into family stress and coping in a decade review of these topics. These authors note that the study of family coping depends on multiple cognitive psychologic theories and sociologic sources. Coping strategies are described in terms of both the individual and the family by Olson et al.[11]

Olson et al.,[12] at the University of Minnesota Department of Family Social Science, have developed a series of instruments called Family Inventories. These inventories consist of nine instruments that measure various aspects of family life, adaptability, cohesion, and coping. Three instruments in particular were developed as part of the Family Stress and Coping Project.

Family Inventory of Life Events and Changes (FILE)

The FILE scale was developed as an index of family stress and records both normative and non-normative life events and changes experienced by the family unit.[13] FILE consists of 72 items, grouped into nine subscales. A high raw score indicates low stress, and a low raw score indicates high stress. One subscale is labeled "losses" and includes the following item: "A parent/spouse died." Responses to each statement are recorded as "yes" or "no," and a total scale score is obtained. The authors suggest that the total scale score be calculated rather than the subscales separate, as the subscale scores are not empirically stable.

Reliability for the overall scale is 0.81 (Cronbach's alpha), with subscale scores varying from 0.30 to 0.73. These scores support use of the total scale score, rather than scoring by individual subscales. Instrument validity was determined by discriminant analyses between low-conflict and high-conflict families ($p < 0.01$).

Adolescent-Family Inventory of Life Events and Changes (A-FILE)

The A-FILE[14] is a 50-item, self-report instrument designed to record normative and non-normative life events and changes as perceived by an adolescent during the immediately preceding 12 months of family life. This instrument measures adolescent-family life changes and records events experienced by any member of the family. The instrument is comprised of six conceptual dimensions, including life transitions. One statement from this dimension is: "Parent started school." Subjects respond yes (coded as 0) or no (coded as 1) to each statement. A high score implies low stress.

The total scale alpha reliabilities for the A-FILE are 0.83 and 0.80 and were determined by two different samples. Validity assessments were made by correlating the conceptual dimensions with two outcome measures, adolescent substance use and adolescent health locus of control ($p < 0.01$). A suggested future use of this instrument is in research with adolescents diagnosed with chronic or catastrophic illnesses.

Family Coping Strategies (F-COPES)

The F-COPES instrument[15] was created to identify effective problem-solving approaches and behaviors used by families in response to problems or difficulties. The F-COPES is a 30-item self-report instrument. Each item is answered on a Likert-type scale, with answers ranging from "strongly disagree" to "strongly agree." One dimension of the F-COPES is to seek spiritual support. An example of one statement from this dimension is: "Attending church services."

The instrument is conceptually organized for Internal Family Coping Patterns (three scales) and External Family Coping Patterns (five scales) (A.J. Thompson, personal communication, October 7, 1993).

Because of the interval nature of the data, scores can be obtained and parametric statistical analyses can be performed on the results. Scores may be obtained for each dimension or the total instrument. Reliability for the F-COPES was determined by Cronbach coefficient alpha (0.86 and 0.87 for two samples) and test–retest.

Family APGAR

The Family APGAR measures personal satisfaction with one's own family function in five parameters: adoption, partnership, growth, affection, and resolve. It is a five-item Likert-type self-report questionnaire. Cronbach's alpha is reported at 0.86.[16]

Two-Part Coping Assessment Scale

Sidel et al. developed a structured, easily scored assessment scale for coping strategies.[17] Their two-part coping scale includes three problem situations for which the subject lists possible approaches or strategies, and a list of ten strategies for coping with the situation is provided. In the second part of this scale, the subject responds, on a seven-point scale, to the likelihood of using each of the 10 strategies. The authors conclude that both free response and ratings are important because they may elicit different sources of information about coping strategies. The validity and reliability of this scale are not addressed. This study is an early attempt to develop a pencil-and-paper measure to learn more about less socially approved ways of coping and is the groundwork for the development of more recent instruments. This tool illustrates the use of vignettes[9] for data collection.

Parental Coping Scale (1962)

Hurwitz et al.[18] sought to develop a tool to assess parent–child relationship patterns in families with juvenile delinquents. Five areas of parental coping are assessed via interviews with both parents, together and separately. These areas are rated immediately after the interviews using a four-point scale ranging from "very constructive" to "very destructive." This type of data collection represents Brailey's[9] fourth method of study, that is, having subjects identify coping responses used in relation to specific events or situations. Hurwitz et al.[18] state that reliability for the scoring of the interviews was determined by Chi-square analysis ($p \leq 0.05$). Validity was achieved by differentiating constructive from destructive parental coping mechanisms.

Parental Coping Scale (1989)

The Parent Coping Scale is an 81-item questionnaire designed for parents of handicapped children.[19] Parents respond in terms of their coping outcomes with their handicapped children, using the preceding week as the time frame. Items employ a five-point frequency scale ranging from "never" (0) to "most of the time" (4). Eight subscales make up this questionnaire. The authors report instrument coefficient alphas ranging from 0.80 to 0.87 for six of the subscales, 0.65 for the subscale Minimization of Threat, and 0.67 for the Self-Blame Subscale.[19]

Coping Health Inventory for Parents (CHIP)

The Coping Health Inventory for Parents assesses the relationship between parental attitudes toward a child's chronic illness and parental coping patterns. Eighty items of coping behavior are operationally defined. Parents are asked to record how helpful (scale of 0 to 3) each behavior is in their family situation.[20] Three subscales are measured. McCubbin[13] reports Cronbach's alphas of 0.97, 0.79, and 0.71 for these subscales, respectively. Coefficient alphas also are reported and range between 0.84 and 0.89 for the three subscales.[21]

Chronicity Impact and Coping Instrument: Parent Questionnaire (CIC:PQ)

Hymovich[22] reports on the CIC:PQ. This instrument was developed to determine the impact of a child's chronic illness on parents and to understand how parents cope. The author describes the results of three tests and the three phases of the instrument.

The current format of the CIC:PQ contains 167 items divided into six sections, including: your child, yourself, your spouse, brothers and sisters, hospitalization, and other. This self-report instrument is completed by parents. There are 60 stressor items, 61 coping items, and 9 value/attitude/belief items. Other items seek demographic information.

Hymovich reports that internal consistency was determined for each of the three revisions of this instrument. The current version of the CIC:PQ has a Hoyt reliability coefficient of 0.95, which the author cautions may be artificially inflated. She states further that the test–retest reliability still needs to be determined. Although this is a relatively new instrument for measuring family coping, its value lies in its ability to determine the impact of chronic disease on parents and their coping practices with chronically ill children and predict the outcome of intervention with these families.

Goldstein Cooper-Avoider Sentence Completion Test (SCT)

Cohen and Lazarus investigated the relationship between the mode of coping with preoperative stress and recovery from surgery.[23] Among the instruments used to gather information was the Goldstein Cooper-Avoider Sentence Completion Test (SCT). This test consists of a series of sentence-completion items and responses are scored by the investigator for either avoidance or coping. An example of one item is: "My greatest fear is. . . ." The authors acknowledge that there may be gender differences in responses. No information is offered on the reliability or validity of this instrument. Nevertheless, this test appears to be easily administered and elicits predictive information about individuals' coping styles before a threatening event. As such, it offers potential value to nursing research.

Preoperative Coping Scale

Another study of surgical patients used a preoperative coping scale to assess the extent to which patients desired and sought information about impending surgery.[24] The preoperative coping scale consists of 15 items that address location and size of incision, length of the operation, expected level of pain, and type of postoperative treatment. Sime[24] reports that quantitative data were derived by assigning a plus or minus to each item and summing across items. The possible range of scores is –15 to 15, with extreme minus scores representing limited information seeking and extreme positive scores indicating extensive information seeking. Very little other information is available about the preoperative coping scale. Validity and reliability are not addressed in Sime's paper.[24] Yet, this scale, too, appears to be a likely instrument for future development in nursing research.

Patient Attitudes of Chronic Illness

Kinsman et al.[25] investigated patient attitudes toward chronic illness in six areas. This 109-item survey is a self-report instrument that offer choices of "agree" or "disagree."

Coping Strategy Questionnaire

The Coping Strategy Questionnaire[26] assesses cognitive and behavioral pain-coping mechanisms in a sample of chronic low-back pain patients. This self-report questionnaire consists of six cognitive coping strategies (e.g., thinking of things that serve to distract one away from the pain) and two behavioral coping strategies (e.g., engaging in active behaviors that divert one's attention away from the pain) when the subject feels pain. Items are scored on a seven-point scale, and the respondent indicates how often he or she uses that particular strategy when feeling pain (0 never, 3 sometimes, and 6 always).

This questionnaire is internally reliable, with an alpha coefficient of 0.71. The authors discuss the predictive value of this questionnaire when working with people experiencing chronic pain. The value of an instrument such as this one to nursing research in a variety of settings is evident.

Respiratory Illness Opinion Survey (RIOS)

Another area of chronic illness that warrants further investigation is respiratory illness. Kinsman et al.[27] use the Respiratory Illness Opinion Survey (RIOS) to measure patient attitudes toward chronic respiratory illness and hospitalization. This survey instrument consists of 78 items to which the subject responds on a scale of 1 to 5 (1 strongly agree, 5 strongly disagree). Six subscales are measured by this tool, including Psychologic Stigma: "A breathing problem makes me feel foolish." An example of one item in the subscale, Negative Staff Regard, is the statement: "This hospital is like a prison." Internal consistency reliabilities are reported as 0.80 and 0.70, and test–retest reliabilities ranged from 0.64 to 0.79.

Response to Illness Questionnaire (RIQ)

Pritchard[28] reports on the development of the Response to Illness Questionnaire (RIQ), a 34-item, self-report survey designed to measure aspects of illness behavior. This instrument was administered to two groups of patients undergoing long-term hemodialysis. The actual instrument is not fully described in this brief report,[28] but temporal reliability was tested. Weighted kappa values ranged from 0.22 to 0.89. The author concludes that the RIQ has a substantial level of temporal reliability and suggests that this is a valuable instrument for studies of illness behavior.

Bedsworth and Molen's Semistructured Interview

To measure the psychologic stress of spouses of myocardial infarction patients immediately after admission to a coronary care unit, Bedsworth and Molen[29] developed a semistructured interview. Four open-ended questions identify perceived threats and perceived coping strategies. These authors identified 45 actual coping strategies and the total actions taken against the perceived threats of a specific group of spouses.

Little information about this semistructured interview is available, yet it appears to be congruent with the second method of data collection described by Brailey,[9] that is, obtaining subjects' responses to vignettes of stressful situations. Bedsworth and Molen[29] do not address issues of validity or reliability, and indeed, one problem with this type of data collection is the potential for selective distortion by the respondent. Nevertheless, identification of actual coping behaviors used by spouses provides valuable information and suggests possible directions for future research.

Coping Strategies Scale

Miller and Nygren[30] used the Coping Strategies Scale developed by Wiesman and Worden[31] to seek descriptive information to evaluate the effects of an education program on the adaptability of chronically ill persons to live with their diseases. This scale was designed to categorize behaviors used by people to cope with concerns and problems. It consists of 15 broad types of behavior frequently observed when a person tries to cope with a specific problem. Miller and Nygren[30] state that efforts to classify how individuals cope are awkward and that the Coping Strategies Scale represents a commendable, yet incomplete, attempt to classify and objectify raw data.

Coping Inventory

Zeitlin[32] used the Coping Inventory, an observation instrument, to assess 48 kinds of coping behaviors of handicapped children. This instrument is used for educational and therapeutic planning and is divided into two categories, self and environment. Items are scored on a scale of 1 to 5, where 1 indicates no or very minimal evidence of competency, and 5 indicates effective behavior. Interobserver reliability of the Coping Inventory ranged from 0.78 to 0.99.[32] Split-half reliability is reported between a group of non-handicapped children and a sample of handicapped children.

Richmond/Hopkins Family Coping Index

Choi et al.[33] revised the instructions for the Richmond/Hopkins Family Coping Index, first reported in 1963, and determined that the accuracy and consistency of this instrument could be enhanced. This instrument measures nine domains of family coping, including emotional competence and family living patterns. It is completed by public health personnel during observations of actual family settings. Scores of the nine subscales range from 1 to 5 ("never" to "always"), and the rater is asked to assess how a family is coping in each of the domains. Interrater reliability was established with the modified instrument by Cronbach's coefficient alpha (0.97). The authors state that the results of improving this scale support its continued use.

California Psychological Inventory (CPI)

Kupst and Schulman[34] used the California Psychological Inventory subscales to measure personal adjustment in families that have a child with leukemia. These are five self-reported scales completed by parents, including work and leisure, in the overall functioning family unit.

Health Attitude Scale

Miller et al.[35] studied coping as adherence to medical regimen in five areas in a group of cardiac patients. Their Health Attitude Scale is a self-report, seven-point bipolar scale that appears to be suitable for measuring attitudes toward coping in a variety of illnesses.

Health-Related Outcomes and Nursing Sources of Coping Instruments

Health-related outcomes have been addressed in family studies of coping, and specific instruments to determine such outcomes are available. The areas explored include measurement of adaptation in specific illnesses and determining coping strategies of patients and families confronting long-term disease problems.

Ways of Coping Checklist (WWC)

The Ways of Coping Checklist (WWC) was developed by Folkman and Lazarus.[36] This 66-item, four-point Likert-type response category checklist assesses behavioral and cognitive coping strategies in eight subscales. This instrument has been widely used in assessing coping in such areas as bereavement, chronic illness, and functional disability. Cronbach's alphas in three studies range from 0.56 to 0.79.[37]

McNett Coping Effectiveness Questionnaire (MCEQ)

Experience and the importance of 14 attributes of coping effectiveness are measured by the McNett Coping Effectiveness Questionnaire (MCEQ). Subjects rate two identical lists of attributes, such as feeling happy, to provide an index of coping effectiveness. Coefficient alphas are reported as 0.82 and 0.89.[38]

Coping Resource Inventory (CRI)

The Coping Resource Inventory (CRI) is a 141-item, self-report questionnaire that measures an individual's coping resources. The coping effectiveness score provides an overall value of how one perceives one's coping methods. Items require a true–false response.[39] Content validity is reported at 90%, and test–retest reliability ranged from 0.59 to 0.87.

Cancer Inventory of Problem Situations

Heinrich and Schag[40] developed an instrument to document day-to-day physical and psychosocial problems confronted by cancer patients. The Cancer Inventory of Problem Situations is a self-report test that takes approximately 20 minutes to complete. It consists of 131 problem statements with a fine-point rating scale. Responses range from "not at all" to "very much." The problem statements are grouped into 27 categories. The instrument evaluates the patient's previous month and how each statement applied to him or her during that time. The content and face validity of this instrument have been established.

Pain Experience Inventory

The Pain Experience Inventory is composed of 37 questions answered on a four-point Likert-type scale ("not at all" to "very much"). It was designed to measure cognitive factors perceived to influence the pain experience. Content analysis by a panel of experts revealed a content validity index of 0.92.[41]

Pain Coping Tool

The Pain Coping Tool measures 14 coping elements, 4 behaviors, and 10 strategies. It is a 28-item tool in which subjects respond to a four-point Likert-type scale ("not at all" to "very much"). Content analysis by a panel of experts revealed a content validity index of 0.94. Cronbach's alpha is reported at 0.71.[41]

Jalowiec Coping Scale

The Jalowiec Coping Scale is a 60-item, self-report psychometric instrument first developed in 1977 by a registered nurse master's student at the University of Illinois, Chicago Medical Center. The respondent rates how often each of the coping strategies is used on an f-point (0–3) rating scale (ranging from "never used" to "often used"). In addition, there is space at the beginning of the questionnaire to list which stressor or stressful event is under investigation. This permits the examination and comparison of situation-specific coping (A. Jalowiec, personal communication, October 18, 1993).

Eight coping styles are identified as descriptive of the coping dimensions represented by the 60 items. The author labels these as: (1) confrontive; (2) evasive; (3) optimistic; (4) fatalistic; (5) emotive; (6) palliative; (7) supportant; and (8) self-reliant (A. Jalowiec, personal communication, October 18, 1993).

This instrument is widely used and has undergone substantial revision in 1987.[42,43] In a summary of 12 studies using the 1987 scale, Cronbach alphas were averaged. The high mean for total scale is reported as 0.97, and low mean as 0.64, with the overall mean alpha as 0.86 (A. Jalowiec, personal communication, October 18, 1993).

Spousal Coping Instrument (SCI)

The SCI is a 118-item, self-report questionnaire that measures coping and factors affecting coping. The respondents are spouses of patients with cardiac disease. This instrument comprises six subscales, and reliability coefficients range from 0.74 to 0.81.[44]

Summary

Both theory testing and clinical instrument development are considered to be important elements in measuring coping. As the concept of coping is better defined and as coping behaviors are more systematically studied, other properties of coping may emerge.[7]

This chapter identified 29 instruments of varying designs for use in the measurement of coping. Self-report scales using Likert-type responses usually facilitate data collection and are amenable to a variety of analytic tests. Not addressed in this chapter are other, more qualitative methods of data collection, including interviews, patient narrative reports, some forms of participant observation, and grounded theory. The reader is encouraged to consider such methods for research into coping, because it is possible to gather much rich, descriptive data through qualitative methods.

Instruments used to measure coping are varied and are derived from many disciplines. As this concept is further understood and empirically measured, its value as a moderator variable in health outcomes should become better documented. Coping represents an area that is ripe for clinical research, and it is anticipated that this summary of instruments that measure coping will be expanded and refined.

Exemplar Studies

Arathuzik, M.D. The appraisal of pain and coping in cancer patients. *West J Nurs Res*, 1991, *13*(6):714-731.

This study identifies that pain presents problems with both the experience of the individual and the management of pain. The dilemma discussed is how one copes with pain. Pain is discussed within a framework of stress. This study uses a correlational descriptive design. A convenience sample of 80 women with metastatic breast cancer was employed to enhance knowledge about the relationship between coping processes and cancer pain. Methods included the use of three instruments: The Pain Experience Inventory, the Pain Coping Tool, which are described in this chapter, and the Multiple Affect Adjective Checklist. Data were analyzed through correlational statistics. Among the results is further understanding of the ways in which cancer patients cope with pain: main coping behaviors were withdrawal and inactivity. This is an exemplar study because of the instruments used and the design. This study deserves replication.

White, N.E., Richter, J.M., & Fry, C. Coping, social support, and adaptation to chronic illness. *West J Nurs Res*, 1992, *14*(2):211-224.

This study was part of a multistage project that examined lifestage transitions of chronically ill women. The sample consisted of 193 adult women who had been diagnosed with diabetes mellitus for at least 1 year. The purpose of this descriptive study was to determine adaptation to illness over a long time. Instruments included the Family Inventory of Life Events (FILE) and the Ways of Coping Questionnaire (described in this chapter). Data were analyzed by multiple regression, which indicated that potential stressors, coping strategies, and social support accounted for a significant amount of the variance. This study contributes to information on the instruments used and is part of an overall larger project.

References

1. Angell, R.C. *The family encounters the depression.* New York: Scribners, 1936.
2. Koos, E.L. *Families in trouble.* New York: King's Crown Press, 1946.
3. Hill, R. *Families under stress.* Norwalk, CT: Greenwood, 1949.
4. McCubbin, H.I., Cauble, A.E., & Patterson, J. (Eds.). *Family stress, coping, and social support.* Springfield, IL: Charles C. Thomas, 1982.
5. Lazarus, R. *Psychological stress and the coping process.* New York: McGraw-Hill, 1966.
6. Lyon, B.L., & Werner, J.S. Stress. *Ann Rev Nurs Res,* 1987, 5:3.
7. Barnfather, J.S. History, Overview, and Project Methodology. In J.S. Barnfather, & B.L. Lyon (Eds.), *Stress and coping: State of the sciences and implications for nursing theory, research and practice.* Indianapolis, IN: Sigma Theta Tau International, 1993.
8. Singer, J.E. Some issues in the study of coping. Proceedings of ACS Workshop on Methodologies in Behavioral Physiological Cancer Research, April 1983. *Cancer,* 1984, 53(suppl):2303.
9. Brailey, L.J. Issues in coping research. *Nurs Papers Perspect Nurs,* 1984, 16(1):5.
10. McCubbin, H.I., Joy, C.B., Cauble, A.E., et al. Family stress and coping: A decade review. *J Marriage Fam,* 1980, 42:855.
11. Olson, D.H.J., McCubbin, H.I., Barnes, H., et al. *Families: What makes them work?* Beverly Hills, CA: Sage, 1983.
12. Olson, D.H., McCubbin, H.I., Barnes, H., et al. *Family inventories.* St. Paul, MN: Family Social Science, University of Minnesota, 1982.
13. McCubbin, H.I., Patterson, D., & Wilson, M. FILE-Family Inventory of Life Events and Changes. In D.H. Olson, H.I. McCubbin, H. Barnes et al. (Eds.), *Family inventories.* St. Paul, MN: Family Social Science, University of Minnesota, 1982, p. 69.
14. McCubbin, H.I., Patterson, J.M., Bauman, E., & Harris, L.H. A-FILE-Adolescent Family Inventory of Life Events and Changes. In D.H. Olson, H.I. McCubbin, H. Barnes et al. (Eds.), *Family inventories.* St. Paul, MN: Family Social Science, University of Minnesota, 1982, p. 89.
15. McCubbin, H.I., Larsen, A.S., & Olson, D.H. F-COPES-Family Coping Strategies. In D.H. Olson, H.I. McCubbin, H. Barnes et al. (Eds.), *Family inventories.* St. Paul, MN: Family Social Science, University of Minnesota, 1982, p. 101.
16. Smith, C.E., Mayer, L.S., Parkhurst, C., et al. Adaptation in families with a member requiring mechanical ventilation at home. *Heart Lung,* 1991, 20(4):349.
17. Sidel, A., Moos, R., Adams, J., & Cady, P. Development of a coping scale. *Arch Gen Psychiatr,* 1969, 20(2):226.
18. Hurwitz, J., Kaplan, D., & Kaiser, E. Designing an instrument to assess parental coping mechanisms. *Soc Casework,* 1962, 43(1):527.
19. Petchel-Damrosch, S., & Perry, L.A. Self-reported adjustment, chronic sorrow, and coping of parents of children with Down Syndrome. *Nurs Res,* 1989, 38(1):31.
20. McCubbin, M. Nursing assessment of parental coping with cystic fibrosis. *West J Nurs Res,* 1984, 6(4):407.
21. Kessner Austin, J., & McDermott, N. Parental attitude and coping behaviors in families of children with epilepsy. *J Neurosci Nurs,* 1988, 20(3):174.
22. Hymovich, D. Development of the Chronicity Impact and Coping Instrument: Parent Questionnaire (CIC:PQ) *Nurs Res,* 1984, 33(4):218.
23. Cohen, F., & Lazarus, R. Active coping processes, coping dispositions, and recovery from surgery. *Psychosom Med,* 1973, 35(5):375.
24. Sime, A.M. Relationship of preoperative fear, type of coping, and information received about surgery to recovery from surgery. *J Person Soc Psychol,* 1976, 34(4):716.
25. Kinsman, R.A., Jones, N.F., et al. Patient variables supporting chronic illness. *J Nerv Ment Dis,* 1976, 163(3):159.
26. Rosentiel, A., & Keefe, F. The use of coping strategies in chronic low back pain patients: Relationship to patient characteristics and current adjustment. *Pain,* 1983, 17(1):33.
27. Kinsman, R., Jones, J., Matus, I., & Schuman, R. A scale for measuring attitudes toward respiratory illness and hospitalization. *J Nerv Ment Dis,* 1976, 163(3):159.
28. Pritchard, M. Temporal reliability of a questionnaire measuring psychological response to illness. *J Psychosom Res,* 1981, 25:63.
29. Bedsworth, J., & Molen, M. Psychological stress in spouses of patients with myocardial infarction. *Heart Lung,* 1982, 11(4):450.
30. Miller, M., & Nygran, C. Living with cancer—Coping behaviors. *Cancer Nurs,* 1978, 1(4):297.
31. Weisman, A.D., & Worden, J.W. Psychosocial analysis of cancer deaths. *Omega: J Death and Dying,* 1975, 6:61-75.
32. Zeitlin, S. Assessing coping behavior. *Am Orthopsychiatry Assoc J,* 1980, 50(1):139.
33. Choi, R., Josten, L.M., & Christensen, M. (1983). Health-specific coping index for noninstitutional care. *Am J Pub Health,* 1983, 73(11):1275.
34. Kupst, J.J., & Schulman, J.L. The CPI subscales as predictors of parental coping with childhood leukemia. *J Clin Psychol,* 1981, 37(2):386.
35. Miller, P., Wikoff, R., et al. Development of a health attitude scale. *Nurs Res,* 1982, 31(3):132.

36. Folkman, S., & Lazarus, R.S. An analysis of coping in a middle-aged community sample. *J Health Soc Behav*, 1980, *21*(3):219-239.

37. Gass, K.A., & Chang, A.S. Appraisals of bereavement, coping, resources, and psychosocial health dysfunction in widows and widowers. *Nurs Res*, 1989, *38*(10):31.

38. Cunningham, McNett, S. Social support, threat, and coping responses and effectiveness in the functionally disabled. *Nurs Res*, 1987, *36*(2):98.

39. Matheny, K., Curlette, W., Aycock, D., et al. *Coping resources inventory*. 1981 [Available from Dr. Kenneth Matheny, Department of Counseling and Psychological Services, Georgia State University, Atlanta, GA].

40. Heinrich, R., & Schag, C. Living with cancer: The Cancer Inventory of Problem Situations. *J Clin Psychol*, 1984, *40*(4):972.

41. Arathuzik, M.D. The appraisal of pain and coping in cancer patients. *West J Nurs Res*, 1991, *13*(6):714.

42. Jalowiec, A., Murphy, S., & Powers, M. Psychometric assessment of the Jalowiec Coping Scale. *Nurs Res*, 1984, *33*(3):157.

43. Jalowiec, A., & Powers, M. Stress and coping in hypertensive and emergency room patients. *Nurs Res*, 1981, *30*(1):10.

44. Nyamathi, A., Jacoby, A., Constancia, P., & Revsevich, S. Coping and adjustment of spouses of critically ill patients with cardiac disease. *Heart Lung*, 1992, *21*(2):160.

Appendix

12A. Summary List of Instruments Used in Research into Coping

Tool	Reliability Information	Validity Information	Population
Two-part Coping Assessment Scale (17)	No	No	Adults
Parental Coping Scale (1962) (18)	Yes	Yes	Parents
FILE (13)	Yes	Yes	Parents
A-FILE (14)	Yes	Yes	Adolescents and parents
F-COPES (15)	Yes	Yes	Adults
Richmond/Hopkins Family Coping Index (33)	Yes	No	Public health personnel
CPI (34)	No	No	Parents
Health Attitude Scale (35)	No	No	Adults
Patient Attitudes of Chronic Illness (25)	No	No	Adults
Chronicity Impact and Coping Instrument (22)	Yes	No	Parents
Goldstein Cooper-Avoider Sentence Completion Test (23)	No	No	Adults
Preoperative Coping Scale (24)	No	No	Adults
Coping Inventory (32)	Yes	No	Handicapped children
Coping Strategy Questionnaire (26)	Yes	No	Adults with low-back pain
Respiratory Illness Opinion Survey (27)	Yes	No	Adults
Response to Illness Questionnaire (28)	Yes	No	Long-term hemodialysis adults
Bedsworth and Molen Semistructured Interview (29)	No	No	Spouses of patients with myocardial infarction
Coping Strategies Scale (30)	No	No	Chronically ill adults
Cancer Inventory of Problem Situations (40)	No	Yes	Adults
Jalowiec Coping Scale	Yes	Yes	Adults
Family APGAR (16)	Yes	No	Adults
Parental Coping Scale (1989) (19)	Yes	No	Parents
Coping Health Inventory for Parents (CHIP) (20, 21)	Yes	No	Parents
Ways of Coping Checklist (WCC) (36)	Yes	No	Adults
Coping Resource Inventory (CRI) (39)	Yes	Yes	Adults
Pain Experience Inventory (41)	No	Yes	Adults
Pain Coping Tool (41)	No	Yes	Adults
Spousal Coping Instrument (SCI) (44)	Yes	No	Adults
McNett Coping Effectiveness Questionnaire (MCEQ)	Yes	No	Adults

Numbers in parentheses correspond to studies cited in the References.

13

Measuring Hope

Martha H. Stoner

Hope, a subtle, if not unconscious, expectation regarding an abstract, but positive, aspect of the future is an important factor influencing the quality and perhaps the quantity of life for people who have life-threatening or chronic illnesses. Health-care professionals have recognized an empirical relationship between the apparent loss of hope and eventual deterioration and death of patients with serious illnesses.[1-5] Practitioners working with persons who have cancer have become interested in the influence of hope and hopelessness on patients' abilities to cope with the uncertainty associated with their diagnosis.[6-15] Interventions designed to maintain and instill hope in patients are described.[16-21] Health professionals continue to try to understand the meaning of hope for themselves as well as for the patients and families for whom they provide care.[22-27] Research studies on hope, including the development of instruments to measure this concept, continue to be reported.[28-60] Hopelessness, frequently considered the polar opposite of hope, also has been measured and researched.[61-65] Because hope is such a complex, abstract phenomenon, a review of the theoretical foundation of the concept, including concept analyses and qualitative studies of hope, is presented. Instruments that measure hope are described.

Theoretical Description of Hope

Hope, thought of as wishful thinking or desire, frequently has been discredited as an impure mode of thought. An exception to this rejection of hope as unworthy of consideration is found in the works of philosopher Gabriel Marcel.[66-68] Marcel described hope as something very real that transcends all particular objects and is more concerned with a person as a being. Central to Marcel's view of hope is the association between hope and captivity and despair and the need to be delivered from some present condition or state. Although described as an inner sense, Marcel believed that there must be an interaction between one who gives and one who receives hope. This intersubjectivity, or bond of love, between self and others, is essential to hope as a mysterious, but important, inner force for human survival.

Lynch also rejected the commonly held view of hope as something vague or negative.[69] Hope was described as something very definite and positive. Hope is an interior sense that needs a response from the outside and has meaning only as it relates to others, that is, an act of collaboration or mutuality. Another similarity Lynch shared with Marcel was the placement of hope in a framework of captivity; the need to imagine a way out of difficulty was central.

Stotland[70] defined hope as the perceived probability of success in obtaining a goal. The person is convinced that the desired goal is truly obtainable. Much of Stotland's analysis was devoted to understanding hope as a psychodynamic force in relation to other factors, such as motivation, achievement, and goal attainment. These philosophical and behavioral science perspectives of hope contributed to a greater understanding of this abstract phenomenon. In addition, they provided conceptual frameworks for the development of measures of hope.

Measurement of Hope

Behavioral scientists and health professionals other than nurses have an interest in hope and have developed instruments to measure this concept. Those instruments are described in the following section.

Gottschalk-Gleser Hope Scale

Gottschalk measured hope as a set of predetermined weighted categories indicating positive or negative levels of hope.[31-33] The method of quantifying hope, one of several scales within the Gottschalk-Gleser Scales, used typescripts of 5-minute tape-recorded speech samples elicited from subjects in response to purposely ambiguous instructions to talk about any interesting or dramatic personal life experience.[31] One positive category consists of reference to self or others getting or receiving help, advice, support, sustenance, confidence, or esteem from others or self. Negative categories reference not being, not wanting, or not seeking to be the recipient of good fortune, good luck, or God's favor or blessing.

Gottschalk reported acceptable construct validity for his Hope Scale and used it in a number of studies.[31,33] In one study of radiation therapy patients, Gottschalk reported that pretreatment hope scores correlated significantly with duration of survival.[31] In a study of the emotional impact of surgery, Gottschalk and Hoigaard[33] found that women having mastectomies had significantly higher hope scores than healthy subjects. The authors concluded that the high hope scores were associated with denial as a coping mechanism. One concern regarding the use of this instrument relates to the measurement of multiple and diverse affects, such as hope, anxiety, and hostility derived the same speech sample.

Erickson, Post, and Paige Hope Scale

Erickson, Post, and Paige[30] developed is a 20-item, self-report instrument based on Stotland's theoretical constructs of hope,[70] that is, the importance of future-oriented goals and the probability of attaining those goals. The goals were focused but not situation-specific in an attempt to reflect goals common to American society. Examples of goals included: "To have enough money for basic needs," "To see my children turn out well," "To have good bodily health."

Subjects rate each goal on a seven-point scale of importance and then indicate the 0% to 100% probability of attaining those same goals. Erickson and associates reported test–retest reliabilities of 0.79 and 0.78 ($p = 0.001$) for importance and probability scales, respectively, when administered one week apart to undergraduate students. In a group of hospitalized psychiatric patients, these researchers found that psychopathology was associated with lower estimates of perceived probability of goal attainment and that effective psychotherapy increased the perceived probability of goal attainment, presumably indicating greater levels of hope.

Hope Index Scale (HIS)

The Hope Index Scale (HIS) defines hope as "a state of mind which results from the positive outcome of ego strength, perceived human family support, religion, education, and economic assets."[71] Obayuwana and associates[71] analyzed Kubler-Ross's five stages of dying and Engel's five characteristics of the giving-up–given-up complex and discovered what they judged to be very similar determinants of hope. They then conducted a telephone survey of randomly selected people ($n = 500$) to learn the meaning of hope. Interviewees were asked to give one-word descriptions of hope, and these words were clustered into themes. The HIS was constructed with 60 yes-no items representing those themes and the resultant definition of hope.[71] Ten of the 60 items test for social desirability and are not included in the scoring. Desirable responses are assigned 10 points for a maximum of 500 points. The HIS was tested with over 3,000 people in a series of studies evaluating the concurrent and predictive validity of the instrument. A significant and high negative correlation (Pearson's $r = -0.88$, $p < 0.001$) was found between the HIS and the Beck Hopelessness Scale. The HIS discriminated between and among normal controls, psychiatric patients, depressed patients without suicide ideation, and suicide attempters. Obayuwana and associates[71] indicate the HIS is suitable for both clinical evaluation of hope and to measure hope for research.

The Hope Index

Staats, a psychologist, developed the Hope Index based on Beck's self-other-world depressive triad and a definition of hope as the "interactions between wishes and expectations."[72,p367] The Hope Index stresses the cognitive rather than the affective aspect of hope and focuses on specific events rather than general optimism. Half of the items ($n = 8$) are self-references such as "To be more competent" and "To have good health." The other eight items focus on others or global circumstances such as "Other people to be more helpful" and "Understanding by my family." The Hope Index is scored by multiplying each "wish score" by each "expect score" and summing them. Scores for Hope-self, Hope-other, Wish, and Expect subscales can be derived. Staats does not reference Stotland's[70] theoretical description of hope as the importance and probability of goal attainment, but the Hope Index seems to reflect a similar theoretical perspective.

Staats evaluated the test–retest reliability of the Hope Index with 101 psychology students. The 9-week test reliability was 0.74. In a second study of college students ($n = 130$) the mean Hope Index score was 257.6 (SD 51.7), but reliability data were not reported. Staats reported that the Hope Index has a future orientation, but one of its limitations is the measurement of a cognitive aspect of hope when the concept has such an affectively laden meaning and use for most people. Another concern about the use of this instrument with diverse populations relates to the fact that items for the Hope Index were derived from a presumably healthy population of students, and all testing of the instrument was done with college students and other adults contacted by students.

Nursing Investigations of Hope: Qualitative Approaches

Nurses continue to investigate hope in an attempt to increase their understanding of this concept for use in research and in clinical practice. These inquiries range from clinicians' recognition of the importance of hope to their patients and a practical need for nursing interventions to support hope, to highly sophisticated research studies of hope using a variety of instruments and methods.

In one of the earliest efforts by a nurse to explicate the concept of hope, Stanley[36] used an existential, phenomenologic method. Her purpose was to isolate discrete, descriptive elements common to the experience of hope in healthy young adults, not to measure levels of hope. Junior and senior college students ($n = 100$) were asked to describe how they felt when they experienced hope in a situation. The phenomenologic analysis identified the following seven elements common to experiencing hope: (1) expectation of a significant future outcome; (2) being "confident" of outcome; (3) taking "action" to effect outcome; (4) experiencing "comfortable feelings"; (5) experiencing "uncomfortable feelings"; (6) having "interpersonal relatedness"; (7) having a quality of "transcendence." These common elements were synthesized into a general structure of hope as follows: "The lived experience of hope is a confident expectation of a significant future outcome, accompanied by a quality of transcendence and interpersonal relatedness and in which action to effect the outcome is initiated."[36,p165]

Thompson[40] investigated hope-related variables identified from the literature as they correlated to the perception of hope in 10 cancer patients. Field study methods with in-depth interviews, responses to scale items, and observation of behavior were used. Scaled items included patient and investigator ratings of hope on a four-point continuum, from lacking hope to hopeful. Findings incorporated a description of hope as "a complex phenomenon involving the variables of love, mutuality, freedom, and newness communicated through a positive orientation."[4,p117] Hope was manifested by a positive orientation and expectations for the future.

In a study of hope in elderly persons with cancer, Dufault used participant observation with 22 women and 13 men between the ages of 65 and 89.[28-29] She reported that her findings support hope as multidimensional and process oriented. Dufault defined hope as "a multi-dimensional dynamic life force characterized by confident yet uncertain anticipation of realistically possible and personally significant desirable future good having implications for action and for interpersonal relatedness."[28,p1821B] Dufault identified two related, but distinct, spheres of hope. Generalized hope included a general sense that future nonspecific developments would be beneficial. The second sphere, particularized hope, concerned the confident expectation of a specific future goal or personally significant future good for self. All subjects spoke of the behavior of significant others as a source of hope. Dufault's conceptualization of hope has influenced the work of other nurse researchers, including serving as a framework to develop instruments to measure hope.[22,26,54,56,57]

The Continuum of Hope

McGee developed a model of hope in which hope and hopelessness represent opposite ends of a continuum.[34] At one extreme is the unjustifiably or totally hopeful person who may be immobilized by feelings of invulnerability. At the other extreme is the unrealistically hopeless person who gives in to what is perceived as inevitable. The desirable balance in this model is achieved by what McGee labels the realistic copers, those people who have a positive outlook on life while accepting areas of actual hopelessness in life.

Most investigations of hope have been with adults facing a life-threatening illness. Adolescents, some well ($n = 17$) and some being treated for substance abuse ($n = 8$), participated in a grounded theory study of hope.[52] Analysis of the data revealed a construct definition of hope for adolescents: "the degree to which an adolescent believes that a personal tomorrow exists; this belief spans four hierarchial levels proceeding from lower to higher levels of believing."[52,p360] In another grounded theory investigation of hope, Hinds and Martin[53,73] learned from adolescents with a variety of cancer diagnoses how they achieve hopefulness and what nursing strategies influenced their hopefulness. Adolescents described four sequential phases to sustain their hopefulness: cognitive discomfort, distraction, cognitive comfort, and personal competence.[53] Nursing strategies positively influencing adolescent hopefulness were embedded in the involvement of the nurse in a personal and committed relationship with the adolescent.[73] The specific strategies identified were: truthful explanations, do something, nursing knowledge of survivors, caring behaviors, cognitive clutter, careful competence, and future focus.

Hall explored the concept of hope as experienced by 11 men with HIV disease.[23] From her own experience of being given a terminal diagnosis and the data from study participants, Hall defined hope as "something all people need until they take their last breath."[23,p178] She further explicates "that life is hope, and that hope, in our culture, is an orientation toward the future that must be maintained in every stage of life, regardless of one's degree of frailty or the potential hazards of an uncertain future."[33,p180] Hall offers a compelling argument that it is just as important to have hope immediately prior to death as it is at other times in life. She supports her position with the knowledge that we will all die and that because some people may have some greater prediction of the timing of their death this should not alter their maintaining hope. Hall urges health professionals not to label the hope expressed by terminally ill people as denial and thus deprive them of the comfort that hope brings to them.

Qualitative inquiries about hope have supported extant theoretical and philosophical conceptualizations of hope. These studies of hope contribute to the understanding of hope and provide further foundation for instrument development.

Nursing Investigations of Hope: Quantitative Approaches

Evidence of the importance of the concept of hope to nurses is apparent in the addition of at least three new instruments to measure hope that have been developed and used by nurse researchers since the first edition of this book. The next sections are devoted to the presentation of hope instruments and a brief discussion of the studies in which they were used.

Time Opinion Survey

Raleigh investigated hope as it was manifested in physically ill adults within the theoretical framework of Rogers' unitary man.[35] She interviewed 45 individuals with a chronic illnesses and 45 with a life-threatening form of cancer. The purposes of the study were to identify and describe attributes of hope as exhibited in the physically ill adult, to describe what these individuals believed to be factors that influenced their hope, and to explore possible relationships among types of illness, degree of hope, personal control, and length of illness. To accomplish her purposes, Raleigh designed a Time Opinion Survey as the measure of hope.

In a subsequent study,[60] Raleigh developed and used a 23-item interview guide, the Sources of Support Interview Schedule, to find out whether oncology patients differed from patients with other chronic illnesses in their sources of hope and their extensions of hope into the future. Respondents indicated how hopeful they were using a 1 to 10 scale. Both types of patients were generally optimistic and able to think positively about their illnesses. Patients used the strategies of (1) getting busy; (2) praying or participating in religious activities; (3) thinking about something else; and (4) talking to others to ease feelings of hopelessness. Nurses were evidently not identified as a specific source of support in this study.

Stoner Hope Scale (SHS)

One of the earliest attempts by a nurse researcher to meet the need for a valid and reliable measure of hope was the Stoner Hope Scale.[37,38] A preliminary form of the SHS adhered closely in both form and content to the scale based on Stotland's theory of hope[70] developed by Erickson and associates.[30] Problems in the use of this form of the scale encountered in a pilot study with 10 cancer patients resulted in modifications. Stotland's[70] conceptualization of hope as the importance and probability of attainment of future-oriented goals was retained. However, the theoretical frameworks of Lynch[69] and Marcel,[66-68] which recognize hope as an interior sense requiring interaction with external resources, had not been adequately reflected. To strengthen this aspect of the scale, generic and specific categories of hope were replaced by three domains of hope representing spheres of involvement. Intrapersonal, interpersonal, and global hope were designated as the three domains of hope. The domains and the goals within them were identified in consultation with nurse clinicians in oncology and psychiatry. Each domain has 10 goals, and subjects are requested to respond to each of the 30 goals on a four-point Likert-type response set, first for the importance of the goal and then for the probability of attainment of each goal. In addition, some items incorporate the conceptualization of hope as a need to escape from some difficulty. An example of this can be seen in the item "to be free from pain."

Intrapersonal hope is defined as the domain of hope grounded on interior resources and beliefs. Although it may be influenced by external stimuli, intrapersonal hope arises from within the person and is not dependent on transaction with another being. One item within the intrapersonal domain is to overcome fears.

Interpersonal hope is the domain of hope in which the sphere of involvement extends beyond the self and is definitely dependent on transactions with external resources. Thus, interpersonal hope occurs or exists because of the connection between individuals. An example of a goal in this domain is to have people seek me out as a friend.

Global hope refers to the broad scope of issues and concerns important to people in a general sense. Global hope goes beyond the person and interpersonal relationships to the sphere of involvement, including hope for the human race, the world, and beyond. One goal in the global hope domain is to see an end to the threat of nuclear war.

Scoring of the SHS was based on Stotland's conceptualization of hope and included both importance and probability as parameters. For each item, the importance score was multiplied by the probability score. These products were then summed to yield subscale scores (intrapersonal, interpersonal, and global) as well as a total hope score, for a maximum total score of 480.

To estimate content validity, three expert judges, all with postgraduate nursing education, independently placed goals into domains, with nearly 100% agreement.[37,74] Concurrent validity of the SHS was assessed through the use of the Beck Hopelessness Scale (BHS) as a criterion measure.[61-62] The BHS was designed to measure hopelessness and provides a measure of the construct hope in the opposite direction. The BHS has a high degree of internal consistency with a KR-20 reliability coefficient of 0.93 reported by Beck et al.[61] for a sample of 294 suicide attempters. The demonstrated negative relationship ($r = -0.47$, $p = 0.001$) between the SHS and the BHS indicates moderate concurrent validity for the SHS.

With a sample of 58 cancer patients, the SHS had a high degree of internal consistency as evidenced by a Cronbach alpha coefficient[75] of 0.93. Item-to-total correlations ranged from 0.37 to 0.65, with a mean interitem correlation of 0.53. When the SHS was subjected to canonical factor analysis,[76] in which the number of factors was limited to one, all 30 of the items loaded positively on the first factor and only four items weighted more heavily on another factor. This suggests that all of the items were measuring a single construct presumed to be hope. The computed reliability coefficient omega for the SHS was 0.94.

In a descriptive, correlational study of hope with 58 people with cancer, Stoner found positive associations between hope and religiosity ($r = 0.37$, $p = 0.01$), social support ($r = 0.34$, $p = 0.01$), and having close contact with other people with cancer ($r = 0.23$, $p = 0.05$).[37] In a further analysis of data from 55 subjects in this study, Stoner and Kaempfer[38] found no significant difference in the level of hope between subjects grouped by phase of illness: (1) no evidence of disease; (2) in active treatment; and (3) terminally ill. People who recalled being given information about their prognosis at the time of diagnosis had significantly lower hope scores than did those who had no recall of being told about their prognosis.

The SHS has been used in a number of studies by nurses, particularly graduate students, and by investigators from other disciplines. In a series of articles Farran and associates[42-44] report on a study of 126 community-living older adults, in which a modified version of the SHS and multiple instruments were used. The modified SHS used only the intra- and interpersonal subscales and only the probability responses were scored. In a report involving 72 of the subjects, a predictive model in which hope was the outcome variable was used. The researchers found that the model was stable over time.[42] Another report describes the association between hope and social support and interpersonal control.[43] The authors suggest that practitioners can influence hope in older people not by denying the losses associated with aging, but by focusing on reality-based hope. They identify the SHS as an appropriate measure for interactive attributes of hope. However, they noted that some items may not represent realistic hope for older adults.[44]

Nowotny Hope Scale (NHS)

The original Nowotny Hope Scale was composed of 47 items within six dimensions of hope identified from the literature.[39,58] The dimensions were (1) orients to future; (2) includes active involvement; (3) comes from within; (4) is possible; (5) relates to or involves others or a higher being; and (6) relates to meaningful outcomes to individuals. Sample items are "In the future I plan to accomplish many things," and "I have difficulty in setting goals."

In a methodologic study, Nowotny asked 306 adults, both well and having a cancer diagnosis, to think of a significant life event that they considered stressful. Subjects then responded to the objective statements using a four-point, scaled response of "strongly agree," "agree," "disagree," and "strongly disagree."

Internal consistency reliability was demonstrated by a Cronbach coefficient alpha of 0.897. A negative correlation coefficient of –0.471 ($p = 0.001$) between the NHS and the BHS indicates moderate concurrent validity. The final NHS consisted of 29 items within six factors: (1) confidence; (2) relating to others; (3) feeling that future is possible; (4) religious faith; (5) active involvement; and (6) the feeling that hope comes from within. The 29-item NHS has a reliability of 0.90, and the subscale alphas and item-to-item correlations were stronger. The mean for NHS was 82.7 (SD = 9.8), with a range of scores of 49 to 104.

Nowotny applies her research in measuring hope to clinical practice by stating that nurses should record their assessment of patients' hope in the medical record.[59] She advocates the use of the NHS as a clinical assessment instrument and suggests nursing interventions to facilitate hope within each of the dimensions measured.

The NHS was used in a study of spiritual well-being, religiousness, and hope in women with breast cancer.[77] In this study of 175 women the coefficient alpha was again 0.90. These women had higher mean hope scores, 95.4 (SD = 9.7), than subjects in Nowotny's study. Hope was positively associated with spiritual well-being.

Herth Hope Scale (HHS) and Herth Hope Index (HHI)

The Herth Hope Scale and an abbreviated version of the scale, the Herth Hope Index, have been used extensively in research with a variety of subjects.[45-51] The original HHS was developed from Lazarus and Folkman's Stress Appraisal and Coping theoretical perspective and Stotland's theory of hope. Hope was defined as "an energized mental state characterized by an action-oriented, positive expectation that goals or needs for self and future are obtainable, and that the present state or situation is temporary."[45,p69] This original 32-item scale used a categorical response set, in which respondents were asked to indicate "applies to me" or "does not apply to me" to items. The HHS was used in a descriptive study to determine the existence and nature of the relationship between hope and coping (Jalowiec Coping Scale) in 120 people with a variety of types of cancer who were receiving chemotherapy. A significant positive association between level of hope and level of coping response was found ($r = 0.80$, $p = 0.001$).

In a later report,[48] Herth described modifications of the HHS in which she incorporates the model of hope by Dufault and Martocchio.[29] Items were conceptualized within the spheres of generalized and particularized hope. Six dimensions of hope were combined into three: (1) cognitive-temporal; (2) affective-behavioral; and (3) affiliative-contextual. An example of a positively worded item is: "I believe a favorable outcome is possible." "My life has little meaning and value" is representative of negatively worded items. Each of the three dimensions had 10 items for a total of 30 items. The response set was modified to a four-point summated rating scale (0 = never applies to 3 = often applies).[48]

The HHS was used in a study of well adults ($n = 185$) to establish normative data on well adults.[49] The mean hope score was 80 (range 60 to 90). A 3-week test–retest with 20 subjects found a correlation coefficient of 0.90. The HHS was negatively correlated ($r = -0.74$) with the Beck Hopelessness Scale.[61] In a similar study to obtain normative data with an elderly population, the HHS was given to 40 randomly selected elderly people.[50] The Cronbach's alpha was 0.94, and a 3-week test–retest reliability coefficient with 20 subjects was 0.89. The mean hope score was 72 (SD = 6.31) and a range of 52 to 88. The HHS and BHS correlation was $r = -0.69$, $p = 0.01$. In a third study of 75 bereaved elderly people,[51] the Cronbach's alpha for the HHS was 0.95, and a 3-week test–retest reliability of 0.91 was obtained with a sample of 20.[51] The mean hope scores were lower at 54 (SD = 5.6) with a range of 29 to 83.[46,51]

Data from these three studies were pooled ($n = 300$) and subjected to factor analysis. Three factors consistent with the theoretical conceptualization of the HHS were supported. The factors were: temporality and future (cognitive-temporal dimension), positive readiness and expectancy (affective-behavioral dimension), and interconnectedness (affiliative-contextual dimension). The alpha coefficients for the subscales were 0.91, 0.90, and 0.87, respectively.

Herth Hope Index (HHI)

Herth developed and evaluated an abbreviated instrument to measure hope, the Herth Hope Index, to meet the need for an instrument to measure hope that is concise, simple, and has acceptable psychometric properties.[49] Because the HHI is intended for clinical application as well as research, the 12 items focus on adults who have an alteration in their health status. Four items in each of the three subscales parallel the conceptual foundation of the HHS. Example items of the HHI are: "I have specific possible short-, intermediate-, or long-range goals," "I see a light in the tunnel," and "I have faith that gives me comfort." The Likert-type response set is retained and each item is scored on an ordinal scale from 1 (strongly disagree) to 4 (strongly agree), with a total range of scores from 12 to 48.

A study to evaluate the psychometric properties of the HHI involved 172 adults from diverse settings, illness status, and backgrounds.[49] Validating instruments included the HHS, the Existential Well-Being Scale (EWS), and the Nowotny Hope Scale for concurrent criterion-related validity and the Hopelessness Scale (HS) to assess divergent validity. Factor analysis confirmed the original conceptualization represented by the three subscales. High correlations were obtained between the HHI and all of the criterion measures, HHI and the HHS ($r = 0.92$), the EWS ($r = 0.84$), and the NHS ($r = 0.81$). The correlation between the HHI and the HS was inverse ($r = -0.73$). All of the instruments attained acceptable Cronbach's alphas, including a 0.97 for the HHI. The respondents used the full range of scores (12 to 48) with a mean HHI score of 32.39 (SD = 9.61). The HHI takes only minutes to administer and is useful for both clinical assessment to facilitate nursing interventions and for research purposes.[49]

Herth has continued to use and evaluate the HHI with other populations.[47,50,51] In a study of terminally ill adults, all of whom were receiving hospice care, the range of scores on the HHI was 16 to 45. The mean score was 39 (SD = 4.34).[47] The mean HHI score of 38 (SD = 3.12), with a range of scores from 12 to 46, was found in a study of 60 older adults residing in one of three settings.[50] Using a similar research protocol, Herth studied family caregivers of terminally ill people ($n = 25$).[51] With this sample the mean HHI score was 37 (SD = 4.11), with a range of scores from 15 to 46. In these three studies, Herth used methodologic triangulation by adding a qualitative interview to enrich her data and validate her findings. The semistructured interviews explored subjects' perception of hope and identified strategies they believed fostered their hope based on their personal experience. Analysis of the interviews increases the understanding of the meaning of hope to diverse segments of the population and provides a framework for nursing interventions based on the categories of hope-fostering strategies. Herth's focused research efforts in developing and evaluating instruments to measure hope have made a significant contribution to the understanding of hope and to its use in both clinical practice and research.

The Miller Hope Scale (MHS)

The Miller Hope Scale is a 40-item instrument with a five-point Likert-type response set (5 representing strong agreement, 1 strong disagreement). The range of possible scores is 40 to 200, with a high score indicating high levels of hope. An example of a positively worded item is "I look forward to an enjoyable future"; "I feel trapped, pinned down" illustrates a negatively worded item. Hope is described as a state of being characterized by an anticipation for a continued good state, an improved state, or a release from a perceived entrapment. The conceptualization of the MHS was based on the works of Dufault,[28,29] Lynch,[69] and Marcel.[66-68] Critical elements of hope identified are: (1) mutuality-affiliation; (2) sense of the possible; (3) avoidance of absolutizing; (4) anticipation; (5) achieving goals; (6) psychologic well-being and coping; (7) purpose and meaning in life; (8) freedom; (9) reality-surveillance-optimism; and (10) mental and physical activity.

In a study to evaluate the psychometric properties of the MHS, 522 college students completed the MHS and construct validation instruments.[56] The Psychological Well-Being Scale (PWBS), the Existential Well-Being Scale (EWBS), and a single-item 10-point self-assessed Hope Scale were used to evaluate criterion-related validity. The Hopelessness Scale (HS) was used to assess discriminant validity. The mean score for the MHS was 164.46 (SD = 16.31) with a range of scores of 105 to 198. Cronbach's alpha on the MHS was 0.93 and with a subsample of 308 students, a 2-week test–retest reliability of 0.82 was obtained. Construct validity was supported by correlation coefficients of 0.71 with the PWBS, 0.82 with the EWBS, and 0.69 with the single-item self-assessment of hope. A negative correlation of 0.67 was found between the MHS and the HS. Factor analysis produced three factors: (1) satisfaction with self, others, and life; (2) avoidance of hope threats; and (3) anticipation of the future. Hope was considered a complex, multidimensional construct, that is, a state of being that is more than goal attainment.

Miller[57] conducted a qualitative descriptive study of hope with a sample of 60 people, aged 38 to 83, who had been critically ill. The purpose of the study was to learn from patients what strategies they used to maintain or increase hope when they felt their existence was threatened. A 20-item structured interview guide was used to generate data analyzed to identify nine categories of hope-inspiring themes. The categories are: (1) cognitive strategies; (2) determinism; (3) worldview; (4) spiritual strategies; (5) relationship with caregivers; (6) family bonds; (7) control; (8) goals; and (9) other. Subjects were less able to identify threats to their hope, perhaps because they felt good because they had survived a recent health crisis. Although, as in other studies, nurses were not specifically identified as a source of hope, Miller identified some strategies for maintaining hope that could guide nursing interventions related to hope.

The Miller Hope Scale was used in a study of hope, self-esteem, and social support in people with multiple sclerosis.[78] Data were gathered on 40 participants, aged 32 to 70 years with a mean age of 48.2. The mean MHS score was 157.9, and scores ranged from 108 to 200. Hope was correlated with both self-esteem ($r = 0.74, p = 0.001$) and social support ($r = 0.68, p = 0.001$). These findings suggest nursing interventions targeting increasing self-esteem and social support also may increase the level of hope in persons with multiple sclerosis.

In a similar study,[79] the MHS was used to evaluate hope in patients with spinal cord injuries. Participants ($n = 77$) were 18 to 73 years of age (mean = 34.79) and had numerous physical impairments. The range of scores on the MHS was 54 to 197 with a mean of 153.51 out of a possible range of 40 to 200. Correlations of 0.908 ($p = 0.001$) between hope and self-esteem and 0.891 ($p = 0.001$) between hope and social support were detected. The authors concluded that nursing care to promote hope in persons with spinal cord injuries is appropriate.

Assessment of hope in psychiatric ($n = 48$) and chemically dependent ($n = 144$) patients was the focus of another research report[80] in which the MHS was used with a convenience sample with a mean age of 38.35. The mean MHS score of 135.73 (SD = 25.17) with this population was statistically significantly lower than Miller's findings with healthy adults.[56] These findings add to the construct validity of the MHS because hope scores were lower at time of admission than just prior to discharge. In addition, this population's hope scores were lower than those of healthy adults.

The Miller Hope Scale was used in a study[81] of functional status and hope in elderly people with ($n = 86$) and without cancer ($n = 88$). The Philadelphia Geriatric Center's

Multilevel Assessment Instrument (MAI) was used to measure functional status. Having cancer was not a threat to hope, but declining physical health and lower socioeconomic status were significantly associated with lower levels of hope.

Progress has been made in the development of valid and reliable instruments to measure hope for research purposes. Efforts to assess hope systematically as a clinical parameter to guide interventions continue to evolve. Perhaps, use of the single-item, 1-to-10 scale to assess levels of hope will become another "vital sign," similar to the 1-to-10 pain assessment scale as a standard of practice.

Summary

Many of the articles on hope are anecdotal descriptions of hope as an important clinical phenomenon. Hope is recognized as a powerful force in the survival of patients confronted by life-threatening and chronic illnesses. Some authors encourage nurses to instill, inspire, and maintain hope as a therapeutic intervention with patients, and others caution against what they label supporting unrealistic hope or denial.

Because hope is a complex, abstract phenomenon, this review of instruments to measure hope includes a discussion of the theoretical analysis from the perspective of philosophy and the behavioral sciences. Themes common to most of the discussion of hope, including theoretical, clinical, and measurement issues are (1) a future orientation; (2) an expectation of attainment of important goals; (3) recognition of hope as an interior sense that is dependent on interaction with others; and (4) a need to escape from some feeling of captivity or despair. Additional research to refine and evaluate the existing instruments for research purposes is ongoing. Progress in developing instruments to be used in collecting data on hope and to direct interventions to maintain hope have been made. Continued research, including replication of studies with different populations, testing of theoretical models, and evaluation of therapeutic interventions to influence levels of hope, is needed.

Exemplar Studies

Stoner, M.H., & Kaempfer, S.H. Recalled life expectancy information, phase of illness and hope in cancer patients. *Res Nurs Health*, 1985, 8:269.

This descriptive, comparative study exemplifies the measurement of hope within a specific theoretical conceptualization and with a defined population, persons with different stages of cancer. Of particular value is the detailed description of the development and evaluation of the Stoner Hope Scale, including the thorough review of the literature for the theoretical formulation of the instrument. Appropriate procedures to ensure and to evaluate the reliability and validity of all instruments used are well described. Analysis of variance revealed a significant main effect of recalled life expectancy on level of hope in 55 cancer patients. Individuals who had no recollection of receiving information regarding their prognosis were more hopeful. This has implications for determining what, how much, when, and how life expectancy information is communicated to patients with a life-threatening diagnosis.

Herth, K. Abbreviated instrument to measure hope: Development and psychometric evaluation. *J Adv Nurs*, 1992, 17:1259.

This methodologic study to evaluate the psychometric properties of an abbreviated hope scale exemplifies a program of research in which an investigator pursues the measurement of a concept, culminating in a refined, abbreviated instrument to measure hope, the Herth Hope Index. A description of the development and evaluation of the longer instrument to measure hope, the Herth Hope Scale, conveys the rigorous methods used in many studies with diverse subjects. The result is a carefully constructed instrument that, although it will require further testing with adolescents, children, and people representing different cultural backgrounds, is useful for clinical screening of patients and for research data. The brevity of the instrument has not diminished its reliability and validity and has increased the potential utility with individuals who might experience fatigue or be reluctant to complete a more time-consuming instrument.

References

1. Engel, G. A life setting conducive to illness: The giving-up given-up complex. *Bull Menninger Clinic,* 1986, 32(2):324.
2. Hyland, J. Death by giving up. *Bull Menninger Clinic,* 1978, 42(4):339.
3. Richter, C.P. On the phenomenon of sudden death in animals and man. *Psychosom Med,* 1957, 19(3):191.
4. Stewart, W.K. Hopelessness following illness in middle age. *Psychosomatics* 1977, 18(2):29.
5. Vaux, K.L. *Will to live, will to die.* Minneapolis, MN: Augsburg Publishing House, 1978.
6. Allen, A. Psychosocial factors in cancer. *Am Fam Phys,* 1981, 23(2):197.
7. Buehler, J.A. What contributes to hope in the cancer patient? *Am J Nurs,* 1975, 75(9):1353.
8. Lange, S.P. Hope. In C.E. Carlson & B. Blackwell (Eds.), *Behavioral concepts and nursing intervention* (2nd ed.) Philadelphia: Lippincott, 1978, p. 171.
9. Miller, J.F. Inspiring hope. *Am J Nurs,* 1985, 85(1):22.
10. Roberts, S.L. *Behavioral concepts and nursing throughout the life span.* Englewood Cliffs, NJ: Prentice-Hall, 1978.
11. Walsi, E. *Hope, a basic nursing concept.* Conference on Teaching Psychiatric Nursing in Baccalaureate Programs, Atlanta, GA: Southern Regional Educational Board, 1967.
12. Ersek, M. The process of maintaining hope in adults undergoing bone marrow transplantation for leukemia. *Oncol Nurs Forum,* 1992, 19(6):883.
13. Hickey, S.S. Enabling hope. *Cancer Nurs,* 1986, 9(3):133.
14. O'Connor, A.P., Wicker, C.A., & Germino, B.B. Understanding the cancer patients's search for meaning. *Cancer Nurs,* 1990, 13(3):167.
15. Scanlon, C. Creating a vision of hope: The challenge of palliative care. *Oncol Nurs Forum,* 1989, 16(4):491.
16. Barckley, V. A visiting nurse specializes in cancer. *Am J Nurs,* 1970, 70(8):1680.
17. Dubfee, M., & Vogelpohl, R. When hope dies: So might the patient. *Am J Nurs,* 1980, 80(6):1046.
18. Laney, M.L. Hope as a healer. *Nurs Outlook,* 1969, 17(1):45.
19. Limandri, B.J., & Boyle, D.W. Instilling hope. *Am J Nurs,* 1978, 78(1):79.
20. Taylor, P.B., & Gideon, M.D. Holding out hope to your dying patient. *Nursing 82,* 1982, 82(2):268.
21. Vaillot, N.C. Hope, the restoration of being. *Am J Nurs,* 1970, 70(2):268.
22. Haase, J.E., Britt, T., Coward, D.D., Leidy, N.K., & Penn, P.E. Simultaneous concept analysis of spiritual perspective, hope, acceptance and self-transcendence. *IMAGE: J Nurs Scholar,* 1992, 24(2):141.
23. Hall, B.A. The struggle of the diagnosed terminally ill person to maintain hope. *Nurs Sci Q,* 1990, 4(3):177.
24. Obayuwana, A.O., & Carter, A.L. The anatomy of hope. *J Nat Med Assoc,* 1982, 74(3):229.
25. Stephenson, C. The concept of hope revisited for nursing. *J Adv Nurs,* 1991, 16(12):1456.
26. Yates, P. Towards a reconceptualization of hope for patients with a diagnosis of cancer. *J Adv Nurs,* 1993, 18(5):701.
27. Campbell, L. Hopelessness. *J Psychosoc Nurs,* 1987, 25(2):18
28. Dufault, K.J. *Hope of elderly persons with cancer* (doctoral dissertation, Case Western Reserve University). *Dissertation Abstracts International,* 1981, 42(05):1820-1b (University Microfilms No. 8118642).
29. Dufault, K.J., & Martocchio, B. Hope: Its spheres and dimensions. *Nurs Clin North Am,* 1985, 20(2):379.
30. Erickson, R.C., Post, R.D., & Paige, A.B. Hope as a psychiatric variable. *J Clin Psychol,* 1975, 31(a):324.
31. Gottschalk, L.A. A hope scale applicable to verbal samples. *Arch Gen Psychiatr,* 1974, 30(6):779.
32. Gottschalk, L.A., Lolas, F., & Viney, L.L. (Eds.). *Content analysis of verbal behavior: Significance in clinical medicine and psychiatry.* New York: Springer-Verlag, 1986.
33. Gottschalk, L.A., & Hoigaard, J. Emotional impact of mastectomy. In L.A. Gottschalk, F. Lolas, & L.L. Viney (Eds.), *Content analysis of verbal behavior: Significance in clinical medicine and psychiatry.* New York: Springer-Verlag, 1986, p. 171.
34. McGee, R.F. Hope: A factor influencing crisis resolution. *Adv Nurs Sci,* 1984, 6(4):34.
35. Raleigh, E.D. *An investigation of hope as manifested in the physically ill adult* (doctoral dissertation, Wayne State University). *Dissertation Abstracts International,* 1980, 41(04):1313B (University Microfilms No. 8022786).
36. Stanley, A.T. *The lived experience of hope: The isolation of discrete descriptive elements common to the experience of hope in healthy young adults* (doctoral dissertation, The Catholic University of America). *Dissertation Abstracts International,* 1978, 39(03):1212B (University Microfilms No. 7816899).
37. Stoner, M.J.H. *Hope and cancer patients* (doctoral dissertation, The University of Colorado). *Dissertation Abstracts International,* 1982, 44(1):115B (University Microfilms No. 8312243).
38. Stoner, M.H., & Kaempfer, S.H. Recalled life expectancy information, phase of illness and hope in cancer patients. *Res Nurs Health,* 1985, 8(3):269.
39. Nowotny, M.L. *Measurement of hope as exhibited by a general adult population after a stressful event.* Doctoral dissertation, Texas Woman's University, Denton, TX, 1986.
40. Thompson, M. *An investigation of the relationship of love, mutuality, freedom, and newness with the perception of hope in patients with the diagnosis of cancer.* Unpublished thesis, California State University, 1980.
41. Grimm, P.M. *Hope, affect, psychological status and the cancer experience* (doctoral dissertation, University of

Maryland at Baltimore) *Dissertation Abstracts International*, 1989 (University Microfilms No. PUZ8924458).

42. Farran, C.J., & McCann, J. Longitudinal analysis of hope in community-based older adults. *Arch Psychiatr Nurs*, 1989, 3(5):272.

43. Farran, C.J., & Popovich, J.M. Hope: A relevant concept for geriatric psychiatry. *Arch Psychiatr Nurs*, 1990, 4(2):124.

44. Farran, C.J., Salloway, J.C., & Clark, D.C. Measurement of hope in a community-based older population. *West J Nurs Res*, 1990, 12(1):42.

45. Herth, K.A. The relationship between level of hope and level of coping response and other variables in patients with cancer. *Oncol Nurs Forum*, 1989, 16(1):67.

46. Herth, K. Relationship of hope, coping styles, concurrent losses, and setting to grief resolution in the elderly widow(er). *Res Nurs Health*, 1990, 13(1):109.

47. Herth, K. Fostering hope in terminally-ill people. *J Adv Nurs*, 1990, 15(11):1250.

48. Herth, K. Development and refinement of an instrument to measure hope. *Scholar Inquiry Nurs Pract Int J*, 1991, 5(1):39.

49. Herth, K. Abbreviated instrument to measure hope: Development and psychometric evaluation, *J Adv Nurs*, 1992, 17(10):1251.

50. Herth, K. Hope in older adults in community and institutional settings. *Issues Ment Health Nurs*, 1993, 14(2):139.

51. Herth, K. Hope in the family caregiver of terminally ill people. *J Adv Nurs*, 1993, 18(4):538.

52. Hinds, P.S. Inducing a definition of "hope" through the use of grounded theory methodology. *J Adv Nurs*, 1984, 9(4):357.

53. Hinds, P.S., & Martin, J. Hopefulness and the self-sustaining process in adolescents with cancer. *Nurs Res*, 1988, 37(6):336.

54. Miller, J.F. Inspiring hope. In J.F. Miller, *Coping with chronic illness: Overcoming powerlessness*. Philadelphia: Davis, 1983.

55. Farran, C.J., Wilken, C., & Popvich, J.M. Clinical assessment of hope. *Issues Ment Health Nurs*, 1992, 13(2):129.

56. Miller, J.F., & Powers, M.J. Development of an instrument to measure hope. *Nurs Res*, 1988, 37(1):6.

57. Miller, J.F. Hope-inspiring strategies of the critically ill. *Appl Nurs Res*, 1989, 2(1):23.

58. Nowotny, M.L. Assessment of hope in patients with cancer: Development of an instrument. *Oncol Nurs Forum*, 1989, 16(1):57.

59. Nowotny, M.L. Every tomorrow, a vision of hope. *J Psychosoc Oncol*, 1991, 9(3):117.

60. Raleigh, E.D.H. Sources of hope in chronic illness. *Oncol Nurs Forum*, 1992, 19(3):443.

61. Beck, A.T., Lester, D., Trexler, L., & Weisman, A. The measurement of pessimism: The hopelessness scale. *J Consult Clin Psychol*, 1974, 42(6):861.

62. Durham, T.W. Norms, reliability, and item analysis of the hopelessness scale in general psychiatric, forensic psychiatric, and college populations. *J Clin Psychol*, 1982, 38(3):597.

63. Carson, V., Soeken, K.L., Shanty, J., & Terry, L. Hope and spiritual well-being: Essentials for living with AIDS. *Perspect Psychiatr Care*, 1990, 26(2):28.

64. Campbell, L. Hopelessness: A concept analysis. *J Psychosoc Nurs*, 1987, 25(2):18.

65. Rideout, E., & Montemuro, M. Hope, morale and adaptation in patients with chronic heart failure. *J Adv Nurs*, 1986, 11(4):429.

66. Marcel, G. *Homo viator* (E. Crawford, trans.). San Francisco, CA: Harper & Row, 1962.

67. Marcel, G. *The mystery of being. vol. 11:* Faith and reality. South Bend, IN: Regnery/Gateway, 1951.

68. Marcel, G. *Desire and hope.* In N. Lawrence & D. O'Connor (Eds.), *Readings in existential phenomenology.* Englewood Cliffs, NJ: Prentice-Hall, 1967, p. 277.

69. Lynch, W.F. *Images of hope.* Baltimore, MD: Helicon, 1965.

70. Stotland, E. *The psychology of hope.* San Francisco, CA: Jossey-Bass, 1969.

71. Obayuwana, A.O., Collins, J.L., Carter, A.L., et al. Hope index scale: An instrument for the objective assessment of hope. *JAMA*, 1982, 74(6):761.

72. Staats, S. Hope: A comparison of two self-report measures for adults. *J Person Assess*, 1989, 53(2):366.

73. Hinds, P.S., Martin, J., & Vogel, R.J. Nursing strategies to influence adolescent hopefulness during oncologic illness. *J Assoc Pediatr Oncol*, 1987, 4(1&2):14.

74. Mitchell, S.K. Interobserver agreement, reliability, and generalizability of data collected in observational studies. *Psychol Bull*, 1979, 86(2):376.

75. Anastasi, A. *Psychological testing* (4th ed.). New York: Macmillan, 1970.

76. Allen, M.P. Construction of composite measures by canonical-factor-regression method. In H.L. Costner (Ed.), *Sociological methodology.* San Francisco, CA: Jossey-Bass, 1974, p. 51.

77. Mickley, J.R., Soeken, K., & Belcher, A. Spiritual well-being, religiousness and hope among women with breast cancer. *IMAGE: J Nurs Scholar*, 1992, 24(4):267.

78. Foote, A.W., Piazza, D., Holcome, J., Paul, P., & Daffin, P. Hope, self-esteem and social support in persons with multiple sclerosis. *J Neurosci Nurs*, 1990, 22(3):155.

79. Piazza, D., Holcombe, J., Foote, A., et al. Hope, social support and self-esteem of patients with spinal cord injuries. *J Neurosci Nurs*, 1991, 23(4):224.

80. Holdcraft, C., & Williamson, C. Assessment of hope in psychiatric and chemically dependent patients. *Appl Nurs Res*, 1991, 4(3):129.

81. McGill, J.S., & Paul, P.B. Functional status and hope in elderly people with and without cancer. *Oncol Nurs Forum*, 1993, 20(8):1207.

14

Instruments to Measure Aspects of Spirituality

Jan M. Ellerhorst-Ryan

Commitment to viewing health care in a holistic manner must include the client's spiritual concerns. Highfield and Cason stated, "We cannot abdicate our responsibility for treating a person's spiritual needs to the chaplain, any more than we can abdicate our responsibility for man's physical needs to the physician, or his psychosocial needs to the psychologist and social worker."[1,p191]

Historically, research on spirituality has focused on religiosity. Moberg and Brusek,[2] in comparing religiosity and spiritual well-being, associate the former with institutional goals and behaviors. Measures of religious practice are not always reliable indicators of spirituality.

Spirituality is more than the sum of the client's religious preference, religious beliefs, and religious practices. It relates to "the totality of man's inner resources, the ultimate concerns around which all other values are focused, the central philosophy of life that guides conduct, and the meaning-giving center of human life which influences all individual and social behavior."[3,p2] It encompasses man's need to find satisfactory answers to questions about the meaning of life, illness, and death.

The Third National Conference on Classification of Nursing Diagnoses recognized the importance of spirituality by including "spiritual concerns," "spiritual distress," and "spiritual despair" in the list of approved nursing diagnoses. In 1980, the Fourth National Conference combined these three diagnoses into one, "spiritual distress," defined as "a disruption in the life principle which pervades a person's entire being and which integrates and transcends one's biological and psychosocial nature."[4] This definition, although a beginning, is vague and does not lend itself easily to research.

Spiritual concepts apply to persons who are religious, nonreligious, or antireligious. Given that both a religious component and a psychosocial component are involved in spiritual concerns, both should be addressed in a tool designed to assess aspects of spirituality.

The concept of "God" does not easily conform to a universal definition. It is, therefore, important to consider ways of eliciting information about the subject's perception of God. Persons holding traditional views of God characterize Him as the ultimate Deity. For others, particularly the nonreligious or antireligious, "God" may be whatever that person values most, the focal point of life, work, family, or community service.

In view of the significant influence that the Judeo-Christian philosophy has had on the development of Western culture, the instruments discussed most often reflect that perspective. Information regarding applicability to persons who have other religious orientations is included when available.

Instruments

Before selecting a measurement tool, the researcher must first decide which aspect of spirituality is to be investigated. Spiritual needs in general may be studied, or the focus may be limited to a specific spiritual need. Four commonly identified spiritual needs include hope, forgiveness, love and relatedness, and meaning and purpose in life. Other related concepts for which measurement tools are available include spiritual well-being, spiritual coping, and religious orientation.

Consideration also must be given to the population under study (e.g., adults vs. children, nurses vs. patients) to ensure appropriate measurement tool selection.

Spiritual Needs: Quantitative Tools

Spiritual Health Inventory (SHI)

The SHI[5] is a 31-item self-report instrument worded in the first person. Respondents rank how often they have experienced the feeling or behavior described on a 1 to 5 Likert scale. SHI content is consistent with the author's definition of spiritual health; that is, having satisfactorily met spiritual needs for self-acceptance; a trusting relationship with self based on a sense of meaning and purpose in life (e.g., "I feel valuable as a person even when I cannot do as much as before"); relationships with others and/or a supreme other characterized by unconditional love, trust, and forgiveness (e.g., "I believe my nurses and doctors care about me," "I feel a need to be forgiven for some of my thoughts and feelings"); and hope (e.g., "I worry about life after death").[5] A ranking of 5 indicates frequent occurrence, and a ranking of 1 indicates infrequent occurrence. Scores are determined by reversing subject-recorded ratings of each negative indicator of spiritual health, then summing ratings for all items. Higher scores are associated with higher levels of spiritual health.

Content and construct validity for the SHI are based on a review of the literature, input from an expert panel, and factor analysis. Three factors, representing the spiritual needs for self-acceptance, relationships, and hope, account for 71.5% of variance. Analysis using 23 subjects produced a Cronbach's alpha of $r = 0.77$.[5]

Spiritual Perspective Scale (SPS)

Formerly titled the Religious Perspective Scale, the SPS contains 10 items that measure the subjects' "perspectives on the extent to which spirituality permeates their lives and (their degree of engagement) in spiritually-related interactions."[6,p337] The SPS can be administered either as a structured interview or questionnaire. Responses are ranked on a 1-to-6 scale. Scores are determined by calculating the arithmetic mean across all items, with higher scores indicating greater spiritual perspective. An example of an item is "In talking with your family or friends, how often do you mention spiritual matters?" with response options ranging from 1, not at all, to 5, about once a day.

Reliability and validity for the SPS have been demonstrated in both healthy and terminally ill adult populations. Internal consistency was measured by Cronbach's alpha, with alpha coefficients ranging from 0.93 to 0.95. Interitem analysis revealed average correlations between 0.57 and 0.68. The fact that subjects who reported having a religious background scored higher on the SPS provided evidence for construct validity.[6,7]

Serenity Scale

The 40-item Serenity Scale is designed to measure serenity, "a spiritual experience of inner peace that is independent of external events."[8] Although related to peace of mind, serenity goes further, bringing comfort to those confronted by harsh circumstances that are difficult and sometimes impossible to change. Attributes of serenity, as discussed by the authors of the scale, include hope, forgiveness, love and relatedness, and meaning and purpose in life.[8]

Items are scored using a Likert scale, with subjects rating frequencies of personal experiences from 1, never, to 6, always. Thirteen of the 40 items are negatively stated and require reverse scoring. Higher scores indicate greater levels of serenity. Examples of test items include "I experience an inner calm even when under pressure" and "I experience an inner quiet that does not depend upon events."

Content validity of the Serenity Scale was established by an expert panel analysis during instrument development. Internal consistency was established by Cronbach's alpha, reported as 0.92. Factor analysis revealed nine factors that explained 58.2% of the variance: inner haven, acceptance, belonging, trust, perspective, contentment, present centered, beneficence, and cognitive restructuring.[8] The authors acknowledge questionable validity with low-literacy subjects.

Serenity transcends formal religious dogma; therefore, the Serenity Scale can be used with subjects holding a variety of religious views, including atheism. Participants in field studies represent a wide range of age and economic groups from both rural and urban areas. The authors note, however, that the scale has been tested on primarily white and well-educated adults.[9]

Spiritual Needs: Qualitative Tools

Interview schedules using open-ended questions may be more useful for qualitative spiritual research. The interview tools described here can be utilized in populations of individuals with diverse religious beliefs and orientations.

Stallwood, Hess,[9,10] and Stoll,[11] well-known for their interest in spiritual concerns of patients, have defined spiritual needs as "any factors necessary to establish and/or maintain a dynamic personal relationship with God (as defined by the individual) and out of that relationship to experience forgiveness, love and relatedness, hope, trust and meaning and purpose in life."[9] Each author has developed an assessment tool useful for interviewing and data collection.

Hess's Spiritual Needs Survey

Hess's Spiritual Needs Survey was designed for use in hospitals or extended care facilities, but could be easily modified for use in other settings.[10] Five questions focus on the patient's awareness of his or her spiritual needs and efforts to address them:

- Were you aware of having a spiritual need at any time during your hospitalization?
- Are you able to describe it? Can you tell me about it?
- With whom did you discuss this need?
- How did you feel about the assistance you received?
- Has your need been met to any degree or is it still present?[10]

Stoll's Guidelines for Spiritual Assessment

Although Stoll's Guidelines for Spiritual Assessment were not designed for use as a research tool, they have been used in conjunction with other measurement scales to evaluate the ability of hospitalized patients to meet their spiritual needs.[11-13] Stoll's Guidelines include 13 questions addressing the person's concept of God, sources of hope and strength, religious practices, and the relationship between spiritual beliefs and health. A sample item is: "To whom do you turn when you need help?"

Fish and Shelly[14] modified Stoll's Guidelines to organize the questions into four categories: understanding a person's beliefs about and involvement with God and religious practice; determining the extent to which a person's religious practices serve as a resource for faith and life; assessing whether resources for hope and strength are founded in reality; and extending an opportunity to accept spiritual help. Excluding the fourth category, which is an invitation for intervention by the interviewer, the remaining three categories make up 11 open-ended questions.

The Reed Interview Schedule

The Reed Interview Schedule is designed to elicit information regarding patient preferences for spiritually related nursing interventions.[15] The schedule consists of one structured item and one open-ended item. The first question, "In what ways could hospital nurses help you in your spiritual needs?" is followed by descriptions of seven spiritually related interventions identified in a review of current nursing literature. Interventions included reading to or with the patient; allowing time for personal prayer or meditation; talking with the patient about beliefs and concerns; providing time for the patients to talk or pray with family members; arranging a visit with a minister, priest, or rabbi; and helping the patients to attend the hospital chapel. Participants may select more than one intervention in response to the question. The second open-ended item invites participants to describe other interventions important to them but not listed in the first item.

Singular Concepts of Spiritual Need

An alternative to investigating spiritual needs is to limit the scope of the study to one or more specific spiritual needs. The concept of hope, meaning and purpose in life, forgiveness and love, and relatedness are discussed in greater detail in Chapter 13; however, each concept is briefly reviewed here, and a measurement tool for each is highlighted.

Hope

Dufault and Martocchio have defined hope as "multidimensional life force characterized by a confident yet uncertain expectation of achieving a future good which . . . is realistically possible and personally significant."[16] These characteristics are clearly demonstrated in the Nowotony Hope Scale (NHS).[17]

The NHS is a 29-item questionnaire that assesses six components of hope: (1) confidence in outcome; (2) relationships with others; (3) belief in the possibility of a future; (4) spiritual beliefs; (5) active involvement; and (6) inner readiness. Responses are recorded using a four-point scale (strongly agree, agree, disagree, strongly disagree). An example of an NHS item is: "Sometimes I feel I am all alone."[17]

Reliability analysis of the NHS using Cronbach's alpha yielded a coefficient of 0.90. Concurrent validity was established by comparing participant scores on NHS with scores on the Beck Hopelessness Scale. Pearson's product moment correlation produced $r = -0.47$ ($p < 0.001$).[17]

Meaning and Purpose in Life

Crumbaugh's Purpose in Life Test (PIL) is designed to measure the degree to which a person experiences a sense of meaning and purpose in life.[18] The tool was developed based on Frankl's concepts of noogenic neurosis that occurs in response to an absence of purpose in life, manifested by "existential frustration" and boredom.[19]

The PIL consists of 20 items to which respondents reply on a seven-point scale. Construct validity was established by comparing scores of healthy subjects with clients undergoing psychiatric therapy. Differences reported were significant and in the direction predicted. Concurrent validity was demonstrated by correlating PIL test scores with therapists' ratings for psychiatric clients and ministers' ratings of healthy subjects. Correlations were 0.37 ($n = 50$) and 0.47 ($n = 120$), respectively. Reliability testing, using split-half correlation ($n = 120$), yielded a coefficient of 0.85, corrected to 0.92 by the Spearman-Brown formula.[20]

Love and Relatedness

Although the definitions of social support vary, factors consistently identified include the perception that one is cared about, loved, esteemed, and valued, and the perception that support is readily available when needed. These elements of love and relatedness are not only essential components of relationships with other people but also present to varying degrees in a person's relationship with God.[21]

Maton's Spiritual Support Scale employs three items to assess perceived support from God. Responses are recorded using a five-point scale, ranging from "not at all accurate" to "completely accurate." The first two items, "I experience God's love and caring on a regular basis" and "I experience a close personal relationship with God," were found in a prior study to predict well-being in a congregational sample and to correlate positively with other measures of intrinsic religion.[22] A third item, "My religious faith helps me cope during times of difficulty," elicits faith aspects of perceived spiritual support. Cronbach's alpha produced a reliability coefficient of 0.92, with test–retest reliability yielding $r = 0.81$ ($n = 66$).[21]

The Spiritual Support Scale has been used to evaluate the relationship between perceived levels of spiritual support and well-being among two groups of high-stress and low-stress individuals.[21] Among recently bereaved parents and adolescents experiencing three or more uncontrollable life events, perceived spiritual support correlated significantly with multiple measures of well-being in the direction predicted. No significant relationships were found between spiritual support and well-being in low-stress populations. Limitations acknowledged by the author in testing the Spiritual Support Scale include small sample size and inadequate minority representation.[21]

Forgiveness

Studkinski has defined forgiveness as a "response to suffering which an individual has incurred at the hands of someone else . . . the choice presented to the sufferer is between harbouring resentment or allowing the healing of forgiveness to take place."[23] Two scales measuring forgiveness were developed by Mauger et al.[24] as part of a project to produce an objective personality inventory that would examine multiple dimensions of behavior related to personality disorders. The scales, Forgiveness of Self (FS) and Forgiveness of Others (FO), are actually subscales of the Behavior Assessment System I (BAS), an inventory consisting of 301 true-false items.[25,26] Each of the forgiveness scales is composed of 15 statements. Items on the FO scale focus on taking revenge, justifying retaliation, and holding grudges: "I would secretly enjoy hearing that someone I dislike had gotten into trouble," and "It is not right to take revenge on a person who tries to take advantage of you." The FS scale assesses feelings of guilt over past mistakes, perceptions of oneself as sinful, and having a variety of negative attitudes toward self: "I am often angry at myself for the stupid things I do" and "It is easy for me to admit that I am wrong."[24]

Test–retest reliability was calculated with 21 graduate students who completed the scales with a 2-week interval between administrations. Reliability for the FO was reported at 0.94, for FS, 0.67. In reviewing these differences, the authors suggest that "forgiveness of others is a stable characteristic across time, but our attitude toward ourselves, as reflected in feelings of guilt, anger at ourselves, and having a negative evaluation of ourselves, fluctuates over time."[24]

Further testing of validity and reliability on the FS and FO was performed using data from 237 outpatient counseling clients from Christian counseling centers. Clients completed both the BAS and the Minnesota Multiphasic Personality Inventory (MMPI) as part of the initial intake process. The authors noted a correlation of 0.37 between scores on the FO and FS, indicating that the scales measure two related, but different, phenomena. In addition, factor analysis revealed different loading patterns for the FO and FS scales. The FO scale loads significantly on a factor labeled Alienation from Others, which includes other scales such as cynicism, negative attitudes toward others, and passive aggressive behavior; the FS scale loads primarily on the factor neurotic immaturity, along with negative self-image, self-control deficit, and motivation deficit scales. Correlations between the forgiveness scales and scales of the MMPI indicate an association between problems with forgiveness and other types of psychopathology, including depression, anxiety, anger, distrust, and negative self-esteem.[24]

Information regarding demographics of subjects involved in validity and reliability testing for the FS and FO is limited to age, sex, and education, with gender being the only variable with clinical significance. Women tended to report slightly more difficulty in forgiving themselves than did men. There are no references in either scale to religious beliefs, which would appear to make the FS and FO useful regardless of religious orientation.

Spiritual Well-Being

An alternative approach to assessing spiritual needs is the evaluation of spiritual well-being (SWB), which has been defined by the National Interfaith Coalition on Aging as "the affirmation of life in a relationship with God, self, community and environment that nurtures and celebrates wholeness."[27]

The universality of SWB was summarized by Moberg:

> A central concern of the Christian faith, if not also of Islam, Judaism, Hinduism, and Buddhism, is to enhance the SWB of people. Although the semantics and theology of this concern vary from one group to another, it is located at the very core of many religious goals. It also is central to the ultimate values of Soviet Marxism, which hopes to shape "the new man" who combines "spiritual richness" with "moral purity."[28,p351]

The Spiritual Well-Being Scale

The Spiritual Well-Being Scale, a 20-item Likert-type tool authored by Ellison and Paloutzian, reflects the belief that SWB involves a vertical and a horizontal dimension. The vertical dimension refers to the sense of well-being in the relationship with God, and the horizontal refers to sense of purpose in and satisfaction with life.[27,29] These two dimensions can be addressed separately using one of the two subscales comprising the SWB scale. The Religious Well-Being (RWB) subscale measures the vertical component, and the Existential Well-Being (EWB) subscale focuses on the horizontal. For example, the statement, "I have a personally meaningful relationship with God" refers to RWB, and "I believe that there is some purpose for my life" refers to EWB.[27] Responses to each item range from "strongly agree" to "strongly disagree."

Factor analysis of the SWB Scale using Varimax rotation was performed on data obtained from 206 students at three colleges having a religious orientation. The items clustered together as expected, with existential items loading into two subfactors, life direction and life satisfaction.[27,29]

The scale was then administered to 100 student volunteers at the University of Idaho. Test–retest reliability coefficients were 0.93 (SWB), 0.96 (RWB), and 0.86 (EWB). Internal consistency was evaluated using coefficient alpha, yielding 0.89 (SWB), 0.87 (RWB), and 0.78 (EWB).[27]

Examination of item content supports the face validity of the scale. In addition, the SWB Scale scores have correlated in predicted ways with other theoretically related measures, including the Purpose in Life Test and Intrinsic Religious Orientation.[27]

The authors of the SWB Scale acknowledge that the tool arises from the Judeo-Christian perception of religious well-being in which God is viewed in personal terms. However, they note that "it is . . . possible that those from eastern religions such as Hinduism and Buddhism may be able to use the scale if they can meaningfully interpret the statements about relationship with God."[27]

Moberg's Indexes of SWB

Moberg's Indexes of SWB, a 45-item questionnaire, include a variety of factors that may influence SWB: social attitudes; self-perceptions; theological and religious contexts; and religious beliefs, opinions, experiences, preferences, and affiliations.[28] Seven indices identified through factor analysis include Christian faith, self-satisfaction, personal piety, subjective SWB, optimism, religious cynicism, and elitism.

Response categories for most items range from "strongly agree" to "strongly disagree." Items in the personal piety index differ in that they require a response that indicates how frequently the subject participates in a particular activity. An example from this tool is: "How often do you pray privately?" (personal piety).[28]

The instrument indexes of SWB are believed to have face validity, as the items were based on information gained through multiple earlier studies performed by the tool's author.[28] Preliminary data support criterion validity of the indices. When scores for evangelical Christians were compared with those of other Christians, differences were in the expected direction. Likewise, scores for Christians were higher than scores for persons professing to be agnostic or atheist.[28] Additional testing with other criterion groups is needed to establish the tool's validity further. Further analysis of the validity of the indices has demonstrated coefficients ranging from 0.60 to 0.86 when scores were correlated with the SWB Scale.

Moberg's indexes of SWB represent a major attempt to demonstrate the multifaceted nature of SWB. However, two characteristics may limit its usefulness in clinical research. The tool in its present form is somewhat lengthy and may not be practical to use with populations with extensive disease who would tire easily. The indexes also are specific to Christianity and could not be used in their present form with patients of Jewish or Eastern orientations.

Spiritual Coping

The importance of religious faith often is overlooked by nurses when routinely assessing how a person copes with disease. Investigating spiritual coping may appear, on the surface, to document the performance of religious activities. In reality, spiritual coping looks beyond the actual behavior to the meaning or significance the behavior holds for the individual.

Patient Spiritual Coping Interview

The Patient Spiritual Coping Interview was developed by McCorkle and Benoliel[30] and adapted for use in a "one-time" interview format by Sodestrom.[31] This semistructured interview contains 30 items that investigate relationship with God or a "higher being," use of spiritual behaviors and/or resource persons, expressions of spiritual needs, and perception of the nurse's role in spiritual care.[31] Questions include "Do you ever watch religious TV or listen to religious radio?," "Have you spoken about your spiritual thoughts or concerns to someone?," and "How do you think nurses can assist you with your spiritual needs?"

The content validity of the interview was established by its consistency with the current literature and an expert panel of judges, three in oncology nursing research and two in theology. All agreed the items included were adequate and appropriate. Reliability was inferred by the assumption that subjects are reliable sources of information pertaining to the use of spiritual coping strategies.[31]

Religious Orientation

Intrinsic Religious Motivation Scale

The importance of spirituality in a person's life also can be evaluated by the Intrinsic Religious Motivation Scale developed by Hoge.[32] An intrinsically motivated person is one whose most central and ultimate motive in life can be found in his or her religious faith. The extrinsically motivated person views his or her religion as subservient to other aspects of life, such as economic or social status.[33] The scale consists of 10 statements to which the participant answers "yes" or "no." "One should seek God's guidance when making every important decision" indicates intrinsic motivation. "It doesn't matter what I believe as long as I lead a moral life" is consistent with extrinsic motivation.[32]

The Intrinsic Religious Motivation Scale was administered to 42 adult Protestants, 21 of whom were judged by their ministers as intrinsically motivated and 21 judged as extrinsically motivated. The initial scale included 30 items. The final scale is composed of the 10 items having highest validity, reliability, item-to-item correlations, and item-to-scale correlations.

All ten items correlated with the ministers' predications in the direction predicted beyond 0.03 level of significance. The reliability of the scale, measured by the Kuder-Richardson formula 20, was 0.901. Item-to-item correlations ranged from 0.132 to 0.716, with 22 of 45 item-to-item correlations greater than 0.5.[32]

The shorter version of the Intrinsic Motivation Scale may be easier to use than the Patient Spiritual Coping Interview. However, the Intrinsic Motivation Scale fails to identify specific behaviors that provide a source of comfort or strength to the subject. Another potential problem with the Intrinsic Motivation Scale lies in the classification of items. Seven of the items are indicative of intrinsic motivation, but only three reflect external motivation. The author has acknowledged this limitation and suggests deletion of the intrinsic item "My faith sometimes restricts my actions." With this change, the Kuder-Richardson score becomes 0.902.[32]

Spiritual Needs of Children

The potential difficulties in obtaining spiritual data from children are summarized by Shelly:

> If sound assessment is crucial to caring for adults, it is even more important in the pediatric setting. Children, especially young children, have a limited ability to communicate, particularly about abstract concepts.[34,p88]

A study of adolescents reported by Elkind and Elkind[35] used only two questions: "When do you feel closest to God?" and "Have you ever had a particular experience when you felt especially close to God?" Responses from 144 ninth-grade students to these items indicated differences between males and females and between honor students and "average" students ($p < 0.05$). Differences also were noted between Protestants, Catholics, and Jews; however, the uncertainty about exact numbers represented in each denomination precluded statistical analysis.

A Nurses Christian Fellowship task force developed a seven-question assessment tool to obtain information about the spiritual needs of children: "How do you feel when you're in trouble?" or "Do you know who God is? What is He like?"[34]

Additional information can be obtained from young children by asking them to draw pictures of God and themselves and/or with significant others. Using this technique requires special skill in interpretation to obtain meaningful data.

Nurse Recognition of Spiritual Needs of Patients

Several tools measure nurses' awareness of and appropriate interventions for spiritual needs. Chadwick devised a seven-item multiple-choice questionnaire to investigate "awareness and preparedness of nurses to meet spiritual needs."[36] Sample questions include: "How long has it been since you last recognized a spiritual need in your patients?" and "Have you ever read the Bible or prayed with a patient?"

Sodestrom developed a Nurse Interview schedule to correspond to the one discussed above for patients. Seventeen items were selected from the patient interview and modified to evaluate nurses' awareness of the spiritual strategies used by patients in coping with disease.[31] Nurse participants answer "yes," "no," or "don't know" to questions such as "Do you know if your patient has spoken to a clergyman?," "Do you know if s/he has read the Bible?," and "Does your patient make reference to guilt feelings related to God?" Reliability and validity for the Nurse Interview are based on the same data as the Patient Spiritual Coping Interview.

Highfield and Cason developed a 49-item questionnaire for their study of nurses' ability to identify behaviors and conditions expressive of spiritual health or spiritual need.[1] Nurse participants are instructed to note whether the behavior or condition described is related to either the spiritual or psychosocial dimension. They also are to rate on a scale of 1 to 5 how frequently each behavior or condition is seen in their patients. Finally, participants are to note each item considered to be a patient problem.

The items contained in the Highfield-Cason questionnaire were identified from the nursing and pastoral care literature and were submitted to a review panel of theology and psychology experts. Although many items in the questionnaire are legitimately a part of the spiritual domain (e.g., "expresses fear of tests and diagnosis," "is unable to pursue creative outlets"), the less specific items could easily represent a psychosocial problem rather than or in addition to a spiritual problem. This ambiguity needs to be addressed by researchers who choose to use the Highfield-Cason questionnaire.

Summary

Clinical research related to spiritual issues has been hampered by a variety of factors including discomfort among health professionals who believe that spirituality and spiritual needs are a private matter; difficulty in distinguishing psychosocial needs from spiritual needs; lack of valid and reliable measurement tools that address spiritual concerns; and confusion about differences between spiritual concerns and religiosity. The tools described here represent a heightened awareness of different aspects of spirituality. The development of new measures and further refinement of tools currently available will enable us to expand our understanding of this underresearched, but important, area.

Exemplar Study

Carson, V., Loeken, K.L., Shanty, J., & Terry, L. Hope and spiritual well-being: Essentials for living with AIDS. *Perspec Psychiatr Care*, 1990, 26:28-34.

The purpose of the study was to evaluate levels of hope and spiritual well-being among HIV-positive homosexual men. Sixty-five subjects were recruited, 25 of whom had been diagnosed with AIDS. Participants completed the Beck Hopelessness Scale and the Spiritual Well-Being Scale (SWBS) while waiting in an outpatient clinic to be seen by the physician. Only four subjects had scores consistent with hopelessness, with half scoring in the range of no or minimal pessimism. Persons with AIDS were found to be significantly more hopeful than those with AIDS-related complex (ARC; $p < 0.05$). SWBS scores were determined for overall SWB, existential well-being (EWB), and religious well-being (RWB). Participants were found to have positive levels of SWB; those with higher SWB scores tended to be more hopeful. A similar pattern was seen with EWB and RWB scores; however, the relationship between hope and EWB was significantly stronger than between hope and RWB.

The authors note that existential well-being enables individuals to respond to a crisis as a challenge and as an opportunity for personal growth. They suggest that EWB's greater contribution to overall SWB reflects feelings of alienation and abandonment experienced from society and from organized religion.

The study is important in that it examines the spiritual health of a group of gay men who are HIV-infected. The findings support those of other studies demonstrating a direct relationship between spiritual well-being and hope.[37,38] Moreover, the results are consistent with subjective observations that homosexual men often are poorly accepted in organized religion. Denying homosexual men access to religious participation (e.g., opportunities to experience RWB) may compromise overall SWB for some, although the population studied may have offset their RWB losses to some degree through EWB enhancement.

References

1. Highfield, M., & Cason, C. Spiritual needs of patients: Are they being recognized? *Cancer Nurs*, 1983, 6(3):187.
2. Moberg, D., & Brusek, P. Spiritual well-being: A neglected subject in quality of life research. *Soc Indicators Res*, 1978, 5(3):303.
3. Moberg, D.O. Development of social indicators of spiritual well-being for quality of life research. In D.O. Moberg (Ed.), *Spiritual well-being: Sociological perspectives.* Washington: University Press of America, 1979, p. 1.
4. Kim, M., & Moritz, D. *Classification of nursing diagnoses: Proceedings of the third and fourth national conferences.* New York: McGraw-Hill, 1980.
5. Highfield, M.F. Spiritual health of oncology patients. *Cancer Nurs*, 1992, 15(1):1.
6. Reed, P.G. Spirituality and well-being in terminally ill hospitalized adults. *Res Nurs Health*, 1987, 10: 335.
7. Reed, P.G. Religiousness in terminally ill and healthy adults. *Res Nurs Health*, 1986, 9:35.
8. Roberts, K.T., & Aspy, C. Development of the serenity scale. *J Nurs Meas*, 1993, 1(2):145-164.
9. Stallwood, J. Spiritual dimensions of nursing practice. In I. Beland & J. Passos (Eds.), *Clinical nursing.* New York: Macmillan, 1975.
10. Hess, J.S. Spiritual needs survey. In S. Fish & J.A. Shelly (Eds.), *Spiritual care: The nurse's role.* Downers Grove, IL. Intervarsity Press, 1983, p. 157.
11. Stoll, R. Guidelines for spiritual assessment. *Am J Nurs*, 1979, 79:1574.
12. Stoll, R. Spiritual assessment: A nursing perspective. Presented at the Spirituality in Nursing workshop, Marquette University, Milwaukee, WI, August 1984.
13. Fordyce, E. *An investigation of television's potential for meeting the spiritual needs of hospitalized persons.* Doctoral dissertation, Catholic University of America, 1981. *Dissertation Abstracts International*, 1982.
14. Fish, S., & Shelly, J.A. *Spiritual care: The nurse's role.* Downers Grove, IL: Intervarsity Press, 1983.
15. Reed, P.G. Preferences for spiritually related nursing interventions among terminally ill and nonterminally ill hospitalized adults and well adults. *App Nurs Res*, 1991, 4(3):122.
16. Dufault, K., & Martocchio, B.C. Hope: Its spheres and dimensions. *Nurs Clin North Am*, 1986, 20(2):379.
17. Nowotony, M.L. Assessment of hope in patients with cancer: Development of an instrument. *Oncol Nurs Forum*, 1989, 16(1):57.
18. Crumbaugh, J.C., & Maholick, L.T. An experimental study in existentialism: The psychometric approach to Frankl's concept of noogenic neurosis. *J Clinical Psychol*, 1964, 20:200.
19. Frankl, V. *Man's search for meaning.* New York: Washington Square Press, 1984.
20. Crumbaugh, J.C. Cross-validation of purpose in life test based on Frankl's concepts. *J Indiv Psychol*, 1968, 24:74.

21. Maton, K.I. Stress-buffering role of spiritual support: Cross-sectional and prospective investigations. *J Sci Study Rel*, 1989, *28*(3):310.

22. Maton, K.I. Empowerment in a religious setting: An exploratory study. Unpublished Master's Thesis, University of Illinois at Urbana-Champaign, IL, 1984.

23. Studzinski, R. Remember and forgive: Psychological dimensions of forgiveness. In C. Floristan & C. Duquoc (Eds.), *Forgiveness*. Edinburgh: T and T Clark, 1986, p. 12.

24. Mauger, P.A., Perry, J.E., Freeman, T., et al. Measurement of forgiveness: Preliminary research. *J Psychol Christian*, 1992, *11*(2):170.

25. Mauger, P.A., Webb, J.H., Davis, R., et al. Development of a multi-dimensional inventory for the diagnosis of personality disorders. Paper presented at the annual meeting of the Southeastern Psychological Association, Atlanta, GA, 1985.

26. Mauger, P.A. *Behavior assessment system I, preliminary manual, version 2.1*. Atlanta, GA: Automated Assessment, 1991.

27. Ellison, C.W. Spiritual well-being: Conceptualization and measurement. *J Psychol Theol*, 1983, *11*(4):330.

28. Moberg, D. Subjective measures of spiritual well-being. *Rev Relig Res*, 1984, *25*(4):351.

29. Paloutzian, R., & Ellison, C.W. Loneliness, spiritual well-being, and the quality of life. In A. Peplau & D. Perlman (Eds.), *Loneliness: A sourcebook of current theory, research, and therapy*. New York: Wiley, 1982, p. 224.

30. McCorkle, R., & Benoliel, J.Q. *Manual of data collection instruments*. Unpublished manual. Seattle: University of Washington, 1981.

31. Sodestrom, K.E., & Martinson, I. Patient's spiritual coping strategies: A study of nurse and patient perspectives. *Oncol Nurs Forum*, 1987, *14*(2):41.

32. Hoge, D.R. Validated intrinsic religious motivation scale. *J Sci Study Rel*, 1972, *11*:369.

33. Soderstrom, D., & Wright, E.W. Religious orientation and meaning in life. *J Clin Psychol*, 1977, *33*(1):65.

34. Shelly, J.A. *Spiritual needs of children*. Downers Grove, IL: Intervarsity Press, 1982.

35. Elkind, D. & Elkind, S. Varieties of religious experience in young adolescents. *J Sci Study Rel*, 1962, *2*(1):102.

36. Chadwick, R. Awareness and preparedness of nurses to meet spiritual needs. In S. Fish & J.A. Shelly (Eds.), *Spiritual care: The nurse's role*. Downers Grove, IL: Intervarsity Press, 1983.

37. Carson, V., Soeken, K.L., & Grimm, P.M. Hope and its relationship to spiritual well-being. *J Psychol Theol*, 1988, *16*(2):159.

38. Mickley, J.R., Soeken, K., & Belcher, A. Spiritual well-being, religiousness, and hope among women with breast cancer. *IMAGE: J Nurs Scholar*, 1992, *24*(2):267.

15

Measuring Body Image

Julie F. Robertson and Judy M. Diekmann

The concept of body image has application in a wide range of disciplines, including medicine, nursing, psychology, physical therapy, dentistry, and dietetics. The importance of body image in our culture is significant. One only has to note the tremendous expenditure of time, effort, and money by people seeking to alter their appearance to resemble an ideal image.

Life events that alter one's body can profoundly affect how one perceives oneself and functions in society. Such alterations can be very disrupting and anxiety provoking. Physical alterations caused by trauma, surgery, or treatment can lead to depression and lowered self-esteem. Health-care professionals encounter patients experiencing a variety of alterations in body image, including changes in body structure and function, deformities, loss of body boundaries, and depersonalization. Whether the consequence of surgery, drugs, sensory deprivation, fatigue, stress, immobility, or anesthesia, adequate assessment of body image change is key to effective intervention that will promote, reestablish, or maintain self-esteem. Health care that successfully assists patients to integrate physical changes can significantly influence adaptation and survival. Quality of life is inextricably linked with body image.

The Concept of Body Image

The concept of body image has been well researched by multiple authors, producing several classic articles on the subject.[1,2] Schilder defined body image as "the picture of our own body which we form in our mind, . . . the way in which the body appears to ourselves."[1] Body image, in this instance, refers to a psychologic experience and focuses on individuals' feelings and attitudes toward their body.[2] Norris believes that body image is a "social creation . . . basic to identity and it has been referred to as the somatic ego."[3] Body image in this case is subjective and is grounded in life experiences.

The concept of body image has been researched from different perspectives, including neurologic, somatic, and psychologic characterizations. Definitions have included both direct perceptions of the body through visual, tactile, and proprioceptive senses and indirect perceptions via attitudes, emotions, and reactions.[4] Body image also has been defined as an adaptive mechanism that perpetuates balance among the physiologic, psychologic, and sociocultural components of the body.[5] Certain behavioral aspects of body image disturbance, such as avoiding social situations that might be associated with food or appearance, also have garnered the attention of researchers.[6] Body image differs from self-concept. Body image refers to perception, whereas self-concept denotes feelings about oneself. These terms have been used interchangeably despite the fact that they are distinct concepts.

Neurologists have observed that patients with selective brain lesions demonstrate a wide range of distorted body images.[4] Such patients were unable to distinguish one side of the body from the other, denied the existence of various body parts, denied the incapacitation of various parts, or falsely attributed new body parts to themselves. It is believed that body image disturbances can occur with brain lesions at any level. However, the parietal region of the minor hemisphere is commonly regarded as a site of special significance because of the relationship that exists between right parietal disease and body image disorders.[2,7]

In the field of psychiatry, investigators have reported that numerous schizophrenic patients demonstrate almost the same range in distortions of body image as that observed in neurologic patients.[8] To substantiate this phenomenon, Fisher and Cleveland[2] reviewed and classified the bizarre body perceptions reported by schizophrenics. They grouped these distortions into several categories. One prominent cluster centers around issues of masculinity and femininity. It includes such distortions as feeling that one has the body parts of the opposite sex or that one is half-man, half-woman. A second group of distortions involves feelings of body disintegration and deterioration. Commonly, these involve sensations that some minor part of the body had been destroyed. Another category refers to feelings of depersonalization. Schizophrenics lose a sense of reality about the existence of body parts or the total body. The person experiences his or her body as if it were alien or belonged to a stranger. The fourth category of distortions proposed by Fisher and Cleveland is a sense of body boundary loss. Schizophrenics with this disorder feel that things happening elsewhere and to other people are happening to them.

The relationship between psychiatric disorders and body image is multiplex. Early research focused on the emotional distress that results from disfigurement. However, this changed when Freud[4] hypothesized that concerns about appearance resulted from psychologic conflict. Social and cultural influences are now believed to significantly affect body image and closely tie body parts and appearance to personality development and socialization.[4]

Much research has been conducted on the relationship between eating disorders and body image. Studies of patients with the syndrome of anorexia nervosa support a relationship between body image distortions and feelings of inadequacy.[7,9] This syndrome is characterized by a negative evaluation of body appearance and the tendency to overestimate or underestimate body size. Increasingly more published research describes the relationship between distorted body image and obesity[10] or bulimia.[9] In 1980, the *Diagnostic and Statistical Manual of Mental Disorders* included body image disturbance as a diagnostic criteria for bulimia and anorexia nervosa.[11]

Research in the area of body image is proliferating. Many investigators have turned from clinical analysis to the analysis of body perception as a psychologic phenomenon in healthy populations. They postulate that the normal person's attitude toward his or her body influences behavior in the same way as attitudes do. Feelings about the body appear to affect decisions at all levels; even decisions relating to survival may be biased by one's prevailing body image. Findings of recent studies demonstrate a strong correlation between body image disturbance and feelings of low self-worth and depression in normal populations. Experts predict that body image disturbance will continue to increase, especially among women, as a result of the emphasis that Western societies place on beauty, youth, and slimness.[11A]

Measuring the Body Image Concept

Although most agree that body image is important, there is little consensus about the best procedure to measure this phenomenon. Theoretical models of body image, although thought-provoking, have not resulted in utilitarian methods to measure this concept. Whether disturbances in body image are functions of direct sensoriperceptual deficits, distortions in thought processes, or distortions in affective experiencing is not clearly defined in the literature.[4,12]

The most popular measurement techniques used for the major dimensions of body image include questionnaires, scales (*see* Appendix 15A), draw-a-person tests, body image boundary determinations, direct measurement of perceived body size, distortion techniques, and videotape feedback (*see* Appendix 15B). When administering the instruments, the assistance of a psychologist or psychiatrist may be helpful in interpreting results.

Since the late 1970s there has been increasing interest among nurses to study the phenomenon of body image in a variety of clinical populations, resulting in the development of a number of measures of body image. Populations studied include pregnant women and their spouses,[13] multiple sclerosis patients,[14] cancer patients,[15,16] ill children,[17] patients with halo braces,[18] immobilized patients,[19] older adults,[20] and patients who have undergone head and neck surgery[21] and cerebral bypass surgery.[22] Nurse developed instruments are shown in Appendix 15A.[19,21,23-45]

Three body measurement techniques used by investigators with increasing frequency are (1) mirror images and other self-representations that measure subjects' internalized picture of their body's physical appearance; (2) videotape recordings which give people an opportunity to scrutinize how they appear to others; and (3) direct video monitoring using a TV screen to assess body image. In several studies, employing direct video monitoring, Gardner et al. found that the use of the TV video was "quite accurate" in determining body size.[10,69] These researchers advocate the use of this methodology because it "allows a direct, simultaneous, and exact assessment of body image"[10] and is a viable technique to use with a variety of populations to include eating disorder individuals and children.[69] Gardner et al. reported that TV video methodology has been found to have acceptable reliability and validity as a measure of body image by several researchers.[69] Examples of these measurement tools are shown in Appendix 15B[46-68].

Summary

There are many instruments available to measure the different aspects of body image. It is important to note that body image is a complex construct that cannot be measured with any single instrument. Most likely, multiple instruments will be necessary. Clinical researchers are in an excellent position to expand the knowledge about body image across the lifespan in both healthy and ill populations. It is evident that continuing work is needed to determine the usefulness, reliability, and validity of each of the instruments described in this chapter. Studies employing a single instrument need to be replicated with various samples to establish psychometric properties.

Exemplar Studies

Gardner, R.M., Morrell, J., Urrutia, R., et al. Judgements of body size following significant weight loss. *J Soc Behav Perspect*, 1989, 4(5):603.

This study exemplifies measurement of body image perception after significant weight loss. Two separate cross-sectional investigations are reported in which subjects responded to a randomized ordering of TV images of their entire body that were either too thin or too wide. Methods are well described and rigorous. This study uses TV video monitoring, which has been documented in the literature to be a reliable and valid method of measuring body image.

Fawcett, J., Bliss-Holtz, V.J., Hass, M.B., et al. Spouses' body image changes during and after pregnancy: A replication and extension. *Nurs Res*, 1986, 35(4):220.

This study exemplifies the measurement of body image changes of spouses during and after pregnancy. This is a longitudinal investigation that replicates and extends work previously done by the first author. Methods are well described, rigorous, and appropriate. Several measures are used, including the Body Attitude Scale (BAS) and the typographic device developed by Fawcett and Frye.[13] All measures used have excellent documented reliability and validity.

References

1. Schilder, P. *Image and appearance of the human body.* New York: International Universities Press, 1950 (originally published in 1935).
2. Fisher, S., & Cleveland, S. *Body image and personality.* New York: Dover, 1968.
3. Norris, C. The professional nurse and body image. In C. Carlson & B. Blackwell (Eds.), *Behavioral concepts and nursing intervention* (2nd ed.). Philadelphia: Lippincott, 1978, p. 5.
4. Lacey, J.H., & Birtchnell, S.A. Body image and its disturbances. *J Psychosom Res*, 1986, 30(6):623.
5. Dropkin, M.J. Change in body image associated with head and neck cancer. In L.B. Marino (Ed.), *Cancer Nursing.* St. Louis: Mosby, 1981, p. 560.
6. Rosen, J.C., Srebnik, D., Saltzberg, E., & Wendt, S. Development of a body image avoidance questionnaire. *Psychol Assess J Consult Clin Psychol*, 1991, 3(1):32.
7. Van Deusen, J. Body image and perceptual dysfunction in adults. Philadelphia: Saunders, 1993.
8. Cash, T.F., & Pruzinsky, T. *Body image: Development, deviance, and change.* New York: The Guilford Press, 1990.
9. Ben-Tovim, D.I., & Walker, M.K. A quantitative study of body-related attitudes in patients with anorexia and bulimia nervosa. *Psychol Med*, 1992, 22:961.
10. Gardner, R.M., Martinez, R., & Espinoza, T. Psychological measurement of body image of self and others in obese subjects. *J Soc Behav Person*, 1987, 2(2):205.
11. American Psychiatric Association. *Diagnostic and statistical manual of mental disorders* (3rd ed.). Washington, DC: American Psychiatric Association, 1980.
11A. Thompson, J.K. Body image disturbance: assessment and treatment, New York: Pergamon Press, 1990.
12. Ben-Tovim, D.I., & Walker, M.K. Women's body attitudes: A review of measurement techniques. *Int J Eating Dis*, 1991, 10(2):155.
13. Fawcett, J., & Frye, S. An exploratory study of body image dimensionality. *Nurs Res*, 1980, 29(5):324.
14. Sammonds, R.J., & Cammermeyer, M. Perceptions of body image in subjects with multiple sclerosis: A pilot study. *J Neurosci Nurs*, 1989, 21(3):191.
15. Padilla, G.V., & Grant, M.M. Quality of life as a cancer nursing outcome variable. *Adv Nurs Sci*, 1985, 8(1):45.
16. Ramer, L. Self-image changes with time in the cancer patient with a colostomy after operation. *J ET Nurs*, 1992, 19(6):195.
17. Beardslee, C., & Neff, J.A. Body-related concerns of children with cancer as compared with the concerns of other children. *Mat Child Nurs J*, 1982, 11:121.
18. Olson, B., Ustanko, L., & Warner, S. The patient in a halo brace: Striving for normalcy in body image and self concept. *Orthopaed Nurs*, 1991, 10(1):44.
19. Baird, S.E. Development of a nursing assessment tool to diagnose altered body image in immobilized patients. *Orthopaed Nurs*, 1985, 4(1):47.
20. Janelli, L.M. The realities of body image. *J Gerontol Nurs*, 1986, 12(10):23.
21. Droughton, M.L., & Verbic, M. Body image reintegration after head and neck surgery: Application and evaluation of three nursing interventions. *J Off Pub Soc Otorhinolaryngol Head-Neck Nurs*, 1988, 6(1):19.
22. Stewart-Amidei, C., & Penckofer, S. Quality of life following cerebral bypass surgery. *J Neurosci Nurs*, 1988, 20(1):50.
23. Fisher, S. *Body experience in fantasy and behavior.* New York: Appleton-Century-Crofts, 1970.
24. Bruchon-Schweitzer, M. Body image and personal-

ity: A French adaptation of Fisher's Body Focus Questionnaire. *Percept Motor Skills*, 1978, *46*:1227.

25. Reihman, J., & Seymour, F. The body focus questionnaire: Interpretive issues. *Percept Motor Skills*, 1984, *58*:356.

26. Ajzen, Y., & Iagolnitzer, E.R. Dimensionality of revisited body awareness. *Percept Motor Skills*, 1985, *60*:455.

27. Gleghorn, A.A., Penner, L.A., Powers, P.S., & Schulman, R. The psychometric properties of several measures of body image. *J Psychopathol Behav Assess*, 1987, *9*(2):203.

28. Gray, S. Social aspects of body image: Perception of normalcy of weight and affect of college undergraduates. *Percept Motor Skills*, 1977, *45*:1035.

29. Leon, G.R., Bemis, K.M., & Melard, M. Changes in body image and other psychological factors after intestinal bypass surgery for massive obesity. *J Behav Med*, 1979, *2*(1):39.

30. Secord, P., & Jourard, S. The appraisal of body cathexis: Body cathexis and self. *J Consult Clin Psychol*, 1953, *17*:343.

31. Jourard, S.M., & Secord, P.F. Body-cathexis and the ideal female figure. *J Abnorm Soc Psychol*, 1955, *50*:243.

32. Mayer, J.D., & Eisenberg, M.G. Body concept: A conceptualization and review of paper-and-pencil measures. *Rehabil Psychol*, 1982, *27*(2):97.

33. Hammond, S.M., & O'Rourke, M.M. A psychometric investigation into the Body Cathexis Scale. *Person Indiv Diff*, 1984, *5*(5):603.

34. Franzoi, S.L., & Shields, S.A. The Body Esteem Scale: Multidimensional structure and sex differences in a college population. *J Person Assess*, 1984, *48*(2):173.

35. Thomas, C.D., & Freeman, R.J. The Body Esteem Scale: Construct validity of the female subscales. *J Person Assess*, 1990, *54*(1&2):204.

36. Secord, P. Objectification of word-association procedures by the use of homonyms: A measure of body cathexis. *J Person*, 1953, *21*:479.

37. Jupp, J.J., & Collins, J.K. Instruments for the measurement of unconscious and conscious aspects of body image. *Aust J Clin Exp Hypnosis*, 1983, *11*(2):89.

38. Winston, B.A., & Case, T.F. Reliability and validity of the Body-Self Relations Questionnaire: A new measure of body image. Paper presented at the meeting of the Southeastern Psychological Association, New Orleans, March 1984.

39. Brown, T.A., Cash, T.F., & Mikuka, P.J. Attitudinal body-image assessment: Factor analysis of the Body–Self Relations Questionnaire. *J Person Assess*, 1990, *55*(1&2):135.

40. Cash, T.F., & Green, G.K. Body weight and body image among college women: Perception, cognition, and affect. *J Person Assess*, 1986, *50*(2):290.

41. Cooper, P.J., Taylor, M.J., Cooper, Z., & Fairburn, C.G. The development and validation of the Body Shape Questionnaire. *Int J Eating Dis*, 1987, *6*(4):485.

42. Hadigan, C.M., & Walsh, B.T. Body shape concerns in bulimia nervosa. *Int J Eating Dis*, 1991, *10*(3):323.

43. Bunnell, D.W., Cooper, P.J., Hertz, S., & Shenker, I.R. Body shape concerns among adolescents. *Int J Eating Dis*, 1992, *11*(1):79.

44. Thompson, J.K., Fabian, L.J., Moulton, D.O., et al. Development and validation of the Physical Appearance Related Teasing Scale. *J Person Assess*, 1991, *56*(3):513.

45. Ben-Tovim, D.I., & Walker, M.K. The development of the Ben-Tovim Walker Body Attitudes Questionnaire (BAQ), a new measure of women's attitudes towards their own bodies. *Psychol Med*, 1991, *21*(3):775.

46. Manchover, K. *Personality projection in the drawing of the human figure*. Springfield, IL: Charles C. Thomas, 1949.

47. Wooley, O.W., & Roll, S. The Color-a-Person Body Dissatisfaction Test: Stability, internal consistency, validity, and factor structure. *J Person Assess*, 1991, *56*(3):395.

48. Askevold, F. Measuring body image: Preliminary report on a new method. *Psychother Psychosom*, 1975, *25*:71.

49. Fichter, M.W., Meister, I., & Koch, H.J. The measurement of body image disturbances in anorexia nervosa: Experimental comparison of different methods. *Br J Psychiatr*, 1986, *148*:453.

50. Thomas, C.D., & Freeman, R.J. Body-Image Marking: Validity of body-width estimates as operational measures of body image. *Behav Modif*, 1991, *15*(2):261.

51. Datson, P.G., & McConnell, O.L. Stability of Rorschach penetration and barrier scores over time. *J Consult Psychol*, 1962, *26*:104.

52. Hartley, R.B. The barrier variable as measured by homonyms. *J Clin Psychol*, 1967, *23*:196.

53. Dillon, D.J. Measurement of perceived body size. *Percept Motor Skills*, 1962, *14*:191.

54. Dillon, D.J. Estimation of bodily dimensions. *Percept Motor Skills*, 1962, *14*:219.

55. Slade, P.D., & Russell, G.F. Awareness of body dimension in anorexia nervosa: Cross-sectional and longitudinal studies. *Psychol Med*, 1973, *3*:188.

56. Meerman, R., Vandereycken, W., & Napierski, C. Methodological problems of body image research in anorexia nervosa patients. *Acta Psychiatr Belgica*, 1986, *86*(1):42.

57. Ruff, G.A., & Barrios, B.A. Realistic assessment of body image. *Behav Assess*, 1986, *8*:237.

58. Mizes, J.S. Validity of the body image detection device. *Addict Behav*, 1991, *16*:411.

59. Fawcett, J., & Chodil, J.J. The topographic device: Development and research. In E. Bauwens (Ed.), *Research for clinical nursing: Its strategies and findings*. Monograph Series 1979: 3. Indianapolis, IN: Sigma Theta Tau, 1980.

60. Traub, A.C., & Orbach, J. Psychophysical studies of body image. *Arch Gen Psychiatr*, 1964, *11*:53.

61. McCrea, C.W., Summerfield, A.B., & Rosen, B. Body image: A selective review of existing measurement techniques. *Br J Med Psychol*, 1982, *55*(3):225.

62. Glucksman, M.L., & Hirsch, J. The response of obese patients to weight reduction. III. The perception of body size. *J Psychosom Med*, 1969, *31*(1):1.

63. Garner, D.M., Garfinkel, P.E., Stancer, H.C., et al. Body image disturbances in anorexia nervosa and obesity. *Psychosom Med*, 1976, *38*(5):327.

64. Gustavson, C.R., Gustavson, J.C., Pulmariega, A.J., et al. Body-image distortion among male and female college and high school students, and eating-disordered patients. *Percept Motor Skills*, 1990, *71*:1003.

65. Allebeck, P., Hallberg, D., & Espmark, S. Body image—An apparatus for measuring disturbances in estimation of size and shape. *J Psychosomat Res*, 1976, *20*:583.
66. Collins, J.K. The objective measurement of body image using a video technique: Reliability and validity studies. *Br J Psychol*, 1986, *77*:199.
67. Collins, J.K. Methodology for the objective measurement of body image. *Intl J Eating Dis*, 1987, *6*(3):393.
68. Williamson, D.A., Davis, C.J., Bennett, S.M., et al. Development of a single procedure for assessing body image disturbances. *Behav Assess*, 1989, *11*:433.
69. Gardner, R.M., Morrell, J., Urrutia, R., & Espinoza, T. Judgements of body size following weight loss. *J Soc Behav Person*, 1989, *4*(5):603.

Appendices

15A. Important Questionnaires and Scales Used in the Measurement of Body Image Dimensions

Instrument	Description	Psychometric Indices
Body Focus Questionnaire Developed by Fisher (23)	Measures attention to various body regions; Fisher believed that amount of attention was linked to intensity of conflict about that body region/part 108 forced-choice alternatives corresponding to paired body region; subject selects the region that at this moment is "most clear in your awareness" 8 subscales represent focal body parts (back/front, right/left, stomach, mouth, eyes, arms, head, heart) Subscale scores determined by number of times an item on that scale is chosen	Adapted in French and showed significant test-retest reliability (24) Validity questioned and not widely used (12,25,26)
Body Distortion Questionnaire (BDQ) Developed by Fisher (23)	Affective measure of body image, identifies abnormal attitudes related to body appearance and function 82-item questionnaire, offers 3-response format (yes, no, undecided)	High Kuder-Richardson reliability (0.95) High convergent correlations with other affective measures of body image (27) Discriminates well between normals and bulimics (27), and anorexics (12)
Gray Questionnaire to Determine Body Affect Developed by Gray (28)	Measures perception and normalcy of weight and affect 10-item, Likert-type scale asking subjects to respond to statements (agree to disagree) Last item asks subjects whether they are underweight, average, or overweight Weight compared to standard for weight normalcy	Reliability and validity not reported
Self-Attitude Scale (SAQ) (29)	Self-administered, 40-item multiple-choice measure Elicits present attitude toward one's body; best and least liked body parts; attitudes about physical and sexual attractiveness, food and eating; interpersonal activities	Not reported
Body Parts Satisfaction Questionnaire (BPSQ) Developed by Berscheid et al. and modified by Gleghorn et al., 1987 (27)	Modified version has 25-items, uses 7-point Likert Scale	High internal consistency (Cronbach's alpha): 0.92 Good convergent correlations with other affective measure of body image Construct validity: known groups technique showed statistically significant differences between normal and bulimic individuals: $F(1,108) = 91.06$, $p < 0.001$ (27)

15A. Important Questionnaires and Scales Used in the Measurement of Body Image Dimensions (*cont.*)

Instrument	Description	Psychometric Indices
Body Cathexis Scales Developed by Secord and Jourard (30)	Measures body cathexis (31) (degree of self-reported satisfaction with one's own body) 2 scales: body cathexis scale: 46 item; self-cathexis (general self-satisfaction); sum of scores indicates body esteem Use expanded to include patients with multiple sclerosis (14), older adults (20), and others	Split-half reliability ($r = 0.81$) (32) Unidimensional, "tight internal structure" when 51-item version used (33); recommended use in researching role of body feelings in self-concept and personality Moderately good test–retest reliability; contains 3–4 factors (12)
Secord and Jourard Modified Body Cathexis Questionnaire (31)	Modified to include 12 body parts, each rated on a 7-point scale (1 "strong, positive feeling" to 7 "strong negative feeling") Scoring: total score divided by 12 to give final score (1–7)	Internal consistency (all subscales), Cronbach's alpha: 0.74 (13)
Body Esteem Scale (BES) Developed by Franzoi and Shields (34)	36-items (23 original Body Cathexis scale items plus 13 new) Body esteem shown to be multidimensional construct differing for males and females Female subscales sound and meaningful, offer potentially useful method for assessing body image in high-risk populations (35)	Factor analysis: Clusters of variables (men: physical attractiveness, upper body strength, physical condition); (females: sexual attractiveness, weight concern, physical condition) Cronbach's alpha: 0.78–0.87 Convergent validity: moderate correlation between self-esteem on Rosenberg Self-Esteem Scale and each of 3 body esteem subscales of BES Discriminant validity established: Wilkes lambda stepwise selection method: "weight concern subscale" discriminates anorexic females from nonanorexic (lambda = 0.86, $p < 0.001$, canonical correlation = 0.37); same means of analysis for male data: upper-body subscale differentiated male weightlifters from nonweightlifters (lambda = 0.90, $p < 0.01$, canonical correlation = 0.34) (34,35)
Secord Homonym Test (36)	Word-association technique eliciting associations to a recited list of 100 homonyms, each with meanings pertaining to body parts/processes, or nonbody meanings Also includes stimulus words Score is number of body reference responses given Taps changes in unconscious body involvement (37)	Interrater reliability: 0.95 Test–retest reliability: 0.94 Split-half reliability: 0.85 (35)

Instrument	Description	Reliability and Validity
Body Self-Relations Questionnaire (BSRQ) (38,39)	Subscale of Multidimensional Body–Self Relations Questionnaire (MBSRQ) (38) 54-item scale using 5-point Likert format ("definitely agree" to "definitely disagree") Measures attitude toward body image related to physical appearance, fitness, health 3 dimensions of attitude: cognitive, affective, behavioral	Cronbach's alpha: 0.83–0.92 Test-retest reliabilities (over 1 month): 0.85–0.91 (40) Convergent and discriminant validity established Factor analysis: 7-factor, stable structure consistent for males and females (39)
Body Shape Questionnaire (BSQ) Developed by Cooper et al. (41)	Measures concerns about body shape, especially "feeling fat" (features of body image distortion) in both bulimia and anorexia nervosa 34-item scale, using a 6-point format ("never" to "always") Subjects asked to respond about feelings toward their appearance over last 4 weeks Valid measure of body shape concerns (42,43)	Validated using 4 samples of women (bulimics, attending family planning clinic, occupational therapy students, undergraduate students) Concurrent validity: moderate to high correlations between BSQ, Eating Disorder Inventory (EDI), and Eating Attitudes Test (EAT) among bulimic patients and students Discriminant validity established (41)
Physical Appearance Related Teasing Scale (PARTS) Developed by Thompson et al. (44)	Measures role teasing plays in development of negative body image and eating disorders 18-item scale, using a 5-point format ("never" to "frequently") 2 subscales: Weight/Size Teasing Scale (W/ST), General Appearance Teasing Scale (GAT)	Internal consistency reliability (coefficient alpha): 0.91 (W/ST) and 0.71 (GAT) Test-retest reliability: 0.86 (W/ST), 0.87 (GAT) Convergent and discriminant validity established: (1) strong relationship between teasing about weight/size and adult eating disturbances and body image dysfunction, (2) GAT statistically significant predictor of bulimic behavior (44)
Ben-Tovim Body Attitudes Questionnaire (BAQ) Developed by Ben-Tovim and Walker (45)	Measures broad range of body-related attitudes held by women 44-item questionnaire 6-factors: feelings of fatness, feelings of disgust with body, perceived physical strength/fitness, importance of weight and shape in one's life, perceived physical attractiveness, feeling of lower body fatness	Normed with large sample of community women ($n = 504$) Factor analysis: 6 factors Kuder-Richardson reliability: 0.92 Test-retest reliability (4-week period): 0.83 Good convergent validity with existing instruments (45)
Body Image Avoidance Questionnaire (BIAQ) Developed by Rosen et al. (6)	Body image viewed as multidimensional construct where negative body image expressed by dysfunctional behaviors related to grooming, dressing, socialization 19-item questionnaire, using 6-point scale Instrument may yield information "above and beyond" typical attitudinal measures of body image" (6)	Internal consistency reliability (Cronbach's alpha): 0.89 Test-retest reliability (2 weeks): 0.87 Concurrent validity established: self-reported behavioral avoidance strongly associated with negative attitudes towards weight and shape (Body Shape Questionnaire): $r(351) = 0.78, p < 0.0001$ (6) Discriminant validity: discriminates between bulimic and normal subjects (6)
Baird Body Image Assessment Tool (BBIAT) Developed by Baird (19)	11-item assessment tool Copy of instrument found in Orthopaedic Nursing (19)	Interrater reliability: adequate for 6/11 items Validation: preliminary work done by comparing to standard Further testing warranted

15A. Important Questionnaires and Scales Used in the Measurement of Body Image Dimensions (*cont.*)

Instrument	Description	Psychometric Indices
Body Image Reintegration Tool (B.I.R.T) Developed by Droughton and Verbic (21)	13-item tool, intended to determine whether certain nursing interventions corrected or minimized patients' alterations in body image "Yes/no" response to description of patient outcomes expected to occur if nursing interventions successful Intervention successful if 11 or more out of 13 responses positive 4 weeks after hospital discharge.	No reliability or validity data reported.

Numbers in parentheses correspond to studies cited in the References.

15B. Important Instruments to Measure Body Image

Instrument	Description	Psychometric Indices
Draw-a-Person Test Developed by Manchover (1949) (46)	Based on belief that individual's spontaneous drawing of human figure represents projection of own body image Subject asked to draw a picture of self Interpretation requires expertise in administering projective tests	Conflicting data as to accuracy Difficult to differentiate aspects of drawing linked to body image, drawing skill, or manner in which drawing obtained (2,12)
Color-a-Person Body Dissatisfaction Test (CAPT) Developed by Wooley and Roll, 1991 (47)	2 gender-appropriate drawings (front and side view of human body) are shown to subjects Subjects asked to indicate level of satisfaction/dissatisfaction with 16 body parts by coloring the 2 drawings: red, very dissatisfied; yellow, dissatisfied; black, neutral; green, satisfied; blue, very satisfied 3 scores calculated: CAPT total (mean of all 16 parts), CAPT score I (mean of abdomen, hips, buttocks, thighs), CAPT score II (mean of remaining parts)	Test–retest reliability: 0.72–0.89 (2- to 4-week intervals, no gender differences) Cronbach's alphas (all): 0.70–0.88 (both normal and subjects with eating disorders) Validity established by correlation with Secord and Jourard's Body Cathexis Scale and Rosenberg's Self-esteem Scale Factor analysis/varimax rotation for 3 groups (female, male college students, eating disorder patients): face, extremities, torso (47)
Askevold Method for Measuring Body Image (Image Marking) (48)	Subject asked to draw specific marks: to measure accuracy of determining dimensions in general; to identify specified body parts while imagining self in mirror (body height, acromioclavicular joints, narrowest waist width, femoral trochanter bones) Investigator assists in marking as well as noting differences in position of actual body parts compared to those marked	Discriminates best between anorexics and controls as compared to video monitor procedure and movable caliper procedure (49) Reliability and validity (tested with group of bulimic and normal women): reliability: 0.72–0.92; construct validity (multitrait-multimethod matrix): met 2 of 3 standards (26) Recent evidence suggests Image Marking may reflect error variance rather than meaningful assessments of body width (50)

Instrument	Description	Reliability/Validity
Body Image Boundary Concept Developed by Fisher and Cleveland, 1958 (2)	Based on hypothesis that people view their bodies as clearly and sharply bounded from nonself objects or as lacking demarcation from the environment Barrier score derived from content analysis of Rorschach inkblot protocol: score = number of responses elicited by an inkblot series characterized by protective, containing, or covering functions of the periphery Penetration score: count of all inkblot responses suggesting destruction, evasion, or by-passing of the boundary	The higher the penetration score, the less definite the body image boundary Interrater reliability: (Pearson's product moment correlation): barrier scores: 0.84; penetration score: 0.79 (51) Barrier score calculation is complicated and time-consuming (52) Best administration by professionals trained in administering psychologic tests
Direct Measurement of Perceived Body Size Developed by Dillon (53)	Directly measures visually perceived body height, width, depth Device constructed of wooden beams; subject asked to adjust beams to form a doorway they can just fit through; subjects estimate dimensions during 10 sessions (vertical, then horizontal, ascending, and descending estimates)	Error of estimate (estimate minus actual measure): no systematic variation except for estimation of knee height (54) Test–retest reliability: 0.85–0.95 Validity coefficients: 0.00–0.95 (significant for full height, mouth height, shoulder height, $r = 0.95$) Gradual increase in reliability and validity as estimate progressed from knee to full height (54)
Slade and Russell Moving Caliper Technique (55)	Apparatus consists of 2 lights mounted on horizontal bar; subjects asked to adjust the lights to estimate the dimensions of body regions Estimates compared to actual dimensions and expressed as ratio or index (perceived × 100 divided by real): 100 corresponds to accurate, <100 shows underestimation of physical size, >100 shows overestimation	Variable reliability estimates (0.25–0.94) (56) Discriminates well between anorexic and normal subjects (27,49) Correlates well with other perceptual measures of body image (27)
Body Image Detection Device (BIDD) Developed by Ruff and Barrios (57)	Modification of Slade and Russell's technique Overhead projector, projecting a 1-cm-wide horizontal band of light used by subjects to estimate widths of 5 body parts by adjusting beam of light 2 measures: Body Perception Index (BPI): difference between actual and perceived body dimensions; Subjective Rating Index (SRI): subjective rating of weight status assigned by the subject to each body site (58)	Respectable reliability for both measures coefficient alphas: BPI, 0.83–0.93; SRI, 0.79–0.81. Test–retest: BPI, 0.75–0.92; SRI, 0.60–0.93 Validity studies inconsistent (58)
Fawcett Measure of Perceived Body Space Originally developed by Schlachter, then modified by Fawcett and Chodil (59)	54-inch square sheet of opaque yellow ochre vinyl on which are superimposed concentric circles ranging in diameter from 11 to 54 inches: each circle is 1 inch larger than the preceding one; each circle is designated by a 2-digit random number; subject asked to position self in center circle and to identify circle that represents space body occupies	Has face validity Test–retest reliability coefficients: 0.89 (3-hour interval) 0.74 (1 week) (13) Requires further testing

15B. Important Instruments to Measure Body Image (*cont.*)

Instrument	Description	Psychometric Indices
Distortion Mirror Developed by Traub and Orbach (60)	Measures internalized picture of body's physical appearance Mirror capable of wide range of distortions in height, width, and shape Subject asked to adjust mirror until it appears undistorted Data consists of 2 numbers (deviations from zero distortion)	Objectivity, face validity Usefulness is disputed: measures direct perception while body image may more accurately involve a recall of the relation of body parts (61)
Distorting Picture Technique (DPT) Developed by Glucksman and Hirsch (62)	Determines response of obese patients to weight reduction Slide photographs of obese and nonobese subjects are projected and systematically distorted in either obese or thin directions: subjects are asked to adjust distorted images to correspond to their body size; slides of a symmetrical vase is shown as instruction, first, accurate, then with successive distortions in the slide. Subjects are asked to correct the screen image to the initial undistorted image.	Study results show: obese subjects increasingly overestimate body size during and after weight loss (this may be limited to small subsection of superobese subjects) (63); nonobese subjects underestimate size during maintenance (62) Test–retest reliability coefficient: 0.61 (27) Significant correlation found with affective measures ($p = 0.05$), suggesting that DPT may not be measuring perceptual component (27)
Body Image Distortion Evaluation Developed by Gustavson et al. 1990 (64)	Evaluates body image distortion using computer image analysis Subjects asked to redraw standardized pictures of a person to look like themselves Distortion scores computed	Does not discriminate between eating disorder and normal people, but small study Calls into question use of body image distortion as a criterion for the diagnosis of certain eating disorders (64)
Allebeck et al. Apparatus for Measuring Disturbances in Size and Shape (65)	Picture of subject or external object displayed on TV monitor; subject adjusts size and height/width proportions Deviations from correct measures read directly by electrical instrumentation	Respectable reliability estimates (56): internal consistency (Cronbach's alpha): 0.87–0.97; test–retest: eating disorder subjects ($r = 0.91$), normal subjects ($r = 0.83$) Validity unclear; does not discriminate between anorexic and control groups (49)
Video Camera Developed by Collins (66)	Polaroid picture of subject distorted by videocamera to provide range of representations from thin to obese Subjects asked to change image on TV screen to match own image of their body	Test–retest reliability (67): 0.83–0.96 (5 consecutive assessments of body image 10 minutes apart); 0.63 (24 hours apart); 0.61 (8 weeks apart) Limited data on construct validity (66, 67)
Body Image Assessment (BIA) Developed by Williamson et al. (68)	Inexpensive, simple measure of body image disturbances in women Subject selects silhouette of female body frames perceived to resemble own current and ideal body size 3 scores: Current Body Size Score (CBS), Ideal Body Size Score (IBS), discrepancy score	Reliability and validity data obtained from large sample ($n = 659$) of eating disorder and normal subjects Test–retest reliability: CBS, discrepancy scores: 0.72–0.93 (1- to 8-week interval); IBS: 0.60 (3- to 8-week interval) Validity: correlates well with 2 other measures of eating disorders; discriminates between eating disorder patients and normals (68) Further studies warranted

Numbers in parentheses correspond to studies cited in the References.

224

16

Measuring Sexuality
Physiologic, Psychologic, and Relationship Dimensions

Saundra E. Saunders, Susan Heame Kaempfer, and Susan Gross Fisher

Human sexuality as a focus of scholarly interest has been reflected in an extensive body of literature since the first half of the twentieth century.[1-3] However, psychometric instrumentation in the realm of human sexuality is relatively recent; formal, serious attempts to measure sexual behavior, function, and adjustment had to await the pioneering efforts of Masters and Johnson in the 1960s.[4] Since then, numerous authors have addressed a multitude of clinical and research perspectives of human sexuality.[5] Interest in this topic has proliferated since the mid-1960s, to the extent that even the general notion of what defines an individual's sexual identity is undergoing radical change.

Human sexuality can be defined as the degree of maleness or femaleness in a person's personality and physique. It also is what defines how we act and react to our world, ourselves, and to each other. Sexuality and resultant sexual behavior are a composite of physiologic, intrapsychic, and interpersonal phenomena. The physiologic dimension represents the function of the organs involved in the biology of the sexual response. The intrapsychic or psychologic dimension represents the private experience of sexual functioning, including knowledge and attitudes about sexuality, level of sexual satisfaction, sexual fantasies, gender role definition, body image, sexual experience, and basically how an individual defines himself or herself as a sexual being. The interpersonal dimensions represent the nature and degree of social, interactive sexual behavior. To be of clinical and scientific merit research on human sexuality requires the development and use of measurement instruments that integrate all three dimensions of sexuality.[6] Operationalization of the construct of sexuality for scientific investigation requires a more refined conceptualization, including attitudes, behaviors, physiologic change, orientation, and relationship issues is needed.

Acknowledgment: The work of the original chapter (1986) was supported in part by National Cancer Institute predoctoral training grant 1F31 CA08000.

225

Research on Human Sexuality

In contrast to the energy that has been devoted to the developmental, social, and epidemologic perspectives of sexuality research, the physiologic or somatic perspective of impaired organic sexual function has been relatively neglected.[7,8] Research on the physiology of sexual function in men is limited, and that on the female sexual response is even more so. However, work to date suggest three avenues of inquiry: neurovascular, psychophysiologic, and gonadal.

Neurovascular Research

Neurovascular research pertains to mechanisms underlying autonomic innervation (glandular and smooth-muscle function), regulation by central nervous system structures (e.g., the limbic system) and neurotransmitters (e.g., peptides and monoamines), and hemodynamics.

Psychophysiologic Research

Psychophysiologic research deals with the grossly observable outcomes of neurovascular mechanisms. Traditionally, this has entailed measuring autonomically mediated effects on such parameters as heart rate, blood pressure, respiration, skin conduction, and papillary response. Such indices are generally not considered to be sufficiently sensitive or discriminating. Instead, genital measures seem to distinguish more reliably sexual arousal from other emotional states. For example, erectile function in males, including determination of penile tumescence, has been demonstrated to correlate with self-reports of sexual arousal. Pelvic vascular competency in male sexual arousal also has been investigated. Alternatively, psychophysiologic research on female sexual response has included measurement of vaginal lubrication and acidity, labia minora temperature, clitoral engorgement, and genital vasoconstriction during sexual arousal. All have failed to demonstrate statistically significant correlation with self-reports of sexual arousal.

Gonadal Research

Sexuality, as reflected by gonadal function, has been approached through endocrine studies (e.g., circulating levels of gonadal steroids, gonadotropins, prolactin, thyroid-stimulating hormone, and thyroid hormones), fertility evaluation (e.g., menstrual history, contraceptive use, gonadal biopsy, semen evaluation), physical assessment of the genitalia and secondary sexual characteristics, and clinical manipulation of the endocrine milieu (e.g., endocrine ablation or replacement therapies).[8]

Psychologic and Interpersonal Research

Psychologic research in sexuality involves psychometric documentation of affect, libido, knowledge, and attitudes toward sexual function and sexual experience. Psychosexual research not only has drawn on standard and well-established psychologic testing methods but also has begun to generate valid and reliable instruments designed specifically to measure the persona or intrapsychic dimensions of sexuality.[9] Research on the interpersonal aspects of sexuality addresses the sexual adjustment of couples. Measurement of sexuality as it relates to dyads is less well developed than either physiologic or psychologic methodologies. However, in the 1990s additional measurements of sexuality as it pertains to couples have been developed, and some await more thorough testing for reliability and validity.[10] Nonpsychometric surveys of interpersonal components of sexuality abound and in general consist of tools for assessment, counseling, and discussion involving premarital, marital, and family interventions in nonresearch settings. Such tools are not and were not intended to be used for scientific investigation.[11] This lack of sophistication highlights the fact that until the organic and intrapersonal nature of human sexuality is more clearly delineated, the constructs that comprise those that are distinctively interpersonal will remain elusive both conceptually and empirically.[9]

Sexual Function

Any illness involving distress, fatigue, pain, fear, anxiety, or depression may affect sexual function. Pathology that impairs anatomic structures alters sexual performance. Sexual drive, however, may still persist in the presence of altered sexual performance, regardless of etiology. In sexual research, it is critical to distinguish between research populations of people complaining of sexual problems and those whose sexuality is being examined in a broader context, such as physical illness.[9] Furthermore, because most psychometric instruments have been developed and used outside the context of the individual suffering from significant medical disorders, their application in these settings requires concurrent reliability and validity determinations.[6]

Measures of sexuality are useful both to evaluate change resulting from therapy or dyadic experience and to conduct research on the relationship between sexual function and other variables.[12] Several reviews of research measures of human sexuality exist and provide a point of departure in organizing one's thinking on this topic.[10-12] Critical reviews of sexuality are found in Appendix 16A.[13-15] The review by Talmadge and Talmadge[10] is especially helpful.

Fundamental to psychosexual assessment, irrespective of setting, is the determination of psychologic constructs or domains that are inherent in sexual behavior, followed by the development of ways to measure them.[16] Construct validation of behaviors, characteristics, or aptitudes important to sexual functioning is in progress and is reflected in the broad range of instruments available for scrutiny. This chapter is limited to a survey of currently available methods of studying empirically the two psychosexual dimensions of human sexuality: the psychologic and the interpersonal.

Instruments are organized according to their originally intended use. An attempt has been made to contact the authors of the psychometric instruments mentioned in the literature to obtain the most current data on their reliability and validity. The results of this survey demonstrated that many instruments are either difficult to access or are no longer available or appropriate for use. Therefore, selected instruments that are of potential practical use to investigators are described in detail, and the remaining tools are summarized in the appendices. This chapter reflects a relatively thorough treatment of research instrumentation of human sexuality However, the discipline of the study of human sexuality is developing rapidly, and new instruments or adaptations of available instruments to different subject populations are continually in progress.

Comprehensive Measures of Sexuality

Sexual Performance Evaluation Questionnaire of the Marriage Council of Philadelphia

Interviews are a commonly used method of obtaining information related to sexual issues. A particularly comprehensive interview guideline is that based on the Sexual Performance Evaluation Questionnaire of the Marriage Council of Philadelphia. Useful in obtaining a sexual history, the lines of inquiry addressed are under the major topic headings of: childhood sexuality; onset of adolescence; orgasmic experiences; feelings about self as masculine/feminine; sexual fantasies and dreams; dating; engagement; marriage; extramarital sex; sex after widowhood, separation, or divorce; sexual deviations; certain effects of sex activities; and use of erotic material. A related sexual performance evaluation outline covers investigation of specific characteristics of an individual's coital activities.[17]

Participation in an interview can be a therapeutic experience for an individual. This method of data collection, however, is very time-consuming, and the resultant findings are often difficult to quantify. Research conclusions obtained in this way, can become extremely tenuous. However, such data can describe phenomena from which concepts can be identified that can lead to the development of more quantifiable instruments.

Derogatis Sexual Function Inventory (DSFI)

The most comprehensive and thoroughly evaluated psychometric instrument to measure sexual function is the Derogatis Sexual Function Inventory (DSFI).[10,16,18] On the assumption that sexuality is comprised of multiple behavioral domains, 10 constructs are operationalized in the subscales of the 245 item DSFI as follows: (1) information (sexual knowledge); (2) experience (sexual behavior); (3) drives (biologically determined and subject to neuroendocrine control); (4) sexual attitudes (liberal versus conservative); (5) psychologic symptoms (such as obsessive-compulsiveness or somatization); (6) affect (such as depression, anxiety, or guilt); (7) gender role definition or identity (relative masculinity or femininity is conceived along a continuum); (8) sexual fantasy (rehearsal and vicarious fulfillment/expression of sexual drives); (9) body image (self-evaluation of physical attractiveness as well as the reflected perceptions of others); and (10) satisfaction (sexual frequency and novelty; achievement of orgasm; communication between partners).

These constructs are designed to permit valid clinical prediction of current sexual functional status and also provide conceptual clarity in deliberations on the nature and breadth of human sexuality as a component of personality and biologic function.

The DSFI has been well tested in a broad variety of populations, including male and female heterosexuals, homosexuals, transsexuals, and sexually dysfunctional individuals. Test–retest reliabilities for the 10 subscales range from 0.42 to 0.96. Internal consistency reliability coefficients range from 0.56 to 0.97. Predictive validity of the DSFI has been demonstrated in populations of individuals suffering from sexual dysfunctions and their partners and in populations consisting of male and female transsexuals. Normed scores from 200 normal and 200 sexually dysfunctional individuals also are available. Factor analysis based on a group of 380 patient and nonpatient subjects revealed seven empirical dimensions that underlie the DSFI: (1) body image; (2) psychologic distress; (3) heterosexual drive; (4) autoeroticism; (5) gender role; (6) sexual satisfaction; and (7) sexual precociousness.

The other psychometric instruments described in this chapter lack the comprehensiveness of the DSFI and instead focus more on the dimension(s) of human sexuality they endeavor to quantify. Except where specified by a specific technique (such as factor analysis), the dimensions measured reflect the conceptual framework of the researcher.

Psychologic Dimension of Sexuality

Sexual Experience, Knowledge, or Attitudes

A number of instruments that assess the different components of sexual experience, knowledge, or attitudes have reported reliability and validity information and are accessible to researchers.[19,20-25] These tools were designed for use in clinical and research settings with normal and dysfunctional individuals. Additional measures of this component of the psychologic dimension of sexuality are summarized in Appendix 16B.

Negative Attitudes toward Masturbation Scale

The Negative Attitudes Toward Masturbation Scales is a 30-item self-report measure that addresses three factors: (1) false beliefs about the harmful nature of masturbation;

(2) positive attitude toward masturbation; and (3) personally experienced negative affects associated with masturbation.[19] Statements are rated on a 5-point scale (from 1 "strongly agree" to 5 "strongly disagree"). Two sample items are: "Masturbation is a normal sexual outlet"; and "After I masturbate, I am disgusted with myself for losing control of my body."

This tool has been tested among psychiatric populations, normal adults, and patients with sexual dysfunctions. The split-half reliability coefficient corrected by the Spearman-Brown prophecy formula was reported to be 0.75. Point biserial correlations ranged from 0.11 to 0.57 with a median of 0.40. Evidence for instrument validity has been provided by its correlation with measures of monthly masturbation frequency for males and females, self-report of negative attitudes toward masturbation and sexual experience, and a measure of sex-related guilt.[20,21]

Mosher Forced-Choice Guilt Inventories (FCGI) and the Revised Mosher Guilt Inventory (RMGI)

As originally developed, the Mosher Forced-Choice Guilt Inventories (FCGI) measured three aspects of guilt: (1) hostility guilt; (2) sex guilt; and (3) morality (guilty) conscience using a completion forced-choice format.[20,21] The Revised Mosher Guilt Inventory[10] is a nonbehavioral self-report inventory that uses a limited comparison format, consisting of 114 items arranged in pairs of responses to the same sentence completion stem. This revision allows for an increase in the range of responses and can be completed in 20 minutes.[10] There are 50 items for Sex Guilt, 42 items for Hostility Guilt, and 22 items for Guilty Conscience. Each of these scales can be used independently. A 7-point Likert scale (0 "Not at all true of (for) me" to 6 "Extremely true of (for) me") is used for responses for statements, such as "When I have sexual desires. . . ."

> "I enjoy it like all healthy human beings."
> "I fight them, for I must have complete control of my body."

Reliabilities of the Revised Mosher Guilt Inventory are the following: Split-half and alpha coefficients of the original FCGI averaged around 0.90. Item analysis showed item subscale total correlations ranging from 0.32 to 0.62, with a median of 0.46.

Sex Anxiety Inventory (SAI)

The purpose of the Sex Anxiety Inventory (SAI)[10] scale is to distinguish guilt from anxiety, assuming that guilt produces self-mediated punishment, whereas anxiety speaks to the expectation of external punishment when normative standards of sexuality are violated. This inventory looks more at general anxiety that is related to broader social/sexual anxiety, whereas the SAI-E is more specific to sexual interactions between partners.[10] The inventory is a self-report measure consisting of 25 forced-choice items that identify behavioral, attitudinal, and affective responses. Studied in undergraduate students, it takes approximately 15 minutes to complete. Scores range from 0 to 2 with a score of 0 for an item that is absent and a score of 1 for an item that is present. Interitem Pearson's product–moment correlations for the 25 items were subjected to a principal factor analysis that yielded three factors: (1) discomfort in social sexual situations (50.8% of the variance); (2) socially unacceptable sexual behaviors (13% of the variance); and (3) sexuality experienced in private (10.2% of the variance). The Kuder-Richardson (KR) coefficient measured internal consistency at 0.86. Test–retest reliability for 10 to 14 days was measured as 0.85 for males and 0.84 for females. For discriminant validity the SAI was correlated with the Mosher Forced-Choice Sex Guilt Inventory with a correlation of 0.67. Usually, this type of information would be assessed by taking a sexual history. However, this instrument could be used individually to identify specific areas for further assessment and intervention with clinical populations.[10]

Other Aspects

Evaluation of Sexuality Curricula

Several instruments have been developed specifically to determine the effects of sex education programs on changes in the sexual knowledge and attitudes of participants.[33-36] In these settings, success is judged by an increase in sexual knowledge and/or change in attitudes reflecting greater permissiveness. Four instruments are presented with psychometric indices in Appendix 16C. Other available measures are summarized in Appendix 16D.[14]

Sexual Orientation Roles

Sexual orientation and sexual roles are viewed from three perspectives; gender role definition, gender identity, and sexual deviancy. Gender role definitions and attitudes are the focus of several instruments.[37-44] Appendix 16E presents the most commonly used instruments.

Sexual Dysfunction

Sexual dysfunction is a broad concept that can encompass both physiologic and psychologic components. Approaches to the medical evaluation of infertility or sterility, as well as problems with sexual performance or response, have been described.[9] This discussion is limited to psychometric determination of the nature and extent of an individual's sexual health. Four important measures are described in Appendix 16F.

Body Perception

Body perception or image is an integral component of an individual's sexuality and can make a significant contribution to sexual health or dysfunction. Because of the growing recognition of and interest in body image disturbance among people suffering from physical illness and disability, it is given separate consideration here. Major instruments are detailed in Appendix 16G.[44-47]

Aging and Developmental Adaptations

The elderly and the developmentally disabled are two special nonpatient populations that have been the focus of psychosexual inquiry.[48-50]

Aging Sexuality Knowledge and Attitudes Scale (ASKAS)

The Aging Sexuality Knowledge and Attitudes Scale (ASKAS)[48] measures sexual attitudes and knowledge in the context of age-related changes and sexuality for the elderly.[48] The 61 items can be either self-administered or administered in interview format. The Knowledge section consists of 35 true–false questions. The Attitude section uses a 7-point Likert scale response format in which the extent of agreement or disagreement with the item statement is determined. Sample items from the ASKAS are: "Males over the age of 65 usually experience a reduction in intensity of orgasm relative to younger males" (Knowledge); or "If family members object to a widowed relative engaging in sexual relations with another resident of a nursing home, it is the obligation of the management and staff to make certain that such sexual activity is prevented" (Attitude). The ASKAS has been used extensively with staff and residents of nursing homes and with aged people in the community and their families. Reported (KR) split-half reliabilities for both sections of the ASKAS range from 0.83 to 0.91. Test–retest reliabilities range from 0.72 to 0.97. Alpha reliabilities range from 0.76 to 0.93. Factor analysis and changed scores before and after a sexual education program among aged subjects, people who work with the aged, and family members of elderly persons have demonstrated the validity of the ASKAS. Furthermore, in contrast to control groups, experimental groups showed significant changes in the direction of greater knowledge and more permissive attitudes.

Sociosexual Knowledge and Attitudes Test (SSKAT)

The Socio-Sexual Knowledge and Attitudes Test (SSKAT) was originally developed to measure the sexual knowledge and attitudes of developmentally disabled adults who are not verbally proficient or whose speech is unintelligible.[49,50] However, the SSKAT also can be used with nonretarded persons provided they have visual and verbal comprehension. A 227-page *Stimulus Picture Book* presents realistic pictures requiring "yes–no" and "point to" responses to questions on 14 sociosexual topic areas, including anatomy, terminology, menstruation, intimacy, intercourse, pregnancy and childbirth, birth control, masturbation, homosexuality, and venereal disease. Sample items from one section of the SSKAT are:

> I. Anatomy terminology:
> *"What is this called?"* point to vulva (naked female, front view)
> *"What is this for?"* point to vulva (naked female, front view) . . . probe once and ask,
> *"Is there anything else this is for?"**

The last question tries to get at the depth of understanding, by giving the individual another chance at defining the concept.

Although content and predictive validity for the SSKAT remain to be established, test–retest reliability for a 7- to 10-day interval in a sample of 100 retarded men and women for both knowledge and attitude subscales ranged from 0.76 to 0.91. In addition, KR reliability coefficients for SSKAT subscale items have ranged from 0.53 to 0.83.

Interpersonal Dimensions of Sexuality

Measures of the interpersonal dimensions of sexuality address marital/dyadic characteristics, including a range of parameters and indicators of adjustment and satisfaction. Measures of this dimension of sexuality are summarized in Appendix 16H.[51-62]

Applications in Specific Clinical Populations

All of the instruments described in this chapter were developed for people of varying age, developmental level, and sexual health, but who were not suffering from a concurrent physical illness or disability. The use of these instruments in special populations requires adaptation of items and evaluation of their reliability and validity. Research into the demands imposed on one's sexuality by the presence of physical illness is being conducted by researchers in a wide variety of disciplines. To illustrate the form this has taken in different realms of clinical expertise, efforts to assess psychosexual impacts in the presence of several types of chronic illness are briefly presented in Appendix 16I.[63-72]

Summary

Psychometric instrumentation in the field of sexuality is a relatively recent phenomenon. The growing recognition of sexuality as an issue of overall health and well-being has permitted the evolution of a growing number of instruments to measure human sexuality in both research and clinical practice. The preceding discussion of instruments available for the measurement of issues related to sexuality is fairly extensive both in breadth and depth of inquiry. A common concern for all but a few designated instruments is that they have typically been normed on college students and have had limited validation with other populations, such as a variety of ages, gender, orientation, educa-

*Courtesy of Stoeling Co., 1350 Kostner Ave., Chicago, IL 60623.

tional background, and socioeconomic class, as well as those who are culturally divergent, and those who are dealing with acute and chronic illness and its impact on their sexuality. Controlled studies using the different instruments with different populations are needed to test reliability and validity. At the same time, researchers will be better able to define more clearly the issues around sexuality that are most important to those they wish to serve.

Since the 1960s the groundwork has been laid not only to question the concepts and issues of sexuality, but also to provide an atmosphere of sensitivity, awareness, and openness that allows for scientific and conscientious study of an individual's sense of his/her sexuality and what impacts it in what way. However, there are possible limitations to research in the field of sexuality. First, because of the sensitive nature of sexuality, it often is quite difficult to obtain objective data from the subject and/or partner. Some people are unwilling to participate in research related to sexual matters because of embarrassment, denial, fear, and/or a desire for privacy. Similarly, people who have sexual problems and are seeking help may self-select themselves to participate in such studies, thus creating a biased sample. Some subjects may respond to inquiries based on what they suppose to be the desirable or socially acceptable response because of reluctance to reveal unusual or nonconventional sexual values and practices.

Still it is hoped that this chapter has provided enough depth to meet the interests of those who would wish to continue the work that has been started in this field. Some of the instruments, though begun as a research tool, are also quite useful as part of an assessment package designed to identify problems and help individuals with specific issues.

For all subjects, the introduction of the topic of sexuality should be both straightforward and sensitive, showing respect for the individuals involved. For patient populations in particular, introduction of sexual assessment early in the diagnostic and therapeutic plan enables the establishment of an environment of openness and comfort in exploring what has been regarded traditionally as a highly personal and sensitive topic.

Exemplar Studies

Rudy, E.B., & Estok, P.J. Running addiction and dyadic adjustment. *Res Nurs Health*, 1990, *13*:219–225.

This study exemplifies the use of the Dyadic Adjustment Scale by Spanier to determine the effects of runner's addiction, as described by the Runners Addiction Scale, on the relationship of the individual and his/her spouse. The sample was 45% of a group of runners who had just completed a marathon with an almost equal sample of males and females and an age range from 25 to 71. The study concept was well researched and led logically to this comparison. A Pearson's product moment correlation was used to determine the relationship between addiction and dyadic adjustment. Dependent *t*-tests were used to analyze the differences between spouses. This study extended the work of Spanier by using the tool with both members of a marital dyad instead of a single member, as had been done previously. The authors showed that there is no significant difference between the members, which supports the accuracy of using the instrument with only one member of a dyad.

Beutler, L.E., et al. Women's satisfaction with partner's penile implant: Inflatable vs noninflatable prosthesis. *Urology*, 1984, *24*(6):552–558.

This study exemplifies the use of the Derogatis Sexual Functioning Inventory in the consideration of the many variables that could effect a partner's sexual satisfaction when a penile prosthesis is being used. The study compares factors on the DSFI with factors on the authors' own scale, the

Arizona Partner Questionnaire, which was specifically designed for this study to evaluate subjective impression of interpersonal satisfaction, rating of current sexual adjustment, report of complications, and problems encountered by virtue of the prosthesis. The methods are fairly well described, and care was taken to ensure reliability and validity. It was determined that the DSFI was the most discriminant instrument in detecting difference between the two groups of women in the area of overall sexual satisfaction.

References

1. Kinsey, A.C., Pomeray, W.B., & Martin, C.E. *Sexual behavior in the human male.* Philadelphia: Saunders, 1948.
2. Kinsey, A.C., et al. *Sexual behavior in the human female.* Philadelphia: Saunders, 1953
3. Thompson, A.P., & Cranwell, F.R. Frequently cited sources in human sexology. *J Sex Mar Ther*, 1984, *10*(1):63.
4. Masters, W.H., Johnson, V.E., & Kolodny, R.C., *Human sexuality.* Boston: Little, Brown, 1982.
5. Woods, N.F. *Human sexuality in health and illness* (3rd ed.). St. Louis: Mosby, 1984.
6. Derogatis, L.R. Response: The measurement of sexual dysfunction in cancer patients. *Cancer*, 1984, *53*(10):2285.
7. Abramson, P.R., Perry, L.B., Rothblatt, A., et al. Negative attitudes toward masturbation and pelvic vasocongestion: A thermographic analysis. *J Res Pers*, 1981, *15*:497.
8. Schiavi, R.C., & Schreiner-Engel, P. Physiologic aspects of sexual function and dysfunction. *Psychiatr Clin North Am*, 1980, *3*(1):81.
9. Greenberg, D.B. The measurement of sexual dysfunction in cancer patients. *Cancer*, 1984, *53*(10):2281.
10. Talmadge, L.D., & Talmadge, W.C. Sexuality assessment measures for clinical use: A review. *Am J Fam Ther*, 1990, *18*(1):80.
11. Sweetland, R.C., & Keyser, D.J. (Eds.). *Tests: A comprehensive reference for assessments in psychology, education, and business.* Kansas City: Test Corporation of America, 1983.
12. Conte, H.R. Development and use of self-report techniques for assessing sexual functioning: A review and critique. *Arch Sex Behav*, 1983, *12*(6):555.
13. Schiavi, R.C., et al. The assessment of sexual function and marital interaction. *J Sex Mar Ther*, 1979, *5*(3):169.
14. Williams, A.M., & Miller, W.R. The design and use of assessment instruments and procedures for sexuality curricula. In N. Rosenzweig and F.P. Pearsall (Eds.), *Sex education for the health professional: A curriculum guide.* New York: Grune & Stratton, 1978, p. 137.
15. Green, R., & Wiener, J. (Eds.). *Methodology in sex research.* Rockville, MD: DHHS, National Institute of Mental Health, 1981.
16. Derogatis, L.R. Psychological assessment of psychosexual function. *Psychiatr Clin North Am*, 1980, *3*(1):113.
17. Group for the Advancement of Psychiatry. *Assessment of sexual function: A guide to interviewing.* New York: Jason Aronson, 1974.
18. Derogatis, L.R., & Melisaratos, N. The DSFI: A multi-dimensional measure of sexual functioning. *J Sex Mar Ther*, 1979, *5*(3):244.
19. Abramson, P.R., & Mosher, D.L. Development of a measure of negative attitudes toward masturbation. *J Consult Clin Psychol*, 1975, *43*(4):485.
20. Mosher, D.L. The development and multitrait-multimethod matrix analysis of three measures of three aspects of guilt. *J Consult Psychol*, 1966, *30*:35.
21. O'Grady, K.E., & Janda, L.H. Factor analysis of the Mosher Forced-Choice Guilt Inventory. *J Consult Clin Psychol*, 1979, *47*:1131.
22. Harbison, J.J.M., Graham, P.J., Quinn, J.T., et al. A questionnaire measure of sexual interest. *Arch Sex Behav*, 1974, *3*(4):357.
23. Hoon, E.F., Hoon, P.W., & Wincze, J.P. An inventory for the measurement of female sexual arousability: The SAI. *Arch Sex Behav*, 1976, *5*(4):291.
24. Chambless, D.L., & Lifshitz, J.L. Self-reported sexual and anxiety arousal: The Expanded Sexual Arousability Inventory. *J Sex Res*, 1984, *20*(3):241.
25. Allen, R.M., & Haupt, T.D. The Sex Inventory: Test–retest reliabilities of scale scores and items. *J Clin Psychol*, 1966, *22*(4):367.
26. Thorne, F.C. The Sex Inventory. *J Clin Psychol*, 1966, *22*(4):367.
27. Thorne, F.C., & Haupt, T.D. The objective measurement of sex attitude and behavior in adult males. *J Clin Psychol*, 1966, *22*(4):395.
28. Fretz, B.R. An attitude measure of sexual behaviors. Paper presented at the American Psychological Association 82 annual convention, New Orleans, Sept. 1974.
29. Perkel, A.K. Development and testing of the AIDS Psychosocial Scale. *Psychol Rep*, 1992, *71*:767.
30. Lief, H.I., Fullard, W., & Devlin, S.J. A new measure of adolescent sexuality: SKAT-A. *J Sex Educ Ther*, 1990, *16*(2):79.
31. Snell, W.E., Jr., Fisher, T.D., & Miller, R.S. Development of the Sexual Awareness Questionnaire: Components, reliability, and validity. *Ann Sex Res*, 1991, *4*:65.
32. Snell, W.E., Jr., Belk, S.S., Papini, D.R., & Clark, S. Development and validation of the Sexual Self-Disclosure Scale. *Ann Sex Res*, 1989, *2*:307.
33. Miller, W.R., & Lief, H.I. The sex knowledge and attitude test (SKAT). *J Sex Mar Ther*, 1979, *5*(3):282.
34. Fisher, S.G., & Levin, D. The sexual knowledge and attitudes of professional nurses caring for oncology patients. *Cancer Nurs*, 1983, *6*(1):55.
35. Zuckerman, M., Tushup, R., & Finner, S. Sexual attitudes and experience: Attitude and personality correlates and changes produced by a course in sexuality. *J Consult Clin Psychol*, 1976, *44*(1):7.
36. Williams, H.A., Wilson, M.E., Hongladorum, G., et al. Nurses' attitudes toward sexuality in cancer patients. *Oncol Nurs Forum*, 1986, *13*(2):39.

37. Bem, S. The measurement of psychological androgyny. *J Consult Clin Psychol*, 1974, 42(2):155.

38. MacDonald, A.P., Jr. Identification and measurement of multidimensional attitudes toward equality between the sexes. *J Homosex*, 1974, 1(2):165.

39. Snell, W.E., Jr., Fisher, T.D., & Schuh, T. Reliability and validity of the Sexuality Scale: A measure of sexual-esteem, sexual-depression, and sexual-preoccupation. *J Sex Res*, 1992, 29(2):261.

40. MacDonald, A.P., Jr., Huggins, J., Young, S., et al. Attitudes toward homosexuality: Preservation of sex morality of the double standard? *J Consult Clin Psychol*, 1973, 40:161.

41. Sambrooks, J.E., & MacCullock, M.J. A modification of the sexual orientation method and an automated technique for presentation and scoring. *Br J Soc Clin Psychol*, 1973, 12(2):163.

42. Berkey, B.R., Perelman-Hall, T., & Kurdek, L.A. The Multidimensional Scale of Sexuality. *J Homosex*, 1990, 19(4):67.

43. Schover, L.R., Friedman, J.M., Weiler, S.J., et al. Multiaxial problem-oriented system for sexual dysfunction. *Arch Gen Psychiatry*, 1982, 39(5):614.

44. Hollender, M.H., Luborsky, L., & Scaramella, T.J. Body contact and sexual enticement. *Arch Gen Psychiatr*, 1969, 20(2):188.

45. Kurtz, R., & Hurt, M. Body attitude and physical health. *J Clin Psychol*, 1970, 26(2):149.

46. Snell, W.E., Jr., & Papini, D.R. The Sexuality Scale: An instrument to measure sexual-esteem, sexual-depression, and sexual-preoccupation. *J Sex Res*, 1989, 26(2):256.

47. Wiederman, M.W., & Allgeier, E.R. The measurement of sexual-esteem: Investigation of Snell and Papini's (1989) Sexuality Scale. *J Res Person*, 1993, 27:88.

48. White, C.B. A scale for the assessment of attitudes and knowledge regarding sexuality in the aged. *Arch Sex Behav*, 1982, 11(6):491.

49. Edmonson, B., & Wish, J. Sex knowledge and attitudes of moderately retarded males. *Am J Ment Defic*, 1975, 80(2):172.

50. Wish, J.R., et al. *The Socio-Sexual Knowledge and Attitude Test: Instruction Manual.* Chicago: Stoelting Co., 1980.

51. Foster, A.L. The sexual compatibility test. *J Consult Clin Psychol*, 1977, 45(2):332.

52. Spainer, G.B. Measuring dyadic adjustment: New scales for assessing the quality of marriage and similar dyads. *J Mar Fam*, 1976, 38(1):15.

53. Reiss, I.L. *The social context of premarital sexual permissiveness.* New York: Holt, Rinehart, and Winston, 1967, p. 211.

54. Barret-Lennard, G.T. The Relationship Inventory: Later developments and adaptations. *JSAS Catalog of "Selected Documents in Psychology,"* 1978, 8:68 (MS No. 1732).

55. Gurland, B.J., Yorkston, N.J., Stone, A.R., et al. The Structured and Scaled Interview to Assess Maladjustment (SSIAM). I. Description, rationale and development. *Arch Gen Psychiatr*, 1972, 27(2):259.

56. Gurland, B.J., Yorkston, N.J., Goldberg, K., et al. The Structured and Scaled Interview to Assess Maladaptation (SSIAM). II. Factor analysis, reliability and validity. *Arch Gen Psychiatr*, 1972, 27(2):264.

57. LoPiccolo, J., & Steger, J. The Sexual Interaction Inventory: A new instrument for assessment of sexual dysfunction. *Arch Sex Behav*, 1974, 3(6):585.

58. McCoy, N.N., & D'Agostino, P.A. Factor analysis of the Sexual Interaction Inventory. *Arch Sex Behav*, 1977, 3(6):25.

59. Noller, P. *Nonverbal communication in marital interactions.* Elmsford, NY: Pergamon, 1984.

60. Bienvenue, M.J., Sr. Measurement of marital communication. *Fam Coord*, 1970, 19(1):26.

61. Schaefer, M.T., & Olson, D.H. Assessing intimacy: The PAIR Inventory. *J Mar Fam Ther*, 1981, 7(1):47.

62. Waring, E.M., & Reddon, J.R. The measurement of intimacy in marriage: The Waring Intimacy Questionnaire. *J Clin Psychol*, 1983, 39(1):53.

63. Wilmoth, M.C. *Development and testing of the sexual behaviors questionnaire.* Warrensburg: Department of Nursing, Central Missouri State University, 1994.

64. Bullard, D.G., Causey, G.C., Newman, A.B., et al. Sexual health care and cancer: A needs assessment. *Front Radiat Ther Oncol*, 1980, 14:55.

65. Harris, R., Good, R.S., & Pollack, L. Sexual behavior of gynecologic cancer patients. *Arch Sex Behav*, 1982, 11(6):503.

66. Waterhouse, J., & Metcalfe, M. Development of the sexual adjustment questionnaire. *Oncol Nurs Forum*, 1986, 13(3):53.

67. Meyer-Bahlburg, H.F.L., & Ehrhardt, A.A. Sexual Behavior Assessment Schedule: Adult (SEBA-A). 1983.

68. Althof, S.E., Coffman, C.B., & Levine, S.B. The effects of coronary bypass surgery on female sexual, psychological and vocational adaptation. *J Sex Mar Ther*, 1984, 10(3):176.

69. Watts, R.J. Sexual functioning, health beliefs and compliance with high blood pressure medications. *Nurs Res*, 1982, 31(5):278.

70. Pieper, B.A., et al. Perceived effect of diabetes on relationship to spouse and sexual function. *J Sex Educ Ther*, 1983, 9(2):46.

71. Jensen, S.B. Diabetic sexual dysfunction. A comprehensive study of 16 insulin-treated diabetic men and women—An age matched control group. *Arch Sex Behav*, 1981, 10:493.

72. Jensen, S.B. Sexual dysfunction in insulin-treated diabetics: A six year follow-up study of 101 patients. *Arch Sex Behav*, 1986, 15(4):271.

Appendices

16A. Critical Reviews of Sexuality

Author	Focus	Comments
Schiavi et al. (13)	Psychometric instruments and measuring more than 1 aspect of sexual activity and marital interaction with heterosexual individuals and dyads	Early overview; provides names, authors, description of instruments, reliability/validity data
Talmadge and Talmadge (10)	Clinical instruments	Excellent reference: describes usefulness of measures of research
Williams and Miller (14)	Criteria for evaluating effectiveness of curricula on sexuality	9 questionnaires summarized
Green and Wiener (15)	Research issues in the study of human sexuality	Sex and aging, sexual dysfunction, heterosexual relationships, rape, neurobiologic components, homosexuality, psychosexual differentiation addressed
Conte (12)	Self-report psychometric measures (Guttman scales, inventories)	Application to heterosexual or homosexual subjects
		Guttman scales: assume unidimensionality of items reflecting sexual behavior (10–20 items), measure narrow range of sexual functioning; inventories are questionnaires that assess a broad range of sexual behaviors (multidimensionality of items).

Numbers in parentheses correspond to studies cited in the References.

16B. Instruments Measuring the Psychologic Dimension of Sexuality

Name	Description	Psychometric Indices
Sexuality Arousability Inventory (SAI) (10,23,24)	Self-report of sexual arousability in women Descriptions of 28 sexual activities and situations are rated on a 7-point Likert scale (−1 "adversely affects arousal" to +5 "always causes sexual arousal")	Discriminates between normal and sexually dysfunctional individuals (from middle and upper-middle socioeconomic class) Cross-validation with 2 different samples; coefficient alphas: 0.91, 0.92 Test–retest reliability coefficient: 0.69 (8-week interval)
Sexual Arousability Inventory-Expanded (SAI-E)	Measures amount of arousal and anxiety experienced during specific sexual behaviors Behavioral self-report 28 items, answered once for arousal and once for anxiety (total 56 items) Scored on 7-point Likert scale (−1 "adversely affects arousal/extremely anxiety provoking" to +5 "extremely arousing/relaxing")	Factor analysis: 5 factors (preparation/participation in intercourse, pornography, nongenital sex play, breast stimulation, other sex play) Split-half Spearman-Brown reliability coefficient (females): 0.92 (arousal), 0.94 (anxiety) Can be used with males regardless of sexual orientation or marital status (10)
Sex Inventory (SI) (25-27)	200 true/false items Self-report measure of sexual attitudes and behavior in adult men 9 subscales (sex drive and interest, sexual maladjustment, neurotic conflict, fixation, repression, loss of control, confidence, homosexuality, promiscuity)	Test–retest reliability: 0.40–0.50 (23) Discriminates between normal and clinical groups and among clinical groups
Sex Attitude Questionnaire (28)	Self-report measure of attitudes toward sexual behaviors and situations Semantic differential 12 concepts evaluated on bipolar dimensions	Test–retest reliability: 0.35–0.67 (concept); 0.52–0.78 (bipolar dimensions) Validity established
Guttman Scale of Sexual Experience (GSSE)	Measures heterosexual behavior/experience Self-report, 30 items (female) or 31 items (male) Forced choice May be less helpful than Zuckerman's Human Sexuality Questionnaire (10)	Reliability: coefficients 0.88 (male) and 0.87 (female) No validity data available
AIDS Psychosocial Scale (29)	Measures self-concept, defenses (denial, repression, rationalization), peer pressure, perceived empowerment (locus of control, self-efficacy) Revised to 28 items, 7 subscales Scored in a 5-point Likert format	Concurrent validity of subscales: eigenvalues >1.00 Cronbach's alpha: 0.84

Instrument	Description	Reliability/validity data
Sexual Function Questionnaire (SFQ) for Heterosexuals (10)	Comprehensive measure of sexual functioning 6 sections (biographic, present sexual experience, past experience, intrapersonal factors, interpersonal factors, medical history)	Lacks normative, reliability, and validity data
Sexual Risk Taking Scale (SERT-A) (30)	Being developed to accompany Sex Knowledge and Attitude Test for Adolescents (SKAT-A) Attempts to measure immediate/future risk of HIV infection, pregnancy, sexually transmitted diseases in teens	No data available
Sexual Awareness Questionnaire (SAQ) (31)	36-item self-report, measuring 4 personality factors (subscales) associated with sexual awareness and assertiveness Scored using a 5-point Likert scale (0–4)	Convergent and discriminant validity established (31) Cronbach's alpha (male, female): sexual consciousness (M, 0.83; F, 0.86); sexual monitoring (M, 0.80; F, 0.82); sex appeal consciousness (M, 0.89; F, 0.92); sexual assertiveness (M, 0.83; F, 0.81)
Sexual Self-Disclosure Scale (SSDS) (32)	Measures sexual communication issues (extent to which an individual would discuss sexual topics) 12 subscales related to sexual esteem, sexual depression, and sexual preoccupation 60-items, 5-point Likert scale Revised (SSDS-R) to include 12 new subscales (sexual behaviors, values preferences, attitudes and feelings); total of 24 subscales 72 items 5-point Likert scale	Internal consistency of 12 subscales: Cronbach's alpha: female therapist: 0.83–0.93 (average 0.90); male therapist 0.84–0.94 (average 0.92) Reliability, validity established

Numbers in parentheses correspond to studies cited in the References.

16C. Major Instruments Used in Evaluating Sexuality Curricula

Name	Description	Psychometric Indices
Sex Knowledge and Attitude Test (SKAT) (33) Developed by Lief and Reed	149 items, self-administered Measures sexual knowledge, attitudes, level of experience in sexual activity Attitude section: 4 subscales (sexual myths, heterosexual relations, abortion, autoeroticism) containing 35 Likert format items Knowledge section: 1 subscale (psychologic, biologic social, psychobiologic), 71 True–false items	Used in wide range of educational settings, including nursing (33) Standardized scores available for comparison (based on results of 850 medical students from 16 U.S. schools tested in 1971)
Sex Knowledge and Attitude Test for Adolescents (SKAT-A)	Comprehensive scale with 3 main sections (knowledge, attitudes, behavior) Identifies behaviors that put adolescent at risk for acquiring/transmitting HIV or becoming parent teenager Knowledge section: 61 items (40 true–false, 21 multiple-choice, randomly placed) Attitude section: 43 statements scored on 5-point Likert scale randomly placed Behavior section: 43 items (yes–no, checklist format)	Factor analysis: 4 subscales in attitude scale (sexual myths, responsibility, sex and its consequences, sexual coercion) Test–retest reliability: 0.804 (knowledge) and 0.916 (attitude scale) Internal consistency: Cronbach's alpha (knowledge): 0.70; (attitude): 0.89 Validity: correlations with KIRBY knowledge and Attitude scales: 0.41–0.60 (similarities in expected areas) SKAT-A explores important attitudes that other measures do not, "consequences" of behavior and "responsibility" toward others (30)
Human Sexual Knowledge and Attitude Inventory (HSKAI)	Designed for use with nurses (34) 163 items (multiple-choice, true–false forced choice, rating scales) Measures biographical information, sexual attitudes and experience Assesses sexual knowledge	Test–retest reliability: 0.84 Construct validity: (sexual knowledge established by jury rating)
Human Sexuality Questionnaire (HSQ) Developed by Zuckerman (can be used only with author's permission)	Focuses on the cumulative heterosexual and homosexual experiences Guttman type behavioral self-report questionnaire Measures sexual experiences and attitudes: 6 experience scales (heterosexual, homosexual, numbers of hetero- or homosexual partners, orgasmic experience, masturbation) Attitudes: scale of items dealing with parental attitudes about children's sexuality and adult heterosexual activities	Coefficients of reproducibility: 0.97 for both males and females Rank-order correlations for male and female items: 0.95 (confirming ordinality of scales, high reliability) (10)

Numbers in parentheses correspond to studies cited in the References.

16D. Instruments Used to Evaluate the Success of Sex Education Curricula

Instrument Name/Author	Number of Items	Response Format	Types of Data Elicited
Minnesota Sexual Attitudes Scales (MSAS)/Held et al.	35	Rating scale	Attitudes toward and feelings about designated groups of people (e.g., married adults) engaging in certain categories of sexual activities
Sexual Attitude and Behavior Survey (SABS)/Kilpatrick; Smith	40	Rating scale	Sexual attitudes and experience. Attitudinal measures elicit reported permissibility/liberality of male, female and personal behavior and fantasy
Test for Assessing Sexual Knowledge and Attitudes (TASKA)/Hawkins	122	True–false; completion; rating scale; forced choice	Biographical information, sexual attitudes, experience, changes in personal behavior, and suggestions for sexuality course development
National Sex Forum Questionnaire/McIlvenna	26	Rating scale	Biographical information; sexual attitudes and experience
Harvard Sex Questionnaire/Nadelson; Shaw	61	True–false; forced choice	Biographical information; sexual attitudes, experience and knowledge
Obstetrics-Gynecology Sexuality Course Evaluation Questionnaire/Montgomery; Singer	6	Likert scale	Emotional discomfort experienced in response to hypothetical clinical situations
Physicians Workshop Questionnaire/Pion	40	Essays; fill-in-blanks; rating scales	Sexual attitudes and knowledge; change in professional behavior; suggestions for sexual course development

Number in parentheses corresponds to studies cited in the References.

Adapted from William, A.M. and Miller, W.R. The design and use of assessment instruments and procedures for sexuality curricula. In N. Rosenzweig and F.P. Pearsall (Eds.) *Sex education for the health professional: A curriculum guide.* New York: Grune & Stratton, 1978.

16E. Measures of Gender Role Definitions and Attitudes

Name	Description	Psychometric Indices
BSM Sex Role Inventory (BSRI) (37)	60 item, self-report of gender role definition Scored on 7-point Likert-scale (masculinity, femininity and androgyny subscale scores, plus social desirability scale)	Test–retest reliability: 0.89–0.93 (4-week interval) Coefficient alpha (3 scales): 0.70–0.86 Concurrent validity with other measures of masculinity, femininity Normative data available
Sex Role Survey (SRS) (38)	53-item, self-report measure of attitudes toward sex roles (4 dimensions: power in the home, sex role-appropriate behavior, equality in business, equal involvement in social/domestic work) 9-point scale	Alpha coefficients: 4 factors and total score: 0.85–0.96 Cross-validation studies have been performed; normative data available Construct validity has been evaluated
AIDS Discussion Strategy Scale (39)	Measures 6 specific types of discussion tactics to persuade a partner to discuss AIDS (rational, manipulative, withdrawal, charm, subtlety, persistence)	Unavailable
AIDS Empathy Scale (39)	Measures the extent to which an individual reports feeling empathy toward a person with AIDS	Unavailable
Attitudes Towards Homosexuality Scale (ATHS) (40)	Measures attitudes towards homosexuality (general, lesbian, male) 28-item, self-report 9-point scale ("strongly agree" to "strongly disagree")	Split-half reliability: 0.93 Alpha coefficients: 0.93–0.94
Sexual Orientation Method (41)	Self-report test of relative hetero-erotic and homoerotic orientation of homosexual men 120 paired questions (half re: attitudes toward men; half re: attitudes toward women) 5-point scale of degree of sex attributes (attractive, interesting, hot, handsome, exciting, pleasurable)	Test–retest reliability: 0.80–0.94 in control subjects of adult males Homosexual scores significantly different from controls
Multidimensional Scale of Sexuality (MSS) (42)	Self-report questionnaire with 9 categories of sexuality (heterosexuality, homosexuality, asexuality plus 6 categories of bisexuality) 45 items, 5 items relating to each category 3 sets of scores for each of the 9 categories: behavior, cognitive/affective, description of oneself	Reliability: chi-square analysis (MSS compared to Kinsey scale) showed significant relationship ($p < 0.001$) Normed using college students Additional research needed to validate categories
Kinsey Heterosexual-Homosexual Scale (42)	Equal interval scale with 7 ratings (entirely heterosexual to entirely homosexual) Bisexuality seen as half heterosexual, half homosexual	Scale based on relative amounts of both overt sexual experience, and psychologic reactions (e.g., sexual fantasies) Has limitations (life situation over time, multiple variables)
Klein Sexual Orientation Grid (KSOG) (42)	Multidimensional, addresses changes in life situations over time time and multiple variables	Unavailable

Numbers in parentheses correspond to studies cited in the References.

16F. Important Measures of Sexual Dysfunction

Name	Description	Psychometric Indices
Multiaxial Problem-Oriented System for Sexual Dysfunction (43)	Comprehensive measure of specific behavioral sexual problems associated with different phases of sexual cycle (e.g., desire, arousal, orgasm, coital pain) (43) Uses history format and produces a normed computerized sexual function profile May be used to classify sexual dysfunction in clinical situations and research	Not available
Sex History Form (Derived from multiaxial problem-oriented system)	28-multiple-choice item questionnaire May be used to classify sexual dysfunction in clinical situations and research	Norms available for sexually well-functioning people
Index of Sexual Satisfaction (ISS)	Used to determine degree of satisfaction and dissatisfaction in a relationship 25-item self-report questionnaire reflecting common problems (12 positively worded, and 13 negatively worded) Items rated on Likert scale; scoring takes 5 to 8 minutes	Normed on large Hawaiian multiethnic sample Reliability alpha coefficients: 0.906–0.925 Test–retest reliability: 0.93 Discriminant validity (compared to IMS and SAS): differed significantly from Index of Marital Satisfaction—IMS ($p < 0.001$) (10)
Sexual Anxiety Scale (SAS)	22 item self-report of sexual and social anxieties Separate gender versions	Reliability 0.92; validity coefficient 0.62 (intensity of sexual dysfunction)
Golombok Rust Inventory of Sexual Satisfaction (GRISS)	Brief and well-organized measure of sexual quality and present function in heterosexuals (10) 28-item self-report questionnaire (male/female versions) Responses on 5-point Likert scale (never to always) Takes 3–8 minutes to complete, 4–10 minutes to score Overall global functioning score (higher score, higher level of dysfunction) 4 subscales: 2 for males (impotence, premature ejaculation), 2 for females (anorgasmia, vaginismus) Other items: lack of sensuality, avoidance, dissatisfaction, infrequency, noncommunication Value in diagnosing potency and helpful in understanding pattern of couple' interrelatedness	Normed on group of sexual therapy clients Split-half reliabilities: 0.94 (female), 0.87 (male) for scales Internal consistencies, all scales: 0.61–0.83 (mean 0.74) Test–retest reliabilities: 0.47–0.84 (mean 0.65) Discriminant validity established

Numbers in parentheses correspond to studies cited in the References.

241

16G. Instruments Used to Measure Body Perception

Name	Description	Psychometric Indices
Body Attitude Scale (BAS) (44,45)	Self-report semantic differential rating scale of attitude towards outer body form 30 different body concepts rated on 7-point, bipolar adjective scale ("most negative" to "most positive") Constructs comprise 3 primary attitude dimensions (evaluative, potency, activit0y)	Generalizability coefficients (both sexes): 0.93–0.98 Individual differences in body attitude score correlate with gross variations in physique Distinguishes between normal and chronically ill subjects
Sexuality Scale (SS) (39,46,47)	Measures concepts of [1] sexual esteem, [2] sexual depression, [3] sexual preoccupation 30-item measure, scored on 5-point Likert scale (+2 agree to –2 disagree) 10 items measure each of 3 concepts Studies comparing SS with people's attitudes, empathy with persons with AIDS to determine predictibility (0.68): significant gender effect only for subscale 3 (M>F) SS subscales compared to measures of locus of control, anxiety, depression, guilt, self-esteem, sexual awareness: Cronbach's alphas high for all. [1], [3] more associated with positive orientation toward sex; [2] accompanied by greater levels of anxiety, depression, and less self-esteem and sexual assertiveness (39)	Cronbach's alpha coefficients for each concept subscale for W (women) and M (men): [1] W: 0.88, M: 0.93, all: 0.92; [2] W: 0.88, M: 0.94, all: 0.90; [3] W: 0.88, M: 0.79, all: 0.88 Test–retest reliability ($p < 0.001$): [1] 0.69–0.74; [2] 0.67–0.76; [3] 0.70–0.76 Significant correlations between subscales: negative between [1] and [2] among both men and women Correlations established in 1 study (46), but the reverse found in a later study (39): positive between [1], [3] in women; positive between [2], [3] in men (46) SS compared to Beck Depression Inventory (BDI) and Rosenberg Self-Esteem Scale (RSE): factor analysis showed inadequate fit in subscale [3]. Deleted items with reliabilities <0.50 and created short form (SF) (5 items for each subscale). Reliabilities for SS-SF improved: reliability coefficients: [1] W: 0.92, M: 0.94; [2] W, M: 0.89; [3] W: 0.96, M: 0.92 Correlations: [1], [2] highly negatively correlated, and unrelated to [3] Question on sexual esteem too narrow, but [1] does differentiate from "self-esteem" (47)

Numbers in parentheses correspond to studies cited in the References.

16H. Measures of the Interpersonal Dimension of Sexuality

Name	Description	Psychometric Indices
Locke-Wallace Marriage Inventory	Self-report measure of marital adjustment 15 items in 4 formats: multiple-choice, 6-point scale (always agree to always disagree), selection of applicable items from a checklist ("very unhappy" to "perfectly happy")	Discriminates between adjusted and maladjusted couples Split-half reliability (Kude-Richardson): 0.90
Sexual Compatibility Test (51)	101-item self-administered measure of sexual activity, attitudes, satisfaction, responsiveness in couples Specific sexual activity rated along 6 dimensions Normative data available	Cronbach's alphas: 0.90–0.96 Product moment correlations: 0.79–0.97 Concurrent validity: omega-squared ranges from 0.08–0.48
Dydadic Adjustment Scale (marital or similar dyads) (52)	32-item self-report measure of dyadic satisfaction, dyadic consensus, dyadic cohesion, affectional expression Items rated on 6-point scale	Cronbach's alpha (total, subscales): 0.73–0.96 Criterion-related and construct validity demonstrated (differentiates between married and divorced people) Correlation coefficients: 0.86 (married) and 0.88 (divorced)
Reiss Premarital Sexuality Permissiveness (PSP) (53)	12 item self-report attitudinal scale Assesses kissing, petting, coitus, each considered under 4 conditions of affection (engagement, no affection, strong affection, love) Rating scale used to show degree of agreement or disagreement	Guttman Scale reliability criteria met with coefficient of reproducibility > 0.90 Coefficient of scalability > 0.65 and pure scale types 50%–60%
Barrett-Lennard Relationship Inventory (RI) (54)	Measures 4 dimensions of interpersonal relationships (congruence, level of regard, empathetic understanding, unconditionality) 64 items (for each dimension, 8 positively and 8 negatively-worded items) Rated from +3 (strongly true) to –3 (strongly not true) Scale scores for each dimension	Split-half and test-retest reliability of each component scale averages 0.85 Correlates with other measures of marital relationship adequacy
Structured and Scaled Interview to Assess Maladjustment (SSIAM) (55,56)	60-item, structured interview format Measures maladjustment in 5 areas (work, family, marriage, sex, social) 11 dimensions for each area rated on a 10-point scale	Interrater reliability established Correlation coefficients of reliability of subscales: 0.78–0.97 Patient self-ratings yielded correlation coefficients 0.20–0.70 compared to ratings of close informants
Sexual Interaction Inventory (SII) (10,57,58)	Self-report inventory of sexual adjustment and satisfaction of heterosexual couples Useful in determining treatment for sexual dysfunction 17 items, with 6 questions on each item, rated on 6-point scale Issues: degree of satisfaction with frequency/range of sexual behaviors, sexual pleasure, self-acceptance, partner acceptance	Test–retest reliability: 0.53–0.90 over 2-week period Cronbach's alpha: 0.85–0.93 Validity established Discriminates between sexually satisfied couples and sexually dysfunctional couples; scales correlate with global ratings of sexual satisfaction

16H. Measures of the Interpersonal Dimension of Sexuality (*cont.*)

Name	Description	Psychometric Indices
Marital Communication Scales (MCS) (59)	Measure of nonverbal communication accuracy Couples participate in dyadic, face-to-face testing situation 16 hypothetical situations presented (8 where 1 member of couple is expresser, other receiver, and 8 with roles reversed)	Discriminates between satisfied and dissatisfied couples Split-half reliability using Spearman-Brown correction: coefficients 0.87 (2 groups)
Marital Communication Inventory (MCI) (60)	Self-report measure of success or failure in marital communication (emotions, feelings, economics, behaviors, communication patterns) 46 items with responses: usually, sometimes, seldom, never Separate male and female versions	Corrected odd-even split-half correlation coefficient: 0.93 (Spearman-Brown correction formula) Mann-Whitney U test: significant difference between matched groups (with and without marital problems)
Personal Assessment of Intimacy in Relationships (PAIR) (61)	75-item measure of 5 types of intimacy: social, emotional, intellectual, sexual, recreational Subjects respond to statements using a 5-point Likert scale in 2 steps: perceived, "as it is now" and expected, "how he or she would like it to be"	Factor analysis and split-half reliabilities of the PAIR have been evaluated Validity demonstrated by its correlation with measures of marital adjustment, self-disclosure, and family environments Cronbach's alpha reliability coefficient for each of 6 subscales of the PAIR: $>= 0.70$
Waring Intimacy Questionnaire (WIQ) (62)	160-item true–false format Assesses 8 components of marital intimacy (sexuality, cohesion, affection, conflict resolution, identity, expressiveness, autonomy, compatibility)	Test–retest reliability: 0.70–0.90 KR 20 reliabilities: 0.52–0.87 High significant correlation with PAIR Inventory (47)
Passionate Love Scale (PLS) (10)	30-item, nonbehavioral self-report questionnaire 9-point Likert format Assesses level of longing for union with another Includes component of sexual desire and profound physiological arousal 3 components of construct: cognitive, emotional, behavioral	Internal consistency: coefficient alphas 0.94 and 0.91 (short version) Uncontaminated by social desirability Convergent validity compared to Rubin's Liking and Loving scales (41): $r = 0.86$, $p < 0.001$ PLS measures romantic, sexual component of love; may be good outcome measure for effectiveness of sexual therapy

Numbers in parentheses correspond to studies cited in the References.

16I. Measures of Sexuality Used in Special Populations

Name	Description	Psychometric Indices
Sexual Behaviors Questionnaire (SBQ) (63) Women with breast cancer	Assesses a broad spectrum of female behaviors 8 scales (original version) scored on Likert scale (communication, appearance, desire, arousal, activity level, techniques, orgasm, satisfaction) Originally tested on convenience sample of healthy women and women having breast cancer for at least 6 months Offers reliable measure of sexuality for both healthy women and women with cancer; can be used in Quality of Life research to assess effects of cancer therapy over time	Index of Content validity: 1.00 Factor analysis: 7 scales (communication, techniques, sexual response, self-touch, body scar, masturbation, relationship) MANOVA: significant differences between healthy women and women with breast cancer, but not difference between women having lumpectomy versus mastectomy Convergent validity tested using Watt's Sexual Functioning Questionnaire Internal consistency: reliability: 0.94 Alpha coefficients: 0.53–0.94 Pearson's correlation coefficients: 0.57–0.87
Bullard et al. Questionnaire (64) Patients with cancer	67-item questionnaire and interview schedule Assesses need for sexual health services as perceived by patients with cancer Likert-type and open-ended questions asked relating to perceived importance, satisfaction, frequency of specific behaviors	Unavailable
Harris et al. Questionnaire (65) Women with gynecologic cancer	63-item sexual behavior questionnaire Explores concerns and perceptions of patient and partner on broad range of topics, including impact of malignancy on sexual functions	Unavailable
Sexual Adjustment Questionnaire (SAQ) (66) Patients with cancer	Measures changes in sexual expression following a cancer diagnosis Subsections: activity level, desire, relationship, arousal, orgasm, techniques	Test–retest reliability: 0.54–0.94 (mean 0.67) Construct validity: scores of patients with cancer significantly lower than nonpatients (activity level, techniques, relationship subsections)
Sexual Behavior Assessment Schedule: Adult (SEBA) (67) Patients with cancer (9)	Interview schedule Assesses sexual orientation, sexual dysfunction, libido, psychosexual development Originally developed to study potential long-term effects of concurrent medical conditions on sexuality	Unavailable
Althof et al. Semi-structured interview (68) Female cardiac surgery patients (68)	Developed to evaluate preoperative and longitudinal post-operative effects on sexuality of women undergoing coronary bypass surgery	Unavailable

245

16I. Measures of Sexuality Used in Special Populations (*cont.*)

Name	Description	Psychometric Indices
Sexual Functioning Questionnaire Patients receiving antihypertensive medications (69)	17-item instrument 5-point Likert rating scale High score indicates positive sexual functioning Assesses major elements of sexual experience	Test-retest reliability: 0.83 (72 hours) Cronbach's alpha: 0.55–0.65
Perception of Diabetes Mellitus Questionnaire (PDM) (70–72) Patients with diabetes mellitus	Assesses perceived impact of diabetes on sexual functioning and relationships with a spouse or partner 7-item relationship score (RS), and 6-item Sexual Function Score (SF) Rated on 7-point scale (1 "minimal effect" to 7 "great effect")	Coefficient alphas: 0.79 (RS), 0.83 (SF)
Jensen Sexual History Form (71,72) Male and female insulin-treated diabetics	Adaptation of the Sexual History Form (from the Multiaxial Problem-Oriented System for Sexual Dysfunction) (43)	Unavailable

Numbers in parentheses correspond to studies cited in the References.

17

Measuring Dietary Intake and Nutritional Outcomes

Nancy A. Stotts and Nancy Bergstrom

Cancer and its treatment often are associated with weight loss and the development of malnutrition. Associated factors include loss of appetite, inability to take in adequate nutrients, increased nutrient losses, and in some cases, cachexia and tumor-induced derangements in host metabolism.[1-3] The degree of alteration in nutritional status is associated with specific cancer sites. For example, patients with lung cancer or cancer of the gastrointestinal tract often develop cachexia, whereas those with breast cancer and sarcoma do not experience significant weight loss.[1,2,4]

Favorable nutritional status has been related to positive outcomes for cancer patients after surgery and other therapy.[5-7] Nutritionally compromised patients have higher morbidity and mortality than persons who have normal nutrition.[1,8,9] In fact, loss of more than 30% to 50% of lean body mass due to malnutrition is predictive of death.[10]

Various approaches have been investigated to mitigate malnutrition in cancer patients. In a randomized clinical trial with patients undergoing cyclic chemotherapy for cancer of the lung (small-cell), ovary, or breast, nutritional counseling increased energy intake but did not result in a significant increase in body weight when the experimental group was compared with the control group.[4] Response to chemotherapy and overall survival did not differ between the groups. In contrast, after 10 weeks of induction therapy in leukemics randomized to intensified oral nutritional intake during a 22-week course of tumor therapy, 68.8% of the patients in the experimental group regained their initial nutritional status, whereas only 31.3% of controls were similarly repleted.[7]

The routine use of enteral and parenteral nutrition is not recommended in cancer patients, and many approaches have been evaluated to increase oral intake. Only stimulation of appetite with megestrol acetate has been reported to have positive effects on severe and persistent anorexia in cancer patients that do not respond to counseling.[3]

Nutrition also is recognized as a risk factor for the development of specific types of cancer. To mitigate this risk, the United States has set two dietary goals for the year 2000: to reduce fat intake so it constitutes no more than 30% of caloric intake and to increase carbohydrate and fiber-containing foods by increasing fruit and vegetable consumption to 5 to 6 servings per day.[11] As society moves toward that goal, evaluation of dietary intake is important to monitor progress.[12] Thus data indicate that nutrition is an important consideration in the prevention and treatment of cancer. Measuring nutritional status and the effects of various nutritional therapies, as well as the effects of non-nutritional interventions on nutritional status, is important in research on cancer patients. Selecting appropriate measures requires understanding the methods employed as well as their validity and reliability.[13]

This chapter addresses the measurement of nutrition, specifically measures of ingestion, clinical evaluation, energy expenditure, biochemical measures, and high-tech approaches. Within each category, various measures will be presented, each measure will be described and its usability, accuracy and precision discussed.

Measures of Ingestion

Various approaches have been used to measure the type and amount of intake. Direct observation and weighing food, diet recall, dietary records or food diary, food frequency records, and dietary scoring are frequently used approaches.

Direct Observation and Weighing Food

Direct observation of food intake and the weighing of food are methods of dietary evaluation that allow valid measurement of nutrients consumed, especially when persons are in institutional settings. Menus from the dietary department provide data on food served, serving size, and variations based on special diets. Recipes are obtained to assist in computer analysis of nutrient intake.[14] The investigator observes the tray just before delivery to the subject to verify the items present. When trays are collected, the amount actually eaten is recorded by the observer after determining that the food was not saved or discarded.

Calorie counts as seen in hospitalized patients are one form of direct observation. Breslow and Sorkin[15] compared 1-day and 3-day calorie counts in hospitalized patients, in hopes that 1-day counts would provide data comparable with 3-day data. Using 30 patients, they found mean 3-day intake (952 ± 91 calories) and first-day intake were similar (918 ± 116 calories). The first day had high sensitivity (calories 96%, protein 93%) and had positive predictive value (calories 100%, protein 96%). These data suggest that the 1-day calorie count may be a valid alternative to the 3-day dietary intake record.

The major advantage of direct observation is that an accurate or valid record of intake can be accomplished. Memory and motivation are not critical to this method. Disadvantages are that having intake observed may precipitate behavior change and thus the recorded intake may not represent the usual intake nor intake under circumstances that do not include direct observation. In addition, this technique is expensive because of the need for a trained observer. Error is present, but neither the amount nor direction of error with this method can be anticipated.[16]

Direct observation of dietary intake in patients in a free-living situation usually is too expensive if collection needs to be conducted for more than 1 day.[16] Thus direct observation is not a technique that can readily be used in large epidemiologic studies, and so weighing of food more frequently is used in the free-living population.[16]

Weighing food involves the individual using a scale to determine the quantity of food taken in. This approach works well in countries where recipes are given by weight rather than volume. Weighing food can be an accurate reflection of intake, but other issues need to be considered, such as whether intake is reduced by the need to weigh and record intake or whether the diet is more homogeneous under these circumstances so the participant has to make fewer measurements.

One approach that has been used to circumvent this threat to validity is the recording of intake using a computerized system. Kretsch and Fong compared food intakes of research volunteers ($n = 9$) recorded on computer with intakes recorded by the metabolic unit dietary staff. In this one group study, mean differences were less than 5% for the two methods of documenting intake and correlations were between 0.81 and 0.92.[17] Further testing of the system is needed with larger samples and among those who are free-living.

The validity of observation or weighing may be questioned because of the effects of being observed. The use of computers hold hope for mitigating this threat.[17] In addition, high interrater reliability for observing and weighing has been established by pairs of observers.[18]

Twenty-Four-Hour Dietary Recall

The work of Burke[19] forms the foundation for dietary recall, a quantitative approach to the assessment of recent diet intake. With this method, subjects are interviewed and asked to recall all the food they consumed in the previous 24 hours, usually from the time of the last snack on the night before until the person goes to bed.[20] The interviewer guides the subject through the day asking questions such as: "What did you eat for lunch?" Specific food items are usually not suggested by the interviewer to avoid leading the subject. The interviewer may stimulate the subject by asking broad questions such as: "Did you eat your toast dry?" The quantity of food is determined by asking the person to describe the amount. Food models and measuring cups and spoons are used to assist the subject in recalling the serving size. The interview takes 30 to 60 minutes when conducted by a trained interviewer.[16]

The advantages[12,21] of the method are that it requires only memory for the past 24 hours and that most people can remember intake over that time. Data are collected rather quickly and may be obtained by telephone interview. In addition, because this method is used only once, there is no training effect.

The disadvantages are numerous.[21,22] The method requires accurate short-term memory, which may be problematic for some elderly people. Subjects may report what they think the researcher wants to hear or may have difficulty estimating portion size. Data analysis can be difficult. This method cannot be used to evaluate the usual dietary intake or adequacy of the diet to meet specific nutritional needs or to assess deficiency states. The inability to diagnose deficiencies has led some investigators to conclude that the 24-hour recall has limited utility.[22] When 24-hour recalls are used to measure the intake of specific nutrients, estimates of reliability have been known to vary widely, necessitating multiple recalls to place subjects in the same quartile for specific nutrients.[71]

Interrater reliability must be established for any investigation where two or more interviewers collect data. The use of a standardized training manual helps investigators to obtain this type of reliability. To assess the validity of the 24-hour recall technique, intake has been observed and recorded and compared to subjects' recall of their intake. High correlation has been found between these two measurement methods, supporting concurrent validity of the recall method. Populations studied using the recall technique include the elderly participating in congregate meal programs,[23] preschool children,[24] children,[25] children in school lunch programs,[26] and hospitalized lactating women.[27]

The Dietary Record or Food Diary

The dietary record or food diary has been used to collect information about what an individual has eaten for 1, 3, or 7 days.[12,13] Subjects are instructed on how to keep the record. Each food or fluid and some measure of quantity are recorded as close to the time of ingestion as possible to reduce memory-related inaccuracies. Subjects may or may not be asked to weigh or evaluate the quantity of food using measuring cups.

The dietary record approach often is used as the gold standard for validating other methods, when observation of food weighing is not possible.[16] Dietary records tend to be most accurate when patients have been trained by a dietician.

The advantages[12,16] of this method include the: (1) limited dependence on memory; (2) accuracy in serving size data if foods are weighed or measured; (3) ability to record data over a prolonged period, thus increasing the representativeness of the data; (4) lack of the need for additional personnel to collect data, thereby minimizing the cost of data gathering.

Major disadvantages[16] of the method are adherence problems, the fact that those who record all food intake may differ from people who do not, and a potential training effect (i.e., intake may change because it is being recorded). In addition, subjects must be highly motivated to record and/or measure their intake, and/or to measure or weigh food. Memory-related errors may be replaced with recording errors, and the generation of copious data requires significant time for analysis.[12] All of these represent potential threats to validity and reliability.

The validity of dietary records has been evaluated over a 2-week period[28] and at 1- and 9-month intervals.[29] Intake was not significantly different when dietary intake for 1 week was compared with that of a second week.[27] Correlations were 0.70 to 0.85 for the 1- and 9-month intervals, supporting the validity and reliability of this technique.[29]

Food Frequency Records

The food frequency record or interview often asks the individual how often a specific food is eaten in a given time frame. Food items are selected with the study purpose in mind (e.g., foods high in saturated fat to study heart disease risk or foods high in calcium when studying osteoporosis). Data usually are analyzed to indicate adequacy of intake in broad categories such as quartiles.[12,16,30]

Advantages[16] of this method include the low cost and representativeness of the data regarding usual intake. Cost-savings methods can include having subjects independently complete records, brief interviews, telephone, or mailed questionnaires. Questionnaires may be easily formatted for computerized scanning. Disadvantages relate to the nature of the food list to be studied. These include the order of the questions, the specificity of the foods listed,[31] and cultural differences in food preferences.[16] These problems can threaten accuracy and specificity. It should be noted that no additional validity is added to the food frequency record by adding portion size to items that do not come in natural units.[32]

Intake estimated using self-administered semiquantitative food frequency record was compared with data obtained from five 2-day diet records in 53 elderly people. The mean intake difference for most nutrients was less than 5% between the two methods. Intake correlations between the diet records and the food frequency record were quite variable. For example, 0.34 for zinc in women to 0.75 for protein, zinc, and calcium in men. For most nutrients, the diet records classified 70% of the subjects in the same quartile as that by the food frequency record. These data suggest that for individuals and groups, the food frequency record can produce data similar to that from 10 days of diet records.[33]

A cross-cultural food frequency record was developed for major epidemiologic study of breast and colorectal cancer in Spain. Subjects completed the food frequency record before and after a 4-day food intake record. Validity varied, with correlations of $r = 0.20$ for vitamin A and $r = 0.88$ for alcohol. Reliability coefficients when measured at 1-year intervals ranged from $r = 0.51$ for saturated fat to $r = 0.88$ for alcohol.[34] These data suggest that culturally specific food frequency records can be created.

Dietary Scoring

The dietary score is a method used to evaluate whether what is consumed represents the composite of foods required to meet an individual's needs. It is based on the premise that various food groups contribute unique nutrients and together meet the individual's nutritional needs. The score is the sum of the points assigned for food items from each group.[35]

The validity of this method has been evaluated by Guthrie and Scheer.[35] They assigned dietary scores to the 24-hour dietary records obtained from 212 university students.[35] Dietary scores were compared with diet records, and a nutrient ratio was calculated. The Recommended Daily Allowance (RDA), using the relevant age and gender chart, was the standard against which the adequacy of the diet was judged. This method is valid as a maximum dietary score of 16 met the RDA for 7 of 12 nutrients, and the remaining 5 nutrients met 80% (an acceptable value) of the RDA.

Data were examined to evaluate 24-hour recalls to determine variety among the 5 major food groups (dairy, meat, grain, fruit, vegetable) using a dietary diversity score.[36] Data showed that age-adjusted mortality was inversely related to the diet diversity score ($p < 0.0009$). The relative risk of death in men and women consuming two or fewer food groups was 1.5 (95%, CI 1.2–1.8) for men and 1.4 (95%, CI 1.1–1.9) for women. Analysis from the same data set showed that African-Americans had lower diet diversity scores than whites and that scores for both groups increased with income and educational preparation.[37]

Reliability of this scoring method has been evaluated by graduate nursing students observing the dietary intake of oncology patients in a demonstration project. Pairs of student observers, student and staff members, and student and patient or family members scored dietary intake. Correlations between pairs of observers were 0.80 or greater, indicating acceptable reliability.[38]

The strengths of dietary scoring are that it can be administered and analyzed by most health-care professionals and many clients and families; it can be modified to assess the needs of specific groups; and data analysis takes only minutes. Limitations are that evaluation of mixed food (e.g., casseroles, ethnic food combinations) requires judgment; it is difficult to rate fast food; the method is not sensitive to portion size, and therefore a wide range of caloric and nutrient levels may be ingested without being accurately reflected in the score.[16]

Analysis of Dietary Intake Data

To analyze nutrient intake data, a computer program generally is used. The critical factor in program selection is the use of established standards for nutrient value calculations. *The U.S. Department of Agriculture (USDA) Bulletin, Nutrient Data Base for Standard Reference*, Full Version, Release 9, Value of Food,[39] is the gold standard. This reference is updated frequently and lists food items, quantities, and nutrient content. The accuracy of this method may be threatened when several foods are mixed together (e.g., stir-fry, casserole) and when the composition of foods is not known. The only more accurate source for data would be a laboratory analysis of specific foods.

Many computer programs can be used to analyze nutrient intake data. Price and program sophistication vary widely, and the user must be sure there is a fit between the planned use and the program selected. Some programs have a limited database and calculate a limited number of nutrients. Others include fast foods, convenience foods, and special diets. Some permit the user to update values, add recipes, or provide supplementary information about specific nutrients. For both research and clinical purposes, evaluation of the nature of the database used in the computer program selected is critical to ensure that the data generated are consistent with the users' purpose.

Nieman et al., compared six microcomputer dietary analysis systems:[40] *DINE Windows*, version 3.1, 1991 (DINE Systems, Amherst, NY); *Food Processor II*, version 3.11 enhanced, 1990 (ESHA Research, Salem, OR); *Minnesota Nutrition Data System*, version 2.2, 1990 (Nutrition Coordinating Center, University of Minnesota, Minneapolis); *Nutri-Calc HD*, version 4.11, 1989 (CAMDE, Tempe, AZ); *Nutritionalist III*, version 7.0, 1991 (N-Squared Computing, Salem, OR); and *Professional Dietician*, version 1.2, 1991 (Wellsource, Clackamas, OR). A 3-day food record with 73 food items was entered into each. Programs varied in the number of foods and nutrients in the database, use of USDA data, the way missing values were managed, and degree of user-friendliness. All microcomputer programs were within 7% of the USDA requirements in energy, protein, total fat, and total carbohydrates; variability in the agreement in the quantity of specific nutrients among the six programs was considerable.[40]

Clinical Evaluation

Clinical evaluation has been the mainstay of nutritional status assessment. Methods of clinical dietary assessment include accurate history and physical examination and anthropometric measures.

History and Physical Examination

The health history and physical examination are the oldest and probably the most widely used evaluation of nutritional status. Numerous texts and journal articles address the techniques for soliciting accurate nutritional assessment.[41]

The health history provides information about events that have led to or have the potential for leading to changes in dietary intake or digestion with implications for nutrition. For example, difficulty swallowing or diarrhea may impact nutritional status. Useful data commonly obtained in the history include usual weight, weight change, change in the pattern or variety of food ingested, changes in appetite, and signs and symptoms of gastrointestinal problems, such as nausea, vomiting, anorexia, and diarrhea.[41] Data from the health history provides the focus for subsequent physical examination.

The physical examination can help to identify nutritional adequacy or deviations. Because signs and symptoms of malnutrition are not frequently seen in the United States, skill and constant vigilance are needed to identify changes in physical findings. An adjunct to physical examination is photographic comparison.[42] When considering the diagnosis of nutritional alterations, there is a need to rule out confounding factors, such as disease process, medication side effects, metabolic abnormality, age, and the half-lives of nutrients suspected as being deficient.

The major advantage of the history and physical examination as a source of nutritional data is its ubiquitous presence in the U.S. health-care system. The practitioner who can identify manifestations of nutritional defects is positioned readily to suggest additional diagnostic services, implement appropriate treatment, and take steps toward prevention in those at high risk.

There are disadvantages in using the health history and physical as a routine means of detecting abnormalities. They include time, money, the need for additional tests to confirm the diagnosis, variations in examiners skills to identify, interpret and diagnose problems, and that deficiencies must be severe and/or persistent to produce visible symptoms.

The accuracy of physical examination has been studied by documenting agreement between objective findings, usually laboratory test findings, and subjective findings, documented by physical examination and history in the clinical impression. Clinical judgments by two surgeons were compared with laboratory data. Correlations for one surgeon were 60% of the cases and the other 65% of the cases.[43] In part, this may be explained by the lack of specificity of laboratory data for various nutritional states.

The reliability of physical examination data has been evaluated in several nutritional studies.[44] These studies suggest there is significant variability in the use of this fundamental measure of nutritional status. However, much of this variability can be mitigated with training and ongoing evaluation.

Anthropometric Measures

Anthropometric measures are easy to perform and have been a cornerstone in the evaluation of nutritional status. Areas addressed include weight, mid-arm muscle circumference, skin fold measures, and head circumference. Knee height and calf circumference also are used to evaluate height and weight in those who are elderly or not ambulatory.

Weight has been used as a measure of nutritional status. It can be used alone or in combination with height or frame size. A loss of 5% of usual weight, weighing less than 90% of ideal body weight, or the loss of 10 pounds in 30 days or less all signal actual or potential nutritional problems. An ongoing controversy in using weight to measure nutritional status is deciding which value to use for comparison, ideal weight, or usual weight. Another problem is that weight standards vary among populations.[45]

Standard tables exist to aid the researcher to evaluate ideal weight for a subject's height. Recent tables to interpret these parameters are based on the National Research Council (NRC) data on weight and height and the dietary guidelines; they also provide data about the ideal body mass index (BMI). The BMI is calculated by dividing weight in kilograms by height in meters and most often is used to diagnose obesity.[39,46,47] It is important to note that body frame size for the NRC tables is based on a ratio of height to wrist circumference,[48] measured on the subject's right hand, just distal to the styloid process. Body frame size is gender specific and categorized as small, medium, or large frame size.

Nowak and Shultz[48] and Frisancho[49] have questioned the use of frame size based on wrist circumference that has been the standard, and new criteria have been developed with frame size based on measurement of elbow breadth. Elbow breadth, quantitated with a special instrument called the Framer, is measured as the distance between the external sites of the medial and lateral epicondyles of the humerus with the subject's arm at 90 degrees.

Arm muscle circumference, as well as skin fold measurement, has been employed in underdeveloped countries to evaluate nutritional status.[50] More recent work has led to the establishment of age-related standards in the United States; standards also have been developed for a limited number of minority populations.[45,51,52]

·Mid-upper-arm circumference is a measure of muscle mass, bone, and skin. It is used to calculate mid-arm muscle circumference as a measure of lean body mass and is derived by the following formula:[50]

Arm Muscle Mass (cm) = Mid-Upper Arm Circumference (cm) – (0.314 × Triceps Skinfold (mm))

Decreases in arm muscle mass can occur because of muscle disease, inactivity, or nutritional deficiencies. Severe depletion is defined as the lowest 5th percentile on established tables, and those in the 6th to 25th percentile are classified as moderately depleted.

Skinfold measures are performed to evaluate fat stores. A skinfold caliper, produced by manufacturers such as Lange, Holtain, or Harpenden, is used to measure skin fold thickness. Many sites can be measured (e.g., scapula, waist, triceps), but the most frequently used site is the triceps. In hospitalized patients where edema may be a consideration, the triceps site often is selected because less edema forms in the upper arm than in the more dependent body parts.

Fat is a concentrated energy store in the body. Because fat stores do not change rapidly, skinfold measures are not a sensitive measure of malnutrition. Depletion generally is indicative of chronic malnutrition or a severe hypermetabolic state leading to rapid fat utilization.[53]

Head circumference is used in children to evaluate growth. Using normative tables, children are classified according to percentiles. Chronic undernutrition results in delayed head growth and its identification and treatment are important to prevent permanent damage.[53]

In nonambulatory or elderly patients who are unable to stand erect, alternative approaches to height and weight measurement are necessary.[54,55] Knee height to evaluate height and calf circumference has been suggested to evaluate weight. Knee height is the distance from the heel of the left foot to the top of the thigh. It is measured with a caliper with the subject supine, on the left leg and at a 90-degree angle. Overall height is then calculated by using the formula:

Height (cm) = 105.9 (±11.6) + 6.48 (±1.81) × sex + 0.988 (±0.24) × knee height (cm)

A nomogram has been constructed based on this formula.[55]

Body weight in the nonambulatory can be calculated using calf circumference. It is measured on the left leg at the widest point with the subject in the supine position. The distance measured as well as knee height, mid-upper-arm circumference and subscapular skinfold are used to derive body weight for a female from the standard formula:

(0.98 × arm circumference) + (1.27 × calf circumference) + (0.4 × subscapular skinfold thickness)
+ (0.87 × knee height) – 62.35

Available coefficients are used to calculate weight in men with a similar formula.[54]

The validity and reliability of anthropometric measures are an important consideration. Instrument accuracy is important. The manufacturer's specifications, reports of previous studies, and personal experience are all important in instrument evaluation. For example, the Lange calipers (Scientific Industries, Cambridge, MA) apply 10 g/mm^2 of pressure to measure skinfold thickness. Accuracy is determined by using a standard calibration block provided by the manufacturer. If the caliper registers 10 mm while resting on the first step and 10 (± 0.5) additional mm on each of the four subsequent steps, its precision is established. If the instrument is not calibrated, it needs to be returned for servicing.

Sources of error in the measurement of skinfold thickness can include the selection of different skin sites, variations in body and hand positions that affect the amount of tissue grasped, and the length of time the caliper is applied before taking a reading.[56] Standardized protocols and adequate training sessions and supervision reduce measurement variability. Planned periodic interrater reliability testing is needed to maintain the stability of measurement techniques over time and to ensure precision.

Energy Expenditure

Energy expenditure reflects the metabolism of substrates. It is measured by direct and indirect calorimetry, doubly labeled water, and oxygen consumption derived from pulmonary artery data.

Direct and Indirect Calorimetry

Direct calorimetry is a measure of heat production. Knowing that specific substrates produce a given amount of heat, energy expenditure can be derived. Direct calorimetry requires that a subject be placed in a chamber where heat production is measured. It is the "gold standard" against which other methods are compared. There is excellent accuracy (1%) and precision (±2–3%).[57] The advantage of direct calorimetry is accuracy. Alternatively, it restricts activity, changes the subject's usual activity patterns, and requires expensive equipment and considerable investigator time.

Indirect calorimetry measures the gas exchange associated with the oxidation of energy substrates. The metabolic cart used for gas measurement can be taken to the subject's bedside. It is less expensive than direct calorimetry. Its disadvantages are primarily that it remains an expensive technique and requires the use of a hood or a mask that the subject may find confining. More recent indirect calorimetry instrumentation allows subjects to be ambulatory and so more closely approximates an actual living situation, while retaining accuracy of 3% and precision of 6%.[58]

Doubly Labeled Water

Energy expenditure can be measured with doubly labeled water. This method involves giving the subject a loading dose of water labeled with the stable isotope deuterium and ^{18}O. The deuterium is eliminated as water and the ^{18}O is disposed of as both carbon dioxide and water and the difference in the two elimination rates is a measure of carbon dioxide production. The rate of isotope elimination, and hence energy expenditure, is measured by collection of urine for isotope analysis. The method is accurate to 1% with precision of 4% to 7%.[59]

The advantage of the doubly labeled water technique is its accuracy. Disadvantages include the need for isotope administration, urine gathering, and need for sophisticated instruments and trained personnel for isotope data analysis. At this time, these limitations restrict its usability.[57]

Oxygen Consumption Measurement via Pulmonary Artery Catheter

Another means to measure energy expenditure is with oxygen consumption measured using a pulmonary artery catheter in critically ill patients. Data show a strong correlation between energy expenditure measured by indirect calorimetry using a metabolic cart and that calculated from the Fick equation with data obtained from a pulmonary artery catheter. There is a strong correlation ($r = 0.83$, $p < 0.001$) between oxygen consumption obtained by the two methods, with a mean difference of 4%. There also is a strong correlation ($r = 0.82$, $p < 0.001$) in energy expenditure between the two methods, but the range of differences is –36% to +40%. These differences reflect a hyperdynamic and metabolically stressed critically ill population. Cardiac output measures tend to be overestimated at higher values and therefore are a potential source of error. Thus when indirect calorimetry is not available, the Fick method can be used to estimate energy expenditure in patients with pulmonary artery line in place if its limitations are kept in mind.[60]

Biochemical Measures

Biochemical parameters reflect the end-product of ingestion, digestion, absorption, and metabolism of nutrients. A simple approach that can be measured with minimal invasive strategies, they often are used to evaluate nutritional status. They involve laboratory techniques and can be performed on blood, serum, plasma, hair, nails, urine, sweat, and stool. They offer an objective measure of nutritional status and in some cases provide data about subclinical deficiencies. Important considerations are selecting the appropriate test, sample collecting and handling, sample analysis, and interpretation of the findings.[61]

Selecting the Measure

Laboratory studies are performed to determine nutrient concentration, nutrient–balance studies, nutrient needs, changes in blood components related to intake, and responses to tests, doses, or loads. The investigator must be familiar with the alternative laboratory tests and determine which tests provide the most direct, valid, and reliable data. Knowing the purpose of the study thus becomes critical in selecting the outcome measure.

Sample Collecting and Handling

Serious consideration needs to be given to sample collection and handling. The timing of sampling may be an important consideration as food and fluid intake influence the results of some tests. Also, some tests are sensitive to circadian rhythms, and so measurement needs to be performed at a consistent time. If it is necessary to fast for the test or a special test meal is required, planning is necessary. For all tests, subjects will require instruction. Special equipment may be needed to collect the sample. For example, specific tubes may be needed, and some tests may require that the tubes be chilled immediately to stop metabolic processes.

Selecting a Clinical Laboratory

Most researchers are required to use a clinical laboratory for at least a portion of the assays required. Labs must be state certified and to remain certified must maintain high standards as patient care decisions are based on the findings. Laboratory test accuracy, precision, and sensitivity should be evaluated. Sensitivity is important when perhaps a thousandth of a milliliter may be crucial to data.[61]

The accuracy of the assay itself can be ensured by using appropriately calibrated equipment and known standards. Results that agree with known standards across a range of values (highest to lowest expected) provide evidence to support the validity of the assay. The precision of the analysis can be evaluated by submitting samples in double or triplicate for analysis and evaluating the agreement between the results generated. The decision as to the degree of variability that is acceptable is the investigator's. Reliability is worthless, however, if the test is not accurate. The laboratory will provide the researcher with information about accuracy, precision, and sensitivity on request; it is important to know the technique used by the laboratory when performing the test so that it can be reported as part of any publication arising from the study.

Interpretation of Laboratory Data

Interpretation of laboratory results requires careful judgements. Clinical laboratories will provide information about acceptable normal values for that specific laboratory. Data about the nature of the sample on whom the sample was normed ideally should be similar to the study population. When using published norms, the rationale for cutoff points created by authors of tables should be clear and acceptable to the investigator.

Example: A Biochemical Measure of Protein Status

An example of the process of selecting a biochemical parameter is the selection of a measure of protein status. The serum proteins are biochemical indicators of malnutrition.[62] They are synthesized by the liver and vary primarily in their rate of turn-over. The following are serum protein measures frequently used to evaluate protein status:

Albumin	Transferrin
Nitrogen balance	Urine creatinine
Prealbumin	3-Methylhistidine
Retinol-binding protein	

For all of them, hydration status is important in their validity; dehydration produces falsely elevated serum levels. It should be noted that posture and circadian rhythm also can affect hydration and the accuracy of the values.

Probably the most frequently measured laboratory evaluation of protein status is serum albumin level. Albumin has a long half-life (18–20 days), is not sensitive to rapid changes in nutritional status, and falls late in malnutrition. It therefore is not appropriate to use low serum albumin to diagnose either recent or mild to moderate malnutrition. Low albumin is associated with increased morbidity and mortality in medical-surgical patients,[8] intensive care patients,[9] and cancer patients.[63]

Transferrin, another frequently used measure of protein status, has a shorter half-life (8–10 days) and a smaller body pool. Its major function is to transport iron. Normally, about one-third of the body transferrin is bound to iron. Although initially recommended as a measure of protein malnutrition, it is affected by many factors other than protein-calorie malnutrition and so is not sufficiently sensitive or specific to be a meaningful measure. For example, an iron deficiency is seen with protein-calorie malnutrition, which stimulates hepatic synthesis, and elevated levels of transferrin are seen. At the other extreme, inflammatory states, liver disease, and some anemias result in depressed transferrin levels.

Prealbumin, another plasma protein, has a short half-life (2 days). It also is known as thyroxin-binding prealbumin and transthyretin. It transports a portion of thyroxine and vitamin A. Because of its short half-life, prealbumin decreases quickly when protein or calorie intake is decreased. In contrast, it responds quickly when nutrients are provided exogenously. This measure provides a better evaluation of nutritional status than intake as prealbumin reflects not only what has been ingested but also what has been able to be absorbed, digested, and metabolized. On the other hand, prealbumin is quite sensitive to inflammatory response and will decrease dramatically because of the decrease in protein synthesis.

Retinol-binding protein has a very short half-life (12 hours) and very low serum levels. It participates with prealbumin in the transport of vitamin A, and its response follows that of prealbumin. Although it has a theoretical advantage over other plasma proteins by virtue of its short half-life, its low normal values and the technical difficulties in measurement have not demonstrated its superiority over other measures of nutrient status.

Another frequently used measure of protein metabolism is urine creatinine. Creatinine is the byproduct of muscle catabolism and so is a measure of lean body mass. Diurnal variations occur, but over a 24-hour period its excretion is relatively constant. Creatine excretion is a theoretically strong measure of nutritional status, but is subject to many threats to validity. It requires normal renal function and urinary output, an accurately collected 24-hour specimen, and adequate hydration. In addition, it is not accurate in patients who have been on prolonged bedrest and those who have had a recent high-protein meal.[53] Normally nutritional status with creatinine is evaluated using a 24-hour urine creatinine excretion divided by normal creatinine for height, producing a creatinine height index. Valid age-specific tables are required to interpret data.

Similarly, 3-methylhistidine is another measure of skeletal muscle breakdown. Its excretion is seen as a sensitive measure of catabolism, however, because there is a large pool of 3-methylhistidine outside of skeletal muscle, it is not a specific test. It is threatened by all of the measures noted for creatinine. In addition, reference tables are lacking for children.

Fundamental to any discussion of protein status is the concept that nitrogen turnover is in balance, that is, intake and loss from the body are carefully regulated and closely approximate each other under normal nutritional circumstances. For anabolism and repair to occur, a positive nitrogen balance is needed. To measure nitrogen balance, protein intake and loss in the urine are measured for a 24-hour period. A standard formula is used to calculate nitrogen balance, and it takes into consideration nonurine nitrogen loss such as stool and skin.

During periods of starvation and concomitant catabolism, intake of nitrogen is not as great as output, and so nitrogen balance is negative. Threats to the validity of this test are posed by liver function, renal function, hydration status, medications, and the accuracy of the 24-hour urine data. It is important to realize that this measure provides no information about nutritional status or protein stores, but rather only about the immediate intake and metabolic balance.[53]

Selection of the measure or measures of protein status first needs to be addressed from a theoretical perspective, that is, what dimension of protein status is of interest and over what period of time. Is it synthesis of plasma proteins, breakdown of exiting protein stores, or nitrogen turnover? Consideration then needs to be given to the accuracy, precision, and sensitivity of the test. Accuracy is evaluated both through the literature and by understanding the accuracy available in the laboratory that you plan to use. It is important when evaluating accuracy in the literature to consider whether the sample studied and the outcome evaluated reflect your situation. One example of this is a study where the ability of anthropometric and biochemical indices to predict death among patients ($n = 294$) in a general medical ward was assessed.[64] Death within 3 months was predicted with a linear discriminant analysis method with a sensitivity of 83% and specificity of 84% using the variables sex, functional ability, urea, total protein, alkaline phosphatase, and albumin-adjusted calcium. The authors report that the anthropometric and biochemical indices did little to improve the accuracy of the prediction and acknowledge that these data contradict findings among surgical patients. The precision of tests also needs to be evaluated based on the literature. Interpretation requires that the researcher consider practical issues, such as the cost and ease of data collection.

High-Tech Measures in Nutrition

Recent data show that nutritional changes in cancer patients do not follow the same wasting distribution as other conditions.[65] These findings have caused researchers to question whether increased attention needs to be given to the evaluation of body composition and whether assessing the body compartments needs to be done with accurate, precise, and sensitive instruments.[66]

A new and sophisticated set of instruments have been applied to nutritional assessment, and they hold hope for increased understanding of the mechanisms of nutritional alternations in humans.[67] Appendix 17A[68-73] describes a number of these techniques. Many of them are complex and expensive and require sophisticated knowledge. Several are invasive and many involve considerable subject burden.

Summary

Serious consideration needs to be given to all available measurement techniques as a study is designed. Future research in the field will require consideration of sophisticated instruments, although their use in studies conducted by nurse researchers at this time is limited. Selection and use of the most appropriate instruments for measurement are pivotal to producing advanced knowledge on which health-care knowledge can be built.

Exemplar Studies

Waltman, N.L., Bergstrom, N., Armstrong, N., Norvell, K., & Braden, B. Nutritional status, pressure sores, and mortality in elderly patients with cancer. *Oncol Nurs Forum*, 1991, *18*(5):867-873.

This study used biochemical, anthropometric, and dietary intake measures to determine differences in nutritional status, incidence of pressure sores, and incidence of mortality between two groups (*n* = 66), institutionalized elderly patients with cancer and a matched group of persons without cancer. Subjects were paired based on age, sex, and pressure sore risk. Protein malnutrition was found in 70% of the subjects with cancer and pressure ulcers versus 21% of the subjects without cancer. The methods were described in detail. The validity and reliability of instruments were addressed or referenced. Issues related to the validity of biochemical measures can be found in the chapter on physiologic measures, and the Braden scale is described in the chapter on skin integrity.

Sami, H., Saint-Aubert, B., Szawlowski, A.W., Astre, C., & Joyeux, H. Home enteral nutrition system: One patient, one daily ration of an "all-in-one" sterile and modular formula in a single container. *J Parenteral Enteral Nutr*, 1990, *14*(2):173-176.

Weight gain, biochemical analysis, how well the feeding was tolerated, rate of rehospitalization, cost, and quality of life were used to assess the benefits of total enteral feeding in two groups of subjects who were unable to take calories orally: one group due to oral and esophageal cancer and a second group without cancer, but esophageal perforation. Nutritional outcomes were measured with classic methods, such as the Harris-Benedict equation, corrected for stress and activity; biochemical analysis; weight gain. Use of nonphysiologic outcomes is a strength of this study. The procedures and description of instruments are sufficiently detailed to allow replication or extension of the study.

References

1. Dewy, W.D., Begg, D., Lavin, P.T., et al. Prognostic effect of weight loss prior to chemotherapy in cancer patients. *Am J Med*, 1980, *69*:491-497.
2. Daly, J.M., Redmond, H.P., & Gallagher, H. Perioperative nutrition in cancer patients. *JPEN*, 1992, *16*(6 suppl):100S-105S.
3. Tchekmedyian, N.S., Zahyna, D., Halpert, C., & Heber, D. Assessment and maintenance of nutrition in older cancer patients. *Oncology*, 1992, *6*(2 suppl): 105-111.
4. Ovesen, L., Allingstrup, L., Hannibal, J., et al. Effect of dietary counseling on food intake, body weight, response rate, survival, and quality of life in cancer patients undergoing chemotherapy: A prospective, randomized study. *J Clin Oncol*, 1993, *11*(10): 2043-2049.
5. Daly, J.M., Lieberman, M.D., Goldfine, J., et al. Enteral nutrition with supplemental arginine, RNA, and omega-3 fatty acid in patients after operation: Immunological, metabolic, and clinical outcome. *Surgery*, 1992, *112*:56-67.
6. Rossi-Fanelli, F., Cascino, A., & Muscaritolo, M. Abnormal substrate metabolism and nutritional strategies in cancer management. *JPEN*, 1991, *15*(6): 680-683.
7. Ollenschlager, G., Thomas, W., Konol, K., et al. Nutritional behavior and quality of life during oncological polychemotherapy: Results of a prospective study on the efficacy of oral nutrition therapy in patients with acute leukemia. *Eur J Clin Invest*, 1992, *22*(8):546-553.
8. Seltzer, M.H., Bastidas, J.A., Cooper, D.M., et al. Instant nutritional assessment. *JPEN*, 1979, *3*(3):157-159.
9. Seltzer, M.H., Fletcher, H.S., Slocum, B.A., & Engler, P.E. Instant nutritional assessment in the intensive care unit. *JPEN*, 1981, *5*(1):70-72.
10. Kotler, D.P., Tierny, A.R., Wang, J., & Pierson, R.N. Jr. Magnitude of body-cell-mass depletion and timing of death from wasting in AIDS. *Am J Clin Nutr*, 1989, *50*:444-447.
11. Byers, T. Dietary trends in the United States. Relevance to cancer prevention. *Cancer*, 1993, *72*(3 suppl):1015-1018.
12. Block, G. Human dietary assessment: Methods and issues. *Prev Med*, 1989, *18*(5):653-660.
13. Lee-Han, H., McGuire, V., & Boyd, N.F. A review of the methods used by studies of dietary measurement. *J Clin Epidemiol*, 1989, *42*(3):269-279.
14. Bergstrom, N., & Weise, N.A. Feeding institutionalized elderly: 3- versus 5-meals a day (unpublished manuscript).
15. Breslow, R.A., & Sorkin, J.D. Comparison of one-day and three-day calorie counts in hospitalized patients: A pilot study. *J Am Geriatr Soc*, 1993, *41*:923-927.
16. Barrett-Connor, E. Nutrition epidemiology: How do we know what they ate? *Am J Clin Nutr*, 1991, *54*:182S-187S.
17. Kretsch, M.J., & Fong, A.K. Validation of a new computerized technique for quantitating individual dietary intake: The Nutritional Evaluation Scale System (NESS) vs. weighed food record. *Am J Clin Nutr*, 1990, *51*(3):477-484.
18. Bergstrom, N. The consistency of diet intake observed weekly among elderly residents in a nursing home (unpublished manuscript).
19. Burke, B.S. The dietary history as a tool in research. *J Am Diet Assoc*, 1947, *23*(12):1041.
20. Freidenreich, C.M., Slimani, N., & Riboli, E. Measurement of past diet: Review of previously proposed methods. *Epidemiol Rev*, 1992, *14*:177-196.
21. Beaton, G.H., Milner, J., Corey, P., et al. Sources of variance in 24 hour dietary recall data: Implications for nutrition study design and interpretation. *Am J Clin Nutr*, 1979, *32*:2456-2459.
22. Willett, W. Nutritional epidemiology: Issues and challenges. *Int J Epidemiol*, 1987, *16*(suppl):312-317.
23. Gersovitz, M., Madden, M.P., & Smiciklas-Wright, H. Validity of the 24-hour recall and seven-day record for group comparisons. *J Am Diet Assoc*, 1978, *73*(1):48-55.
24. Treiber, F.A., Leonard, S.B., Frank, G., et al. Dietary assessment instruments for pre-school children: Reliability of parental responses to the 24-hour recall and a food frequency questionnaire. *J Am Diet Assoc*, 1990, *90*(6):814-820.
25. Lytle, L.A., Nichaman, M.Z., Obarzanek, E., et al. Validation of 24-hour recalls assisted by food records in third-grade children. The CATCH Collaborative Group. *J Am Diet Assoc*, 1993, *93*(12):1431-1436.
26. Meredith, A., Matthews, A., Zickefoose, M., et al. How well do school children recall what they have eaten? *J Am Diet Assoc*, 1951, *27*(9):749.
27. Linusson, E.F.I., Sanjur, D., & Erikson, E.C. Validating the 24-hour recall method as a dietary survey tool. *Arch Latinoam Nutr*, 1975, *24*:277.
28. Adelson, S. Some problems in collecting dietary data from individuals. *J Am Diet Assoc*, 1960, *36*(5):453-460.
29. Heady, J.A. Diets of bank clerks. Development of a method of classifying the diets of individuals for use in epidemiological studies. *J Res Stat Soc [A]*, 1961, *124*:336.
30. Block, G. & Hartman, A.M. Issues in reproducibility and validity of dietary studies. *Am J Clin Nutr*, 1989, *50*:1133-1338.
31. Sertoli, M., Beers, T., Coates, R., et al. Assessing consumption of high-fat foods: The effect of grouping foods into single questions. *Epidemiology*, 1992, *3*(6): 503-508.
32. Jonneland, A.T., Haraldsdottir, J., Overvad, K., et al. Influence of individually estimated portion size on the validity of a semiquantitative food frequency questionnaire. *Int J Epidemiol*, 1992, *21*(4):770-777.
33. Horwath, C.C. Validity of a short food frequency questionnaire for estimating nutrient intake in elderly people. *Br J Nutr*, 1993, *70*(1):3-14.
34. Martin-Moreno, J.M., Boyle, P., Gorgojo, L., et al. Development and validation of a food frequency questionnaire in Spain. *Int J Epidemiol*, 1993, *22*(3):512-519.
35. Guthrie, H.A., & Scheer, J.C. Validity of a dietary score for assessing nutrient adequacy. *J Am Diet Assoc*, 1981, *78*(3):240-242.
36. Kant, A.K., Schatzkin, A., Harris, T.B., et al. Dietary diversity and subsequent mortality in the First National Health and Nutrition Examination Survey

Epidemiologic follow-up study. *Am J Clin Nutr*, 1993, *57*(3):434-440.

37. Kant, A.K., Block, G., Schatzkin, A., et al. Dietary diversity in the U.S. population, NHANES II, 1976–1980. *J Am Diet Assoc*, 1991, *91*(12):1526-1531.

38. Bergstrom, N. Quantifying dietary intake of cancer patients: A quick and reliable method. Proceedings of the Ninth Annual Congress of the Oncology Nursing Society, 1984.

39. U.S. Department of Agriculture, U.S. Department of Health and Human Services. *Nutrition and your health, dietary guidelines for Americans*. Home and Garden Bulletin No. 232 (3rd ed.). Washington, DC, U.S. Government Printing Office, 1990.

40. Nieman, D.C., Butterworth, D.E., Nieman, C.N., et al. Comparison of six microcomputer dietary analysis systems with the USDA Nutrient Data Base for standard reference. *J Am Diet Assoc*, 1992, *92*(1):48-56.

41. Stotts, N.A., & Washington, D.F. Nutrition: A critical component of wound healing. *AACN Clin Issues Crit Care*, 1990, *1*(3):585-594.

42. Fitzpatrick, T.B., Johnson, R.A., Polano, M.K., Suurmond, D., & Wolff, K. (Eds.). *Color atlas and synopsis of clinical dermatology: Common and serious diseases* (2nd ed.). New York, McGraw-Hill, 1992.

43. Baker, J.P., Detsky, A.S., Wesson, D.E., et al. Nutritional assessment: A comparison of clinical judgement and objective measures. *N Eng J Med*, 1982, *306*(16):969-972.

44. Pettigrew, R.A., Charlesworth P.M., Farmilo, R.W., & Hill, G.L. Assessment of nutritional depletion and immune competence: A comparison of clinical examination and objective measurements. *JPEN*, 1984, *8*(1):21-24.

45. Ireton-Jones, C.S., & Turner, W.W., Jr. Actual or ideal body weight: Which should be used to predict energy expenditure? *J Am Diet Assoc*, 1991, *91*(2):193-195.

46. Food and Nutrition Board, Committee on Diet and Health, National Academy of Sciences-National Research Council. *Diet and health: Implications for reducing chronic disease risk*. Washington, DC, U.S. Government Printing Office, 1990.

47. Bray, G.A. Pathophysiology of obesity. *Am J Clin Nutr*, 1992, *55*(2 suppl):448S-494S.

48. Nowak, R.K., & Schultz, L.O. A comparison of two methods for the determination of body frame size. *J Am Diet Assoc*, 1987, *87*(3):339-341.

49. Frisancho, A.R. Nutritional anthropometry. *J Am Diet Assoc*, 1988, *88*(5):553-555.

50. Jeliffe, D.B. Direct nutritional assessment of human groups. In *The assessment of nutritional status of the community*. Monograph No. 53. Geneva Switzerland, World Health Organization, 1966, pp. 238-239.

51. Frisancho, A.R. New standards of weight and body composition by frame size and height for assessment of nutritional status of adults and the elderly. *Am J Clin Nutr*, 1984, *40*:808-819.

52. Gray, G.E., & Gray, L.K. Validity of anthropometric norms used in the assessment of hospitalized patients. *JPEN*, 1979, *3*:366-368.

53. Benjamin, D.R. Laboratory tests and nutritional assessment. *Ped Clin North Am*, 1989, *36*(1):139-160.

54. Chumlea, W.C., et al. Prediction of body weight for the nonambulatory elderly from anthropometry. *J Am Diet Assoc*, 1988, *88*(5):564-568.

55. Haboubi, N.Y., Hudson, P.R., & Pathy, M.S. Measurement of height in the elderly. *J Am Geriatr Soc*, 1990, *38*(9):1008-1010.

56. Burkinshaw, L., Jones, P.R., & Krupowicz, D.W. Observer error in skinfold thickness measurements. *Human Biol*, 1973, *45*(2):273-279.

57. Schoeller, D.A., & Racette, S.B. A review of field techniques for the assessment of energy expenditure. *J Nutr*, 1990, *120*:1492-1495.

58. McNeill, G., Gox, M.D., & Rovers, J.P.W. The Oxylog oxygen consumption meter: A portable device for measurement of energy expenditure. *Am J Clin Nutr*, 1982, *45*:1415-1419.

59. Schoeller, D.A. Measurement of energy expenditure in free-living humans by using doubly labeled water. *J Nutr*, 1988, *118*:1278-1289.

60. Corbean, R.A., Gentillo, L.M., Parker, A., et al. Nutritional assessment using a pulmonary artery catheter. *J Trauma*, 1992, *33*(3):452-456.

61. DeKeyser, F.G., & Pugh, L.C. Approaches to physiologic measurement. In C. Waltz, O. Strickland, & E. Lentz (Eds.), *Measurement in nursing* (2nd ed.). Philadelphia: Davis, 1991, pp. 387-412.

62. Stotts, N.A. Nutrition: Current bases for practice. In S.G. Funk, E.M. Tournquist, M.T. Champagne, L.A. Copp, & R.A. Wiese (Eds.), *Key aspects of recovery: Improving nutrition, rest and mobility*. New York: Springer, 1990, pp. 32-45.

63. Mullen, J.L., Gerter, M.H., Buzby, G.P., et al. Implications of malnutrition in the surgical patient. *Arch Surg*, 1979, *114*(2):121-125.

64. Woo, J., Mak, Y.T., Lau, J., & Swaminathan, R. Prediction of mortality in patients in acute medical wards using basic laboratory and anthropometric data. *Postgrad Med J*, 1992, *68*(806):954-960.

65. Burkinshaw, L. Some aspects of body composition in cancer. *Infusiontherapie*, 1990, *17*(suppl 3):57-58.

66. Burkinshaw, L., Hedge, A.P., King, R.F.J.G., & Cohn, S.H. Models of the distribution of protein, water and electrolytes in the human body. *Infusiontherapie*, 1990, *17*(suppl 3):21-25.

67. Williams, S.R. *Nutrition and diet therapy* (7th ed.). St. Louis: Mosby, 1993.

68. Jensen, M.D. Research techniques for body composition assessment. *J Am Diet Assoc*, 1992, *92*(4):454-460.

69. Heymsfield, S., Wang, J., Lichtman, S., et al. Body composition in elderly subjects: A critical appraisal of clinical methodology. *Am J Clin Nutr*, 1989, *50*:1167-1175.

70. Bacheri-Bauman, P., Guckel, F., Sellmer, W., & Lorenz, W.J. Principles of in vivo magnetic resonance spectroscopy in whole-body magnetic resonance systems. *Infusionstherapie*, 1990, *17*(suppl. 3):39-42.

71. Gunkel, R., Bacheri-Baumann, P., Semmler, W., et al. MR tomography and multinuclear MR spectroscopy in a whole-body MR system—Applications in cancer research. *Infusionstherapie*, 1990, *17*(suppl 3):43-47.

72. Shizgal, H.M. Nutritional assessment with body composition measurements by multiple isotope dilution. *Infusionstherapie*, 1990, *17*(suppl 3):9-17.

73. Hill, G.L. Clinical body composition using in vivo neutron activation analysis. *Infusionstherapie*, 1990, *17*(suppl 3):18-20.

Appendix

17A. High-Tech Measures of Nutrition

Instrument/ Aspect Measured	Description	Psychometric Testing/Limitations
Bioelectric impedence analysis Measure of lean body mass (LBM)	Alternating current introduced into the body at a distal site (e.g., hands or feet) Resistance measured by proximal electrodes so that fat-free mass can be calculated by prediction equations of LBM Test may be insensitive to different tissue composition in trunk as electrical resistance is primarily affected by the limbs Method is quick, safe, noninvasive, and can be performed at bedside	Bioelectrical impedence analysis highly correlated with total body water: (1) cross-validation analysis: suggests LBM estimates can be enhanced by use of gender-specific and body type-specific equations; (2) technique may be improved by using multiple frequencies to differentiate extracellular and total body water Limitations: experience required for estimating levels of obesity and acute changes in electrolyte balance (68)
Computed tomography (CT) Distinguishes adipose from nonadipose tissue	Patients placed within special scanner Dose of radioactive tracer administered, creating signal detected by scanner Visual image of adipose and nonadipose tissues produced within body sections	Limitations (68): very obese subjects do not fit in scanner; requires subject to remain immobile for >30 minutes; subject may become claustrophobic; unsuitable for subjects with metallic substances in the body (e.g., pacemaker); exposure to radiation and cost
Densitometry Direct measures of body composition	Calculated by underwater weighing (69): submerged body weight = body fat + fat-free body mass, corrected for amount of air in lungs Standard equations used to estimate LBM Advantages: noninvasive, precise technique used in healthy, cooperative subjects	Limitations: changes in densitometry may not always reflect a physiologically meaningful compartment (fat-free mass includes LBM and total body water); subject must be submerged in water, so inappropriate for uncooperative or ill subjects; measurements must be repeated to obtain the mean of the three highest densities; residual lung volume must be corrected for buoyancy Inaccurate in elderly population (changes in bone density related to aging) Accuracy of method in doubt (density of fat-free mass may be inconsistent between individuals)
Dual photon absorptiometry Identifies body tissue composition	Specialized body scanner divides body weight into soft-tissue mass and bone ash using gadolinium (^{153}Gd) Absorbance of different energy level photons is linearly related to fat in soft tissues Sodium iodide crystals in scanner detect differential attenuation of bone and soft tissue (at 2 gamma-ray energy levels)	Precision is 1% Limitations: exam tables narrow, so appropriate only for individuals weighing <150% of ideal body weight; subjects must be brought to machine; exposure to radiation precludes use in pregnant women and children (68)

	Neutron activation analysis further identifies protein, fat, and water components Advantages: takes 10–70 minutes to complete; provides picture of body tissue composition	
Infared interactance Determines tissue composition	Probe measures subcutaneous depot (about 1 cm deep) using reflected energy	Less valid than ultrasonography (68) Unlikely that measurement of single area is representative of entire body
Magnetic resonance imaging (MRI) Estimates total body fat	Identifies abnormalities by creating sectional images of body: provides clear body images in response to magnetic field; chemical shift effect used to identify chemical groups and compounds (70); provides visual image of adipose and nonfat tissue (71) Volume of adipose summed in each section to estimate total body fat	Both fat and nonfat tissue present in areas surrounded by fat included in estimate leads to overestimation of total fat, greater than that obtained by densitometry More accurate than other methods, except CT scanning Limitations: subject must lie still for multiple body scans; MRI scans do not accommodate very obese subjects; May cause claustrophobia (68)
Neutron activation analysis Measures total body fat, protein, minerals, and carbohydrates	Uses deuterium-tritium neutron generator Some of body's nitrogen, chloride, calcium changed to radioactive isotopes by heavy water; decay then measured by a scanner Body composition measured independent of age or health (72,73) Tritiated water injected, and gamma-radiation decay measured Used to measure response to nutritional therapy LBM is the active, oxidizing, work-performing tissue (72) Ideal parameter to use to correct metabolic activity	Precision 2% (68) Limitation: available in only a few medical centers; significant radiation exposure
Total body electroconductivity Measures LBM	Subject placed in a large cylindrical coil that generates an electrical current at a specific radio frequency Hydrated lean tissue and extracellular water conduct electrical energy when subjected to specific radio frequencies (68) Rapid, safe, comfortable technique	Accuracy and precision related to methods used to develop prediction equations Concurrent validity established by comparison with underwater weighing, total body water, and body potassium counting Limitations: patients must be transported to device; fluid and electrolyte changes due to illness can influence accuracy; expensive instrument
Ultrasonography Estimates total body fat	Scans taken of several body areas Estimation of total body fat similar to that used for skinfold thicknesses Low cost and risk	Lacks precision and accuracy (68)

Key: LBM = Lean Body Mass, IBW = Ideal Body Weight, CT = Computed Tomograph, MRI = Magnetic Resonance Imaging
Numbers in parentheses correspond to studies cited in the References.

18

Measuring Sleep

Felissa L. Cohen

Sleep is an active, rather than passive, process that is part of a cyclic circadian alternation of sleep and wakefulness.[1] This sleep–wake rhythm is regulated by neural systems that include a neural pacemaker and various neurochemical systems. It is influenced by other factors and conditions, such as light and darkness.[1]

In humans, sleep consists of two major states: rapid-eye-movement (REM) sleep, and non-REM (NREM) sleep. REM sleep usually is not divided into stages, but various stages have been identified in NREM sleep. NREM sleep is subdivided in stages from 1 to 4 corresponding to an approximate continuum of depth of sleep from light to deep. Each of these stages have distinct electroencephalographic (EEG) characteristics.[2] NREM sleep is controlled by multiple neuronal groups and systems involving the hypothalamus, basal forebrain, midbrain, pons and medulla, but REM sleep is controlled by systems located mainly in the pons.[3]

In normal adults, there is a cyclical alternation of REM and NREM sleep, with NREM sleep occurring first in the transition from wakefulness to sleep. The first sleep cycle is usually shorter, both NREM and REM sleep normally alternate in cycles averaging approximately 90 to 110 (but ranging from 70 to 120) minutes through the night. A normal adult will have between four and six cycles per night. REM sleep occupies about 20% to 25% of total sleep, and NREM sleep accounts for 75% to 80% of total sleep in normal young adults.[1] Various factors influence sleep stages, including age, circadian rhythms, temperature, drugs, and pathologic alterations.[2]

Typically, in adults, in the first part of the night, NREM sleep predominates; and as the night wears on, REM sleep occupies an increasing proportion of the approximate 90-minute cycle. Sleep normally begins with NREM stage 1 sleep (drowsiness), which is a transitional state between wakefulness and deeper levels of sleep. It usually comprises only 5% to 10% of normal sleep time. Persons can be easily aroused from this stage. Stage 2 NREM sleep (light sleep) usually follows and comprises the greatest proportion (45%–55%) of adult sleep. As stage 2 sleep continues, the EEG shows slow-wave activity that eventually meets the criteria for stage 3 sleep. Stages 3 and 4 sleep typically follow. NREM stages 3 and 4 sleep often are called slow-wave, delta, or deep sleep. NREM stage 3 sleep comprises 4% to 6% of total sleep time, usually appearing in the first third of the sleep episode.

In the first sleep cycle, NREM stage 4 sleep lasts about 20 to 40 minutes. NREM stage 4 sleep represents 12% to 15% of sleep time, and slow-wave sleep predominates. Then, usually, sleep returns to stages 3 and 2. From stage 2 sleep, REM sleep may be entered, preceded by a series of body movements. REM sleep normally appears after a full cycle of NREM sleep has occurred. The REM sleep stage has spontaneous, rapid eye movements with high brain activity and metabolism. Dreaming occurs during this stage. NREM sleep stages 3 and 4 usually predominate during the first half of the sleep period and are reduced later. REM sleep occurs more in the second half of the sleep period, usually alternating with NREM stage 2 sleep. As the night or sleep period wears on, the cycles repeat, but the REM periods become longer, and NREM sleep may reach only stages 2 or 3.[4-7]

Variation in sleep patterns are characteristically associated with age. Newborns spend about half of their sleep in the REM stage; this percentage is higher in premature infants.[8] Slow-wave sleep is at a maximum in children and decreases with age. In some older individuals, stage 4 sleep may be absent.[1,2] Other observed changes in the elderly are shorter total sleep times (although in one survey, older respondents reported more sleep than younger ones[9]), increased night awakenings, and increased fragmentation of sleep. The nighttime awakenings are sometimes due to physical problems, such as the need to urinate or pain.[10] The elderly frequently take medications to help them sleep. An inadequate amount of sleep or poor sleep quality often are reflected in daytime napping, lack of alertness, and fatigue.[11]

In the United States approximately 40 million people have chronic sleep disorders, and 20 to 30 million have intermittent sleep problems.[1] Sleep disorders affect infants (e.g., sudden infant death syndrome), children, adults (e.g., sleep apnea, insomnia, circadian rhythm disorders due to shift work), the elderly (>50% of those 65 years and older), and individuals with medical and/or psychiatric illness.

Disorders of sleep and arousal have been variously classified. In 1990, the new International Classification of Sleep Disorders, produced by the American Sleep Disorders Association was released.[12] This detailed classification system summarizes diagnostic and coding information. An outline of this system is shown:[12]

1. Dyssomnias
   Intrinsic sleep disorders
   Extrinsic sleep disorders
   Circadian rhythm sleep disorders
2. Parasomnias
   Arousal disorders
   Sleep–wake transition disorders
   Parasomnias usually associated with REM sleep
   Other parasomnias
3. Sleep disorders associated with medical/psychiatric disorders
   Associated with mental disorders
   Associated with neurologic disorders
   Associated with other medical disorders
4. Proposed sleep disorders

The first category, the dyssomnias, includes many of the disorders commonly associated with either insomnia (difficulty in initiating or maintaining sleep) or excessive sleepiness. Dyssomnias are a heterogeneous grouping that include the major primary sleep disorders associated with either disrupted nocturnal sleep or impaired wakefulness and excessive sleepiness.[12] Included are intrinsic sleep disorders (those in which the primary cause is an internal abnormality originating within the body, such as narcolepsy or central sleep apnea syndrome); extrinsic sleep disorders (those in which the primary cause is outside the body such as environmental sleep disorder or hypnotic-dependent sleep disorder); and circadian rhythm disorders in which the underlying problem is chronophysiologic, such as shift work sleep disorder.[12]

The second category, parasomnias, are undesirable physical phenomena that usually occur during, or are exacerbated by, sleep. These may occur during REM sleep, arousal, or the transition from sleep to awakening or vice-versa, and include such disorders as bruxism (teeth grinding), sleepwalking, rhythmic movement disorder, night terrors, nightmares, and sudden infant death syndrome.[12]

The third category consists of sleep disorders associated with medical/psychiatric disorders and may include alcoholism, psychoses, parkinsonism, sleep-related asthma, and peptic ulcer disease. The final category is called "proposed sleep disorders" and includes short sleeper and pregnancy-associated sleep disorder.[12]

Issues in the Measurement of Sleep

Selecting a measure of sleep depends on the problem being investigated and the purpose of the investigation. Is the investigator interested in the problem from a research or a clinical perspective? Is the aim of the investigation diagnostic, evaluation of management and treatment, or assessment of a given sleep parameter under different conditions? Because *sleep* is a general term, the investigator must determine in advance what parameters or variables are of interest for the particular study. Possible variables and parameters related to sleep are:

Time spent in bed
Sleep quantity or total sleep time
Time and percentage spent in various stages of sleep
Number of sleep stage shifts
Sleep onset latency (time from "lights out" to sleep)
"Lights out" time
Time of falling asleep
Difficulty/ease in falling asleep
Quality of sleep
Bedtime rituals
Use of medications to promote sleep
Sleep arousals per night (number, length, time of night, circumstance [e.g., urination], difficulty/ease in falling back to sleep)
Sleep sufficiency
Sleep efficiency
Sleep fragmentation
Soundness of sleep
Satisfaction with sleep
Time of arising
Difficulty/ease in awakening in the morning
Feeling rested or refreshed after sleep
Moods or feelings on awakening
Occurrence of parasomnias or sleep-related symptoms
Dreams
Daytime sleepiness/alertness
Napping during the day (time of day, number, duration, circumstances)

Certain aspects of sleep can be measured objectively provided that instrumentation is calibrated correctly, the results are examined by a skilled interpreter, and reliability and validity issues, including the appropriateness of the measure for the problem, are addressed. Aspects of sleep that lend themselves to measurement by instrumentation include the time spent in each stage of sleep, sleep latency, total sleep time, number of arousals or awakenings, time of awakening, amount and type of movement, and the like. However, if an investigator wishes to assess the prevalence of general sleep problems in relation to another parameter in a large population, he/she may choose survey research methodology and devise one or two questions related to sleep as discussed later in this chapter.

Objective techniques are useful for many purposes, but it often is of interest to know how respondents perceive their sleep. In some ways, measuring sleep perception is similar to measuring pain perception in that there are important subjective perceptions to assess. These can include sleep quality, whether sleep was "good" or not, and whether the person felt "rested" upon awakening. Other considerations that guide the choice of measurement include budget; the number of professionals participating in the project; the availability of specialized equipment or space; expertise of the investigator or consultants; the size of the sample; the anticipated cooperation of subjects and any inconvenience to them; and time constraints. The "gold standard" for traditional sleep studies is polysomnography, but this method may not be available to all investigators. Furthermore, it may not provide the type of information desired and may provide data not necessary to the particular study. Instrumentation also has been used to indirectly assess sleep states through activity monitoring or movement.

Another approach to assess sleep has been the use of questionnaires. These can be particularly useful for screening, triage, and assessing the effects of treatment. They are inexpensive, nonintrusive, and may subjectively assess the respondent's perceptions. Instruments with credible reliability and validity are desirable. Unfortunately, many questionnaires developed to measure sleep have not predefined the aspects of sleep they measure; the reference time of the inquiry may be unclear; psychometric information may not be available; scoring information may be absent; intentional and unintentional bias may be present;[13] data are usually retrospective, and recall bias may play a significant role; and the population on which the tool was normed may be homogeneous, leading to problems of generalization (e.g., age, sex, ethnic group). Many questionnaires have been developed by an author for a specific study and have not been tested again. Questionnaires may be administered by self-report and interview. Because few researchers, even in studies using single sleep-related questions, have used consistent wording in the question and response choices, it is difficult to make cross-study comparisons.

Instruments such as sleep diaries and sleep logs have been used as self-reports or as charts completed by observers. Sleep diaries permit comparison between sleep parameters and other events of interest over a continuous period but can be burdensome. Observational techniques, such as those by health-care providers, bed partners, or parents, have been used alone or in conjunction with instrumentation and self-reports and may include the use of time-lapse photography or video/audio recording. Indirect measures of sleep have been through daytime performance testing, or psychologic testing. These are discussed later in this chapter.

A brief discussion of the relationship between subjective and objective measures of sleep is warranted. Results have varied, and ultimately the relationship between objectively measured and subjectively perceived parameters, such as length of time slept, may depend on the definition of the variable; the extent and significance of the variation of the parameter; factors related to the individual subject, such as age, mood, drug use, cognition, and disease state; instrument-related factors, such as question wording; selection of the objective and subjective measures; unintentional investigator bias; and the method used to compare the objective and subjective measures. Furthermore, although an overnight sleep study may objectively indicate restlessness and arousals, a subject may report "good" sleep and indeed may feel rested. Both results are useful.

Some researchers[14] have documented that persons can accurately describe at least some sleep parameters, but other researchers comparing other sleep parameters with electrophysiologic monitoring have found less reliability with estimates of depth of sleep and the number of brief awakenings.[14] Turner and Ascher reported a correlation of 0.84 between roommate report and self-report on sleep latency.[15] Researchers finding acceptable correlations between various variables measured by objective and subjective counterparts are numerous,[16,17] as are those who find questionable relationships between the two approaches.[18] Others find variation within the same experimental setting.[19] Thus, it cannot be assumed that all subjective measures are invalid and that subjective assessments do provide unique information, but caution is needed in instrument selection and interpretation.

This chapter is organized by instrumentation; questionnaires (including rating scales) and interviews; single- and few-item survey-type questions; sleep diaries and logs; observation; and performance and psychologic testing.

Instrumentation Used to Measure Sleep

Polysomnography (PSG)

The "gold standard" for monitoring sleep is polysomnography. A sleep study is usually done overnight in a sleep laboratory and employs a standardized scoring method.[20] Monitoring may include the recording of sleep-related physiologic parameters, such as respiratory, neuromuscular, cardiac, genitourinary, gastrointestinal, and/or endocrine functions.[21] An individualized, tailored protocol may be designed for a given person based on the type of problem suspected. The electroencephalogram (EEG) is the core of polysomnography, but other standardly assessed measures include the continuous monitoring of (1) eye movement activity by electrooculogram (EOG); (2) cardiac rhythm monitoring by electrocardiogram (ECG); (3) muscle monitoring by electromyogram (EMG); and (4) respiratory parameters. At least one channel of EEG is monitored (e.g., C3/A2 or C4/A1). More extensive monitoring may be desirable to evaluate seizures or the parasomnias. The EOG records eye movement activity during sleep and is particularly useful in detecting REM sleep (distinguished by bursts of rapid eye movements), sleep onset, and transition into NREM stage 1 (when slow rolling eye movements may be seen). At least two channels are recommended. For the EMG, usually the muscles beneath the chin (mentalis/submentalis muscles) are monitored. However, additional muscle monitoring specific to a particular interest may be added. For example, the anterior tibialis muscles are of particular interest in detecting periodic leg movements or restless legs syndrome. To monitor bruxism, the masseter muscle may be an EMG location. Other parameters may be added, including respiratory parameters, core temperature determinations, heart rate, blood pressure, penile tumescence, and esophageal pH. The minimal respiratory parameters necessary to evaluate breathing disorders during sleep, such as in sleep apnea, include airflow or exchange monitoring through the nose and mouth; respiratory effort; and a measure of oxygen saturation (usually oximetry).

These concurrent measurements should be recorded and interpreted by certified experts, using standardized procedures and scoring.[22] Sleep-stage scoring techniques have been well developed and standardized.[20] The standard for scoring remains the visual interpretation, although computer-aided systems are expected to become the norm in the near future.

Audio and video monitoring during the overnight recording, combined with behavioral observation, are useful to characterize arousal disorders, assess seizure activity, and observe body position and movement during sleep.[22] After the person has "settled in," electrodes are applied, and the mechanical apparatus is calibrated. Recording is usually done on chart paper 300 mm wide recorded at a chart speed of 10 or 15 mm/second. To begin PSG, the lights should be turned off as close to the person's regular bedtime as possible; testing should be concluded as close to the normal time of arising as possible. These times should be marked on the chart paper. A technologist usually observes the patient throughout the procedure. If possible, 8 hours of recording (and at least 6.5 hours) should be done. Sleep recordings are commonly scored by dividing the paper tracing into segments or epochs. The most commonly used epoch lengths are 20 or 30 seconds. A "first night" effect has been described for adaptation to the sleep laboratory. Some researchers believe that even after several adaptation nights, an accurate assessment of the subject's usual asleep is not possible; hence the interest in at-home measures and other ways of assessment.[23]

Multiple Sleep Latency Test (MSLT)

The Multiple Sleep Latency Test (MSLT) consists of polygraphic monitoring with a standard recording montage that usually includes EEG, EOG, EMG, ECG, respiratory flow, and respiratory sounds. The major purposes of the MSLT are to assess readiness to fall asleep, detect daytime sleepiness, and detect sleep-onset REM episodes (SOREMPs). SOREMPs do not usually occur in normal adults, as sleep usually begins with NREM sleep. The MSLT can be used: (1) to diagnose narcolepsy; (2) to assess responses to drug therapy; and (3) to evaluate the experimental effects of different drugs, the manipulation of dosages or changing nighttime sleep schedules.[24] The MSLT generally is done on the day following overnight polysomnography. The subject should have kept sleep diaries for one to two weeks before admission because values on the MSLT can be influenced by previous sleep. Drugs influencing sleep (e.g., caffeine, alcohol, hypnotics, amphetamines, sedatives, antihistamines, and others) must be withdrawn 2 weeks prior to this test. The patient is in street clothes and between tests is not in bed. To begin the test, the recording equipment is attached to the patient. Specific standardized instructions are given. The patient lies down in a dark room with a nonstimulating environment and is given the opportunity to nap at 2-hour intervals for four to five times during the day. The usual times are 10:00 A.M., noon, 2:00 P.M., 4:00 P.M., and 6:00 P.M. These nap periods are usually 20 minutes long. The time to sleep onset (sleep latency) and the types of sleep are monitored. In normal persons, sleep onset usually is 10 minutes or more. The mean sleep latency is shorter in persons with narcolepsy, usually averaging less than 5 minutes. Normal people usually begin REM sleep 75 to 90 minutes after going to sleep; sleep onset does not normally begin with REM sleep. REM sleep usually is not experienced during a short nap period. The occurrence of two or more SOREMPs during the MSLT nap period is virtually diagnostic of narcolepsy, especially if other causes of early onset of REM sleep, such as severe sleep deprivation, have been ruled out. The MSLT is said to have a sensitivity of 84% and specificity of 99% using narcoleptic diagnosis criteria of less than 5 minutes to fall asleep and at least 2 SOREMPS.[22,24,25] Studies of the use of nasal continuous positive airway pressure (CPAP) for both chronic snorers and sleep apneics showed an improvement in MSLT scores with CPAP administration,[26] suggesting validity of the MSLT. Other research has demonstrated that the MSLT scores are related to the amount of sleep on one or more previous nights, time of day, and other variables in normal subjects.[27] One study in six insomniacs demonstrated a test–retest reliability over 3 to 90 weeks of 0.65.[28] Another study demonstrated that the MSLT is highly reliable in testing daytime sleepiness in normal subjects even over periods exceeding a year. However, these researchers cautioned that at least three and preferably four MSLTs were necessary for good reliability. For four tests, the test–retest reliability in 14 normal subjects was reported as 0.97 by Zwyghuizen-Doorenbos and colleagues.[29] The MSLT has also been used to investigate sleep latency in persons undergoing smoking cessation.[30] The MSLT shows promise for being carried out in an ambulatory setting, although its use is not yet widespread.[31] The MSLT has been called "the accepted clinical standard" for the diagnosis of daytime sleepiness.[24]

Maintenance of Wakefulness Test (MWT)

The Maintenance of Wakefulness Test (MWT) evolved from the MSLT. It also is a polysomnographic procedure in which the variables monitored include EEG, EOG, EMG, ECG, and respiratory parameters. The MWT uses a multiple-nap approach but measures the subject's ability to stay awake rather than to fall asleep. Subjects are instructed to "try to stay awake for as long as possible" while sitting in a comfortable chair in a dark room for five 20-minute trials between 10:00 A.M. and 6:00 P.M.[32] This procedure evaluates the degree of alertness and can detect sleep tendency at inappropriate times.[22]

Another test, said to be similar to the MWT, has been referred to as "lapses." It consists of a 10-minute tapping test, 5 minutes with the eyes open and 5 minutes with the eyes closed. The person is instructed to stay awake during tapping, and a lapse is scored if the time between taps is longer than 3 seconds. The number of lapses in the 10 minutes is scored and used as a measure of sleepiness. Freeman et al. found a negative correlation of 0.51 between lapses and the MSLT.[33]

Repeated Test of Sustained Wakefulness (RTSW)

The Repeated Test of Sustained Wakefulness (RTSW) also is a polygraphic test and examines the effects of treatment on the ability to sustain wakefulness in persons who are excessively sleepy.[34] The subject lies in bed in a dimly lit room and is instructed to remain awake. Some researchers believe that the MWT and RTSW are more sensitive to nighttime changes in sleepiness and alertness than the MSLT and in one study discriminated between subjects in "nap," "no-nap" conditions.[34]

Modified Assessment of Sleepiness Test (MAST)

The Modified Assessment of Sleepiness Test (MAST) is a modification of the MSLT. Subjects are studied in alternating conditions in both a "bed nap" setting and a "chair nap" setting. The researchers[35] believe that the "chair" setting has face validity and that the MAST may provide a sensitive measure, particularly in the assessment of sleepiness in patients with some type of hypersomnia.[35]

Home or Ambulatory Monitoring

Among the disadvantages of polysomnography is the expense, including an overnight stay in the sleep laboratory and the need for all-night technologists and for specialized equipment and facilities.[36] In addition, recorded sleep may be influenced by of the unnatural environment. Technologic advances have resulted in some ambulatory and home-monitoring devices that allow the recording of sleep and associated physiologic parameters outside the sleep laboratory.[21] Advantages include allowing data collection in a more natural environment, less expense, round-the-clock data collection, and in ambulatory monitoring the person is allowed free movement. Disadvantages include the potential for the monitoring device to develop a "glitch"; for the patient to misunderstand the instructions; uncontrolled conditions; and the lack of immediate medical backup if needed. Ambulatory or home monitoring may be particularly suited to document disorders occurring sporadically, such as the parasomnias or seizures.[31] Some systems allow for transmission of the home-collected sleep data by telephone lines directly to the sleep laboratory.[37] Both analog ambulatory recorders (e.g., Medilog 9000 system, Oxford Medical Systems, Clearwater, FL); and digital systems (e.g., the Vitalog portable recorder, Vitalog Corporation, Palo Alto, CA) can be used for home monitoring. Each has certain suitabilities and advantages and disadvantages. Sewitch and Kupfer compared analog ambulatory and laboratory recordings to monitor sleep in normal persons and found that the results were essentially the same.[38] However, a consensus statement issued by the American Thoracic Society has not recommended home monitoring devices for the diagnosis of sleep-related respiratory problems at this time.[39]

Pupillometry

Pupillometry is a nonintrusive technique that evaluates the ability of the subject to maintain alertness by measuring pupillary constriction. The behavior of the pupil reflects autonomic activity; the sympathetic nervous system predominates in maintaining alertness, and the parasympathetic system is associated with sleep. In pupillometry an infrared pupillograph is used to measure the length of time a person maintains a large and stable pupillary diameter (characteristic of alertness) when the subject is seated in a dark room. Persons who are sleepy, such as in narcolepsy, may show progressive pupillary constriction or miosis over the 15-minute testing period and/or marked variation in pupillary diameter or oscillations called hippus.[40]

Pupillometry has been used to follow patients under various types of treatment for insomnia. Some studies have reported that parameters, such as baseline pupil diameter, pupillary light reflex and the pupillary orienting response, do not differentiate between normal individuals and those with narcolepsy.[41] Other studies have shown that pupillometry can distinguish sleep-deprived normals from controls or those with narcolepsy from normals and can accurately measure inalertness during attempts to stay awake.[42]

Pupillometry is relatively inexpensive and is not as time-consuming as polysomnography. However, standardization has not been accomplished, and the recognition of and procedure for dealing with artifacts such as involuntary eyeblinks remain an issue.[43]

Activity Measurement

An indirect method of studying sleep is by examining activity or motility. In sleep, major body movements occur mainly before and after REM sleep, long periods of immobility are associated with NREM sleep, and small body movements have been found to be associated with REM sleep.[44] The latter has been demonstrated by combining time–lapse videorecording with electrophysiologic monitoring.[44] Movement-sensing devices to measure sleep or wakefulness have been applied to studies of sleep in humans.[45] The actigraph is a small box containing a movement detector and memory storage that can be worn by subjects on the wrist or ankle. It allows continuous recording for several days during normal activities in the home. The internal piezoelectric sensor in the actigraph records movement and interpretation is based on the fact that fewer limb movements occur during sleep than during wakefulness.[46] Thus, it is used to infer sleep and wake periods. The time-based recording system uses various time periods or epochs such as 5, 30, or 60 seconds, for measurement. Various models are available, such as the Motionlogger and the Actillume (both from Ambulatory Monitoring, Inc., Ardsley, NY, 10502; 914-693-9240). Scoring may be accomplished by various methods, including a hand-scoring method, a computer-scoring system called Sleepest that has several options,[46] Actigraphic Scoring Analysis, and the "Action" algorithm supplied with the actigraph. Appendix 18A presents research activities to demonstrate correlation of the actigraph with EEG.[45-59]

In summary, the actigraph is useful because it can provide data over time in the home environment, is relatively inexpensive, appears more accurate than sleep logs, and for some parameters, particularly the distinction between sleep and wakefulness and total sleep time, correlates well with data from polysomnography. The method of scoring and characteristics of the population influence the accuracy of the results obtained. Other monitoring devices are highlighted in Appendix 18B.

Questionnaires and Interviews

A variety of questionnaires have been devised to measure various aspects of sleep and sleep-related behavior. As discussed, the self-report questionnaires are largely subjective and have both advantages and disadvantages. In some cases, questionnaires are wholly concerned with sleep, but in other cases, sleep is only one of several parameters investigated. A number of questionnaires will be discussed fully, and the other are detailed in Appendix 18C.

The Stanford Sleepiness Scale (SSS)

The Stanford Sleepiness Scale (SSS) is a self-rating scale in which subjects are asked to record the number corresponding to the statement best describing their degree of sleepiness.[60] The SSS is administered every 15 minutes during waking activities and may be averaged over the hour. When averaged in this way, a decrease of approximately three scale values indicates a significant decrease in performance in those affected by sleep loss. Validity ratings of mean SSS values using the Wilkinson Addition Test and the Wilkinson Vigilance Test was reported at a correlation of 0.68; and correlation on an abridged version of the Williams Word Memory test was reported at 0.47. Reliability using alternate forms has been reported at 0.88.[60] The SSS is said to measure feelings of sleepiness or tiredness at a particular point in time. It is more often used in research protocols than in clinical evaluation and diagnosis.[24]

Two early validity studies were done. One found the SSS sensitive to total acute sleep deprivation.[61] Correlations were low and/or variable with level of performance and sleep deprivation, and therefore the elevated sleep ratings were not predictive of performance efficiency for individual subjects on the Wilkinson Auditory Vigilance test, a four-choice serial RT test, a visual simple RT test, anagrams, and the Wisconsin Card Sorting test.[62]

In another investigation using four-short duration performance tasks and the Wilkinson Auditory Vigilance task along with the SSS, Glenville and Broughton[63] found that the SSS was a reliable indicator of acute sleepiness and that there were significant (but unreported) correlations between the SSS and a decrease in performance on vigilance, choice reaction, and simple reaction time, but not with short-term memory and handwriting.[63] Reliability of the SSS in chronically sleep-deprived patients and those with cumulative partial sleep deprivation, as well as in narcoleptics, has been questioned.[64] When comparing a group of normal subjects with a group of patients with sleep apnea and excessive daytime sleepiness, Roth and colleagues did not find differences in SSS scores.[65]

The Epworth Sleepiness Scale (ESS)

The Epworth Sleepiness Scale (ESS) measures general levels of sleep propensity, defined as the probability of falling asleep at a particular time.[66] Sleep propensity will vary by time of day and from day to day depending on activity, drugs, sleep deprivation, pathology, and cognitive and affective state. Average sleep propensity over a prolonged period, (for example, a week), can be calculated.[66] In terms of validity, the ESS was said to distinguish significantly among patients with disorders of excessive daytime sleepiness and those without and was significantly correlated with the multiple sleep latency test and with polysomnography. The test–retest reliability of the ESS in a group of medical students in one study was 0.82. Patients with sleep apnea showed ESS scores that were statistically significantly lower after treatment than before treatment was started, as would be expected with successful treatment. Internal consistency reliability showed Cronbach's alphas of 0.88 for the patients and 0.73 for the students, showing a reasonably high consistency. A factor analysis was performed on the ESS scores of 150 patients and 104 students; one main factor was identified for each group. The ESS is reliable, internally consistent, and has one main dimension in its variance.[67] It has been used to assess sleep-disordered breathing in Hispanics and non-Hispanics.[68]

For this paper-and-pencil questionnaire, the subject is asked to rate on a scale of 0 (low) to 3 (high) the chances that they would doze in certain situations. Thus, when the 8-item scores are summed, the individual's score can range from 0 (abnormally low sleepiness) to 24 (very high level of sleepiness).

The Pittsburgh Sleep Quality Index (PSQI)

The Pittsburgh Sleep Quality Index (PSQI) measures subjective sleep quality. This subjective, self-rated, paper-and-pencil questionnaire consists of 19 items. In addition, clinical information is assessed by the bed partner in 5 additional questions that are not used in the scoring. Responses to the 19 items are grouped into 7 component scores that are weighted equally on a 0-to-3 scale, as some components consist of one question and others have several questions. The 7 components of the PSQI are sleep quality, sleep latency, sleep duration, habitual sleep efficiency, sleep disturbances, use of sleeping medication, and daytime dysfunction. The 7 component scores also can be summed to produce a global PSQI score that can range from 0 to 21. Higher scores indicate more severe complaints and worse sleep quality.[69] A geriatric version has been used to examine sleep in older adults in various fitness programs.[70]

Internal consistency reliability for each individual component via Cronbach's alpha ranged from 0.35 to 0.76, with an overall reliability coefficient of 0.83. Test–retest reliability for 91 patients revealed a correlation for global scores of 0.85, and individual components ranged from 0.65 to 0.84. In regard to validity, global PSQI scores were compared across controls, depressives, and two groups of persons with sleep disorders. Patients were discriminated from controls, and concurrent polysomnographic findings supported the questionnaire findings. A global PSQI score above 5 was said to have a diagnostic sensitivity of 89.6% and specificity of 86.5% in differentiating good from poor sleepers.[69] Other instruments to measure sleep are found in Appendix 18C.[71-109]

Other Instruments

Single- or Few-Item Sleep Surveys

A number of investigators have examined various aspects of sleep either singularly or as part of multidimensional studies of health in large populations. The latter studies usually include instruments with one or a few sleep-related items that are obtained by mailed survey or as part of large-scale telephone or face-to-face interviews.[110,111] Single-item inquiries about sleep often have less sensitivity and specificity than do composite scales.[74] Results from survey questions often can be difficult to compare because methodologic differences, variations in the question phraseology, and differences in the type and wording of response choices.

Sleep Diaries/Sleep Logs/Charts

Polysomnographic recordings provide objective information about sleep, its stages, awakenings, and the like, but information about how individuals evaluate their sleep is not obtained in that manner. Sleep diaries are usually self-reports of sleep, are obtained daily, and, although subjective, they may be less biased than retrospective recalls obtained on an infrequent basis. Generally these day-to-day reports of sleep activities may be used not only at bedtime, but also to give a 24-hour picture of sleep–wake activities and patterns over a period of time, such as a week. Diaries are clinically relevant and over time may provide insights into patterns affecting sleep and the degree of disruption experienced by the patient. For example, in examining nocturnal enuresis in a child, the daily log may indicate that this occurred on nights when the child's daily nap was skipped, thus suggesting a possible cause-and-effect relationship and opportunity for intervention.[112]

Advantages of sleep diaries include their ease of use, convenience, low expense, reflection of the natural setting, relative nonobtrusiveness, and recording of the person's perceived sleep experience.[13] Diaries may be used independently or in conjunction with polysomnography to obtain a picture of usual behavior. They may be used to monitor adherence to therapy, such as scheduled naps; facilitate longitudinal data collection (such as in shift workers); evaluate treatment progress; monitor symptoms; and promote self-management.[113] Problems include the fact that they can be burdensome, are subject to intentional and unintentional bias, subjects may not keep them daily and thus fill them in just before collection, and that they are subjective. Sleep diaries may have a single focus, such as recording the number of minutes required to fall asleep in the previous night;[114] may combine this information with other data to judge the success of a relaxation treatment for long sleep-onset periods; or they may have multiple purposes. Depending on why the diary is being kept, daytime activities that influence sleep, such as caffeine intake, alcohol or drug use, smoking, meals and snacks, medication use, and exercise may be recorded. Sometimes a sleep log may be kept by an observer, such as in the case of a child.[113]

A major question regarding the use of self-reported sleep diaries or logs concerns reliability and validity. Haythornthwaite and colleagues[115] examined the use of diaries to study sleep in patients with chronic pain. The reliability of coefficients of stability was examined among subjects, as were reliability coefficients across four nights. They reported item ranges of 0.38 to 0.62 for coefficients of stability. Using the Spearman-Brown prophesy formula for reliability coefficients across four nights, they reported ranges of 0.69 to 0.87. Regarding validity they noted that subjects accurately discriminated different aspects of sleep behavior and reported adequate concurrent and convergent validity with individual items relative to sleep in other instruments. Rogers and colleague[16] compared recordings in a sleep diary about nocturnal sleep and the time and duration of daytime naps with ambulatory polysomnographic recordings in 25 normal and 25 narcoleptic subjects. Agreement between the sleep diaries and polysomnographic data for these parameters was reportedly high (kappa = 0.87), as was the sensitivity (92.3%) and specificity (95.6%). They concluded that sleep diaries were reliable for collecting information about sleep–wake patterns in most subjects. Subjects with fluctuations in daytime vigilance were said to require greater sensitivity to detect short frequent naps.[16] In studies of sleep diaries, estimates of sleep latency were compared with observer estimates from the same night. Correlations have ranged from 0.84 to 0.99.[15,116] Other methods include daily sleep diary and spouse sleep diaries,[117] sleep card,[118] and a modified sleep card.[119]

Observation

Observation of sleep and wakefulness may occur through several methods, including direct behavioral observations by one or more observers (such as roommates, bedpartners, or nurses);[10] video,[44,120] and time-lapse photography, or motion pictures.[121] The latter is now used less frequently. Observation by a trained observer and/or by audio and video recording may accompany polysomnography. The issue of reliability is important. Direct observation often involves the use of a variety of investigator-developed protocols, descriptors, and/or forms. Often, these are developed according to what it is that the investigator wishes to observe. Thus, as in survey methodology, it often is difficult to make comparisons across studies.

Visual Analog and Rating Scales

Visual analog scales (VAS) and adjective checklists often are used to assess subjective parameters, such as sleep, pain, fatigue, dyspnea, and moods. Detailed discussions may be found elsewhere.[122-125]

Performance and Psychologic Tests

Performance, vigilance, and psychologic tests sometimes are used as indirect measures of alertness or sleepiness. A consequence of impaired nighttime sleep and the use of certain medications, such as depressants, are decreased alertness, increased daytime sleepiness, and altered mood states.[126] As a result, daytime performance can decline.[127] Consistency has been demonstrated between objectively measured sleepiness, performance, vigilance, and certain moods.[126] Some of the most commonly used tests to measure performance or vigilance that have been used in regard to increased sleepiness and decreased alertness include the Wilkinson four-choice reaction time; Wilkinson addition test; the Trailmaking test; the digit-symbol substitution test; symbol copying test; tracking tasks; auditory reaction time; complex visual reaction time; tapping rates; Serial 7 Subtraction; the Shipley-Hartford Abstraction Scale; Sentence Completion Test; card sorting; the Wechsler Memory Scale and other short- and long-term memory tests; reaction time tests; manual dexterity tests; and paired-associates tests.[127] Determining the psychologic parameters affected by sleep, such as mood, anxiety, hopelessness, and depression, also is common in conjunction with sleep-related measures. Commonly used tests in sleep-related studies have included mood-related visual analog scales; the Profile of Mood States; the Multiple Affect Adjective Checklist; the Crown-Marlowe Social Desirability Scale; the Rotter Locus of Control; the Beck Depression Inventory; the Spielberger State/Trait Anxiety test; Minnesota Multiphasic Personality Inventory (MMPI);

the California Personality Inventory; and the Cornell Index. A discussion of these tests is beyond the scope of this chapter.

Summary

A variety of methods are available to measure the broad area of sleep. The choice of instrument and method depends on the purpose of the study, the aspect of sleep being studied, available resources, and the expertise of the investigator. Any choice of instrument should consider the issues of validity and reliability. Many of the more recently developed questionnaires have paid more attention to these issues. Promising advances have been made in less expensive instrumentation and in ambulatory monitoring. These approaches may offer more options for future studies.

References

1. National Commission on Sleep Disorders. *Research report. Vol. 1. Executive summary and executive report.* Bethesda, MD: National Institutes of Health, 1993.

2. Carskadon, M.A., & Dement, W.C. Normal human sleep: An overview. In M.H. Kryger, T. Roth, & W.C. Dement (Eds.). *Principles and practice of sleep medicine* (2nd ed.). Philadelphia, Saunders, 1994, pp. 16-25.

3. Siegel, J.M. Mechanisms of sleep control. *J Clin Neurophysiol*, 1990, 7(1):49-65.

4. Thorpy, M.J. (Ed.). *Handbook of sleep disorders.* New York, Marcel Dekker, 1990.

5. Thorpy, M.J., & Yager, J. *The encyclopedia of sleep and sleep disorders.* New York, Facts on File, 1991.

6. Pressman, M.R., & Fry, J.M. What is normal sleep in the elderly? *Clin Geriatr Med*, 1988, 4(1):71-81.

7. Kryger, M.H., Roth, T., & Dement, W.C. (Eds.). *Principles and practice of sleep medicine* (2nd ed.). Philadelphia, Saunders, 1994.

8. Horne, J. Annotation: Sleep and its disorders in children. *J Child Psychol Psychiatr All Disc*, 1992, 33(3):473-487.

9. Kripke, D.F., Simons, R.N., Garfinkel, L., & Hammond, E.C. Short and long sleep and sleeping pills. Is increased mortality associated? *Arch Gen Psychiatr*, 1979, 36(1):103-116.

10. Webb, W.B., & Swinburne, H. An observational study of sleep of the aged. *Percept Motor Skills*, 1971, 32(3):895-898.

11. Prinz, P.N., Vitiello, M.V., Raskind, M.A., & Thorpy, M.J. Geriatrics: Sleep disorders and aging. *N Eng J Med*, 1990, 323(8):520-526.

12. Diagnostic Classification Steering Committee (Thorpy, M.J., Chairman). *International classification of sleep disorders: Diagnostic and coding manual.* Rochester, MN: American Sleep Disorders Association, 1990.

13. Bootzin, R.R., & Engle-Friedman, M. The assessment of insomnia. *Behav Assess*, 1981, 3:107-126.

14. Browman, C.P., & Tepas, D.I. The effects of presleep activity on all-night sleep. *Psychophysiology*, 1976, 13(6):536-540.

15. Turner, R.M., & Ascher, L.M. Controlled comparison of progressive relaxation, stimulus control and paradoxical intention therapies for insomnia. *J Consult Clin Psychol*, 1979, 47(3):500-508.

16. Rogers, A.E., Caruso, C.C., & Aldrich, M.S. Reliability of sleep diaries for assessment of sleep/wake patterns. *Nurs Res*, 1993, 42(6):368-372.

17. Edwards, G.B., & Schuring, L.M. Pilot study: Validating staff nurses' observations of sleep and wake states among critically ill patients, using polysomnography. *Am J Crit Care*, 1993, 2(2):125-131.

18. Weiss, B.L., McPartland, R.J., & Kupfer, D.J. Once more: The inaccuracy of non-EEG estimations of sleep. *Am J Psychiatr*, 1973, 130(11):1282-1285.

19. Monroe, L.J. Psychological and physiological differences between good and poor sleepers. *J Abn Psychol*, 1967, 72(3):255-264.

20. Rechtschaffen, A., & Kales, A. (Eds.). *A manual of standardized terminology, techniques and scoring system for sleep stages of human subjects.* NIH Publication No. 204. Washington, DC, Public Health Service, U.S. Government Printing Office, 1968.

21. Kayed, K. Use of home monitoring in a sleep disorders clinic. In L.E. Miles and R.J. Broughton (Eds.), *Medical monitoring in the home and work environment.* New York, Raven, 1990, pp. 245-254.

22. American Electroencephalographic Society guidelines for polygraphic assessment of sleep-related disorders (polysomnography). *J Clin Neurophysiol*, 1992, 9(1):88-96.

23. Johns, M.W., & Dore, C. Sleep at home and in the sleep laboratory: Disturbance by recording procedures. *Ergonomics*, 1978, 21(5):325-330.

24. Carskadon, M.A. (1994). Measuring daytime sleepiness. In M.H. Kryger, T. Roth, & W.C. Dement (Eds.). *Principles and practice of sleep medicine* (2nd ed.). Philadelphia, Saunders, 1994, pp. 961-962.

25. Carskadon, M.A., Dement, W.C., Mitler, M.M., et al. Guidelines for the multiple sleep latency test (MSLT): A standard measure of sleepiness. *Sleep*, 1986, 9(4): 519-524.

26. DiPhillipo, M.A., Fry, J.M., & Pressman, M.R. Objective measurement of daytime sleepiness following treatment of obstructive sleep apnea with nasal CPAP. *Sleep Res*, 1988, 17:167.

27. Richardson, G.S., Carskadon, M.A., Orav, E.J., & Dement, W.C. Circadian variation of sleep tendency in elderly and young adult subjects. *Sleep*, 1982, 5(suppl 2):S82-S94.

28. Seidel, W.F., & Dement, W.C. The Multiple Sleep Latency Test: Test–retest reliability. *Sleep Res*, 1981, 10:284.

29. Zwyghuizen-Doorenbos, A., Roehrs, T., Schaefer, M., & Roth, T. Test–retest reliability of the MSLT. *Sleep*, 1988, 11(6):562-565.

30. Prosise, G.L., Bonnet, M., Berry, R.B., & Dickelj, M.J. Effects of abstinence from smoking on sleep and daytime sleepiness. *Chest*, 1994, 105(4):1136-1141.

31. Broughton, R.J. Ambulant home monitoring of sleep and its disorders. In M.H. Kryger, T. Roth, & W.C. Dement (Eds.), *Principles and practice of sleep medicine* (2nd ed.). Philadelphia, Saunders, 1994, pp. 978-983.

32. Mitler, M.M., Gujavarty, K.S., & Browman, C.P. Maintenance of wakefulness test: A polysomnographic technique for evaluating treatment efficacy in patients with excessive somnolence. *Electroencephalogr Clin Neurophysiol*, 1982, 53(6):658-661.

33. Freeman, C.R., Johnson, L.C., Spinweber, C.L., & Gomez, S.A. The relationship among four measures of sleepiness. *Sleep Res*, 1988, 17:334.

34. Sugerman, J.L., & Walsh, J.K. Physiological sleep tendency and ability to maintain alertness at night. *Sleep*, 1989, 12(2):106-112.

35. Erman, M.K., Beckham, B., Gardner, D.A., & Roffwarg, H.P. The modified assessment of sleepiness test (MAST). *Sleep Res*, 1987, 16:550.

36. Ancoli-Israel, S. Evaluating sleep apnea with the portable modified Medilog/Respitrace system. In L.E. Miles & R.J. Broughton (Eds.), *Medical monitoring in the home and work environment*. New York, Raven Press, 1990, pp. 275-283.

37. Sewitch, D.E. Evaluation of commercially available home recording systems for all-night sleep recordings: The telediagnostic and Oxford Medilog 9000 systems. In L.E. Miles, & R.J. Broughton, *Medical monitoring in the home and work environment*. New York, Raven, 1990, pp. 231-243.

38. Sewitch, D.E., & Kupfer, D.G. Polysomnographic telemetry using Telediagnostic and Oxford Medilog 9000 systems. *Sleep*, 1985, 8(3):288-293.

39. American Thoracic Society Consensus Conference on Indications and Standards for Cardiopulmonary Sleep Studies. *Am Rev Resp Dis*, 1989, 139(2):559-568.

40. McLaren, J.W., Erie, J.C., & Brubaker, R.F. Computerized analysis of pupillograms in studies of alertness. *Invest Ophthalmol Vis Sci*, 1992, 33(3):671-676.

41. Newman, J., & Broughton, R. Pupillometric assessment of excessive daytime sleepiness in narcolepsy-cataplexy. *Sleep*, 1991, 14(2):121-129.

42. Yoss, R.E., Moyer, N.J., & Ogle, K.N. The pupillogram and narcolepsy. A method to measure decreased levels of wakefulness. *Neurology*, 1969, 19(10):921-928.

43. Eshler, B., Mercer, P., Merritt, S., & Cohen, F.L. Three methods of handling invalid pupillometry data. *Sleep Res*, 1992, 21:338.

44. Aaronson, S.T., Rashed, S., Biber, M.P., & Hobson, J.A. Brain state and body position. *Arch Gen Psychiatr*, 1982, 39(3):330-335.

45. Kripke, D.F., Mullaney, D.J., Messin, S., & Wyborney, V.G. Wrist actigraphic measures of sleep and rhythms. *Electroencephalogr Clin Neurophysiol*, 1978, 44(5):674-676.

46. Hauri, P.J., & Wisbey, J. Wrist actigraphy in insomnia. *Sleep*, 1992, 15(4):293-301.

47. Mullaney, D.J., Kripke, D.F., & Messin, S. Wrist-actigraphic estimation of sleep time. *Sleep*, 1980, 3(1):83-92.

48. Sadeh, A., Lavie, P., Scher, A., et al. Actigraphic home-monitoring sleep-disturbed and control infants and young children: A new method for pediatric assessment of sleep-wake patterns. *Pediatrics*, 1991, 87(4):494-499.

49. Pollmaecher, T., & Schulz, H. The relation between wrist-actigraphic measures and sleep stages. *Sleep Res*, 1987, 16:55.

50. Urbach, D., Lavie, P., & Alster, J. Screening for sleep disorders by actigraphic recordings. *Sleep Res*, 1988, 17:357.

51. Newman, J., Stampi, C., Dunham, D.W., & Broughton, R. Does wrist-actigraphy approximate traditional polysomnographic detection of sleep and wakefulness in narcolepsy-cataplexy? *Sleep Res*, 1988, 17:343.

52. Borbely, A.A. New techniques for the analysis of the human sleep-wake cycle. *Brain Devel*, 1986, 8(4):482-488.

53. Stampi, C., & Broughton, R. Ultrashort sleep-wake schedule: Detection of sleep state through wrist-actigraph measures. *Sleep Res*, 1988, 17:100.

54. van Hilten, J.J., Braat, E.A.M., van der Velde, E.A., et al., Ambulatory activity monitoring during sleep: An evaluation of internight and intrasubject variability in healthy persons aged 50–98 years. *Sleep*, 1993, 16(2):146-150.

55. Thoman, E.B., & Glazier, R.C. Computer scoring of motility patterns for states of sleep and wakefulness: Human infants. *Sleep*, 1987, 10(2):122-129.

56. Lichstein, K.L., Nickel, R., Hoelscher, T.J., & Kelley, J.E. Clinical validation of a sleep assessment device. *Behav Res Ther*, 1982, 20(3):292-297.

57. Keefe, M.R., Kotzer, A.M., Reuss, J.L., & Sander, L.W. Development of a system for monitoring infant state behavior. *Nurs Res*, 1989, 38(6):344-347.

58. Korner, A.F., Thoman, E.B., & Glick, J.H. A system for monitoring crying and noncrying, large, medium and small neonatal movements. *Child Dev*, 1974, 45(4):946-952.

59. Keefe, M.R. Comparison of neonatal nighttime sleep-wake patterns in nursery versus rooming-in environments. *Nurs Res*, 1987, 36(3):140-144.

60. Hoddes, E., Zarcone, V., & Dement, W.C. Cross-validation of the Stanford sleepiness scale. *Sleep Res*, 1972, 1:91.

61. Glenville, M., & Broughton, R. Reliability of the Stanford Sleepiness Scale compared to short duration performance tests and the Wilkinson auditory vigilance task. In P. Passouant, & I. Oswald, (Eds.), *Pharmacology of the states of alertness*. Oxford, Pergamon, 1979, pp. 235-244.

62. Herscovitch, J., & Broughton, R. Sensitivity of the Stanford Sleepiness Scale to the effects of cumulative partial sleep deprivation and recovery oversleeping. *Sleep*, 1981, 4(1):83-92.

63. Glenville, M., & Broughton, R. Reliability of the Stanford Sleepiness Scale compared to short duration performance tests and the Wilkinson auditory vigilance task. *Sleep Res*, 1982, 5:S135.

64. Broughton, R. Performance and evoked potential measures of various states of daytime sleepiness. *Sleep*, 5(suppl 2):S135-S146.

65. Roth, T., Hartse, K.M., Zorick, F., & Conway, W. Multiple naps and the evaluation of daytime sleepiness in patients with upper airway sleep apnea. *Sleep*, 1980, 3(3-4):425-439.

66. Johns, M.W. Daytime sleepiness, snoring, and obstructive sleep apnea. The Epworth Sleepiness Scale. *Chest*, 1993, 103(1):30-36.

67. Johns, M.W. Reliability and factor analysis of the Epworth Sleepiness Scale. *Sleep*, 1991, 15(4):376-381.

68. Sitton, S., & Chediak, A.D. The Epworth Sleepiness Scale correlates with indices of sleep disordered breathing in a population of Hispanics and Nonhispanics with obstructive sleep apnea. *Sleep Res*, 1994, 23:328.

69. Buysse, D.J., Reynolds, C.F., III, Monk, T.H., et al. The Pittsburgh Sleep Quality Index: A new instrument for psychiatric practice and research. *Psychiatr Res*, 1989, 28(2):193-213.

70. Vitiello, M.V., Prinz, P.N., & Schwartz, R.S. The subjective sleep quality of healthy older men and women is enhanced by participation in two fitness training programs: A nonspecific effect. *Sleep Res*, 1994, 23:148.

71. Jenkins, C.D., Stanton, B.A., Savageau, J.A., et al. Physical, psychological, social and economic outcomes six months after cardiac valve surgery. *Arch Int Med*, 1983, 143(11):2107-2113.

72. Croog, S.H., Levine, S., Testa, M.A., et al. The effects of antihypertensive therapy on the quality of life. *N Engl J Med*, 1986, 314(26):1657-1664.

73. Jenkins, C.D., Stanton, B.A., Niemcryk, S.J., & Rose, R.M. A scale for the estimation of sleep problems in clinical research. *J Clin Epidemiol*, 1988, 41(4):313-321.

74. Rose, R.M., Jenkins, C.D., & Hurst, M.W. Health change in air traffic controllers: A prospective study I. Background and description. *Psychosom Med*, 1978, 40(2):142-165.

75. Zomer, J., Peled, R., Rubin, A-H.E., & Lavie, P. Mini Sleep Questionnaire (MSQ) for screening large populations for EDS complaints. In W.P. Koella, E. Ruther, & H. Schulz (Eds.), *Sleep '84*. Stuttgart, Gustav Fischer Verlag, 1985, pp. 467-470.

76. Ellis, B.W., Johns, M.W., Lancaster, R., et al. The St. Mary's Hospital Sleep Questionnaire: A study of reliability. *Sleep*, 1981, 4(1):93-97.

77. Leigh, T.J., Bird, H.A., Hindmarch, I., et al. Factor analysis of the St. Mary's Hospital Sleep Questionnaire. *Sleep*, 1988, 11(5):448-453.

78. Ellis, B.W., Harris, R.I., Hayward, S.J., et al. Factors in the sleep of preoperative patients. *Br J Surg*, 1982, 69(5):281-282.

79. Parrott, A.C. & Hindmarch, I. The Leeds Sleep Evaluation Questionnaire in psychopharmacological investigations—A review. *Psychopharmacology*, 1980, 71(2):173-179.

80. Kronholm, E., & Hyyppa, M.T. Age-related sleep habits and retirement. *Ann Clin Res*, 1985, 17(5):257-264.

81. Hyyppa, M.T., Lindholm, T., Kronholm, E., & Lehtinen, V. Functional insomnia in relation to alexithymic features and cortisol hypersecretion in a community sample. *Stress Med*, 1990, 6(2):277-283.

82. Hyyppa, M.T., & Kronholm, E. Quality of sleep and chronic illnesses. *J Clin Epidemiol*, 1989, 42(7):633-638.

83. Douglass, A.B., Bornstein, R., Nino-Murcia, G., & Keenan, S. Creation of the "ASDC Sleep Disorders Questionnaire." *Sleep Res*, 1986, 15:117.

84. Douglass, A.B., Bornstein, R., Nino-Murcia, G., et al. The Sleep Disorders Questionnaire I. Creation and multivariate structure of SDQ. *Sleep*, 1994, 17(5):160-167.

85. Douglass, A.B., Bornstein, R., Nino-Murcia, G., et al. Test–retest reliability of the Sleep Disorders Questionnaire (SDQ). *Sleep Res*, 1990, 19:215.

86. Lee, K.A. Self-reported sleep disturbances in employed women. *Sleep*, 1992, 15(6):493-498.

87. Schramm, E., Hohagen, F., Grasshoff, U., et al. Test–retest reliability and validity of the structured interview for sleep disorders according to DSM-III-R. *Am J Psychiatr*, 1993, 150(6):867-872.

88. Reynolds, C.F., III, Giles, D.E., Buysse, D.J., et al. The structured interview for sleep disorders according to DSM-III-R. *Am J Psychiatr*, 1993, 150(6):857-858.

89. Rumble, R., & Morgan, K. Hypnotics, sleep and mortality in elderly people. *J Am Geriatr Soc*, 1992, 40(8):787-791.

90. Johnson, J.E. Progressive relaxation and the sleep of older men and women. *J Comm Health Nurs*, 1993, 10(1):31-38.

91. Snyder-Halpern, R., & Verran, J.A. Instrumentation to describe subjective sleep characteristics in healthy subjects. *Res Nurs Health*, 1987, 10(3):155-163.

92. Verran, J., & Snyder-Halpern, R. Do patients sleep in the hospital? *Appl Nurs Res*, 1988, 1(2):95.

93. Verran, J. Personal correspondence, March, 1994.

94. Richards, K. Techniques for measurement of sleep in critical care. *Focus Crit Care*, 1987, 14(4):34-40.

95. McDonald, D.G., & King, E.A. Measures of sleep disturbance in psychiatric patients. *Br J Med Psychol*, 1975, 48(1):49-53.

96. Nicassio, P.M., Mendlowitz, D.R., Fussell, J.J., & Petras, L. The phenomenology of the pre-sleep state: The development of the pre-sleep arousal scale. *Behav Res Ther*, 1985, 23(3):263-271.

97. Coren, S. Prediction of insomnia from arousability predisposition scores: Scale development and cross-validation. *Behav Res Ther*, 1988, 26(5):415-420.

98. Bootzin, R.R., Shoham, V., & Kuo, T.F. Sleep anticipatory anxiety questionnaire: A measure of anxiety about sleep. *Sleep Res*, 1994, 23:188.

99. van Diest, R. Subjective sleep characteristics as coronary risk factors, their association with type A behaviour and vital exhaustion. *J Psychosom Res*, 1990, 34(4):415-426.

100. Kapuniai, L.E., Andrew, D.J., Crowell, D.H., & Pearce, J.W. Identifying sleep apnea from self-reports. *Sleep*, 1988, 11:430-436.

101. Webb, W.B., Bonnet, M., & Blume, G. A post-sleep inventory. *Percept Motor Skills*, 1976, 43(3, part 1):987-993.

102. Domino, G., Blair, G., & Bridges, A. Subjective assessment of sleep by sleep questionnaire. *Percept Motor Skills*, 1984, 59(1):163-170.

103. Hunt, S.M., et al. A quantitative approach to perceived health status. *J Epidemiol Comm Health*, 1980, 34(4):281-286.

104. Alonso, J., Anto, J.M., Gonzalez, M., et al. Measurement of general health status of non-oxygen–dependent chronic obstructive pulmonary disease patients. *Med Care*, 1992, *30*(suppl 5):MS125-MS135.

105. McKenna, S.P., Hunt, S.M., & McEwen, J. Weighting the seriousness of perceived health problems using Thurstone's method of paired comparisons. *Int J Epidemiol*, 1981, *10*(1):93-97.

106. McKenna, S.P., McEwen, J., Hunt, S.M., & Papp, E. Changes in the perceived health of patients recovering from fractures. *Publ Health Lond*, 1984, *98*(2):97-102.

107. Hunt, S.D., McEwen, J., McKenna, S.P., et al. Subjective health status of patients with peripheral vascular disease, *Practitioner*, 1982, *226*(1363):133-136.

108. McDowell, I., & Newell, C. (Eds.). *Measuring health: A guide to rating scales and questionnaires*, New York, Oxford University Press, 1987.

109. Acebo, C., Sadeh, A., Seifer, R., et al. Mothers' assessment of sleep behaviors in young children: Scale reliability and validation during actigraphy. *Sleep Res*, 1994, *23*:96.

110. Morgan, K., Dallosso, H., Ebrahim, S., et al. Characteristics of subjective insomnia in the elderly living at home. *Age and ageing*, 1988, *17*(1):1-7.

111. Morgan, K., Dallosso, H., Ebrahim, S., et al. Prevalence, frequency, and duration of hypnotic drug use among the elderly living at home. *Br Med J*, 1988, *296*(6622):601-602.

112. Ferber, R. *Solve your childs sleep problems*. New York, Simon & Schuster, 1985.

113. Douglass, A.B., Carskadon, M., & Houser, R. Historical data base, questionnaires, sleep and life cycle diaries. In L.E. Miles & R.J. Broughton (Eds.), *Medical monitoring in the home and work environment*. New York, Raven, 1990, pp. 17-28.

114. Borkovec, T.D., & Weerts, T.C. Effects of progressive relaxation on sleep disturbance: An electroencephalographic evaluation. *Psychosom Med*, 1976, *38*(3):173-180.

115. Haythornthwaite, J.A., Hegel, M.T., & Sterns, R.D. (1991). Development of a sleep diary for chronic pain patients. *J Pain Symptom Man*, 1991, *6*(2):65-72.

116. Tokarz, T., & Lawrence, P. An analysis of temporal and stimulus factors in the treatment of insomnia. In R.R. Bootzin, & M. Engle-Friedman, The assessment of insomnia. *Behav Assess*, 1981, *3*:107-126.

117. Coates, T.J., Killen, J.D., George, J., et al. Estimating sleep parameters: A multitrait-multimethod analysis. *J Consult Clin Psychol*, 1982, *50*(3):345-352.

118. Lewis, H.E., Matthew, H., Proudfoot, A.T., et al. Nitrazepam—A safe hypnotic. *Lancet*, 1957, *2*(7008): 1262-1266.

119. Tune, G.S. The influence of age and temperament on the adult human sleep–wakefulness pattern. *Br J Psychol*, 1969, *60*(4):431-441.

120. Anders, T.F., Keener, M.A., & Kraemer, H. Sleep–wake state organization, neonatal assessment and development in premature infants during the first year of life. II. *Sleep*, 1985, *8*(3):193-206.

121. Kligman, D., Smyrl, R., & Emde, R.N. A "nonintrusive" longitudinal study of infant sleep. *Psychosom Med*, 1975, *37*(5):448-453.

122. Herbert, M., Johns, M.W., & Dore, C. Factor analysis of analogue scales measuring feelings before and after sleep. *Br J Med Psychol*, 1976, *49*(4):373-379.

123. Gift, A. Visual analogue scales: Measurement of subjective phenomena. *Nurs Res*, 1989, *38*(5):286-288.

124. Cline, M.E., Herman, J., Shaw, E.R., & Morton, R.D. Standardization of the visual analogue scale. *Nurs Res*, 1992, *41*(6):378-380.

125. Wewers, M.W., & Lowe, N.K. A critical review of visual analogue scales in the measurement of clinical phenomena. *Res Nurs Health*, 1990, *13*(4):227-238.

126. Roth, T., Roehrs, T., & Zorick, F. Sleepiness: Its measurement and determinants. *Sleep*, 1982, *5*(suppl 2):S128-S134.

127. Johnson, L.C., Spinweber, C.L., Gomez, S.A., & Matteson, L.T. Daytime sleepiness, performance, mood, nocturnal sleep: The effect of benzodiazepine and caffeine on their relationship. *Sleep*, 1990, *13*(2):121-135.

Appendices

18A. Studies Illustrating the Accuracy of Actigraphy

Author	Study Description	Results
Kripke et al. (45)	Compared EEG and actigraph (24 hours; $n = 5$)	Positive correlation for total sleep time (0.98)
		Positive correlation of minutes for wake time (0.85)
Hauri and Wisbey (46)	Compared duration of sleep data in insomniacs (1 week, $n = 36$)	Wrist actigraphy more exact than sleep logs but less exact than polysomnography
Mullaney et al. (47)	Wrist actigraph compared to EEG ($n = 85$)	Positive correlation for total sleep time (0.89)
		Positive correlation for wakening after sleep onset (0.70)
		Positive correlation for mid-sleep awakenings (0.25)
Sadeh et al. (48)	Compared sleep-disturbed and normal children (leg actigraph)	Discriminated between 2 groups
		Correct assignment rate 79.4% (sleep-disturbed) and 91.2% (control)
Pollmaecher and Schulz (49)	Compared EEG and actigraph ($n = 26$)	Excellent agreement in deeper sleep stages
		Poor agreement in transition from wakefulness and sleep (insomniacs or supine subjects)
Urbach et al. (50)	Efficacy of treatment for elder insomnia	Actigraph sensitive to treatment effects; reliably distinguishes sleep apnea from insomnia; distinguishes between sleep and wake states in narcolepsy
Newman et al. (51)		
Borbely (52)	Usefulness of wrist activity to examine medication course of action	Measured motor activity and to document sleep attacks in narcolepsy patient
Stampi and Broughton (53)	Compared wrist actigraph and polysomnography ($n = 1$)	Excellent agreement on total sleep time (baseline 99% and recovery 96.1%)
		Less agreement for ultrashort sleep (78.8%)
van Hilten et al. (54)	6 nights of study	Much intrasubject variability; varying results depending on subject and sleep parameter

Numbers in parentheses correspond to studies cited in the References.

18B. Instrumentation Measuring Sleep: Other Monitoring Devices

Name/Description	Psychometrics	Comments
Static charge–sensitive bed (SCSB, Biomatt, Biorec, Inc.) Flexible, sensitive plate placed under mattress	Not widely tested or used in the U.S.	Used to study heart, respiratory, and body movements during sleep Can combine with other assessments Inexpensive
Home monitoring system (HMS) Uses pressure-sensitive mattress pad, signals from respiration and body movements are transmitted Patterns of signals identify sleep, wakefulness, respiratory events, leg movements	Signal scoring procedure reliable and valid (55)	Has been used with elderly and infants
Pressure-sensitive mattress with capacitance-type sensor/amplifier (electronic monitors)	Tandberg instrument recorded 5 states of sleep, computer results compared to observer (55)	Used to study infants
Holter ECG with ear oximetry and breath sound monitoring	In obstructive sleep apnea, there is progressive bradycardia associated with apnea followed by abrupt tachycardia	Used to measure cyclic variation of heart rate and snoring Inexpensive ($100)
Medilog/Respitrace recording system (Ambulatory Monitoring, Inc.)	Wrist actigraph transducer distinguishes sleep from waking (36)	Respirations recorded on Respitrace bands; combined with tibialis EMG
Sleep assessment device (SAD) (Farrall Instruments, Inc., Grand Is, Nebraska)	Compared to EEG recording and sleep questionnaire: percent agreement 83.3%–100% (56)	If awake, subject verbally acknowledges soft tone played every 10 minutes (tape recorded)
Infant state bassinet monitor consists of foam cell air mattress connected via tube to stratham pressure unit (Burwin baby monitor) with output sent to digital event recorder	High correlation with standard sleep polygraph (57) Infant respiratory patterns and movements can be assessed (57)	Pressure-sensitive foot mat to detect caregiver can be added (58) Modified version used to categorize infant movements (59)

Numbers in parentheses correspond to studies cited in the References.

18C. Other Questionnaires and Interviews to Measure Sleep

Name/Description	Psychometric Indices	Comments
Sleep Dysfunction Scale/Sleep Problems Scale 4 questions to ascertain the number of days the subject has problems: falling asleep, staying asleep, awakening early, or tired Coding is a 0–5 Likert-type scale (ATC) or 1–4 Scores may be summed: lower scores, less sleep disturbance	Cronbach's alpha: 0.79 (ATC) and 0.63 (CSRS) (71); 0.79 (72) Test–retest reliability: 0.59 (73) Concurrent validity (taking or not taking certain medications)	Developed from Air Traffic Controllers (ATC) and Cardiac Surgery Recovery Study (CSRS) (71,74) Called Sleep Problems Questionnaire by Jenkins et al. (73)
MiniSleep Questionnaire (MSQ) Contains 7 items Scaled from 1 (never) to 7 (always)	Mean scores for each item and for total MSQ can be determined "Outstanding stability" (75)	Developed to assess excessive daytime somnolence in large populations Work continues on refining selection criteria
St. Mary's Hospital Sleep Questionnaire 14 items evaluate sleep and early-morning behavior in past 24 hours 3 variables (sleep latency, sleep period time, awake onset latency) High score means "good sleep"	"Good" test–retest reliability Factor analysis showed no completely clear structure (77) 2 factors emerged: sleep latency and sleep quality	Evaluates sleep in hospitalized patients Has been used to detect changes in sleep of hospitalized surgical patients (78) and to compare the sleep of patients with arthritic diseases
Leeds Sleep Evaluation Questionnaire (SEQ) Consists of 10 questions, with responses on a visual analog scale (10-cm line with words denoting extremes at each end) subject is asked to mark the line where it approximates his answer	Factor analysis revealed 4 factors corresponding to the 4 areas questioned Reasonable degree of reliability and validity (79)	Formerly known as Sleep Evaluation Questionnaire Used to monitor self-reported perceptions of sleep during drug treatment for sleep problems Questions explore 4 areas: getting to sleep, quality of sleep, awakening, and behavior following wakefulness
Rehabilitation Research Center Sleep Habit Questionnaire (RRC-SHQ) Originally consisted of 65 multiple-choice items Scoring has several indices (additive and dichotomous	2 factors: depression-related insomnia and satisfaction with sleep (account for 39% of variance) (80) Good test–retest stability (81) "Acceptable validity and reliability" (82)	Questions relate to sleep environment, behavior, subjective feelings re: wakefulness, satisfaction with sleep quality, daytime sleepiness, initiating and maintaining sleep, dreams, other (82)
Sleep Questionnaire and Assessment of Wakefulness (SQAW) 863 items (multiple-choice, dichotomous, and fill-in)	No data found	Developed by Laughton Miles at Stanford University Clinical screening tool No scoring information available

ASDC Sleep Disorders Questionnaire 165 variables		Shortened version of SQAW Designed to predict, polysomnographic diagnosis (83)
Sleep Disorders Questionnaire Intent to develop "triage" questionnaire with diagnostic point of view 175 items plus body mass index, at 8th-grade reading level Response choices 1 to 5 on Likert-type scale Scoring manual being developed (84)	Reliability 0.7 overall correlation (2 weeks) (85) Canonical discriminant function analysis performed Criterion validity: related polysomnography and MSLT results to the specific group	Derived from SQAW May serve as a database and screening tool for referrals to sleep laboratory (83,85) Specific diagnostic scales developed were: sleep apnea, narcolepsy, psychiatric sleep disorder, and periodic leg movements
General Sleep Disturbance Scale (GSDS) 21 items Self-rated 10-point scale from 0 (never) to 9 (all the time) Can be broken down into 7 subscales Score: summed from 0 to 189 Higher score, more severely disturbed sleep (86)	Cronbach's alpha: overall 0.88 3 subscales: (1) use of sleep aids: 0.62; (2) sleep quality: 0.79; (3) sleepiness: 0.82 Validity: developed refined from SQAW and statistical difference between permanent and rotating shift nurses	Developed by Lee, a nurse investigator Items address sleep quality, quantity, initiating sleep, fatigue, alertness at work, use of drugs for sleep, others
Structured Interview for Sleep Disorders (DSM-III-R) (SIS-D) Structured clinical interview: semistructured section (e.g., health, meds), structured (sleep disorder symptoms) Takes 20–30 minutes Summary score sheet Instruction manual (87)	Validity: concordance between consensus diagnosis and polysomnographic data (90% confirmation) Test–retest reliability (Cohen's kappa: mean: 0.77) Reliability: 0.56–0.89 Interrater reliability 97%–100% (87)	Fits with forthcoming DSM-IV criteria (88) Used to screen and diagnose sleep disorders Useful screening instrument (88)
Nottingham Longitudinal Study of Activity and Aging Profiles health, well-being and assesses sleep and sleep meds	Not reported	Begun in 1985 to collect baseline data No significant relationships between mortality and subjective insomnia or sleep duration (89)
Baekland, Hoy: Unnamed Sleep Log Modified from Antrobus et al. (86) Also known as "sleep pattern questionnaire" 2-week log of: (A) state of mind, fatigue before retiring, on awakening (3 items); and (B) 8 items completed on awakening (time fell asleep, number of awakenings, state of sleep, dreams)	No composite scoring Test–retest reliability: (A) 0.84, and (B) 0.97 only 7 items (90) Theta reliability: 0.76 (91)	Questionnaire results similar to EEG (14)

18C. Other Questionnaires and Interviews to Measure Sleep (*cont.*)

Name/Description	Psychometric Indices	Comments
Veran and Snyder-Halpern (VSH) Sleep Scale Uses visual analog scale (91,92) Author-modified original scale (8 items sleep, 2 dreams)	Original scale compared to St. Mary's Hospital's Sleep Q and Baekland/Hoy log: theta reliability coefficient: 0.82; factor analysis and correlations showed validity	New scale has 15 items (disturbance, effectiveness, supplementation) Can calculate total sleep period (TSP) Ongoing testing in U.S. and Taiwanese populations (93)
Richards-Campbell Sleep Questionnaire (94) 5-item VAS (e.g., to sleep depth, quality), 0 (poorest quality) to 100 (optimal)	Content construct validity Cronbach's alpha (internal consistency reliability): 0.82	Revised instrument requires further testing (94)
Complaints of Sleep Disturbance Scale (CSD) 20 items from the MMPI (sleep, fatigue, dreams)	Correlation between sleep monitor and CSD score: 0.62 (95)	Distinguishes between subjects with high and low sleep motility
Pre-sleep Arousal Scale (PSAS) (96) 16 item, self-report 2 subscales: (A) somatic; and (B) cognitive Subscale scores range from 8 to 40	Face validity 100% Somatic subscale (A) correlates significantly with CSAQ (0.36), as does cognitive subscale (B) (0.49) Construct validity Internal consistency reliability (A) 0.79–0.84, and (B) 0.67–0.88 Test–retest correlations (over 3 weeks): 0.76 (A) and 0.72 (B)	Discriminates among normal sleepers and insomniacs
Arousal Predisposition Scale (APS) Premise is that insomniacs have higher levels of autonomic activity (19,97) Initial 70 items reduced to 12 Items summed for composite score (higher scores show greater arousal)	Internal consistency reliability: 0.83–0.84 Validation studies conducted; "valid and reliable indicator of a pattern of sleep disruptions and insomnia"	Value: predicts tendency toward sleep disruption in general population (97)
Sleep Anticipatory Anxiety Questionnaire (SAAQ) (98) Assesses presleep anxiety 10 items Higher scores indicate more anxiety	Cronbach's alpha for internal consistency: 0.83 Factor analysis: (1) overall degree of presleep anxiety, (2) extent of cognitive experience as opposed to somatic arousal	Construct validity currently being evaluated

Instrument	Properties	Comments
Sleep Wake Experience List (SWEL) 15 items	Screening quality: average to high (kappa: 52.3%–90.3%) (99) Diagnostic/prognostic: average (K = 51.1%–78.0%) (99)	Also used to assess snoring, napping, and sleep duration
Apnea Score Derived from Hawaii Sleep Questionnaire (100) 2 items	Said to be 10% effective in identifying individuals with moderate to severe sleep apnea by polysomnography	2 items refer to (1) presence of loud snoring and (2) stopping breathing during sleep
Post Sleep Inventory (101) 29 items, bipolar anchor endpoints 13-point scale	Orthogonal rotation, principal component analysis: 7 factors High construct validity Sensitive measure	3 categories of items
Sleep Questionnaire 55 items Choices are Likert-type Scoring not described	Test-retest reliability (10 weeks): 0.79 (102) Internal consistency reliability, Cronbach's alpha: 0.76 (median) Factor analysis: 7 factors (71.7% of variance)	Clinical judgment and factor scales undergoing further testing
Nottingham Health Profile (103) Self-report, 2-part questionnaire 5 sleep-related items (yes-no) Weighted score or summed score (104,105)	Questionnaire valid, reproducible, sensitive to change (104,106) Face, content and criterion validity established (103) Test-retest reliability: 0.75–0.88 (107,108)	
Child Sleep Habits Questionnaire (SHQ) Parental assessment of child sleep habits 63 items, 5 scales	High test-retest reliability; good internal consistency for "bedtime" scale, moderate reliability for remainder (109)	Scales are bedtime problems, sleep problems, night waking, daytime sleepiness, morning problems

Numbers in parentheses correspond to studies cited in the References.

19

Attitudes Toward Chronic Illness

Rebecca F. Cohen

Chronic illness is the number-one health problem in the United States. Between 1900 and 1970, a shift was seen in mortality patterns. Death from acute infections was supplanted by an increase of more than 250% in mortality rates from major chronic diseases. These changes have brought about the need for a new arrangement of values and priorities in health-care policy, finance, and management.[1]

Traditionally, professionals approached chronic symptom management in terms of compliance and service utilization and attempted to engineer the patient to the health team's treatment goals. However, it has been noted that this approach fails to incorporate an appreciation of the role of personality variables in the development and outcome of chronic illness, as well as how chronic illness affects the individual emotionally and psychologically.

If health-care providers are to influence the patient's adaptation to chronic illness, they must acknowledge the lay perception of illness and understand what the patient sees as relevant. A strong relationship has been shown between coping styles and attitudes and treatment results. This is important to remember because ineffective coping styles and damaging attitudes can adversely affect treatment outcomes and, therefore, need to be identified early. By studying coping styles, perception, attitudes, beliefs, and illness behavior, we may be able not only to affect treatment outcomes (including mortality rates) and adaptation to chronic illness, but also the initial development of the illness process itself.[1]

There has been a proliferation of chronic illness studies from a variety of perspectives designed to evaluate the outcome of physical illness and its treatments, as well as the patient's response to physical disease.[2] Some of the instruments used to measure a patient's attitudes toward chronic disease discussed in this chapter also appear in other chapters. In terms of function, this overlap of instruments should be considered when determining which tool to use for a research project. Chronic illness affects an individual in many ways: physically, psychologically, spiritually, emotionally. Often, what appears simple on the surface really is quite complicated (e.g., when measuring disability).

It is important not only to consider what the patient cannot do, but also what he or she *will* not do, for each may result in the same degree of confinement. As we learn more about the human mind and body, the measurement tools used grow more comprehensive in terms of approaching the patient as a whole rather than as a discrete entity. This chapter points out, and emphasizes, the growth that has occurred in the development of tools to measure patient attitudes.

Measures of Ability to Function

With the increasing numbers of elderly in our society, and a similar increase in the need for long-term care, there have been many instruments developed to measure physical functioning to determine the patient's needs so that they can be assigned to the appropriate level of care. These instruments also assess the adequacy and composition of staff and determine how patients respond to various modes of treatment. Some scales, such as the Sickness Impact Profile[3] and Rand Measures of Health Status,[4] measure health status, that is, the patient's overall health as described by diagnoses, doctor visits, days in bed, number of therapeutic drugs, self-assessed health, pain, and other variables, including the ability to perform everyday activities. Other measures, such as the Cumulative Illness Rating Scale,[5] measure impairment, that is, the extent of organic pathologic change determined by a physician. Disability, or how limitations of activities and functioning affect a person, often is measured by using the Barthel Index[6,7] and the Evaluation of Levels of Subsistence.[8]

Parts of scales that measure disability can be divided further into items that specifically measure either activities of daily living (ADL) or instrumental activities of daily living (IADL). Examples of ADL scales include the Index of ADL[9] and the Physical Self-Maintenance Scale.[10] Examples of IADL scales are the Instrumental Activities of Daily Living Scale[10] and a subscale of the Multidimensional Functional Assessment (OARS) Scale. Some scales combine ADL and IADL items or may include other health status variables.[11]

Linn and Linn[11] point out that in institutions most functional status tests are completed by nurses or nursing attendants according to their observations of the patients. When used in the community, rating systems are often self-report inventories. Scales vary regarding the numbers of response choices, ranging from simple dichotomous (yes–no) scales to the 11-point Sickness Impact Profile Scale. Although the purpose of the yes–no response is to allow untrained persons to rate the answers reliably, one disadvantage is that less variance in behavior can be described, and, thus, the scale may not be sensitive to treatment changes or to discrimination in levels of functioning. On the other hand, even trained raters find it difficult to distinguish between 11 different levels of an item such as bathing. Generally, scales that maintain the best discrimination—and are easy to administer—involve only four to seven responses.

Another problem with most of the instruments available to measure physical functioning is that they lack definition specificity and can be unreliable. For example, does one measure whether an activity "is" or "can be" performed? A person may be physically able to dress unassisted, but does not do so because of severe depression. One observer could rate the subject as able to dress without assistance, and another could rate the subject as requiring full assistance. Another source of discrepancy arises from the lack of specificity about conditions for making assessments. The scale may not indicate whether the person is to be evaluated with or without glasses, a hearing aid, or other prostheses.[11]

The following four instruments measure the impact of chronic illness on the patient's ability to function and offer unique, broad approaches to the concept of human health. The Rapid Disability Rating Scale-2 and Simplified Disability Assessment Scales are geared toward what the patient actually does, not what they are able to do, as well as certain psychologic functioning. The Sickness Impact Profile (SIP) measures the impact of illness in terms of dysfunction, not levels of positive functioning, and evaluates psychosocial and physical health. The Arthritis Impact Measurement Scale measures physical health and emotional well-being.

Rapid Disability Rating Scale-2

In response to the limitations of available instruments, Linn and Linn[11] revised Linn's Rapid Disability Rating Scale[12] into the Rapid Disability Rating Scale-2 (RDRS-2). Ratings in the RDRS-2 are based on what the person does and not on what he or she is able to do. There are 18 items, with four-point scales ranging from no assistance or disability to severe. The first group of items measures the ADL, and later items assess related disabilities and special problems of confusion, depression, and uncooperativeness to provide clues concerning the reasons for disability.

Items on the RDRS-2 are scored from 1 (none) to 4 (severe). Total scores can range from 18 (no disability) to 72 (if the responses are all chosen from the most severe disabilities). Item definitions and instructions for ratings appear on the scale, so that little training is needed in making assessments. The scale can be used by any person who knows the subject to be rated and who has observed him or her performing ADL.[11]

Intraclass correlations between the findings of two nurses who independently rated the same 100 patients were found to range from $r = 0.62$ to a high of $r = 0.98$; all were statistically significant. Reliability also was shown by testing the same 50 patients twice within a 3-day period. Test–retest values ranged from $r = 0.58$ to $r = 0.96$ between the first and second ratings by Pearson's product–moment correlations.[11]

Rating scale measurements using both the RDRS-2 and the Maryland-Barthel Disability Index[7] found that the test of functional status usefully predicts outcome. Items on the RDRS-2 were used to predict mortality in a stepwise multiple regression analysis as well as by discriminant function analysis. All items together reached an r of 0.20, with the best predictors of mortality being the need for assistance with eating, incontinence, time in bed, diet, and depression. For accuracy of classification, the scale held a 72% accuracy rate in mortality prediction.[11]

Rapid Disability Assessment Scale

A simplified test for the evaluation of patients with chronic illness developed by Sett[13] is an attempt to simplify the measurement of disability in hospitalized patients. Although developed quite some time ago, it can still serve as a useful tool in caring for patients with chronic illnesses and should be expanded beyond its use with cerebrovascular accident (CVA) patients.

Sett[13] studied other disability instruments and chose among ADL three areas he considered the most essential factors for patient independence for self-care at home: ambulation, self-care, and communication. Four examiners separately performed the testing procedures on 20 patients who had had a CVA. They were instructed not to communicate their findings until each had tested the patient in the designated ADL areas. The chi-square test was applied to the data to determine the statistical significance. The p value was less than 0.01 in all three areas. This simplified disability test was conducted in the following manner:[13,p1096]

Ambulation. The patient was asked to demonstrate his ability to walk or perform a transfer to or from a wheelchair. A five-point scale (0 patient is confined to bed to 5 patient walks without assistance) was used.

Self-care. The self-care item tested the patient's ability to carry out ADL such as eating, dressing, bathing, and toilet care. Seven questions plus observation were used to rate the patient on a five-point scale (0 patient is unable to perform any of the ADL without assistance to 5 patient performs ADL using both upper extremities).

Communication. Scores on nine questions ranged from 0 (patient has severe expressive-receptive [global] aphasia) to 5 (patient has neither aphasia nor dysarthria). The test was a modification of the Schuell technique.

Sickness Impact Profile (SIP)

The Sickness Impact Profile (SIP) was developed to provide a measure of perceived health status sensitive enough to detect changes or differences in health status occurring over time or between groups. It is useful for a variety of illness types and severity, as well as demographic and cultural subgroups. Furthermore, the SIP, which measures the behavioral impact of illness in terms of dysfunction, not levels of positive functioning, is intended to provide a measure of the efforts or outcomes of health care that can be used for evaluation, program planning, and policy formulation.

The instrument contains 136 questions answered in a yes–no format and takes 15 to 35 minutes to complete. It can be administered by an interviewer or self-administered. In completing the SIP, the subject must check only those statements that describe him on a given day and are related to his health.[14] Each item is weighted. The instrument has 12 subscales, seven of which aggregate into two dimensions, physical (ambulation, mobility, body care, and movement) and psychosocial (alertness and emotional behaviors, social activities, communication). A global score (the seven subscales plus eating, recreation, home maintenance, sleep, and rest) is calculated as the weighted sum of all items.[15]

The test–retest reliability of the SIP had an r of 0.92, internal consistency had an r of 0.94, and overall reliability in terms of score was high ($r = 0.75$–0.92) Reliability did not appear to be significantly affected by the variables examined, and results suggest that the SIP is potentially useful for measuring dysfunction under a variety of administrative conditions and with a variety of subjects.[16]

The SIP has been used widely in health services and clinical research since the 1970s. It is considered one of the most responsive instruments used to measure the impact of joint arthroplasty on quality of life[15] and also has been used with persons that have a variety of chronic diseases[17-23] In addition, Sanders[24] tested the instrument on subjects with chronic low-back pain in six different culture groups including Americans, Japanese, Mexicans, Colombians, Italians, and New Zealanders. Findings from their study indicate that the SIP is useful in identifying important cross-cultural differences in chronic pain patients' self-perceived level of dysfunction. American patients were found to be the most dysfunctional, and various explanations for this difference were suggested by the authors. A French version of the original U.S. version of the SIP also has been created because it was felt that a simple, direct translation of the scale was inadequate.[25]

The SIP shows good correlations with other health status and functional status measures and appears to be a reliable instrument with sufficient content validity, but a number of questions regarding its effectiveness remain unanswered. DeBruin et al.[26] conducted a review of the literature on the SIP and found that these unresolved questions related to the theoretical implications of the construct of sickness, the effect of age and gender on SIP scores, the construct validity judged by factor analysis, the responsiveness of the instrument, and whether the list can be shortened and the scoring procedure simplified. They suggest that further evaluation of the methodologic and theoretical aspects of the instrument needs to be done if it is to be used as an international standard measure of functional status.

An interesting question about the results of the SIP Scale, as useful as it may be, is that of the reliability of self-ratings versus ratings by service providers when analyzing disability or dysfunction. Kivela[27] points out that there are three main methods by which disability can be measured: clinical assessment of the individual's performance; questioning the individual about the level of daily performance; and standard tests of individual performance conducted by a trained observer. This study compared a questionnaire-based measure of disability with evaluations by health-care professionals. A total of 205 chronic patients and elderly persons receiving home nursing or home help services or both were included in the study. A questionnaire was developed that used the activities listed in standardized measurements of ADL and IADL. Comparisons between the self-report and rater assessments of performance were then made for individual activities of self-care and domestic duties, including the following six activities: dressing, eating, daily washing, bathing or sauna, cooking, and cleaning.[27]

Results indicated that agreement between the questionnaire-based and the provider ratings was high for basic self-care activities but not high for housework. Kivela[27] points out that the extent of the observer's earlier knowledge about the patient's performance and about their environment may have affected the results, as may have the differences in the educational levels of the observers.

Arthritis Impact Measurement Scales (AIMS)

Meenan et al.[28] developed the Arthritis Impact Measurement Scales (AIMS) to measure three areas of human health (physical, emotional, and social well-being) and to meet the need for a reliable, valid, and comprehensive measure of the health of patients with arthritis.

AIMS built on two previously tested health status measures: Bush's Index of Well-Being and the Rand Health Insurance Study batteries. The Index of Well-Being is a behaviorally based scale that includes three function/dysfunction scales (mobility, physical activity, social activity) and a symptom-problem complex. The Rand approach combines the three behavioral components of the Index of Well-Being with psychologic scales for anxiety and depression. Both approaches have undergone extensive testing and refinement.[28]

AIMS consists of demographic and health status items arranged into nine scale groups as follows: mobility (5 items); physical activity (5); social activity (9); social role (7); activities of daily living (5); pain (5); dexterity (5); anxiety (8); and depression (6). The remaining 11 items related to health perceptions and overall estimates of functional status and arthritis severity.[28] These nine subscales can be aggregated into three health status dimensions: physical function, psychologic function, and pain. Each dimension has a range of 0 to 10, with a higher score indicating more limitation and lower health status.[29]

Shortened forms of the AIMS have been tested on patients with rheumatoid arthritis or total hip replacement. Lorish et al.[30] found that, after reducing the 45-item AIMS to 22 items, alpha reliabilities and test–retest correlations indicated that the full and short scales were comparably reliable on all scales except for pain. Although the convergent validity coefficients were comparable between the short and full versions, the short mobility, pain, depression, and anxiety scales were not comparable to the full scales in detecting changes from baseline. Thus, if minimizing the number of items used with the AIMS is desired, while maximizing reliability and validity, the short versions of physical activity, household activity, dexterity, ADL, and social activity should be used with the full version of mobility, pain, depression, and anxiety. Katz et al.[15] used a shortened version of the AIMS (sAIMS), which was an 18-item questionnaire divided into 9 subscales, on 54 patients undergoing total hip replacement. Two of the five items from each subscale of the original AIMS that had the highest internal consistency and correlation with the total AIMS score were selected. Results from their study indicated that the sAIMS was sensitive to clinical change on the global dimension, but not on the physical dimension.

In the initial research conducted by Meenan et al.,[28] individual health status items showed an impressive degree of disease impact in the study group. The AIMS instrument was found to be easily completed by patients; the scales had face validity and were easy to score in either Guttman or Likert format; and, after deleting some questions that led to confusion or had low item–total correlation, all of the scales, with the exception of Social Activity, fulfilled a number of generally accepted criteria for reliability and scalability. The significance of the correlations held for both patient-generated and physician-generated health status proxies.

A later study of patients with osteoarthritis, conducted by Weinberger et al.,[31] found that both exposure to stressors and low self-esteem support were associated with increased disability along all AIMS dimensions. Physical disability was associated with being older and having less "tangible" support; psychologic disability with being younger, Caucasian, and having less "belonging" support; and pain with being younger, Caucasian, and having less education. Self-esteem was the most consistent social support dimension when predicting functional status. Thus, the AIMS instrument was found to be practical, simple, and dependable and should prove useful for evaluating a wide variety of interventions in the field of rheumatology.[28]

Measures of Illness Behavior

The concepts of *illness behavior* and *sick role* have tremendous implications for public health programs, estimated needs for medical care, medical economics, and our understanding of health and illness in general. For example, what is the influence of various norms, values, fears, and expected rewards and punishments on how a symptomatic person behaves? What makes one person "suffer in silence," whereas another seeks immediate health care for the slightest discomfort? Are there systematic differences in illness behavior in given populations, and, if so, what effect would these differences have on the provision of educational and informational programs? All of these questions have been addressed in various research investigations through three very important instruments: Dimensions of the Sick Role, the Illness Behavior Questionnaire (IBQ), and the Illness Self-Concept Repertory Grid.

Dimensions of the Sick Role

The term *illness behavior* refers to the ways in which symptoms may be differentially perceived, evaluated, and acted (or not acted) upon by different kinds of persons. Kassebaum and Baumann[32] conducted research more than 20 years ago to study the sick role and illness behavior in patients with chronic illness.

Patients with one or more primary diagnoses of chronic illness respond to 20 statements with stipulated response alternatives ranging from "strongly disagree" to "strongly agree" on a seven-point Likert-type scale. Factor analysis was selected because it permits subjects to "group" items cognitively. A scale was constructed for each factor, using the factor's most highly loaded items. Each respondent was given a sum score on each factor's scale. The distribution of scores for each factor scale was trichotomized into "high," "medium," and "low" categories. Factor analysis yielded four distinct dimensions underlying sick role expectations: dependence, reciprocity, role-performance, and denial.

High scores on individual dimensions of the sick role varied with age, sex, ethnic origin, education, occupational category, and diagnosis. Chronic illness, the investigators suggested, may, therefore, be regarded as one subtype of sick role, having special characteristics. Patients with chronic illness are likely to perceive the structure of the sick role along dimensions that differ from those perceived by patients with acute, temporary illness. Also, within the broad classification of chronic illness, they found that different diagnoses had different consequences for people (e.g., patients with arteriosclerotic heart disease were found to have almost double the number of high scores on the dimensions of dependence, reciprocity, role performance and denial than patients with diabetes; diabetics were distinguished from other diseases studied by their low level of denial). For this reason, the authors suggested further research into the concept of the sick role and illness behavior in terms of different types of illness, different social settings and different segments of the population.[32] The Illness Behavior Questionnaire was later developed to serve as a useful tool in such research efforts.

Illness Behavior Questionnaire (IBQ)

To better understand the concept of illness behavior in relation to a specific symptom (in this case, pain), Pilowsky and Spence[33] conducted a research study with unselected patients (48 men, 52 women with a mean age of 49.1 years) referred to either the pain clinic or the psychiatric service of a large metropolitan hospital for the management of intractable pain. They developed the 52-item Illness Behavior Questionnaire (IBQ) to determine the patient's attitudes and feelings about illness, perception of the reactions of significant others in the environment (including doctors) to self and illness, and the patient's own view of his current psychosocial situation. Pain is addressed in another chapter, but this questionnaire is discussed in the section on Chronic Illness Measurements because of its potential for a variety of medical illnesses and/or symptoms and its importance in trying to understand how patients feel about their illness/symptoms.

The seven subscales of the IBQ are general hypochondriasis, disease conviction, psychologic versus somatic perception of illness, affective inhibition, affective disturbance, denial of problems, and irritability.[33]

The results of data analysis showed six principal clusters of patients, each with definite illness behavior characteristics. Groups 1 to 3 had a relatively non-neurotic, reality-oriented attitude toward illness indicated by low scores on the first three scales. The symptom (pain) experience seemed as an adaptive reaction to stress, but one that obscured all other aspects of the stress response. Groups 4 to 6 related more clearly to the syndrome of "abnormal illness behavior." The symptom (pain) was interwoven with and was symptomatic of a personality disorder or an essentially maladaptive response to psychologic stress.[33]

The IBQ, in addition to being used with patients with pain, has been used to assess behavior in patients with neurologic diseases, psychiatric disorders, cancer, and a variety of other diseases including "EI," environmental illness.[34] It is interesting to note the study by Tatarelli et al.[34] of patients with gynecologic cancer. Findings suggest that illness behavior is almost totally involved in a belief dimension: cultural stereotypes of cancer as a fatal illness influence patients' reactions to the disease as well as their delay in seeking care.

Illness Self-Concept Repertory Grid (ISCRG)

In an attempt to extend use of the IBQ, Large[35] used a repertory grid technique involving various self-concepts as "elements" and concepts drawn from the IBQ as "constructs." It was expected that, because they presumably conceived of themselves as being ill, subjects scoring high on the disease conviction scale of the IBQ would similarly rate themselves toward the ill pole of the "illness construct" of the grid. Because illness is considered undesirable, one might expect a considerable difference on this construct between the patient's actual self-concept and his ideal self-concept. The patients with the greatest discrepancy between actual self-concept and ideal self-concept were hypothesized to have the most self-dissatisfaction and, therefore, would have the most motivation toward treatment and show the greatest improvement.

The grid is constructed using *elements* ("as I am, as I would like to be, as others see me, as my doctor sees me") and bipolar constructs.[35] In the original study done by Large,[35] 18 patients with chronic musculoskeletal pain were told that the purpose of the study was to gain some insight into their views of themselves and their world and, therefore, they were being asked to complete a questionnaire. The repertory grids were then completed by each patient during an initial interview in which the subject was exposed to biofeedback. A second grid was completed at the final interview (post-trial), using identical elements and constructs.

The grids were analyzed by means of the principal component analysis devised by Slater for use with individual grids. The main focus of interest was the distance between element 1 (as I am) or "self" and element 2 (as I would like to be) or "ideal self," derived from the initial grid for each subject. The Spearman rank-correlation coefficient was computed between three rankings: changes in pain scores calculated pre- and post-trial; distances between element 1 ("self") and 2 ("ideal-self"); and correlations between electromyelogram activity ratings and pain scores. The rank correlation between pain score changes and element 1 to 2 distances was $r = 0.43$, ($p < 0.05$). Thus, the greater the distance between elements 1 and 2, the greater the decline in pain scores.[35]

In a study by Large,[36] the effect of participation in a pain-management program on self-concept and attitudes toward illness was investigated. It was found that, despite the fact that no change in symptoms was seen, differences between the pre- and postrepertory grids showed a significant increase in the distance between "as I would like to be" and "like a physically ill person." This suggested that physical illness had become less desirable after participation in the pain-management program. It appeared that the program helped the patients to adopt a more balanced view of physical illness as being undesirable and as including both physical and emotional factors. He hypothesized that the findings indicate that attitudes may be more important than symptoms in determining subsequent illness behavior. Large and James,[37] investigating the use of hypnosis for pain, suggest from their results that pain relief may so powerfully alter self-concept that a shift occurs in self-view from illness to wellness. However, it also is possible that a fixed self-view of illness may neutralize treatments such as hypnosis.

The ISCRG is, therefore, a useful research tool because of its flexibility and ability to produce quantifiable data that allow comparison across both individuals and time. The tool provides insight into the individual and can be used to guide the clinician in evaluating and planning treatment because of its ability to identify clinically meaningful changes in self-concept. The grid could be useful as an instrument to predict the optimum timing of treatment, to predict when the patient is ready to respond to treatment, but further testing is needed to determine whether some of the instability found in measurement is due to treatment effects.[37]

Measures of Locus Control

Closely related to the concept of illness behavior are beliefs about internal versus external control. Through comprehensive investigation of how patients with chronic illness feel about themselves, the world around them, and the relationship between the two, techniques can be tailored to individual expectancies to increase the possibility of a successful treatment outcome. Two different reinforcement patterns lead to either the general expectancy that rewards are contingent on internal resources (such as effort) or the general expectancy that rewards are externally related to things such as luck, chance, fate, or powerful others. General expectancy is referred to as "locus of control." The Health Locus of Control (HLC) Scale, Health Specific Locus of Control Beliefs Questionnaire, and the Attribution Interview Schedule are three instruments related to locus of control. These measures are described in Appendix 19A.[38-46]

Although the presence of attributional thinking in everyday life has been supported in numerous studies, the assumption that it always occurs in important or unexpected life situations was not as readily evident. Lowery et al.,[47] wanting to investigate the finding that some patients search for a cause to their illness while others do not, compared a sample of chronically ill and acutely ill patients to determine differences in causal search. Chronic patients had either diabetes, arthritis, or hypertension, and acute patients were hospitalized with stable myocardial infarction.

The results of this study indicated that more than half of each sample had not thought "Why me?" These subjects, in both acute and chronic illness groups, had better affect scores and higher expectations for recovery than those who had engaged in causal thinking. The length of time an individual had had a chronic illness also was not related to their having thought about the question "Why me?"[47]

Thus, contrary to Weiner's theoretical contention that causal thinking is pervasive, differences in affect were not found between those who had and those who had not come up with a cause. Rather, it was the element of the search itself that was associated with affective and expectancy differences, not the construction of a cause.[47] These results also were verified in a study conducted by Weaver and Narsavage[48] with patients with chronic obstructive pulmonary disease. Findings from both studies suggested that causal search may not be the first step in adjustment to a problem and may, in fact, not be the best adjustment mechanism in acute and chronic illness situations. Contemplating causal questions appears to play a significant role in functional status by producing discontentment and disappointment in illness situations where answers are not well defined. Preoccupation with causal search may limit problem solving, thus interfering with the adjustment process.[47,48]

Measures Related to Children with Chronic Diseases

Although many instruments have been developed to evaluate how the patient with a chronic illness feels and thinks, there are few geared specifically to assessing the perceptions of parents who have children with chronic disease. The Chronicity Impact and Coping Instrument: Parent Questionnaire is used to evaluate the effect of chronic disease on the family and to gain information related to how parents cope with the difficulties encountered as a result of their child's illness. Another tool, the Roberts Apperception Test for Children (RATC) has been used to assess the presence of serious emotional disturbances in children. Its use has been extended to help identify maladaptive coping mechanisms in children with chronic diseases. Both are described in Appendix 19B.[49-51]

Appendix 19C presents other available measures.[52-64] These tools are different from those previously discussed in that they tend to be less conceptual and more straightforward concerning attitudes toward chronic disease and characteristics of individuals with chronic disease. Some were tested only on well subjects, and others included well subjects, but they all have many implications for use with patients with chronic disease.

Summary

This chapter has reviewed concepts underlying the development of instruments to measure the impact of chronic illness on patients and in the case of children, on their parents. Specific instruments have been discussed, and others presented for reference.

Exemplar Studies

Large, R. Self-concepts and illness attitudes in chronic pain. A repertory grid study of a pain management program. *Pain*, 1985, *23*(2):113-119.

This study exemplifies the measurement of attitudes toward chronic illness. The Illness Self-Concept Repertory Grid and Illness Behavior Questionnaire was used to determine the impact of an outpatient pain-management program on pain levels in patients with chronic pain. Although no changes in the symptom inventories or in daily visual measurements of pain were shown, the repertory grids showed a significant change in self-concept. The main impact of the program, therefore, was on the patient's attitudes toward illness rather than on symptoms. Methods used for the study are described, and the Illness Self-Concept Repertory Grid is shown in detail. Results indicated a significant difference between pre- and postprogram self-concept measurements and suggest that exposure to such a program can have a significant effect on an individual's attitudes toward illness.

Muhlenkamp, A.F., & Joyner, J.A. Arthritis patients' self-reported affective states and their caregivers' perceptions. *Nurs Res*, 1986, *35*(1):24-27.

This study exemplifies the measurement of attitudes toward chronic illness and the many variables that affect the patient's attitude. The methods are explained in detail, and the various tools used, including the Multiple Affect Adjective Check List (MAACL), are described. The MAACL has been previously tested for reliability and validity. The study attempted to identify the affective states of hospitalized arthritis patients, as reported by the patients, and to compare the self-report to an assessment made by the caregiver. The study found a discrepancy between patient and caregiver perceptions of the patient's affective state, which the authors suggest may be explained by the "requirement of mourning" in the caregiver. The requirement of mourning states that the fortunate person (i.e., the caregiver) tends to insist that the lot of the disabled person (i.e., the patient with a chronic illness) is unfortunate because the fortunate person needs to safeguard his or her values. This is especially true when diagnosis and disability are perceived by caregivers as life-threatening. Caregivers' perceptions of the affective state and attitudes of the patient also related significantly with the patient's education, occupation, and social position. Finally, results appeared to indicate that the meaning of the diagnosis to the patient and number of hospitalizations also created differences in attitudes between patients with various chronic diseases.

References

1. Forsyth, G.L., Delaney, K.D., & Gresham, M.L. Vying for a winning position: Management style of the chronically ill. *Res Nurs Health*, 1984, 7(3):181.

2. Morrow, G.R., Chiarello, R.J., & Derogatis, L.R. A new scale for assessing patient's psychosocial adjustment to medical illness. *Psychol Med*, 1978, 8:605.

3. Bergner, M., Bobbitt, R.A., Carter, W.B., & Gilson, B.S. The sickness impact profile: Development and final revision of a health status measure. *Med Care*, 1981, 19(8):784.

4. Brook, R.H., Ware, J.E., Davies-Avery, A., et al. Overview of adult health status measures fielded in Rand's health insurance study. *Med Care*, 1979, 17(suppl):entire issue.

5. Linn, B.S., Linn, M.W., & Gurel, L. Cumulative illness rating scale. *J Am Geriatr Soc*, 1968, 16:622.

6. Mahoney, R.I., & Barthel, D.W. Functional evaluation: The Barthel index. *Maryland State Med J*, 1965, 14:61.

7. Wylie, C.M., & White, B.K. A measure of disability. *Arch Environ Health*, 1964, 8:834.

8. Gauger, A.B., Brownwell, W.M., Russell, W.W., et al. Evaluation of levels of substance. *Arch Phys Med Rehab*, 1964, 45:286.

9. Katz, S., Ford, A.B., Moskowitz, R.W., et al. Studies of illness in the aged. The index of ADL: A standardized measure of biological and psychosocial function. *JAMA*, 1963, 185:914.

10. Lawton, M.P., & Brody, E. Assessment of older people: Self-maintaining and instrumental activities of daily living. *Gerontologist*, 1969, 9:179.

11. Linn, M.W., & Linn, B.S. The rapid disability rating scale-2. *J Am Geriatr Soc*, 1982, 30(6):378.

12. Linn, M.W. A rapid disability rating scale. *J Am Geriatr Soc*, 1967, 15:211.

13. Sett, R.F. Simplified tests for evaluation of patients with chronic illness (cerebrovascular accidents). *J Am Geriatr Soc*, 1963, 11:1095.

14. Carter, W.B., Bobbitt, R.A., Bergner, M., & Gilson, B.S. Validation of an interval scaling: The sickness impact profile. *Health Serv Res*, 1976, 11(4):516.

15. Katz, J.N., Larson, M.G., Phillips, C.B., et al. Comparative measurement sensitivity of short and longer health status instruments. *Med Care*, 1992, 30(10):917.

16. Pollard, W.E., Bobbitt, R.A., Bergner, M., et al. The sickness impact profile: Reliability of a health status measure. *Med Care*, 1976, 14(2):146.

17. Drossman, D.A., Leserman, J., Li, Z.M., et al. The rating form of IBD patient concerns: A new measure of health status. *Psychosom Med*, 1991, 53(6):701.

18. Fox, E., McDowall, J., Neale, T.J., et al. Cognitive function and quality of life in end-stage renal failure. *Ren Failure*, 1993, 15(2):211.

19. Juniper, E.F., Guyatt, G.H., Ferrie, P.J. & Griffith, L.E. Measuring quality of life in asthma. *Am Rev Resp Dis*, 1993, 147(4):832.

20. Schuling, J., Greidanus, J., & Meyboom de Jong, B. Measuring functional status of stroke patients with the sickness impact profile. *Disab Rehab*, 1993, 15(1):19.

21. Baker, C.A. Factors associated with rehabilitation in head and neck cancer. *Cancer Nurs*, 1992, 15(6):395.

22. Granger, C.V., Cotter, A.C., Hamilton, B.B., & Fiedler, R.C. Functional assessment scales: A study of persons after stroke. *Arch Phys Med Rehab*, 1993, 74(2):133.

23. Syrjala, K.L., Chapko, M.K., Vitaliano, P.P., et al. Recovery after allogeneic marrow transplantation: Prospective study of predictors of long-term physical and psychosocial functioning. *Bone Marrow Transplant*, 1993, 11:319.

24. Sanders, S.H., Brena, S.F., Spier, C.J., et al. Chronic low back pain patients around the world: Cross-cultural similarities and differences. *Clin J Pain*, 1992, 8(4):317.

25. Chwalow, A.J., Lurie, A., Bean, K., et al. French version of the sickness impact profile: Stages in the cross cultural validation of a generic quality of life scale. *Fund Clin Pharmacol*, 1992, 6(7):319.

26. DeBruin, A.F., DeWitte, L.P., Stevens, F., & Diederiks, J.P. Sickness impact profile: The state of the art of a generic functional status measure. *Soc Sci Med*, 1992, 35(8):1003.

27. Kivela, S.L. Measuring disability—Do self-ratings and service provider ratings compare? *J Chron Dis*, 1984, 37(2):115.

28. Meenan, R.F., Gertman, P.M., & Mason, J.H. Measuring health status in arthritis. *Arthrit Rheum*, 1980, 23(2):146.

29. Burckhardt, C.S., Woods, S.L., Schultz, A.A., & Ziebarth, D.M. Quality of life of adults with chronic illness: A psychometric study. *Res Nurs Health*, 1989, 12(6):347.

30. Lorish, C.D., Abraham, N., Austin, J.S., et al. A comparison of the full and short versions of the arthritis impact measurement scales. *Arthrit Care Res*, 1991, 4(4):168.

31. Weinberger, M., Tierney, W.M., Booher, P., & Hiner, S.L. Social support, stress and functional status in patients with osteoarthritis. *Soc Sci Med*, 1990, 30(4):503.

32. Kassebaum, G.G., & Baumann, B.O. Dimensions of the sick role in chronic illness. *J Health Hum Behav*, 1965, 6(1):16.

33. Pilowsky, I., & Spence, N.D. Illness behavior syndromes associated with intractable pain. *Pain*, 1976, 2(1):61.

34. Tatarelli, R., Atlante, G., dePisa, E., et al. Illness behavior in a sample of patients with gynecological cancer compared to other benign pathologies. *New Trends Exp Clin Psychiatr*, 1991, 7(4):187.

35. Large, R.G. Prediction of treatment response in pain patients: The illness self- concept repertory grid and EMG feedback. *Pain*, 1985, 21(3):279.

36. Large, R. Self-concepts and illness attitudes in chronic pain: A repertory grid study of a pain management programme. *Pain*, 1985, 23(2):113.

37. Large, R.G., & James, F.R. Personalized evaluation of self-hypnosis as a treatment of chronic pain: A repertory grid analysis. *Pain*, 1988, 35(1):155.

38. Lowery, B.J. Misconceptions and limitation of locus of control and the I-E scale. *Nurs Res*, 1981, 30(5)294.

39. Wallston, B.S., Wallston, H.A., Kaplan, G.D., & Maides, S.A. Development and validation of the

health locus of control (HLC) scale. *J Consult Clin Psychol*, 1976, *44*(4):580.

40. Rock, D.L., Meyerowitz, B.E., Maisto, S.A., & Wallston, K.A. The derivation and validation of six multidimensional health locus of control scale clusters. *Res Nurs Health*, 1987, *10*(3):185.

41. Strickland, B.R. Internal-external expectancies and health-related behavior. *J Consult Clin Psychol*, 1978, *46*(6):1192.

42. Wallston, K.A., Maides, S., & Wallston, B.S. Health-related information seeking as a function of health-related locus of control and health value. *J Res Person*, 1976, *10*(2):215.

43. Sugarek, N.J., Deyo, R.A., & Holmes, B.C. Locus of control and beliefs about cancer in a multi-ethnic clinic population. *Oncol Nurs Forum*, 1988, *15*(4): 481.

44. Lau, R.R., & Ware, J.F. Refinements in the measurement of health-specific locus-of-control beliefs. *Med Care*, 1981, *19*(11):1147.

45. Nagy, V.T., & Wolfe, G.R. Cognitive predictors of compliance in chronic disease patients. *Med Care*, 22(10):912.

46. Lowery, B.J., & Jacobsen, B.S. Attributional analysis of chronic illness outcomes. *Nurs Res*, 1985, *34*(2):82.

47. Lowery, B.J., Jacobsen, B.S., & Murphy, B.B. An exploratory investigation of causal thinking of arthritics. *Nurs Res*, 1983, *32*(3):157.

48. Weaver, T.E., & Narsavage, G.L. Physiological and psychological variables related to functional status in chronic obstructive pulmonary disease. *Nurs Res*, 1992, *41*(5):286.

49. Hymovich, D.P. The chronicity impact and coping instrument: Parent questionnaire. *Nurs Res*, 1983, *32*(5):275.

50. Humovich, D.P., & Baker, C.D. The needs, concerns and coping of parents of children with cystic fibrosis. Family Relations: *J Appl Fam Child Stud*, 1985, *34*(1):91

51. Palomares, R.S., Crowley, S.L., Worchell, F.F., et al. The factor analytic structure of the Roberts apperception test for children: A comparison of the standardization sample with a sample of chronically ill children. *J Person Assess*, 1991, *56*(3):414.

52. Counte, M.A., Bieliauskas, L.A., & Pavlou, M. Stress and personal attitudes in chronic illness. *Arch Phys Med Rehab*, 1983, *64*(6):272.

53. Pollock, S.E., & Duffy, M.E. The Health Related Hardiness Scale: Development and psychometric analysis. *Nurs Res*, 1990, *39*(4):218.

54. Viney, L.L., & Westbrook, M.T. Patterns of anxiety in the chronically ill. *Br J Med Psychol*, 1982, *55*:87.

55. Rahe, R.H., & Holmes, T.H. The social readjustment rating scale. *J Psychosom Res*, 1967, *11*:213.

56. DeVon, H.A., & Powers, M.J. Health beliefs, adjustment to illness, and control of hypertension. *Res Nurs Health*, 1984, *7*(1):10.

57. Viney, L.L. & Westbrook, M.T. Coping with chronic illness: Strategy preferences, changes in preferences and associated emotional reactions. *J Chron Dis*, 1984, *37*(6):489.

58. Cantril, H. A study of aspirations. *Sci Am*, 1963, *8*(2):41.

59. Laborde, J.M., & Powers, M.J. Life satisfaction, health control orientation, and illness-related factors in persons with osteoarthritis. *Res Nurs Health*, 1985, *8*(2):183.

60. Lubin, B., Rahaim, S., Rinck, C.M., & Nickel, E.J. MMPI experimental scale correlates of the MAACL-R with male alcoholics. *Psychol Rep*, 1991, *69*(2):460.

61. Stevenson, J.S. Construction of a scale to measure load, power and margin in life. *Nurs Res*, 1982, *31*(4):22.

62. Rosenberg, S.J., Hayes, J.R., & Peterson, R.A. Revising the seriousness of illness rating scale: Modernization and re-standardization. *Int J Psychiatr Med*, 1987, *17*(1):85.

63. Sacks, C.R., Peterson, R.A., & Kimmel, P.L. Perception of illness and depression in chronic renal disease. *Am J Kidney Dis*, 1990, *15*(1):31.

64. Milne, B.J., Logan, A.G., & Flanagan, P.T. Alterations in health perception and life-style in treated hypertensives. *J Chron Dis*, 38(1):37.

Appendices

19A. Instruments Used to Determine Locus of Control

Instrument	Description	Psychometric Indices
Multidimensional Health Locus of Control Scale (MHLC) (38–41)	3 subscales of locus of control beliefs: (1) Internal Scale (IS) assesses degree to which individual believes own behavior responsible for health (H) or illness (I); (2) Chance Scale (CS): assesses belief that level of H or I is a function of luck, fate, or uncontrollable factors; (3) Powerful Others (PO): assesses belief that degree of H or I is determined by important figures (e.g., physician) Scaled on 6-point, Likert-type scale: externally worded items: 1 "strongly disagree" to 6 "strongly agree" and internally worded items: reverse scored; range 11 (most internal) to 66 (most external)	Alpha reliability: 0.72 Concurrent validity: 0.33 correlation ($p < 0.01$) with Rotter's Internal–External scale Wallston et al. found correlation of 0.25 (42) Tested in culturally diverse populations (43) using revised MHLC scale: test–retest reliability of Spanish locus of control scale: IS (0.68), CS (0.36), PO (0.61); Cronbach's alpha: IS (0.20–0.40), CS (0.46), PO (0.61–0.72) Suggests that poorly educated people need greater direction to take active role in health maintenance (43)
Health Specific Locus of Control Beliefs Questionnaire Developed by Lau and Ware (44)	Measures person's beliefs about self-control over health, provider control over health, chance health outcomes, general health threat, health-care attitudes, health status perceptions, and value placed on health 28-items: statement of opinion about control over health with 7-point response scale (strongly agree to strongly disagree) 4 dimensions (subscales): self-care, provider control, chance, general health threat (independent of others)	Test–retest (3-week interval) performed Internal consistency reliability estimates (alpha) performed Factor analysis performed
Nagy and Wolfe's Compliance Tool (45)	Authors used health locus of control construct and Health Belief Model to predict compliance with medical regimen in chronically ill patients Reemphasizes multidimensional nature of compliance and suggests cognitive variables in general, and health locus of control beliefs specifically, play limited role in determining compliance in chronic illness	Found lack of relationship between health locus of control scales and compliance measures
Attribution Interview Scale (46)	Uses Weiner's Attribution Model (causal explanations predict behavioral and emotional reactions to life events) Weiner found that causes fall into 3 dimensions: (1) locus (cause internal or external to person); (2) stability (whether or not cause is changeable); (3) control (whether cause is under volitional control or controlled by outside forces) Self-esteem found to be linked to locus dimension	Reliability coefficients (for 3 dimensions): (1) 0.72, (2) 0.86, (3) 0.89

Numbers in parentheses correspond to studies cited in the References.

19B. Instruments Used to Assess the Impact of Chronic Illness in Children or Their Parents

Instrument	Description	Psychometric Indices
Chronicity Impact and Coping Instrument: Parent Questionnaire (CICI:PQ) (49,50)	167-item self-administered measure of the impact of chronic, childhood illness on parents; parental coping; parental perception of needs Items include: (A) demographic data; (B) parent relationships; (C) hospitalization experiences; (D) concerns of oneself (Self-concern) and spouse (Spouse concern); (E) help wanted for child and siblings (Help); (F) coping strategies of self (Self cope) and spouse (Spouse cope); (G) communication with siblings (Sib talk); (H) beliefs (Belief) Responses scaled using Likert-format	Internal reliability of subscales (Cronbach's alpha) Help, Self-Concern, Spouse concern scales combined to form Stressor scale Scale: (number of items) reliability (r): Help (23) $r = 0.95$; Self-concern (16) $r = 0.89$; Spouse concern (15) $r = 0.91$; Self cope (40) $r = 0.80$; Spouse cope (15) $r = 0.80$; Sib talk (9) $r = 0.84$; Beliefs (9) $r = 0.43$; Stressor (54) $r = 0.72$ CICI:PQ helps parents express their concerns to health professionals (50)
Roberts Apperception Test for Children (RATC) (51)	Story-telling technique combining a projective technique with a standardized scoring system Children (6–15 years old) are presented with card series depicting common childhood situations involving parents, peers, and schools 13 scales: 8 adaptive and 5 clinical scales Scored on adaptive (e.g., resolution) and clinical (e.g., depression) scales Helps in identifying children with serious emotional disturbance (SED)	LISREL analysis Chi-square goodness of fit used to evaluate 3-factor solution Cluster analysis of chronically ill sample resulted in 2 cluster solution based on T scores for each scale

Numbers in parentheses correspond to studies cited in the References.

19C. Selected Other Instruments Measuring Attitudes toward Chronic Disease

Instrument	Description	Psychometric Indices
Multiple Sclerosis Adjustment Scale (52)	Used to identify the multiple sclerosis (MS) patient's capacity to maintain distress within manageable limits, to invest emotional concern and energy in non-MS areas, to reevaluate life value and priorities, and to maintain optimism and interest in the future Self-report scale Statements scored in either a positive (good adaptation) or a negative (poor adaptation) direction on a Likert-type scale Can be used to determine ability to adapt to "life with disease" and disease exacerbations in patients with other chronic illness	Testing done on 97 adult MS patients in a treatment center Reliability = –0.79
Health Related Hardiness Scale (53)	51-item, self-report measure of commitment (15 items), challenge (15), and control (21) Target population: adults with multiple sclerosis, hypertension, rheumatoid arthritis, diabetes Items scored on 6-point Likert scale Higher scores indicate greater hardiness	High internal consistency (alpha coefficient): 0.91 Test-retest Pearson: $r = 0.90$ (2 week); $r = 0.80$ (3 months) Content and construct validity established
Total Anxiety Scale (54)	Interview format with tape recorded responses Patient asked questions about feelings related to: death: fears of dying; mutilation: fears; separation: loneliness, loss; guilt: moral disapproval, criticism; shame: self-criticism; diffuse: tension, vague fears	Reliability and validity tested using canonical correlation to analyze relationship between each set of continuously measured variables Can be used to study relationship between anxiety patterns in chronically ill patients and indices of rehabilitation
Social Readjustment Rating Scale (SRRS) (55)	Self-report using a yes–no checklist of 43 life changes (life change assigned value based on adjustment required for each change during prior year): high stress: SRSS > 300 Can be used to study relationship between event and onset of medical illness	Correlation coefficients between discrete groups (Pearson's r) > 0.90, except for relationship between white and black subjects (0.82) Kendall's coefficient of concordance $(W) = 0.477$ $(p < 0.0005)$
Psychosocial Adjustment to Medical Illness (PAIS) (2,56)	45 multiple-choice items in a self-report questionnaire 7 independent domains (Health-care orientation; Sexual relationships; Role function (vocational and domestic environments); Social support (extended family relationships and social environment); and Intrapsychic functioning (psychological distress) Scored using 4-point Likert scale then summed for each domain, and overall adjustment score calculated	Reliability: interrater reliability coefficients significant (>0.50) for all except Family domain (0.33) Validity established except for vocational and family domains
Coping With Chronic Illness: A Self-Appraisal Device (57)	Subject presented with 6 clusters of coping strategies on 6 separate cards Statement given to patients indicating use of the strategy: (1) action; (2) control; (3) escape; (4) fatalism; (5) optimism; (6) interpersonal coping Asked to rank strategies from (1) the one they were most likely to use to (6) the one least likely to use Context and structure of interview schedule described as pertaining to their illness and its implications for them	Tested in 3 separate studies: (1) 92 ill *vs.* well subjects to determine differences in coping strategies (in hospital); (2) 46 chronically ill subjects to determine differences in strategy preferences among patients with different types of chronic illness in different situations (in-hospital and at home); (3) chronically ill patients to determine associations between preferences for coping strategies and emotional reactions to chronic illness (in hospital and at home)

Instrument	Description	Reliability/Validity
	Administered in interview format Useful in determining the extent to which certain factors are related to preferences for different coping strategies (e.g., demographic characteristics, lifestyles, illness roles, degree of disability, perceived handicap and achievement of rehabilitation goals)	Reliability coefficient ($n = 45$, few stresses and relatively stable lives over 1 month): 0.70 (1) action: 0.43; (2) control: 0.30; (3) escape: 0.30' (4) fatalism: 0.50; (5) optimism: 0.38; (6) interpersonal: 0.54 Reliability coefficient over 1 day ($n = 10$) shows higher estimates Overall $r = 0.90$ (range 0.79–0.92 for all clusters)
Cantril's Self-Anchoring Striving Scale (58)	Used in variety of research exploring life satisfaction 10-step ladder to assess a person's general sense of well-being at three points in time: past, present, future Subject asked to describe the best possible life for him/her and the worst possible life Shown drawing of ladder with 10 rungs: (top best possible life, bottom worst life) Asked to show on the ladder where they stand now; where they stood 5 years ago; where they hope to be 5 years from now Interview format Scoring; answers are coded into meaningful categories to enable comparison of different groups Further study with a variety of diseases and populations to determine the effect of chronic illness	End points of scale are self-defined and numerical ratings reflect individual criteria Traditional notions of reliability may not be applicable Extremes are personal, and the meaning of endpoints remains relatively constant for a given individual over time, thereby minimizing error variance Test–retest reliability coefficient (sample of 378 community residents over 2-year period): 0.65 (59) Face validity supported by overt relationship between the nature of the instrument and life satisfaction
Multiple Affect Adjective Check List (MAACL) and revised form (MAACL-R) (60)	Measure of an individual's mood as it varies day to day Self-report check list of 132 adjectives best reflecting feelings that day Subscales: MAACL: 3 negative effects: anxiety, depression, hostility; MAACL-R: above 3 plus positive affect, sensation seeking, dysphoria	Reliability: MAACL: 0.65–0.92; MAACL-R: acceptable internal and test–retest reliabilities Validity: MAACL: 0.41–0.79; MAACL-R: concurrent and discriminant validity confirmed
Margin in Life Scale (MIL) (61)	94-item, self-report measure of vitality or freedom a person has to continue living (McClusky's construct of Margin of Life) Subjects rate load, power, and importance of each item 6 subscales (Self, Family, Religiosity/Spirituality, Body, Extra-Familial Relationships, Environment) Higher scores mean greater innate vitality or margin in life	Validity established through factor analysis and known-groups approach to construct validity Test–retest reliability: stability Cronbach's alpha reliability coefficients: body (0.87), self (0.84), family (0.69), religiosity (0.67), other human relationships (0.37), environment (−0.16)
Seriousness of Illness Rating Scale (revised) (SIRS-R) (62)	SIRS-R is an ordinal-level scale that reliably measures current views on the severity of illness and can be used with a variety of subjects and in psychosomatic research Examines the relationship of biologic, psychologic, and social variables to disease prevention, diagnosis, and treatment Used extensively in health psychology research to examine the link between the occurrence of stressful life events and onset of illness, mediating effects of personality on illness, and emotional factors in medical inpatients Original SIRS has 126 disease items evaluated by magnitude estimates of seriousness, ranked in quantitative order	Geometric mean score determined ranking of each disorder Kendall's coefficient of concordance (W) signifies extent of interrater reliability in rank-ordering of disease items: Kendall's $W = 0.716$ ($p < 0.00001$); Mann-Whitney U test used to test differences in rankings of each disorder among the 3 levels of raters; homogeneity of disease item rating shown within the sample

19C. Selected Other Instruments Measuring Attitudes toward Chronic Disease (*cont.*)

Instrument	Description	Psychometric Indices
SIRS-R (*cont.*)	SIRS-R (revised) includes recently discovered disorders (e.g., AIDS) for final list of 137 Self-report questionnaire Scoring: 1st page requests biographical information, gives scoring instructions; diseases listed are rated by the subject as to relative illness; peptic ulcer given a rating of 500, and each disease was rated in relation to that number	
Illness Effects Questionnaire (IEQ) (63)	20-item questionnaire measuring perception of illness-related effects on personal and social behavior 7-point Likert scale with scores ranging from 0 to 140	Internal reliability alpha: 0.93 Test–retest reliability: 0.99 Scale score correlates moderately with depression in medical patients and changes in depression among patients receiving treatment for chronic pain
Hypertensive Interview Schedule (64)	Used to determine the effect of being treated for hypertension on health perception and lifestyle and the duration of any alterations after first being diagnosed 3 sections addressed: (1) Measures of Health Perception: health status: 9-point scale (1 poorest health, 9 best health); presence of symptoms: asked to identify symptoms from a list of 16, and to rate frequency (1 never to 7 always), individual symptom scores summed to produce total score; worry about health: 9-point scale (1 no worry, 9 most worried possible) (2) Lifestyle: participation in physical and social activities; ability to participate: 9-point scale (1 no worry, 9 most worried possible); self-care behaviors (list) (3) Problems and Beliefs (list): interview format	Tested on 100 adult hypertensives and 50 normotensive controls Reliability and validity: between-group comparisons: Yate's chi square test of Fisher's exact proportions test used to assess nominal level data Mann-Whitney U test for ordinal- or interval-level data Kendall's tau used to measure strength of association between pairs of variables Analysis of variance used to test for differences between groups

Numbers in parentheses correspond to studies cited in the References.

20

Selecting a Tool for Measuring Cancer Attitudes

Nancy Burns

The word *cancer* generates in all of us a terror that we have difficulty defining. The illogical, unspoken, and often unrecognized attitudes or beliefs that lead to this intense emotion occur to some degree in everyone, regardless of rationality, sophistication, or education. These attitudes or beliefs occur in cancer patients and their family members and also in health professionals and the community at large.

Impact of Attitudes and Beliefs on the Cancer Situation

Concern about the attitudes or beliefs about cancer comes from their impact on the cancer situation. The dictionary definition of *situation* is "a state of affairs of special or critical significance" and also "the aggregate of biological, psychological, and sociocultural factors acting on an individual or group to condition behavioral patterns."[1] Experiencing the risk of having cancer, the diagnosis of cancer, or of living through the event of having cancer or of a significant other having cancer is a state of affairs of critical significance affecting in a holistic way the behavioral patterns of the individual and those within the social environment of the individual. The phrase *cancer situation* describes this phenomenon, which affects not only the person with cancer, but also family members, social support systems, and the health professionals providing care.

Attitudes and beliefs drive psychosocial responses to the threat and diagnosis of cancer. Recently, a number of basic research findings have made a compelling case for a link between psychosocial responses and cancer survival.[2] Variations in measures of natural killer (NK) cells and other dimensions of immunologic functioning have been linked to variations in psychosocial variables, such as stress,[3,4] depression,[5] interpersonal relationships,[6] marital disruption,[7] and social support.[8] When the person with cancer experiences high levels of psychosocial distress, particularly in the absence of an effective support system, the level of NK cells decreases. Longitudinally, levels of NK cells vary inversely with the level of psychosocial distress.[9] The level of NK cells is more predictive of the probability of metastasis and survival length than any other variable, including medical treatment. This explanation of the link between psychosocial and physiologic elements in cancer is referred to as the psychoneuroimmunology model. The model explains relationships among variables that have been demonstrated through research for many years but were not understood.

Decision making also is influenced by attitudes and beliefs. Treatment decisions are made by patient/family units, society, and health professionals and may have a major impact on the healthiness of the response to the cancer situation.

Patient/Family Decisions

Patient and family decisions influenced by cancer beliefs may include decisions about lifestyles, self-examination, participation in cancer-screening activities, speed with which symptoms are reported to a health professional, decisions related to initiating and adhering to treatment regimens, and decisions related to self-esteem, quality of life, and degree of hopefulness. Plans for the future by the family or family members, such as job changes, purchasing of new homes or other large expenditures, sending children to college, moving to another region of the country, are often heavily influenced by attitudes about cancer.

Societal Decisions

The social treatment of a person with cancer by his or her family, and of the patient and family by the community, is related to beliefs about cancer. The loss of social support and the abandonment of the patient/family unit by the community, which often occur in the cancer situation, may have serious long-term consequences, not only for the person with cancer but also for the present and future mental health of family members. Negative community attitudes also influence social and political systems. The fear and horror associated with cancer have generated a demand that something be done to prevent it or cure it. These negative attitudes have been helpful in compelling Congress and private foundations to provide increased funding for cancer research. However, they also have led to problems related to rehabilitation, insurability, and employability. Persons who have had cancer often are labeled as "cancer patients" for the rest of their life, a stigmatizing label affecting self-esteem and social functioning.

Health Professionals' Decisions

The decisions of health professionals are influenced by their personal attitudes about cancer. Concern has been expressed about this repeatedly in the nursing and medical literature, and a number of studies have been conducted to examine the impact of cancer attitudes on practice.[10-12] Also of concern is the impact of various educational approaches on cancer attitudes and subsequent practice decisions. Although links have been established between cancer attitudes and the use of prevention and screening interventions for cancer, the impact on other areas of practice remain essentially unstudied. Given the nature of primary care, the issues of concern are difficult to measure and often require self-report strategies that, given the topic, lend themselves to a number of biases. To decrease the risk of biases, Osborn et al.[13] used a medical record audit to examine the primary care activities of physicians and medical educators. Creative strategies will need to be used to understand situations in which negative cancer attitudes affect clinical decisions and interventions that can improve primary care outcomes. A number of primary care situations might be influenced by negative cancer attitudes. For example, a primary care provider with negative cancer attitudes may believe that a cancer diagnosis is a presage of death and might react by refusing to consider the possibility that a patient might have this "horrible" disease. Such an attitude can influence the interpretation of physical examination findings, resulting in signs and symptoms of cancer being overlooked, minimized, or discounted; lumps may be watched for months. When cancer is diagnosed or considered a possibility, negative cancer attitudes may influence choices of referral sources and selection of appropriate treatments. The relationship between the health professional and the client may be altered by a health provider's negative attitudes about cancer as such providers have difficulty addressing the emotional reactions of the patient and family members to a cancer diagnosis and initiate avoidance strategies. If a caregiver's attitudes about cancer are unrealistically negative, he or she may provide physical care but not psychologic care, and rehabilitative strategies may not be considered. Personal closeness with the patient may be avoided. Such caregivers may remain unaware of the feelings and problems faced by the patient/family unit and thus deprive them of needed care. A number of the instruments described in this chapter were developed to address some of these concerns.

Choices about a career in the health professions can be related to cancer attitudes. Such decisions often are made early in one's professional career. In one study, beginning student nurses had more negative beliefs about cancer than any other group tested.[14] These beliefs became even more negative during the nursing school experience. Students reported avoiding the selection of cancer patients to care for and feeling helpless to make a difference in the patient's status. Nursing staff on general medical-surgical units were perceived by the students to provide only minimal care to cancer patients. Few students were assigned to oncology units for clinical experiences. Nursing faculty seemed to avoid clinical contact with cancer patients and tended to limit the number of hours of classroom content related to cancer nursing. These behaviors clearly influenced career decisions by the new graduate.

Beliefs, Attitudes, and Values:
A Theoretical Perspective

Beliefs, attitudes, and values are related ideas but are not the same. Most theorists make clear distinctions among the three. According to Michael Rokeach, *beliefs* reflect an individual's perception of reality.[15] Scheibe proposes that beliefs allow the person to make inferences about what expectations he or she can have in a given situation.[16] Thus, a belief reflects what a person expects to happen in the external world in a given situation. Beliefs often develop during childhood, tend to be unconscious, and cannot be directly observed. Therefore, beliefs must be measured by indirect means.[13] Carl Jung saw beliefs as part of the collective unconscious and thus as acquired from one's culture but also influencing one's culture.[17] Antonovsky considered beliefs as important factors that influence a person's sense of coherence and thus his or her state of health.[18] Caplan thinks that beliefs are important in determining whether a person responds in an effective or ineffective way to a crisis situation.[19]

Rokeach sees *attitudes* as emerging from the belief system.[15] Attitudes involve the joining together of several beliefs. Attitudes are more likely to be conscious and, therefore, can be obtained by direct measurement.

Values are defined by Rokeach as a special type of belief, an abstract idea about ideal ways of behaving and ideal goals of life.[15] For example, values would be involved in determining the beliefs a health-care provider "should" have about cancer. It would be possible, then, to compare the ideal belief with the actual belief.

Ajzen and Fishbein have developed a theory of reasoned action that suggests relationships between beliefs, attitudes, intentions, and behavior.[20] They believe that humans are rational rather than driven by uncontrollable desires and that behavior is carefully reasoned as opposed to automatic. They propose that beliefs (that a certain behavior will lead to a certain outcome) lead to attitudes about that behavior, that attitudes about the behavior lead to intentions to perform a specific behavior, and that intentions are highly predictive of the actual behavior of an individual.

Berrenberg proposes three models that may explain the effects of attitudes toward cancer on behavior.[21] The first model, the *Familiarity Model*, is derived from research demonstrating that contact with minority group members leads to more positive attitudes toward that group.[22] These findings are explained by proposing that contact reduces fear and negative stereotyping. Berrenberg proposes that contact with a disease such as cancer may have a similar effect—more positive attitudes toward cancer.

Second, the *Vulnerability Model* suggests that attitudes toward a disease may not operate in the same way as attitudes toward minorities. Increased contact with cancer may increase the sense of aversion to it by familiarizing the individual with the ravages of the disease. Personal experiences with cancer and contact with cancer patients might increase the person's sense of vulnerability. If this model is correct, one could predict that increasingly negative attitudes would occur with greater experience with cancer. Berrenberg suggests that the Familiarity Model and the Vulnerability Model can be conceptualized as linear functions between experience with cancer and cancer attitudes.

Last, the *Dual Process Model* predicts that the most positive cancer attitudes will be found among those with the highest levels of cancer experience—those with a personal history of cancer. This explanation derives from the Familiarity Model. However, the Dual Process Model goes beyond this to suggest that experience with cancer may result in the individual finding renewed meaning in life. In addition, the cancer experience may enhance a person's sense of competence as a result of achieving mastery in coping with a traumatic life event. Unlike the Familiarity and Vulnerability Models, the Dual Process Model proposes that individuals with moderate levels of cancer experience, such as family members of persons with cancer, will have the most negative cancer attitudes. This proposition is derived from Coyne's social learning theory of depression.[23] Coyne suggests that the social needs of the depressed person over time alienates others and thus elicits negative social feedback and leads ultimately to social rejection. This rejection occurs because repeated attempts to relieve the depressed person fail, producing frustration. Berrenberg suggests that there are similarities between the social interactions of cancer patients and those of depressives.[21] She supports this proposition with the research of Wortman and Dunkel-Schetter, who found that the awkward nature of interpersonal contact with cancer patients can increase negative feelings and therefore increase the tendency to derogate the patient.[24] Negative feelings generated from a single experience with a cancer patient tend to be generalized to the disease itself. Thus, the Dual Process Model proposes a curvilinear relationship between cancer attitudes and cancer experience. Those with personal cancer experience will hold the most positive attitudes, and those having the familial experience with cancer will hold the most negative attitudes. Individuals with minimal experience with cancer should have attitudes somewhere in between these two groups. Berrenberg does not address where health professionals fit in on this attitude curve. Berrenberg has developed an instrument to measure cancer attitudes and conducted studies to test the three models. These are described later in the chapter. The study findings are consistent with the predictions of the proposed Dual Process Model.

Measurement of Beliefs and Attitudes

There is not yet a generally accepted conceptual definition within the body of knowledge of the essential elements of beliefs or attitudes about cancer. Therefore, each scientist has operationalized the concept using somewhat different criteria. A number of methods for measuring beliefs and attitudes about cancer have been developed, but few have been used repeatedly in studies. Many of the existing tools need further work to develop validity and reliability.

Gaps in the Literature

Research examining attitudes and beliefs about cancer has not been a focus of studies in recent years. A high priority of psychosocial oncology research has been the examination of variations in quality of life as a consequence of treatment strategies. However, attitudes and beliefs most likely influence many of the dimensions of quality of life, and this probable relationship needs to be studied. Studies also are needed to document the impact of cancer attitudes and beliefs of the patient, family members, and social support groups on the quality of life of persons with cancer.

The examination of cancer attitudes and beliefs in healthy populations also is important because of the shift in today's health-care delivery system from an illness orientation to the promotion of health and prevention of illness. Research is needed to understand how cancer attitudes influence health choices. It is not known whether beliefs and attitudes about cancer, which tend to be acquired early in life and thus may be entrenched, can be changed or if changes are short term or long term. It is important to identify (1) situations in which unrealistic negative beliefs occur; (2) activities that can modify beliefs; and (3) the impact of revised beliefs on responses to the cancer situation.

Studies are needed to examine the current cancer attitudes of faculty who educate health-care professionals and their students and to assess the effectiveness of teaching strategies designed to promote positive attitudes. The cancer attitudes of students must be examined longitudinally and correlated with relevant clinical experiences during their education. A number of studies have examined cancer attitudes before and after continuing education programs related to cancer care.[25-29] However, many of these studies have not been well designed. Attitude measurement immediately following a program in which the desired attitudes have been discussed introduces a social desirability problem in that the participants will tend to respond by giving the desired response rather than their actual attitude. The lack of comparison groups in many of these studies also is problematic. The cancer attitudes of health-care providers need to be examined longitudinally by taking repeated measures.[25] For example, attitudes might be measured at the time of initial employment in an oncology setting, during a staff-development program about oncology, and at set intervals thereafter.

Correlational studies to examine the relationship of cancer beliefs to other variables of interest in the cancer situation are needed. Studies to specifically examine the validity and reliability of existing tools will make a valuable contribution to the current level of knowledge about such tools. The cultural sensitivity of existing instruments needs to be examined and the cultural sensitivity of new instruments developed to measure cancer attitudes should be reported.[30] Theoretical studies of cancer beliefs and attitudes are badly needed. Corner, in a review of measures of cancer attitudes, suggests that there has been little progress toward understanding the influences that create such pessimism toward cancer.[31]

Selection of a Belief or Attitude Tool

Selecting a belief or attitude tool involves deciding how well the tool measures the dimensions of attitudes or beliefs about cancer, the established validity and reliability of the tool, time required to administer the tool, ease in completing and scoring the tool, and the complexity of data analysis. It also is important to determine whether the tool fits conceptually with the researcher's perception of cancer beliefs or attitudes and the theoretical framework of the study.

Researchers have used a variety of techniques to measure cancer beliefs and attitudes. Early measurement strategies used open-ended interviews.[32] Other studies use stimulus stories followed by questions.[33] A qualitative research approach grounded in symbolic interaction theory has been used to examine cancer attitudes in other countries.[34] Questions related to knowledge about cancer, hopelessness, and self-esteem have been used in many studies to reflect indirectly cancer attitudes.[35] However, the use of quantitative questionnaires and scales to measure cancer beliefs and attitudes is more common.

American Cancer Society Studies

The measurement of cancer attitudes using questionnaires was initiated by the American Cancer Society. The American Cancer Society questionnaire includes items about how likely the respondent believes a patient is to tell people he or she has cancer, their willingness to work next to someone who has cancer, their belief that cancer is curable, their belief that cancer is contagious, that cancer is the worst thing that could happen to a person, that a diagnosis of cancer is a death sentence, any tendency to read news releases about cancer, the expectation that a cure for cancer will be found, and the desire to be informed of a diagnosis of cancer. Two instruments are reviewed in depth. Additional measures are presented in Appendix 20A.

The Haley Cancer Attitude Survey

In 1968, Haley et al. developed a tool to measure the cancer attitudes of medical students.[36] The tool evolved from 600 statements that expressed attitudes toward cancer and the care of cancer patients. From these statements, a preliminary form with 33 questions was developed and given to 163 physicians, 89 medical students, and 13 laypersons. Responses were examined using factor analysis, from which three dimensions of cancer attitude were identified: "(a) attitudes toward the patient's inner resources to cope with serious illness such as cancer (CAS I); (b) attitudes toward the value of early diagnosis and aggressive treatment (CAS II); and attitudes toward personal immortality and preparation for and acceptance of death (CAS III)."[28a,p501]

A second sample of 94 physicians was used to develop the tool further. Correlational analysis of the new data led to the subdivision of CAS II into two subscales: CAS IIa, early diagnosis, and CAS IIb, aggressive treatment. The instrument used a nine-point Likert-type scale with responses ranging from "strongly disagree" to "strongly agree." Scoring used –4 for "strongly disagree," 0 for "no opinion," and +4 for "strongly agree." Completion of the instrument requires approximately 15 minutes.

Examples from the survey include:

- A physician can be so discouraged by the low cure rate of cancer that he will not feel the need to do routine "cancer tests," especially when he is so busy working with sick patients.
- Aggressive treatment of cancer frequently subjects the patient to illness, pain, and expense without much actual benefit to him.
- The dying patient has to be kept happy since he has nothing to look forward to.

Reliability data for this instrument were not reported. Face validity and content validity must be inferred from the tool-development process. Initial steps toward construct validity were obtained through factor analysis and the formation of clearly defined factors. However, no report was given of the constancy of the factors across samples.

The tool was used in a study reported by Haley et al. in 1977 as part of a battery of tests given to examine the cancer-related attitudes of medical students.[28a] Findings indicated that cancer attitudes evolved throughout medical school and were unrelated to the student's intellectual ability or to personal needs associated with daily interactions with others. Cancer attitudes were associated with values in life and the degree of openness to others. Responses tended to be neutral early in medical education but definite attitudes emerged as medical education and experience progressed. There were increases in CAS I, decreases in CAS IIa and CAS IIb, and increases in CAS III. The cancer attitudes of medical students were different from those found in a comparison group of physicians. Medical students had more positive values on CAS I (the patient's psychologic resources) and less positive values on CAS IIa (early diagnosis) and CAS IIb (aggressive treatment) than the practicing physicians. In 1981, the tool was revised by Blanchard et al.[29] Twenty-seven new items were added to address changes in medical practice and modifications in the doctor–patient relationship since the original tool had been developed. The structure of the original tool was kept intact, and the new items were added to the end of the instrument. Using only the original 33 questions, Blanchard failed to replicate the original factor structure reported by Haley. Responses demonstrated a high degree of variability, and only 50% of the variance could be explained by the eight factors. In 1982, Cohen et al. used the revised tool in a comparative study of the responses of cancer patients, medical students, medical residents, physicians, and medical cancer educators.[37] The sample was purposely selected to allow comparison with Haley's original sample. However, factor analysis apparently was not performed on the new data, and, therefore, no additional information on the factor structure is available from this study.

In 1986, Raina et al. reported the use of the CAS over several years to examine the cancer attitudes of medical students and found that it yielded inconsistent results and discriminated poorly.[38] They report "a rigorous analysis of the three subscales based on the CAS showed them lacking in reliability and internal consistency." Peters et al. used the CAS in 1987 in a study of the effect of a course in cancer prevention on medical student's attitudes and clinical behavior.[26] Students and a control group were followed for 3 years after completing the course. The authors found little change in attitude scores over time as measured by the CAS. Corner and Wilson-Barnett used the CAS on a sample of newly registered nurses in London in 1992.[25] They reported that the CAS did not appear to be particularly responsive to changes in attitudes among subjects. Responses to the CAS were compared to data on attitudes collected during interviews, using questions relating to each of the factors of the CAS. In contrast to the CAS, the interview questions did provide evidence of changes in attitude.

The Burns' Cancer Beliefs Scales

The Burns' Cancer Beliefs Scales were developed between 1977 and 1981 as part of a doctoral dissertation.[39] A concept analysis of cancer beliefs was performed, and the essential elements were obtained from the literature and personal experience. A semantic differential format was used to develop the instrument. Therefore, each item is considered a separate scale. The semantic differential was designed to measure meaning. It tends to capture the affective component of meaning rather than factual meaning. It uses strategies similar to word association used by psychotherapists to reflect the unconscious. Thus, the significance of the responses go far beyond the simple dictionary definition of the word used in the instrument. It provides a link with the unconscious belief structure of the individual. The intensity of the response and the correlation of groupings of scales reflects experience or thought that often cannot be expressed directly.

The instrument was first tested on 13 family members of cancer patients participating in a family support group. Then four groups (n = 153) were selected to test the instrument: American Cancer Society volunteers, high school teachers, beginning nursing students, and members of a Baptist church. It was hypothesized that the American Cancer Society volunteers would score highest, high school teachers and beginning nursing students would have moderate scores, and the Baptist church members would score lowest. American Cancer Society volunteers scored highest and beginning nursing students had the lowest scores. Using analysis of variance (ANOVA) the group scores showed a statistically significant difference at the 0.001 level. To examine further the structure of the instrument, factor analysis was performed. Three distinct factors emerged and were labeled, Fear of the Cancer Situation, Hopelessness, and Stigma.

Researchers using the tool were requested to send their data to Burns to allow further examination of the instrument structure, validity, and reliability. Data from the original study and from various additional sources were pooled, resulting in a diverse sample of 767 subjects. Using this sample, correlations between the factor scores and other variables of interest were examined. Factor analysis was performed on this sample with the same factors emerging. Items with a factor loading of 0.4 or greater were selected for inclusion in each factor. All of the items loaded on one of the three factors. There were no secondary loadings. However, because subjects from the original sample were included in the sample, validation of the factor structure will require additional work, including a confirmatory factor analysis. Weights on the items in each factor are available, as well as normative values, such as means and other statistical data for each scale from the 767 subjects.

The Burns' Cancer Beliefs Scales contain 23 semantic differential scales consisting of bipolar adjectives or descriptive terms associated with beliefs about cancer. Each opposing set of descriptive terms is placed at opposite ends of a seven-point scale. Positive and negative responses to an item are randomly assigned to the right or left side of the scale to diminish the probability of global scoring by the respondent. Instructions for completing the scale are included on the instrument form. Individuals are instructed to respond quickly with their initial gut reaction to the descriptive terms by marking one space on each scale.

- *Factor I, Fear of the Cancer Situation* consists of the following scales: painless to severe constant untreatable pain; no fear to terror; body mutilation to no body changes; pleasant odors to foul odors; independency to dependency; no life changes to sudden overwhelming life changes; extreme suffering to no suffering; nourished to wasting away; certain future to uncertain future; and destructive uncontained growth to normal growth.
- *Factor II, Hopelessness* consists of the following scales: punishment to no punishment; worthlessness to worth; shame to pride; acceptance to rejection; alienation to belonging; being wanted to not being wanted; unloved to loved; and abandoned to cared for.
- *Factor III, Stigma* consists of the following scales: hopefulness to hopelessness; certain death to being cured; helplessness to control; optimism to pessimism; and unknown to known.

Instrument administration is fairly simple and should take only 5 to 10 minutes. Participants must be instructed to respond quickly and spontaneously with as little thought as possible to each item. Completion of the tool can generate emotional responses in patients and family members; therefore, it is recommended that a health professional be present at the time the tool is used with these groups.

Scoring is performed by rating the most negative response as 1 and increasing each space by 1 to the most positive response, which is rated as 7. The lowest possible score is 23, and the highest possible score is 161. Added insight can be obtained by calculating factor scores for each of the three factors.

Internal consistency estimates were examined using the alpha coefficient. Alpha coefficients for the three factors range from 0.76 to 0.91. These statistics indicate an acceptable level of internal consistency for the tool.

Content validity was developed through literature review and concept analysis. The instrument was reviewed by family members of cancer patients, nurses practicing oncology, and nursing doctoral students and revised based on their suggestions.

Construct validity was examined using factor analysis. The grouping of the concepts that form the scales leads to the formation of a higher construct defined by the factor. Factor structure has been further examined using a sample of 767 subjects, providing some evidence of factorial validity.

Concurrent validity was obtained by administering the tool to a sample of people concurrently with other instruments thought to measure the same concept. The Hoffmeister Cancer Attitudes Questionnaire and the Beck Hopelessness Scale[40] were administered with the Burns' Cancer Beliefs Scales to 58 subjects. Factor scores of the Beck scale and the Hoffmeister questionnaire were correlated with factor scores of the Burns scales, using Pearson's product–moment correlations. All three factors of the Burns scales correlated significantly ($p < 0.001$) with the factors of the Hoffmeister questionnaire. The pessimism factor in the Beck scale correlated beyond the 0.001 level with all factors of the Burns scales. Correlations of the other two factors in the Beck scale (factor 2, Loss of Motivation, and factor 3, Future Expectations) with the Burns factors and the Hoffmeister clusters indicated no significant correlations. The two factors from the Beck scale apparently measure a phenomenon not related to cancer attitudes and beliefs. The results of the correlations indicate concurrent validity for both the Burns scale and the Hoffmeister questionnaire.

Divergent validity was examined by correlating the three factors on the Burns scale with the Cancer Optimism Cluster in the Hoffmeister questionnaire. The two scores were significantly negatively correlated, suggesting divergent validity.

Ash et al. used the instrument in 1988 in a cancer-prevention and -detection course for 14 nurses in developing countries.[41] They report that the mean score (83.64) compared favorably with Burns's sample of 767 subjects (99.78). Additional measures of cancer attitudes can be found in Appendix 20A.

Summary

Attitudes toward cancer influence emotional health and behavior in the cancer situation. A number of methods for measuring cancer attitudes have been developed, but few have been used repeatedly in studies. Many of the existing tools need further work to develop validity and reliability. Research examining attitudes about cancer has not been the focus of studies in recent years. A high priority in psychosocial oncology research has been the examination of variations in quality of life as a consequence of various treatment strategies. However, attitudes and beliefs influence many of the dimensions of quality of life. The examination of cancer attitudes in health populations also is important because of the shift in our health-care delivery system to promotion of health and prevention of illness. Studies are needed to examine current attitudes about cancer among health professions' faculty and students and to evaluate the effectiveness of teaching strategies designed to promote more positive attitudes about cancer.

Exemplar Studies

Corner, J., & Wilson-Barnett J. The newly registered nurse and the cancer patient: An educational evaluation. *Intl J Nurs Stud*, 1992, *29*(2):177-190.

This study exemplifies a design sufficient to assess the outcomes of an educational intervention aimed at developing an understanding of the attitudes, knowledge, confidence, and educational needs of newly registered nurses in relation to cancer care. A carefully constructed framework for the study was described. Two educational programs were assessed with 127 nurses working in two general hospitals and compared to a control group. Measurements were taken before, after, and 3 months following the intervention using measurement methods described in this chapter (Haley et al.[36]; Craytor et al.[44]) Measurement methods included self-report instruments and taped interviews. Triangulation was used in interpreting results. The reliability and validity of measures were evaluated for the sample. The researchers observed that Haley's CAS was not sensitive to attitude change over time, a finding made possible by comparing the CAS with interview data that did show changes over time.

Peters, A.S., Schimpfhauser, F.T., Cheng, J., et al. Effect of a course in cancer prevention on students' attitudes and clinical behavior. *J Med Educ*, 1987, *62*(7):592-600.

This study exemplifies a longitudinal design with triangulation used to assess the effectiveness of a course in cancer prevention for first-year medical students. Groups of students who took the course and control groups were given a test of knowledge of cancer, the CAS, a clinical practice survey, and a course evaluation. Their clinical behavior was observed, videotaped, and coded during interviews with patients. Self-report measures were repeated during the student's junior and senior year. The researchers acknowledged that follow-up after the students graduated and were practicing medicine would have allowed a more adequate determination of the extent of clinical application of the course content.

References

1. Stein, J. *The Random House dictionary of the English language*, New York: Random House, 1967, p. 1333.
2. Sabbioni, M.E.E. Psychoneuroimmunological issues. *Cancer Invest*, 1993, *11*(4):440-450.
3. Levy, S.M., Herberman, R.B., Maluish, A.M., et al. Prognostic risk assessment in primary breast cancer by behavioral and immunological parameters. *Health Psychol*, 1985, *4*(2):99-113.
4. Khansari, D.N., & Murgo, Faith, R.E. Effects of stress on the immune system, *Immunol Today*, 1990, *11*(5):170-175.
5. Calabrese, J.R., Kling, M.A., & Gold, P.W. Alterations in immunocompetence during stress, bereavement, and depression: Focus on neuroendocrine regulation. *Am J Psychiatr*, 1987, *144*(9):1123-1134.
6. Kennedy, S., Kiecolt-Glaser, J.K., & Glaser, R. Immunological consequences of acute and chronic stressors: Mediating role of interpersonal relationships. *Br J Med Psychol*, 1988, *61*(1):77-85.
7. Kiecolt-Glaser, J.K., Fisher, L.D., Ogrocki, P., et al. Marital quality, marital disruption, and immune function. *Psychosom Med*, 1987, *49*(1):13-34.
8. Levy, S.M., Herberman, R.B., Whiteside, T., et al. Perceived social support and tumor estrogen/progesterone receptor status as predictors of natural killer cell activity in breast cancer patients. *Psychosom Med*, 1990, *52*(1):73-85.
9. Glaser, R., Rice, J., Sheridan, J., et al. Stress-related immune suppression: Health implications. *Brain, Behav Immun*, 1987, *1*(1):7-20.
10. Liberati, A., Apolone, G., Nicolucci, A., et al. The role of attitudes, beliefs, and personal characteristics of Italian physicians in the surgical treatment of early breast cancer. *Am J Pub Health*, 1990, *81*(1):38-42.
11. Bostick, R.M., Spraffka, J.M., Virnig, B.A., et al. Knowledge, attitudes, and personal practices regarding prevention and early detection of cancer. *Prev Med*, 1993, *22*(1):65-85.

12. Chlebowski, R.T., Sayre, J., Frank-Stromborg, M., et al. Current attitudes and practice of American Society of Clinical Oncology-member clinical oncologists regarding cancer prevention and control. *J Clin Oncol*, 1992, *10*(1):164-169.

13. Osborn, E.H., Bird, J.A., McPhee, S.J., et al. Cancer screening by primary care physicians. Can we explain the differences? *J Fam Pract*, 1991, *32*(5):465-471.

14. Burns, N. Development of the Burns' Cancer Beliefs Scales, *Proceedings of the American Cancer Society Third West Coast Cancer Nursing Research Conference*, August 4–5, 1983, Portland, OR.

15. Rokeach, M. *Beliefs, attitudes and values*. San Francisco: Jossey-Bass, 1968.

16. Scheibe, K.E. *Beliefs and values*. New York: Holt, Rinehart, & Winston, 1970.

17. Read, H., Fordham, M., & Adler, G. (Eds.). *The collected works of C. G. Jung*. New York: Pantheon, 1960.

18. Antonovsky, A. *Health, stress, and coping*. San Francisco: Jossey-Bass, 1979.

19. Caplan, G. *Support systems and community mental health*. New York: Grune & Stratton, 1976.

20. Ajzen, I., & Fishbein, M. *Understanding attitudes and predicting social behavior*. Englewood Cliffs, N.J.: Prentice-Hall, 1980.

21. Berrenberg, J.L. Attitudes towards cancer as a function of experience with the disease: A test of three models. *Psychol Health*, 1989, *3*(4):233-243.

22. Amir, Y. The contact hypothesis in ethnic relations. *Psychol Bull*, 1969, *71*(5):319-342.

23. Coyne, J.C. Depression and the response of others. *J Abnorm Psychol*, 1976, *85*(2):186-193.

24. Wortman, C.B., & Dunkel-Schetter, C. Interpersonal relationships and cancer: A theoretical analysis. *J Soc Issues*, 1979, *35*(1):120-155.

25. Alexander, M.A. Evaluation of a training program in breast cancer nursing. *J Cont Ed Nurs*, 1990, *21*(6):260-266.

26. Peters, A.S., Schimpfhauser, F.T., Cheng, J., et al. Effect of a course in cancer prevention on students' attitudes and clinical behavior. *J Med Ed*, 1987, *62*(7):592-600.

27. Scott, C.S., & Neighbor, W.E. Preventive care attitudes of medical students, *Soc Sci Med*, 1985, *21*(3):299-305.

28. Schmelkin, L.P., Wachtel, A.B., Hecht, D., et al. Cancer opinionnaire: Medical students' attitudes toward psychosocial cancer care. *Cancer*, 1986, *58*(3):801-806.

28a. Haley, H.B., Huynh, H., Paiva, R.E., & Juan, I.R. Students' attitudes towards cancer: Changes in medical school. *J Med Educ*, 1977, *52*(6):500-507.

29. Blanchard, C.G., Ruckdeschel, J.C., Cohen, R.E., et al. Attitudes toward cancer: The impact of a comprehensive oncology course on second-year medical students. *Cancer*, 1981, *47*(11):2756-2762.

30. Nielsen, B.B., McMillan, S., & Diaz, E. Instruments that measure beliefs about cancer from a cultural perspective. *Cancer Nurs*, 1992, *15*(2):109-115.

31. Corner, J. L. Assessment of nurses' attitudes towards cancer: A critical review of research methods, *J Adv Nurs*, 1988, *13*(5):640-648.

32. Mitchell, G.W., & Glicksman, A.S. Cancer patients: Knowledge and attitudes. *Cancer*, 1977, *40*(1):61-66.

33. Sloan, R.P., & Gruman, J.C. Beliefs about cancer, heart disease, and their victims. *Psychol Rep*, 1983, *52*(2):415-424.

34. Dodd, M.J., Chen, S., Lindsey, A.M., et al. Attitudes of patients living in Taiwan about cancer and its treatment. *Cancer Nurs*, 1985, *8*(4):214-220.

35. Blinov, N.N., Komiakov, I.P., & Shipovnikov, N.B. Cancer research in Russia, II: patients' attitudes to the diagnosis of cancer. *Soc Work Soc Sci Rev*, 1993, *4*(1):83-87.

36. Haley, H.B., Juan, I.R., & Galen, J.F. Factor-analytic approach to attitude scale construction. *J Med Educ*, 1968, *43*(3):331-336.

37. Cohen, R.E., Ruckdeschel, J.C., Blanchard, C.G., et al. Attitudes Towards Cancer: A comparative analysis of cancer patients, medical students, medical residents, physicians and cancer educators. *Cancer*, 1982, *50*(6):1218-1223.

38. Raina, S., Alger, E.A., Stolman, C., et al. Limitations in testing for attitudes toward cancer. *J Cancer Educ*, 1986, *1*(3), 153-160.

39. Burns, N. *Evaluation of a supportive-expressive group for families of cancer patients*. Unpublished Dissertation, Texas Woman's University, 1981.

40. Beck, A., Weissman, A., Lester, D., et al. The measurement of pessimism: The hopelessness scale. *J Consult Clin Psychol*, 1974, *42*(6):861-865.

41. Ash, C.R., McCorkle, R., & Tiffany, R. Cancer prevention and detection course for nurses in developing countries. *Cancer Nurs*, 1988, *11*(4):230-236.

42. Hochloch, F.J., & Coulson, M.E. Developing an attitude inventory. *J Nurs Ed*, 1968, *7*(3):9-13.

43. Sherif, C.W., Sherif, M., & Nebergall, R.E. *Attitudes and attitude change*, Philadelphia: Saunders, 1965.

44. Craytor, J.K., Brown, J.K., & Morrow, G.R. Assessing learning needs of nurses who care for persons with cancer. *Cancer Nurs*, 1978, *1*(3):211-220.

45. Hoffmeister, J. *First year evaluation results: Test development information, oncology nursing project*. Contract #1-CN-65185. University of Pittsburgh, 1976.

46. Lebovits, A.H., Croen, L.G., & Goetzel, R.Z. Attitudes towards cancer: Development of the Cancer Attitudes Questionnaire. *Cancer*, 1984, *54*(6):1124-1129.

47. Damrosch, S., Denicoff, A.M., St. Germain, D., et al. Oncology nurse and physician attitudes toward aggressive cancer treatment. *Cancer Nurs*, 1993, *16*(2): 107-112.

48. Davison, R.L. Opinion of nurses on cancer, its treatment and curability—A survey among nurses in Public Health Service. *Br J Prevent Sociol Med*, 1965, *19*(1):24-29.

49. Whelan, J. Oncology nurses' attitudes toward cancer treatment and survival. *Cancer Nurs*, 1984, *7*(5): 375-383.

50. Fanslow, J. Attitudes of nurses toward cancer and cancer therapies. *Oncology Nurs Forum*, 1985, *12*(1): 43-47.

51. Donovan, M., Yasko, J., Wolpert, P., et al. *Cancer attitude survey*. Contract #1-CN-55186-07. Pittsburgh, University of Pittsburgh National Cancer Institute, 1977.

52. Gutteling, J.M., Seydel, E.R., & Wiegman, O. Perceptions of cancer. *J Psychosoc Oncol*, 1986, *4*(3):77-93.

53. Becker, M.H., Haefner, D.P., Kasl, S.V., et al. Selected psychosocial models and correlates of individual health related behaviors. *Med Care*, 1977, *15*(suppl 5):27-46.

54. Hailey, B.J., & Lalor, K.M. Perceptions about breast cancer patients: The effect of the type of relationship

with the patient. *J Psychosoc Oncol*, 1990, *8*(1):119-132.

55. Domino, G., Affonso, D.A., & Hannah, M.T. Assessing the imagery of cancer: The Cancer Metaphors Test. *J Psychosoc Oncol*, 1991, *9*(4):103-121.

56. Domino, G., & Lin, J. Images of cancer: China and the United States. *J Psychosoc Oncol*, 1991, *9*(3):67-78.

57. Domino, G., & Lin, W. Cancer metaphors: Taiwan and the United States. *Int J Psychol*, 1993, *28*(1):45-56.

58. Domino, G., Fragoso, A., & Moreno, H. Cross-cultural investigations of the imagery of cancer in Mexican nationals. *Hisp J Behav Sci*, 1991, *13*(4):422-435.

59. Berrenberg, J.L. The Cancer Attitude Inventory: Development and validation. *J Psychosoc Oncol*, 1991, *9*(2):35-44.

60. Rounds, J.B., & Zevon, M.A. Cancer stereotypes: A multidimensional scaling analysis. *J Behav Med*, 1993, *16*(5):485-496.

61. Berman, S.H., & Wandersman, A., Measuring knowledge of cancer. *Soc Sci Med*, 1991, *32*(11):1245-1255.

62. Derogatis, I.R. *SCL-90-R.* Towson, MD, Clinical Psychometric Research, 1992.

63. Pettingale, K.W., Burgess, C., & Greer, S. Psychological response to cancer diagnosis—I. Correlations with prognostic variables. *J Psychosom Res*, 1988, *32*(3):255-261.

64. Greer, S., Morris, T., Pettingale, K.W., et al. Psychological response to breast cancer and 15-year outcome. *Lancet*, 1990, *335*(8680): 49-50.

65. Nelson, D.V., Friedman, L.C., Baer, P.E., et al. Attitudes to cancer: Psychometric properties of fighting spirit and denial. *J Behav Med*, 1989, *12*(4):341-355.

66. Frank-Stromborg, M. Reaction to the diagnosis of cancer questionnaire: Development and psychometric evaluation. *Nurs Res*, 1989, *38*(6):364-369.

67. Frank-Stromborg, M., Wright, P., Segalla, M., et al. Psychological impact of the cancer diagnosis. *Oncol Nurs Forum*, 1984, *11*(3):16-22.

Appendix

20A. Additional Important Measures of Cancer Attitudes

Instrument	Description	Psychometric Indices
Cancer Attitude Inventory Developed by Hocloch and Coulson, 1968 (42)	Measure of nursing students' attitudes toward cancer based on Sherif's conceptual framework of attitude change (43) 36-item, Likert-type scale	Content validity established Test–retest reliability: 0.96
Craytor's Oncology Nursing Questionnaire Developed by Craytor et al., 1978 (44)	Measures attitudes and learning needs of nurses caring for cancer patients Nurses asked to respond to item in 2 ways: (1) importance of cancer patient care activities; (2) how successfully activity performed Modified as cancer nursing skills have changed over time	Reliability data not given Validity: factor analyses for 2 factors: psychosocial care and physical care
The Cancer Attitudes Questionnaire Developed by Hoffmeister, 1976 (45)	21-item measure of cancer attitudes using 5-point Likert-type format Cluster analysis revealed 4 clusters: fatalism, optimism, cancer phobia, stigma	Reliability: test-retest (1-week interval) performed Validity: cluster characteristics of the measure indicate clusters valid (internal consistency) Face-content validity established
Croen and Lebovits's Cancer Attitudes Questionnaire Developed by Lebovits et al., 1984 (46,47)	28-items representing seven attitudinal dimensions (3–6 in each dimension) 50% of items in each dimension expressed negatively, and 50% positively 6-point Likert forced choice scale (no undecided or neutral responses) Instrument modified to contain 5 factors (47)	Construct validity: established by expert panel Factor analysis performed Reliability: interrater: determined by repeated-measures; ANOVA internal consistency: alpha coefficient: 0.96
Nurses' Attitude Questionnaire Modified from the original (48) by Whelan, 1984 (49)	14-multiple choice question measure used to compare cancer attitudes of nurses in the U.S. and England	No reliability or validity data available
Fanslow's Cancer Attitudes Instrument Developed by Fanslow, 1985 (50)	49-item measure derived from American Cancer Society Questionnaire and Crayton's Oncology Nursing Questionnaire 15 items address attitudes about skills in cancer nursing 34 items address cancer-related myths and knowledge 5-point Likert scale used (5 most positive, 1 most negative) Higher total score reflects more positive attitude towards cancer	Internal consistency satisfactory: alpha 0.9 (skill), 0.9 (knowledge) Face and content validity established Higher scores may relate to nurse's ability to effectively care for patients with cancer and knowledge about cancer
Yasko and Power's Cancer Attitude Survey Developed by Donovan et al., 1977 (51)	38-item measure using a forced-choice 4-point Likert-type scale for responses Derived from previous questionnaires; items added	Reliability reported to be 0.80

20A. Additional Important Measures of Cancer Attitudes (*cont.*)

Instrument	Description	Psychometric Indices
Cancer Opinionnaire Developed by Schmelkin et al., 1986 (28)	Developed to measure medical students' attitudes toward psychosocial cancer care Revised to total 50, then 38, items with 6-point Likert-type response scale 5 subscales: (1) outcome expectations (10 items); (2) candor (10); (3) interest in treating cancer (6); (4) psychosocial concerns: role of physician (7); (5) psychosocial concerns: importance to the patient (5)	Principle axis factor analysis performed and 5 factor solution selected: oblique factor rotation indicated factors not correlated; varimax rotation used for item inclusion on subscales Alpha coefficients: (1) 0.79; (2) 0.82; (3) 0.75; (4) 0.68; (5) 0.68
Perceptions of Cancer Developed by Gutteling et al., 1986 (52)	Based on Health Belief Model (53) 4 subscales: (1) cancer knowledge (15 multiple-choice items); (2) health attitudes (11 statements with 5-point Likert scaled responses); (3) behavioral intention (items ask subjects to rate probability of behaving in a particular way to 5 daily situations); (4) fear of cancer (same situations as in (3) but subjects rate reactions on a 5-point scale)	Reliability and validity of subscales tested: (1) Cronbach's alpha: 0.73; item-total correlations averaged 0.34; (2) factor analyses used; principal component analysis revealed 4 factors (eigenvalues > 1.0, accounting for 57.9% of variance); (3) Cronbach's alpha: 0.64; item-total correlation averaged 0.40; (4) Cronbach's alpha: 0.90; item-total correlation averaged 0.58
Cancer Perception Vignettes Developed by Hailey and Lalor (54)	3 one-paragraph vignettes describing a breast cancer patient who recently received a mastectomy Subject asked to imagine what it would be like to visit her Relationship changes in each vignette: 1st is mother; 2nd is close family friend; and 3rd is a distant neighbor 12-item questionnaire then completed by subject concerning perceptions of patient and reactions to her 5 possible responses for each item (5 most negative; 1 most positive); higher total score, more pessimistic attitude toward patient	Factor analysis for 4 factors with eigenvalues >1, accounting for 59% of variance: (1) Reactions and attitudes of others; (2) Psychological effects; (3) Noticeable effects of illness; (4) Optimistic vs. pessimistic attitudes towards illness
Cancer Metaphors Test (CMT) Developed in 1991 (55)	Developed to assess image of cancer Subject asked to indicate the appropriateness of 32 metaphors in giving an image of what cancer is ("very appropriate" to "very inappropriate") Factors identified in factor analysis: (1) Total Pessimism (33.8% variance); (2) Future Optimism (14.2%); (3) Natural Disaster (10.3%); (4) Foreign Intruder (8.3%) Instrument used to compare images in China (56), Taiwan (57), Mexico (58)	Test–retest reliability (10- to 12-week interval) >0.70 Convergent and discriminant validity: factor analysis for 4 factors (25 of 32 metaphors, and 66.6% total variance); 4 factors statistically differentiated Health Locus of Control from CMT Internal consistency reliability of factors: (1) 0.85; (2) 0.88; (3) 0.79; (4) 0.73 Significant correlations with Health locus of control, Quality of life index

Instrument	Description	Reliability/Validity
Berrenberg's Cancer Attitude Inventory (CAI) Developed in 1989 (59)	Developed to test the 3 models explaining cancer attitudes: Familiarity, Vulnerability, and Dual process. Final 41-item inventory, derived from extensive review of the literature, questionnaire survey of 54 cancer survivors, and studies examining cancer attitudes	Reliability and validity tested on 302 undergraduate students. Factor analysis for 2 factors, analyzed by varimax rotation; factor structure could not be defined suggesting unidimensional scale. Cronbach's alpha: 0.91. Test–retest in 2 samples: 0.90, 0.91
Measure of Cancer Stereotypes Developed by Rounds and Zevon, 1993 (60)	Measures preconceptions or stereotypes of general public and cancer patients. Intended to identify the attributes most salient to cancer stereotype to develop strategies to alter the public's view of the cancer patient. Identified attributes important to organization of perception of a medical condition: such as severity, visibility, familiarity, comfort in socialization with affected person. Subject asked to rate each attribute on a 7-point scale and to also rate these attributes for 11 other illnesses as well as cancer, and finally, asked to make comparisons of similarity between pairs of illnesses	Sample tested: 68 physically healthy psychology students. Multidimensional scaling analyses for 2-dimensional solution I: Physical-functional health; II: Normality. Cancer was perceived as normal but having the most extreme physical impact. Responses to cancer clearly distinct from other illnesses. Further research on structure of illness stereotypes warranted
Fear of Cancer Index (FCI) Developed by Berman and Wandersman, 1992 (61)	Indirect measure of fear of cancer by asking subjects to interpret meanings of various physical symptoms. Can also be used to explain health-seeking behavior related to cancer prevention and screening. Composite score: distress ratings of 25 items from Symptom Checklist (SCL-90-R) (62) including 7 Warning Signs of Cancer, and 25 items from the Knowledge of Cancer Warning Signs Inventory (KCWSI) (61,63). Scoring: summed cross product values between each of identical KCWSI and SCL-90-R items (max score 300)	Reliability not addressed. Validity testing (correlation and regression analysis) demonstrated construct validity. Warrants further study
Cancer Adjustment Survey Developed by Nelson et al., 1989 (65)	Developed to measure the concepts of denial and "fighting spirit," reported to extend cancer survival (31,64). Eight 5-point Likert scale items used	Factor analysis for 3 factors: (1) Fighting spirit; (2) Information seeking; (3) Denial (weak). Test–retest reliability performed in samples with breast cancer (BC), and other cancers (OC): (1) BC: 0.71, OC: 0.51; (2) BC: 0.75, OC: 0.81; (3) BC: 0.57, OC: 0.35. Convergent and discriminant validity: suggest "Fighting spirit" has 2 components (fighting back, information seeking). Denial is weak factor requiring further study

20A. Additional Important Measures of Cancer Attitudes (*cont.*)

Instrument	Description	Psychometric Indices
Reaction to the Diagnosis of Cancer Questionnaire (RDCQ) Developed by Frank-Stromborg, 1989 (66)	Developed to assess initial reactions of persons diagnosed with cancer, from work begun in 1984 (67) Initial RDCQ comprised of 19 items, either distress or confronting responses, using yes–no format Revised RDCQ contains 17 items using 5 choice modified Likert format Further revised to improve internal consistency of the 2 groups of items, resulting ultimately in a 28-item instrument	Internal consistency reliability, coefficient alphas: (1) 17-item, initial revised RDCQ: 0.89 (confronting response items 0.72); (2) final 28-item RDCQ: 0.90 (confronting subscale, 0.82, distress subscale, 0.91) Factor analysis confirmed the multidimensional construct measured by the RDCQ Test–retest (2-week interval): 0.89 (distress scale 0.92; confronting scale 0.87)

Numbers in parentheses correspond to studies cited in the References.

21

Measuring Family Outcomes

Betty R. Ferrell and Michelle Rhiner

Cancer, an often chronic illness with significant physical and psychosocial consequences, has an impact on the whole family. It is estimated that two of every three individuals will have a family member who receives a cancer diagnosis.[1] Oncology nurses recognize the integral role of the family in caring for the person with cancer and have contributed significantly to the research related to cancer's impact on the family.

Any discussion on measuring family outcomes must begin with definitions of both *family* and *outcomes*. There is consensus that *family* is best defined by the individual patient, rather than interpretations of family limited to blood relations or those related by marriage. Family is a broad term and may include any significant relationship, such as friend, life partner, lover, relative, or spouse.

Family theorists agree that the family is more than the sum of its individuals. Family is viewed as a social system. Germino, a major contributor to conceptualization of family outcomes in oncology, defined family as a social system in which members have ties to each other, are interdependent, have some common history, and share some goals.[1]

Health-care research has emphasized the need to measure outcomes of nursing and medical interventions. This focus on outcomes has recently been extended to family research. In a thorough review of the methodologic and conceptual issues in family research, Feetham defines family outcomes as "the changes or stabilization in family functioning as an endpoint of nursing practice, or the abilities/functions of the family (at the family system or family member level) as an endpoint of nursing practice."[2,p106]

Thus, the measurement of family outcomes is best guided by a broad definition of family and by selecting outcomes that result from nursing care of the patient and family across the spectrum of illness and disease. The inclusion of family outcomes in health-care research is imperative; yet the theoretical and methodologic challenges of this research are significant.

Theories to Guide Research

Several authors have acknowledged the lack of family theories to guide research.[3-7] Research often is conducted on individual roles or relationships, such as family caregiving in chronic illness, but these studies seldom use a family framework.

Researchers frequently have used nursing theories that include concepts of social support, family, or social well-being to guide family research. These theories or conceptual models, however, are generally individual-specific models with reference to the interaction between patient and family. Feetham promotes the need for research that adds to our knowledge of family functioning and structure and contributes family theories to science.[2]

Methodologic Challenges

Increased attention to family outcomes is timely, particularly in light of health-care reforms that have transferred both acute and chronic care to family members. The burden on family members to provide health care occurs at a time when care also has become complex—high-tech care in the living room. Decreased hospital stays and increased outpatient care have resulted in family members' assuming responsibilities that are both physically and psychologically taxing.

Nursing has historically included family members in interventions such as teaching.[8] However, family members often have been viewed only as components of the patient's environment, rather than recipients of nursing care or as critical outcomes of such care.

Historically, family members often were included in research as proxy measures of patient outcomes. Proxy measures, however, lack validity for most patient variables. More recently, nurse researchers have recognized the importance of family outcomes as distinct and valuable outcome measures of nursing care. Research has demonstrated that care which benefits patients, such as improved pain management, may occur at the risk of creating significant burden on family caregivers.[9,10]

Feetham observes that there has been limited research expertise in family outcomes research, family research, and research involving the interaction of practitioners and families.[2] She also recognizes the need to identify predictors of family outcomes in light of diminishing health-care resources to identify high- and low-risk families.[2] For example, it is important to identify families most in need of assistance following outpatient surgery to best distribute resources for home care.

A critical measurement issue in family outcomes research is the identification of the unit of analysis. Outcomes may focus on an individual family member or be applicable to several family members. Some experiences will be similar for the patient and family members, whereas other experiences will be unique or contradict other ones. Some outcomes focus on the concept of caregiving and thus are primarily concerned with the individual(s) most involved in direct care. Other outcomes, such as family coping, require an analysis of the total family experience and involve multiple family members.

Dimensions of the Concept

Family outcomes has been explored in oncology as a multidimensional concept. Several key variables frequently surface. One of the most common is family communication. Investigators have evaluated the effect of cancer on patterns of communication, generally citing the difficulties imposed by a cancer diagnosis.[11] This variable illustrates the dynamic nature of the concept of family outcomes as family communication varies across the illness trajectory from initial diagnosis, to treatment, remission, relapse, and terminal illness.

An additional variable frequently explored in family research is the need for information.[12] Descriptive and exploratory investigations have assessed the need for education, particularly in the area of home care. A closely related variable is the need for support services. Coping and social support often have been extracted from patient outcomes research and applied to family members.[1,12,13]

Several researchers have identified caregiving demands associated with cancer care.[13-16] Laizner and colleagues[17] reviewed 14 studies between 1982 and 1993 that evaluated caregiver needs. Three general areas of need were identified: (1) personal needs (bathing, self-care); (2) instrumental needs (meals, housework, transportation); and (3) administrative needs (financial and legal). The authors stressed the importance of assessing caregiving demands over time adequately to address the changing nature and intensity of caregiving.

The importance of selecting appropriate concepts for measurement resounds throughout the family research literature. The initial response of family members to a cancer diagnosis may be best measured by concepts such as anxiety or coping but may later focus on entirely different concepts, such as anticipatory grief or loss.[18] Other concepts, such as hope or the need for information, may remain relevant concepts over time, yet take on altered meaning over the course of the illness.[19]

Despite global definitions of family, most family research has remained focused on individual members. The impact of the diagnosis on the spouse has been the predominant area of research.[19,20] The greatest methodologic challenge for the future is to broaden the scope of research to include multiple family members and measurement of the total family experience. Accomplishing this goal requires an interdisciplinary approach in which all researchers benefit from the involvement of other disciplines,[6] attention to the methodologic issues,[2] as described above, and a critical evaluation of the instruments currently used with individuals for their applicability to other family members or to family system outcomes.

Issues Involved in Selecting Instruments

Feetham[4] provides an excellent review of the methodologic issues involved in measuring family outcomes. Researchers recognize that reliability issues are important in family research, as the family system is dynamic and outcomes are expected to change significantly over time. Validity issues are a challenge in family outcome research because researchers need to evaluate the relevance of using outcomes borrowed from patient research in family outcomes analyses. The content of instruments that measure anxiety, coping, or hope may in fact be quite different in the context of the family. Likewise, issues of construct validity are challenged when applied to family caregivers as issues such as the relationship of the individual family member to the patient may in fact have a significant impact on the validity of that concept. For example, the concepts of grief or loss vary greatly in family members caring for a child versus a grandparent with cancer.

Germino has addressed the pragmatic issues of measuring family outcomes. She discusses issues such as respondent burden in relation to family members.[21] Family members may be both physically and psychologically exhausted, and in fact the burden on family caregivers may exceed the needs of the patient. Germino recognizes the difficulties associated with recruiting family subjects. Gaining access to family members outside of the clinic setting and arranging appropriate sites for data collection may be more difficult than in patient research.

Numerous cultural considerations also must be considered in any evaluation of family outcomes. The cultural meanings associated with family, religion, family traditions, and ethnic influences are very relevant in family research.[22]

Family outcomes research is not simply a replication of the outcomes and variables in patient research to families. Many concepts and outcomes are appropriate, but recognizing the unique nature of the family requires careful analysis and selection of outcomes. A clear understanding of the meaning of family and of the family as a system requires both qualitative and quantitative approaches.[23] The research conducted by Clarke-Steffen as summarized at the end of the chapter[23] is an excellent example of the value of qualitative research to garner insight into the meaning of family in the context of childhood cancer.

Most limitations of family research concern sample selection. Most family research has been conducted on highly articulate family members with advanced education and high socioeconomic status. The inclusion of family members from diverse backgrounds and skills requires attention to the readability and the total appropriateness of evaluation methodologies. Several investigators have noted differences in family outcomes based on individual characteristics such as gender[14,24] and age.[25,26] Further exploration of these individual characteristics should enhance our understanding of family outcomes.

Clark and Gwin[12] advocate the identification of additional variables of interest, including the health of the family caregivers, the marital relationship, and adaptation of the children of adults with cancer. Survivorship in pediatric cancer also challenges researchers to explore outcomes of interest for this population.[27-29] The diagnosis of cancer in a child has a significant impact on the entire family over time and on the child into adulthood.[27-29]

Instruments Available for Measuring Family Outcomes

Instruments that have been used in family outcomes research are described in Appendix 21A.[30-50] The concepts measured include family functioning, social support, coping, caregiving demands, caregiver reactions, marital adjustment, quality of life, and others. The reader should note that many other instruments and concepts presented in this text also are relevant for family outcomes research.

Summary

Changes in the health-care environment continue to thrust the burden of caregiving onto the family and emphasize the need for careful evaluation of caregiver needs or burden for effective intervention. A variety of instruments can measure the impact of medical and nursing interventions on family outcomes. However, clearly, additional instrument development and refinement are needed.

Exemplar Study

Clarke-Steffen, L. A model of the family transition to living with childhood cancer. *Cancer Pract*, 1993, *1*(N 4):285–292.

This longitudinal, grounded theory study described family transition in response to everyday life with childhood cancer from the family's point of view when a child is diagnosed with cancer with a favorable prognosis. Favorable prognosis was defined as a long-term survival rate greater than 60%. A convenience sample consisting of 40 members of seven families with a child recently diagnosed with cancer was recruited for the study. Data collection consisted of three tape-recorded, semistructured interviews with family members in the home.

Family transition was characterized in four stages as: (1) a fracturing of reality at the realization of the malignant nature of the illness; (2) a period of limbo, characterized by uncertainty after the diagnosis; (3) a utilization of strategies to reconstruct reality; and (4) a construction of a "new normal" for the family, during which the nature of uncertainty changed, but persisted. A model of family transition in response to the diagnosis of childhood cancer was developed.

This study is exemplar for several reasons. The investigator uses multiple family members to develop a model of family transition in living with childhood cancer. The study also includes longitudinal measures and interviews families at three points in time. The interviews occurred over a 5-month period. This study resulted in the initial development of a theoretical model for explaining family transition to living with childhood cancer. It illustrates how qualitative research can direct future research.

The approach identified important concepts studied in the past and for which existing instruments were known. For example, the model identifies concepts such as uncertainty, vulnerability, helplessness, and meaning in illness that can now be incorporated in future family research in this area. An additional strength of this study is that it included interviews of the individual family members as well as a group interview with all family members. The author concludes by suggesting that research is needed to relate family variables and care variables to both family functioning and medical outcomes.

References

1. Germino, B. Cancer and the family. In S.B. Baird, R. McCorkle, & M. Grant (Eds.), *Cancer nursing: A comprehensive textbook.* Philadelphia: Saunders, 1991, pp. 38-44.

2. Feetham, S.B. *Family outcomes: Conceptual and methodological issues.* NIH Publication No. 93-3411. Washington, DC: Department of Health and Human Services, 1992, pp. 103-111.

3. Feetham, S.L. Family research: Issues and directions for nursing. In H. Werley & J.J. Fitzpatrick (Eds.), *Annual review of nursing research* (2nd ed.). New York: Springer, 1984, pp. 3-25.

4. Feetham, S.L. Conceptual and methodological issues in research of families. In A.L. Whall & J. Fawcett (Eds.), *Family theory development in nursing: State of the science and art.* Philadelphia: Davis, 1991, pp. 43-58.

5. Burr, W.R., Herrin, D.A., Day, R.D., et al. Epistemologies that lead to primary explanations in family science. *Fam Sci Rev,* 1988, 1(3):185-210.

6. Knafl, K. Family outcomes: Practitioner/family interface. In P. Moritz (Ed.), *Patient outcomes research: Examining the effectiveness of nursing practice.* Rockville, MD: National Center for Nursing Research, 1992.

7. Gilliss, C.L. Family nursing research, theory and practice. *IMAGE: J Nurs Scholar,* 1991, 22(4):19-22.

8. Craft, M., & Willadsen, J.A. Interventions related to family. *Nurs Clin North Am,* 1992, 27(2):517-540.

9. Ferrell, B.R., Rhiner, M., Cohen, M.Z., & Grant, M. Pain as a metaphor for illness. Part I: Impact of cancer pain on family caregivers. *Oncol Nurs Forum,* 1991, 18(8):1303-1309.

10. Ferrell, B.R., Cohen, M.Z., Rhiner, M., & Grant, M. Pain as a metaphor for illness. Part II: Family caregivers' management of pain. *Oncol Nurs Forum,* 1991, 18(8):1315-1321.

11. Cassileth, B.R., & Hamilton, J. The family with cancer. In B.R. Cassileth (Ed.), *The cancer patient: Social and medical aspects of care.* Philadelphia: Lea & Febiger, 1979, pp. 233-247.

12. Clark, J.C., & Gwin, R.R. Psychosocial Responses of the Family. In S.L. Groenwald, M.H. Frogge, M. Goodman, & C.H. Yarbro (Eds.), *Cancer nursing principles and practice* (3rd Ed.). Sudbury, MA: Jones & Bartlett, 1993, pp. 468-483.

13. Oberst, M.T., Thomas, S.E., Gass, K.A., & Ward, S.E. Caregiving demands and appraisal of stress among family caregivers. *Cancer Nurs,* 1989, 12(4):209-215.

14. Stetz, K. Caregiving demands during advanced cancer. *Cancer Nurs,* 1987, 10:260-268.

15. Oberst, M.I., & Scott, D.W. Postdischarge distress in surgically treated cancer patients and their spouses. *Res Nurs Health,* 1988, 11(4):223-233.

16. Hinds, C. The needs of families who care for patients with cancer at home: Are we meeting them? *J Adv Nurs,* 1985, 10(6):575-581.

17. Laizner, A.M., Shegda Yost, L.M., Barg, F.K., & McCorkle, R. Needs of family caregivers of persons with cancer: A review. *Sem Oncol Nurs,* 1993, 9(2):114-120.

18. Frank-Stromborg, M., & Wright, P. Ambulatory cancer patients' perceptions of the physical and psychosocial changes in their lives since the diagnosis of cancer. *Cancer Nurs,* 1984, 7(2):117-129.

19. Gotay, C. The experience of cancer during early and advanced stages: The view of patients and their mates. *Soc Sci Med,* 1984, 18(7):605-613.

20. Northouse, L.L. The impact of breast cancer on patients and husbands. *Cancer Nurs,* 1989, 12(5):276-284.

21. Germino, B.B. Quality of life for families with cancer: Research issues. *Meniscus Health Care Comm, Qual Life—Nurs Chall,* 1993, 2(2):39-45.

22. Johnson, J.L., & Lane, C.A. Helping families respond to cancer. In S.B. Baird, R. McCorkle, & M. Grant (Eds.), *Cancer nursing: A comprehensive textbook.* Philadelphia: Saunders, 1991, pp. 921-931.

23. Clarke-Steffen, L. A model of the family transition to living with childhood cancer. *Cancer Pract,* 1993, 1(4):285-292.

24. Siegel, K., Raveis, V.H., Mor V., et al. The relationship of spousal caregiver burden to patient disease and treatment-related conditions. *Ann Oncol*, 1991, *2*(7):511-516.

25. Carey, P.J., Oberst, M.T., McCubbin, M.A., & Hughes, S.H. Appraisal and caregiving burden in family members caring for patients receiving chemotherapy. *Oncol Nurs Forum*, 1991, *18*(8):1341-1348.

26. Hileman, J.W., Lackey, N.R., & Hassanein, R.S. Identifying the needs of patients with cancer. *Oncol Nurs Forum*, 1992, *19*(5):771-777.

27. Lichtman, R.R., Taylor, S.E., Wood, J.V., et al. Relations with children after breast cancer: The mother–daughter relationship at risk. *J Psychosoc Oncol*, 1984, *2*:1-19.

28. Birenbaum, L.K., & Yancey, D. Children's response to parent's cancer. *Second National Conference on Cancer Nursing Research*, Baltimore, MD: American Cancer Society, 1992.

29. Baird, S.B. The effect of cancer in a parent on role relationships with the nurse/daughter. *Cancer Nurs*, 1988, *11*(1):9-17.

30. Roberts, C.S., & Feetham, S.L. Assessing family functioning across three areas of relationship. *Nurs Res*, 1982, *3*(4):231-235.

31. Knafl, K., Gallo, A., Breitmayer, B., et al. One approach to conceptualizing family response to illness. In S. Feetham, S. Meister, J. Bell, & K. Gilliss (Eds.), *The nursing of families*. Newbury Park, CA: Sage, 1992, pp. 70-78.

32. Norbeck, J.S., Lindsey, A.M., & Carrieri, V.L. The development of an instrument to measure social support. *Nurs Res*, 1981, *30*(5):264-269.

33. Norbeck, J.S., Lindsey, A.M., & Carrieri, V.L. Further development of the Norbeck Social Support Questionnaire: Normative data and validity testing. *Nurs Res*, 1983, *32*(1):4-9.

34. Lewis, F.M., Woods, N.F., Hough, E.E., & Bensley, L.S. The family's functioning with chronic illness in the mother: The spouse's perspective. *Soc Sci Med*, 1989, *29*(11):1261-1269.

35. Lewis, F.M., & Hammond, M. Psychosocial adjustment of the family to breast cancer: A longitudinal analysis. *JAMA*, 1992, *47*(5):194-200.

36. Lewis, F.M., Hammond, M., & Woods, N.F. The family's functioning with newly diagnosed breast cancer in the mother: The development of an explanatory model. *J Behav Med*, 1993, *16*(4):351-370.

37. Woods, N.F., Haberman, M., & Packard, N.J. Demands of illness and individual, dyadic and family

adaptation in chronic illness. *Western J Nurs Res*, 1993, *15*(1):10-30.

38. Stetz, K.M. The Experience of spouse caregiving during advanced cancer. Unpublished Doctoral Dissertation. Seattle: University of Washington, 1986.

39. Stetz, K.M. The relationship among background characteristics, purpose in life, and health in spouse caregivers. *Sch Inq Nurs Pract*, 1989, *3*(2):133-153.

40. Given, C.W., Given, B., Stommel, M., et al. The caregiver reaction assessment (CRA) for caregivers to persons with chronic physical and mental impairments. *Res Nurs Health*, 1992, *15*(4):271-283.

41. Stommel, M., Wang, S., Given, C.W., & Given, B. Focus on Psychometrics Confirmatory Factor Analysis (CFA) as a method to assess measurement equivalence. *Res Nurs Health*, *15*(5):399-405.

42. Ferrell, B., Rhiner, M., & Rivera, L.M. Development and Evaluation of the Family Pain Questionnaire. *J Psychosoc Oncol*, 1993, *10*(4):21-35.

43. Ferrell, B.R., Grant, G., Chan, J., et al. The impact of pain education on family caregivers of elderly patients. *Oncology Nursing Forum*, 1995, *22*(8):1211-1218.

44. Robinson, B. Validation of a caregiver strain index. *J Gerontol*, *38*(3):344-348.

45. Smilkstein, G., Ashworth, C., & Montano, D. Validity and reliability of the family APGAR as a test of family function. *J Fam Pract*, 1982, *15*(2):303-311.

46. Spanier, G.B. Measuring dyadic adjustment: New scales for assessing the quality of marriage and similar dyad. *J Marr Fam*, 1976, *31*:15-28.

47. McCubbin, H.I., & Comeau, J. FIRM: Family inventory of resources for management. In H.I. McCubbin, A.I. Thompson (Eds.), *Family assessment inventories for research and practice*. Madison, WI: University of Wisconsin-Madison, Family Stress Coping and Health Project, 1987, pp. 145-160.

48. McCubbin, H., & Patterson, J. FILE: family inventory of life events and changes. In H. McCubbin & A. Thompson (Eds.), *Family assessment inventories for research and practice*. Madison, WI: University of Wisconsin Press, 1987, pp. 81-100.

49. Olson, D.H., Portner, J., & Bell, R. Family adaptability and cohesion evaluation scales (FACES II). St. Paul, University of Minnesota, Family Social Services, 1982.

50. Olson, D.H., Sprenkle, D.H., & Russell, C.S. Circumplex model of marital and family systems. I. cohesion and adaptability dimensions, family types and clinical applications. *Fam Proc*, 1979, *18*(1):3-28.

Appendix

21A. Instruments to Measure Family Outcomes

Instrument/ Target Population	Dimensions/Description	Psychometric Indices
Feetham Family Functioning Survey (FFFS) (3,30) Family's ability to function as a unit within the community and their internal system	21-item, self-report measure of 3 constructs: (1) family interactions with the community; (2) family relationship to various subsystems; (3) reciprocal relationships within the family structure Subjects answer 3 questions on each item on a 7-point Likert scale (1 little, 7 much): (1) "How much is there now?"; (2) "How much should there be?" and (3) "How important is it to me?"	Cronbach's alpha for the 3 measures: 0.66–0.84 Test-retest reliability: 2-week interval: 0.93; 5-week interval: 0.83 Correlations between scores of husbands and wives: 0.72
Defining and Managing Chronic Illness Parent Interviews #1, #2 Child's Interviews #1, #2 Sibling's Interviews #1, #2 (31) Target population: families with a child diagnosed with a chronic illness	Interview guides developed to tape-record the child with a chronic illness, the parents and siblings, covering topics of: history of illness; course of illness; child's condition, medication, and treatment; how the family takes care of the illness; school situation; health-care situation; family events from the parents', child's, and siblings' perspective	None described
Norbeck Social Support Questionnaire (NSSQ) (32,33) Measures social support from all sources, including family members	Respondent asked to list each significant person, and relationship (9 questions measure the perceived support with regard to functional properties of social support) Uses 5-point Likert scale (1 not at all, 5 a great deal) Self-administered to groups or by mail; takes about 10 minutes to complete Separate score for family support can be calculated; allows for cultural variation as studies show the most effective sources of support may differ among cultural groups	Tested on nursing students Test-retest reliability $n = 67$ with 2-week interval: 0.85–0.92 Kendall tau B correlation coefficients: number of categories of persons lost: 0.83 ($p < 0.001$); amount of support lost: 0.71 ($p < 0.001$) Internal consistency tested through intercorrelations among all items: 2 affect items: 0.97; 2 affirmation items: 0.96; 2 aid items: 0.89 3 network property items: 0.88–0.96; correlations highly related to affect and affirmation (0.88–0.97) and moderately related to aid (0.69–0.80) Validity: did not correlate with Marlowe-Crowne Test of Social Desirability-SF Concurrent validity testing: parallels between tangible support (Social Support Questionnaire) and aid and informational support and affect Construct validity: low but significant relationship with Profile of Mood States depression and confusion subscales and NSSQ total loss subscale

21A. Instruments to Measure Family Outcomes (*cont.*)

Instrument/Target Population	Dimensions/Description	Psychometric Indices
F-COPES (34-36) Women with breast cancer and their family	49-question measure of psychosocial adjustment of the family to breast cancer Uses 5-point Likert scale (1 never, 5 almost always) Families interviewed by a 2-person interview team; partners independently complete the self-report questionnaire	Internal consistency reliabilities (coefficient alpha): women and partner's measures: ≥ 0.83 (most 0.90); mother's measure of quality of mother–child relationship: 0.74 Stability reliability coefficients: (4-month interval): 0.58–0.83 Depression and experienced illness demands changing the most over time
Demands of Illness Inventory (DOII) (37) Families with chronic illness	125-question measure of psychosocial adjustment of the family to diabetes and breast cancer Questionnaire can identify demands associated with a recent diagnosis of a chronic illness and with long-term adaptation Questions assess 7 subscales: (1) physical symptoms; (2) personal meaning; (3) family functioning; (4) social relationships; (5) self-image; (6) monitoring symptoms; (7) treatment issues Parallel instrument for partners Employs 4-point Likert scale (1 not at all, 4 extremely) Families interviewed at home; partners complete self-report questionnaire	Internal consistency reliability (alpha coefficients) of 7 dimensions (subscales): demands experienced (0.78–0.91); intensity of demands (0.86–0.92) Cronbach's alphas (total score): number score (0.96); intensity score (0.97)

Caregiving Demands Scale (CDS) (38,39)
Caregivers of individuals with chronic illness in the home
	Self-report questionnaire
	3 dimensions measured: (1) physical care; (2) role alterations; (3) financial alterations
	All scales/dimensions have one or more subscales
	All scales have 2 conceptually different components for measuring demands: (1) caregiving actions or behaviors; (2) perceived level of difficulty on carrying out that behavior
	5-point Likert scale used (1 not at all difficult, 5 extremely difficult)
		Physical care scale
		  Alpha coefficient, total scale: 0.78
		  Internal consistency reliability: meals (0.69); intimate care (0.71); walking/transfers (0.80); meds/treatment (0.60); supervision (0.94); new skill acquisition (0.60); rest (0.45)
		  Content validity established
		Role alteration
		  Alpha coefficient (total score): 0.78
		  Internal consistency reliability coefficients: social participation (0.66); interpersonal relationships (0.83)
		Financial alterations
		  Reliability not established
		  Overall validity confirmed using sample procedures of other 2 scales

Instrument / Population / Description	Psychometric Properties
Caregiver Reaction Assessment (CRA) (40,41) Caregivers of the elderly with physical impairments or dementia in the home 24-item measure of differences in the reactions of various groups of caregivers and how their reactions change over time 5 subscales: caregiver esteem, lack of family support, impact on finances, impact on schedule, impact on health 5-point Likert scale used (1 strongly agree, 5 strongly disagree) Measure completed during an in-person interview with repeat administration over time to assess change	Internal consistency of subscales calculated using Cronbach's alpha All items forming each subscale loaded within 20 points or less of one another (lowest scores 0.60) Loadings range for Impact on Health Scale: 0.91–0.52
Family Pain Questionnaire (FPQ) (42) Caregivers managing chronic cancer pain at home 14-item linear analog measure of knowledge of a family caregiver in managing chronic cancer pain Administered by mail or in person	Established reliability (test–retest, internal consistency) and validity (content, construct, concurrent) content validity: CVI > 0.90 construct validity: ANOVA, $p < 0.05$ concurrent validity: ($r > 0.60$, $p < 0.05$) factor analysis: 2 subscales of knowledge and experience test–retest reliability ($r > 0.80$) with retest or caregivers ($n = 67$)
Quality of Life (family version) (43) Caregivers of persons with cancer in the home 20-item linear analog measure of quality of life of a family member caring for a patient with cancer Subscales include: physical well-being; psychologic well-being; social well-being; spiritual well-being Administered by mail or in person	Psychometric analysis in progress with 60 subjects, 180 observations
Caregiver Strain Index (CSI) (44) Caregivers 13-item, ordinal scale that measures family caregiver's strain in providing various degrees of care to patients at home Administered by mail or in person	Internal consistency (Cronbach's alpha): 0.86 (81 cases) Evidence of construct validity obtained in 3 areas: (1) patient characteristics; (2) subjective perceptions of the caretaking relationship by caregivers; (3) emotional health of caregivers
Family APGAR (45) Individual's perception of family function 5-item questionnaire that measures a family member's perception of family function 5 parameters measured: adaptation; partnership; growth; affection; resolve 3-point ordinal scale (0–2) used for each item Self-administered	Correlated with previously validated instrument, Pless-Satterwhite Family Index and with estimates made by psychotherapists of family function: APGAR/Pless-Satterwhite correlation: 0.80; APGAR/Therapist correlation: 0.64 Family APGAR scores of married graduate students (mean = 8.24) significantly higher than scores of community mental health clinic patients (mean = 5.89)
Dyadic Adjustment Scale (DAS) (46) Married or unmarried, cohabiting couples Spanier DAS is a 32-item questionnaire measuring a family member's perception of family function 5 parameters measured: adaptation; partnership; growth; affection; resolve Uses 5-point Likert scale (1 always disagrees, 5 always agree) Tool useful for assessing marital adjustment Self-administered or can be adapted for interview use	Cronbach coefficient alpha (total DAS and component subscales): 0.73–0.96 Criterion-related and construct validity established (tool's ability to differentiate between married and divorced people) Correlation coefficient (Locke-Wallace Marriage Inventory): 0.86 (married individuals), 0.88 (divorced individuals)

21A. Instruments to Measure Family Outcomes (*cont.*)

Instrument/ Target Population	Dimensions/Description	Psychometric Indices
Family Inventory of resources for Management (FIRM) (47) Patients and family members, including all adults and children	69-item questionnaire measuring family's ability to deal with stressors 4 factors evaluated: (1) family strengths (esteem and communication); (2) family strengths (mastery and health); (3) extended family social support; (4) family well-being 4-point Likert scale used (1 not at all, 4 very well) Self-report	Cronbach's alpha: 0.89 (4 primary subscales: 0.62–0.85) Total FIRM scores correlated with measures of: family cohesion (0.46); expressiveness (0.27); conflict (0.30); organization (0.25)
Family Inventory of Life Events and Changes (FILE) (48) Adult family members	71-item measure designed for adult members of the family unit Items ask family members to check all events experienced by any member of the family over a 1-year period Individual family score is compared to the norm in the appropriate stage and is a means of classifying the family into a high-stress, moderate-stress, or low-stress group Self-report	No data available at this time
Family Adaptability and Cohesion Evaluation Scales (FACES) (49,50) Family members	FACES II is a 20-item questionnaire designed to classify families into 3 general and 16 specific types on adaptability and cohesion dimensions Subjects rate the frequency of a behavior on a 5-point scale (1 almost never, 5 almost always) Family cohesion is measured as a means of evaluating family's ability to adapt/adjust during illness Self-report and should be completed independently	Cronbach's alpha (estimated): cohesion (0.77); adaptability (0.67); total scale (0.68) Scores between family members ranged from 0.30 to 0.40

Numbers in parentheses correspond to studies cited in the References.

22

Measuring Anxiety

Patricia M. Grimm

Anxiety is a word that is familiar to everyone. Depending on usage, anxiety can be considered a normal response to contemporary life stresses and strains, an expected reaction to the demands of illness, an intrinsic personality characteristic, or a psychiatric diagnosis. The measurement of anxiety, therefore, depends on the researcher's perspective and purpose. This chapter reviews the conceptualizations of anxiety, both historical and contemporary, issues in the selection of a measure of anxiety, available instruments, and current trends in anxiety research.

Definition

Anxiety can be defined as "an unpleasant subjective experience associated with the perception of real or imagined threat."[1,p511] Or, more comprehensively, "an emotion that signifies the presence of danger that cannot be identified, or if identified, is not sufficiently threatening to justify the intensity of the emotion."[2,p3] The word *anxiety* comes from the Greek word *agon*, from which we derive the terms anguish and agony. *Agon* also relates to the German word *Angst*, used in modern times by the existential philosophers Kierkegaard and Sartre to describe painful feelings of terror and dread.[2,3] In contemporary psychologic thinking, anxiety is seen as playing a central role in the functioning of personality. We all experience some degree of anxiety to foster creativity and face daily challenges; however, anxiety can also impair cognitive and intellectual functioning as well as interfere with effective problem solving.[3] The origins of anxiety, and the human responses defined as anxiety, have evolved over time and within the social context of those times.

Conceptualization

Since Greco-Roman times and before, anxiety has been associated with ideas of self-awareness and individuality. The philosophic beliefs of those times can be interpreted as systems of thought designed to deal with the threat of anxiety. Stoics believed that anxiety was the result of too great an investment in personal accomplishments. Christianity suggested that guilt was the source of anxiety, specifically guilt about failing to live up to one's high moral ideals. The existential philosophers of the mid nineteenth century associated guilt with personal freedom of choice. Anxiety existed because individuals had not only the freedom to choose, but also the responsibility to do so.[4]

Scientific thinkers of the nineteenth century interpreted anxiety as an adaptive response to a threat that was present in all species. Freud differentiated anxiety as objective, a reaction to the external environment, or neurotic, the intrapsychic struggle that exists within each individual.[4] His extensive work laid the cornerstone for much of our contemporary thinking about anxiety and defined it as a clinical, diagnostic entity. Later psychiatric theorists believed that anxiety had its basis in dependency needs, security needs, or the need for power.[4] Spielberger et al. delineated the influence of both intrapsychic and environmental processes by defining trait and state dimensions of anxiety.[5]

Contemporary conceptualizations of anxiety incorporate a stimulus–response model. Response-oriented theorists define anxiety as the neurophysiologic response to a stimulus. This response, not the stimulus itself, is the focus of their work.[4] Hoehn-Saric and McLeod comprehensively discussed the physiology of anxiety.[6] In contrast, stimulus-oriented theories, such as the cognitive approaches of Lazarus[7] and Beck,[4] approach anxiety as a behavioral response to a pattern of thoughts, feelings, and situations that is unique to the individual. Their focus is on the stimuli and serves as the basis for most clinical work with anxiety.

In summary, anxiety has been described as an experience with psychologic, somatic, and behavioral components. This experience can be characterized as an enduring personality characteristic, a situational response to life events, or a psychiatric diagnosis. The complexity and diversity of these interpretations of anxiety has implications for its measurement.

Issues in Measuring Anxiety

There are several important issues to address when selecting an instrument to measure anxiety. The first is to choose an instrument that is congruent with one's research question and conceptual framework. Questions to consider include how anxiety is defined in the framework of choice. Is it seen as a personality characteristic corresponding to anxiety proneness, as a change in response to an event/experience, or as a diagnostic indicator of psychopathology?[1] The latter question is important because specific measures exist for each definition.

Another important conceptual question to consider is the specificity of measurement required by the research question and the research design. Historically there exists a progression in instrument development from more specific measures of anxiety to more global indices of psychologic health or distress that include anxiety as one dimension. Early instruments, such as the Taylor Manifest Anxiety Scale[8] and the Hamilton Anxiety Scale,[9] were specific measures of anxiety and only anxiety. Instruments such as the Brief Symptom Inventory[10] and the Profile of Mood States[11] are more global assessments of psychologic status and include anxiety as one component. Some clinicians believe it is difficult to differentiate between the affective symptoms of anxiety and those of depression. This concern has resulted in the development of anxiety/depression models[12] and instruments such as the Hospital Anxiety and Depression Scale.[13]

A third consideration is the target population to be studied. Characteristics such as age, psychologic and physical health status, language, education, and reading level must be considered. In terms of age, all the instruments in this chapter assess anxiety in adults. The reader is referred elsewhere for a comprehensive discussion of the measurement of anxiety in children and adolescents.[14,15] Several measures of anxiety assess or differentiate diagnostic anxiety disorders in psychiatric patient populations. Depending on the existence of psychometric data to support their use with other groups, they may or may not be appropriate for nonpsychiatric use.

The preexistence of a physical illness, acute or chronic, presents an interesting dilemma. Many disease processes and their treatment may result in symptoms that are similar to those considered as physiologic indicators of anxiety: changes in pulse rate, respiratory rate and blood pressure; alterations in eating and sleeping patterns; nausea, vomiting, and diarrhea; or fatigue and restlessness.[16] This is particularly true with individuals who have cardiac disease, respiratory disease, cancer, endocrine disorders, or hematologic disorders such as anemia.[4] Certain metabolic states, specific medications, and poorly controlled pain can all result in physical symptoms that mimic anxiety.[17] The choice of an instrument that minimizes or eliminates such indicators of anxiety is an important consideration with medically ill populations. The issues of primary language and educational or reading level also must be addressed. Several of the instruments to be presented were developed in countries other than the United States, therefore close review is necessary to be sure that the language used and cultural context are congruent with the researcher's target population.

A final issue is the method of measurement. Three main approaches are represented by the instruments: structured diagnostic interviews, observational rating scales, and self-report paper-and-pencil instruments. Content analysis of verbal data also is reviewed. In conclusion, the choice of conceptual framework, research design, and target population, as well as the knowledge and expertise of the researcher, all influence the choice of measurement approach.

Instruments

The discussion of instruments developed to measure anxiety is organized in terms of their specificity. Anxiety-specific measures are presented first, followed by those that measure anxiety and depression. Global indices of psychological health or distress are then presented.

Taylor Manifest Anxiety Scale

The Taylor Manifest Anxiety Scale, originally developed in 1950, is a screening test for the identification of research subjects. Taylor[8] describes its development as an alternative to the use of experimental manipulation, such as electric shock or stress-producing situations, to select subjects with varied levels of anxiety. This self-report scale consists of 50-item statements, indicative of anxiety, from the Minnesota Multiphasic Personality Inventory (MMPI). The response format is true–false. Additional items have been added to control for social desirability, lying, and rigidity of responses. Test–retest reliability has been reported as 0.81 to 0.88. Content judges established face validity, and the Taylor scale was found to have a correlation of 0.85 with the administration of the MMPI. This instrument was originally tested on college students and psychiatric patients. Its use has been expanded to include adults in general.

Hamilton Anxiety Scale (HAS)

Another older instrument, the Hamilton Anxiety Scale (HAS) was developed in 1959 as a clinical interview rating scale of the psychic and somatic aspects of anxiety. The scale consists of 14 items or clinical symptoms with a 5-point rating response ranging from 0 (not present) to 4 (very severe). The original form did not include descriptive statements of these rating responses. However, Bech et al.[9] have developed a list of item definitions for each response choice. For example, Item 5, Intellectual Retardation, is defined by:

0   The patient exhibits normal intellectual activity.

1   The patient has to make an effort to concentrate on his work.

2   Even with major effort it is difficult for the patient to concentrate on his work. Less initiative than usual. The patient at an early state experiences brain fatigue.

3   Marked difficulties with concentration, initiative and decision making. The patient needs many breaks even when performing simple, routine jobs.

4   It is difficult for the patient to follow normal conversation, and he cannot read a newspaper or watch television.

In addition, they have developed a scoring system to differentiate generalized anxiety from panic anxiety. The Hamilton Anxiety Scale has been used extensively since its development. An interrater reliability Spearman test correlation of 0.78 has been reported for the revised form, with strong item-to-total score correlations. Validity data is reported with global assessment measures of anxiety used as the criterion.[8] Originally designed to be used with psychiatric patients diagnosed with anxiety disorders, its use has expanded to adult patients and nonpatients, including a study of preoperative and postoperative anxiety experienced by cardiac surgery patients.[8]

State-Trait Anxiety Inventory (STAI)

Probably the most extensively used measure of anxiety, the State-Trait Anxiety Inventory (STAI), is comprised of separate self-report scales for measuring two distinct anxiety concepts: state and trait. *State anxiety* is defined as "a transitory emotional state or condition," whereas *trait anxiety* is defined as "relatively stable individual differences in anxiety proneness."[5,p3] Each scale consists of 20 statements that the subject rates to describe how they generally feel (trait) or how they feel at a particular moment in time (state). The subject responds on a 4-point scale, from 1 (not at all) to 4 (very much so). In studies conducted by Spielberger,[5] test–retest reliability coefficients of 0.73 to 0.86 and 0.86 to 0.92 have been reported for the trait subscale and coefficients of 0.16 to 0.54 and 0.83 to 0.92 for the state subscale.[5] Alpha coefficient values obtained to measure internal consistency ranged from 0.83 to 0.92 for state and 0.86 to 0.92 for trait.[18] Concurrent validity was supported by correlating the STAI with the Taylor and IPAT Anxiety Scales (0.79 to 0.83 and 0.75 to 0.76, respectively). Construct validity was determined by comparing like subjects under stressful and nonstressful situations.[5] The STAI has been successfully used with high school and college students,[5] psychiatric patients,[5] medical and surgical patients,[18-23] obstetrical patients,[24,25] the chronically ill,[26,27] and the elderly.[28] The STAI is written at a fifth-grade reading level, and a children's version also is available.

Anxiety Status Inventory (ASI/SAS)

Developed by Zung,[29] the Anxiety Status Inventory is actually two measures, the ASI and the Self-rating Anxiety Scale (SAS). The former is a 20-item observer rating scale, and the latter, as implied in its name, is a 20-item self-report scale. The ASI uses a 4-point rating scale to evaluate the severity of anxiety symptoms observed, during a clinical interview, from 1 (none) to 4 (severe). The SAS consists of positively and negatively worded statements that the respondent rates as having experienced within the last week from 1 (none or a little of the time) to 4 (most or all of the time). Both scales measure clinical anxiety in psychiatric patients. However, the author also reports studies that have included individuals without psychiatric illnesses.

The reliability coefficient comparing the ASI with the SAS is 0.66. Split-half coefficients for these scales were 0.83 and 0.71, respectively. Concurrent validity correlations with the TMAS were 0.33 for the ASI and 0.30 for the SAS. Discriminant validity was supported in comparison studies of anxiety disorder patients and controls.[29]

Brief Scale for Anxiety

Developed by Tyrer et al.,[30] the Brief Scale for Anxiety is another clinical interview rating scale designed to assess the psychologic and somatic symptoms of anxiety. The interviewer rates the subject on each of 10 symptoms on a 7-point scale from 0 (no occurrence of the symptom) to 7 (incapacitation by/lack of control of the symptom). The instrument was originally created to identify anxiety in psychiatric patients who did not have a primary anxiety disorder, but the author indicates that this measure could also be used with medical and neurologic patients.[30] It also can be used to monitor changes in symptoms. Limited reliability and validity data are available.

Anxiety Scale (Gottschalk-Gleser Content Analysis Scales)

For a qualitative approach to the examination of anxiety, Gottschalk and Bechtel have developed a computer-based scale to analyze verbal samples.[31] The scale consists of six types of anxiety: death, mutilation, separation, guilt, shame, and diffuse/nonspecific, with three or four weighted choices under each type: self, animate others, inanimate objects, and denial. For example:

> *Shame anxiety.* References to ridicule, inadequacy, shame, embarrassment, humiliation, overexposure of deficiencies or private details, or threat of such experienced by:
>   a. Self
>   b. Animate others
>   c. Denial

Reliability coefficients for the computerized version and hand coding were 0.85 for the total scale and 0.58 to 0.92 for the individual items. Validity data were not reported.

Hospital Anxiety and Depression Scale (HADS)

Developed by Zigmond and Swaith, this 14-item measure of anxiety and depression is unique in that it was specifically designed to assess these disorders in medically ill patients by excluding items related to somatic symptoms.[13] Using a 4-point rating format, the respondent assesses how he or she has felt during the past week. The HADS has been used in studies involving general medical outpatients, individuals experiencing chronic illnesses such as cancer[32] and cardiac conditions, and nonpatient community volunteers.[1] The authors report that the HADS can be used to monitor change over time. Item-to-subscale reliability correlations are reported as being 0.41 to 0.76 for the anxiety items and 0.30 to 0.60 for the depression items. Spearman correlations between the scales and psychiatric ratings were 0.70 and 0.74 for anxiety and depression, respectively. The Hospital Anxiety and Depression Scale has been translated into several languages, including Arabic, Dutch, French, German, Hebrew, Swedish, Italian, and Spanish.

Prototypical Anxiety and Depression Scales

Koeter and VanDenBrink developed the prototypical anxiety and depression scales to determine the existence of anxiety disorders among nonpsychotic psychiatric patients.[12] Twenty-one items were drawn from the more comprehensive 148-item Present State Examination-E, eight anxiety items and 13 depression items. The resulting scales are rated based on a clinical interview. The authors report high interrater reliability and internal consistency alpha coefficients of 0.59 to 0.60 for anxiety and 0.77 to 0.81 for depression. The validity of the scales was evaluated using the Hamilton Anxiety Scale and the

Hamilton Depression Scale. Correlations for anxiety were 0.56 to 0.79 and 0.47 to 0.78 for depression.[12] The use of this measurement with other than psychiatric patients has not been reported.

Courtauld Emotional Control Scale (CECS)

Unlike any other scale presented here, the Courtauld Emotional Control Scale was developed to measure emotional control of anxiety, anger, and depressed mood. This 21-item self-report scale assesses the extent to which respondents control their emotional responses to stress. The anxiety, anger, and depressed mood subscales consist of item statements that require rating on a 4-point scale. Watson and Greer report the use of the CECS with adult female cancer patients, male nonpatients, and personality Type A cardiac patients.[33] Test–retest reliability correlations have been reported as 0.84 to 0.95 for the total scale and 0.84 for anxiety, with internal consistency alpha coefficients of 0.86 to 0.88 for the total scale and 0.88 for anxiety. Concurrent validity has been determined using the STAI for the anxiety subscale. It was found that individuals who scored high on the CECS tended to score low on direct measures of anxiety.[33]

Symptom Checklist-90-Revised (SCL-90-R)

As developed by Derogatis et al., the Symptom Checklist 90 was designed primarily to reflect the psychologic symptom patterns of psychiatric and medical patients.[34] In 1976, based on clinical experiences and psychometric analyses, the original instrument was modified and is now the SCL-90-R.[35] This self-report 90-item scale measures nine primary dimensions of psychologic status: (1) somatization; (2) obsessive-compulsive; (3) interpersonal sensitivity; (4) depression; (5) anxiety; (6) hostility; (7) phobic anxiety; (8) paranoid ideation; and (9) psychoticism. It also measures three global indices of overall distress. The respondent is asked to report how much he or she was distressed by the symptoms identified in the item statements. The 5-point responses range from 0 (not at all) to 4 (extremely). "Nervousness or shakiness inside" is an example of an item.

A companion observation rating scale, the SCL-90 Analogue, also is available. This scale consists of nine dimension-specific 100-mm visual analog scales with the anchor "not at all" at one end and "extremely" at the other. Brief defining paragraphs facilitate rating. Interrater reliability correlations are reported as 0.81 to 0.94 for all dimensions and 0.86 for anxiety. The authors report that the SCL-90-R is sensitive to the evaluation of intervention/drug studies. Test–retest reliability coefficients have been reported as 0.55 to 0.94 for the total scale and 0.80 to 0.84 for the anxiety dimension. The internal consistency alpha coefficient for the anxiety dimension was reported as 0.85.[35] The author reports face validity and concurrent validity with the MMPI. The SCL-90-R has been widely used to assess global distress and its specific dimensions.[36] Target populations have included psychiatric patients[35,37] patients without a psychiatric illness,[35] and cancer patients.[38,39] Clinical profiles for the major psychiatric diagnoses exist.[35] Rief and Fichter suggested that modification of the dimension subscales has shown greater discriminant validity in identifying psychiatric disorders.[37] The SCL-90-R is available in Spanish.

Brief Symptom Inventory (BSI)

The Brief Symptom Inventory is a 53-item self-report version of the SCL-90-R.[40] It has the same dimension and global indices structure as its parent measure, and it is administered and scored similarly.[10] The authors report that the BSI can be used in a narrative form if the respondent is unable to read. The reliability test–retest correlations for the dimensions of the BSI are reported as 0.68 to 0.91, with internal consistency alpha coefficients of 0.71 to 0.83. Convergent validity of the BSI was determined using the clinical scales of the MMPI with correlations ranging from 0.30 to 0.72. Correlations ranged from 0.32 to 0.49 over the nine dimensions.[40] Like its parent instrument, the BSI has been used extensively.[10,41] Target populations have included psychiatric patients and individuals without a diagnosed psychiatric illness,[40,10] medical patients, including individuals with asthma,[26] cancer,[42,43] hypertension,[10] HIV/AIDS,[10] and caregivers of individuals with dementia.[44]

General Health Questionnaire (GHQ-28)

The General Health Questionnaire was originally developed as a 60-item self-report designed to detect the presence of general psychiatric disorders in the primary care setting. This measure contains 4 subscales: (1) somatic symptoms; (2) anxiety and insomnia; (3) social dysfunction; and (4) severe depression. Goldberg and Hillier developed a 28-item version of the original scale.[45] The respondents rate their experience of symptoms over the past few weeks. The phrases used for the 4-point rating scales vary with each item statement. The authors recognize the differences in language between Great Britain and the United States and provide the American user with suggested word substitutions for four of the items.[45] The following are examples of the anxiety items: "Been feeling run down and out of sorts?" and "Been getting a feeling of tightness or pressure in your head?" Concurrent validity for the revised GHQ-28 was determined through comparison with clinical interviews. Correlations were 0.51 to 0.75 for the subscales with a total scale correlation of 0.76. Predictive validity also was evaluated. Reliability data were not reported.[45] The GHQ-28 has been used with target populations of patients in primary care and general practice, particularly those experiencing acute psychiatric disorders.[46]

Affects Balance Scale (ABS)

Developed by Derogatis, the Affects Balance Scale is a 40-item self-report checklist that describes affect status in terms of four positive and four negative dimensions.[47] The positive dimensions are joy, contentment, vigor, and affection, and the negative dimensions are anxiety, depression, guilt, and hostility. For each descriptive adjective the respondent indicates on a 5-point scale the extent to which the adjective describes him or her, from 0 (never) to 4 (always). Examples of the adjectives included on the ABS are: nervous, timid, energetic, tense, anxious. The author has reported internal consistency reliability coefficients of 0.78 to 0.92. The construct validity of the ABS has been evaluated using group comparisons.[48] Sangal et al.[48] reported significantly less negative affects among improved anxiety disorder patients than unimproved patients. Long-term survivors of breast cancer had significantly higher negative affect scores than short-term survivors.[49] Target populations for this instrument have included anxiety disorder patients[48,49] and cancer patients.[39] A global, balanced measure of affect, the Affect Balance Index, also can be calculated.

General Well-Being Schedule (GWB)

The General Well-Being Schedule is an 18-item self-report measure of subjective feelings of psychologic well-being and distress.[46] The scale reflects both positive and negative feelings. Six dimensions cover anxiety, depression, general health, positive well-being, self-control, and vitality. The first 14 items use 6-point response scales representing intensity and frequency, and respondents rate their experience over the last month. An example of one of these items is "Have you been bothered by nervousness or your nerves?" The remaining four items use 0 to 10 rating scales defined by adjectives at each end, such as "How *relaxed* or *tense* have you been?"

Test–retest reliability coefficients have been reported as 0.68 to 0.85, with an internal consistency reliability of the total scale of 0.91 to 0.95. The average concurrent validity correlation with three independent anxiety scales was 0.64.[46] The GWB has been successfully used with psychiatric day patients and adults who do not have a diagnosed psychiatric illness.

Profile of Mood States (POMS)

McNair et al. developed the Profile of Mood States to measure six identifiable mood or affective states: (1) Tension-Anxiety; (2) Depression-Dejection; (3) Anger-Hostility; (4) Vigor-Activity; (5) Fatigue-Inertia; and (6) Confusion-Bewilderment.[11] The POMS is a 65-item, self-report adjective rating scale, with a 5-point response from 0 (not at all) to 4 (extremely). The respondents describe their feelings over the past week. A total Mood Disturbance Score also can be calculated. Examples of the adjectives include: shaky, on edge, panicky, and uneasy.

A test–retest reliability coefficient of 0.70 has been reported for the Tension-Anxiety subscale. Internal consistency reliability coefficients for this subscale are reported as 0.90 to 0.92 and 0.93 for the total scale. Concurrent validity of the POMS has been reported with a correlation of 0.80 between this instrument and the Hopkins Symptom Distress Scales (SCL-90, BSI).[11] Target populations for the use of the POMS have been outpatient psychiatric patients, healthy adults, and cardiac surgery patients.[21]

Brief Profile of Mood States (Brief POMS)

Cella et al.[50] developed an 11-item short form of the POMS as a reliable measure of general mood disturbance or distress. The result is the Brief POMS. Through extensive psychometric evaluation, the authors identified the best indicators of overall distress resulting in a Total Mood Disturbance score. There are no somatic item statements in this measure.[51] The 5-point response format has been retained. The internal consistency reliability of the Brief POMS is reported as 0.92. Correlation with the POMS is 0.93. Significant group differences were found between pancreatic cancer and gastric cancer patients, supporting the discriminant validity of the Brief POMS. Although this measure was developed for use with cancer patients during all stages of treatment, the authors suggest that it could be used with individuals experiencing other chronic diseases.

Summary of Research Findings

A comprehensive summary of the current research findings on anxiety is beyond the scope of this chapter. An overview of the trends in recently published anxiety research, with discussion of selected studies, will provide the reader some sense of this area of inquiry. Trends include the general assessment of anxiety, or anxiety as part of global distress, in specific populations; anxiety as a causal factor; anxiety as the direct focus of an intervention; and anxiety as a component of the outcome of an intervention.

General Assessment of Anxiety or Distress in Specific Populations

The assessment of anxiety specifically, or as a component of the global assessment of distress, is a common theme in the current research literature. In a much-cited study, Derogatis and his associates conducted a multi-site assessment of the presence of psychiatric disorders among 215 newly admitted cancer patients.[38] Using a psychiatric interview and standardized psychologic tests, including the SCL-90-R, they found that 44% of their subjects manifested a clinical psychiatric diagnosis. Of this group, approximately

85% experienced a disorder with depression or anxiety as the central symptom. In a similar study, Stefanek et al. assessed the psychologic status of 126 oncology outpatients.[42] Using the Brief Symptom Inventory (BSI), they reported that approximately one-third of the patients expressed moderate to high levels of depression and anxiety.

Gift[26] sought to describe the psychologic and physiologic aspects of acute dyspnea in asthmatics. Anxiety, as one component of psychologic status, was measured with the State scale of the State-Trait Anxiety Inventory (STAI). See the end of the chapter for a summary of her study and its findings. Levels of anxiety and self-confidence experienced by pregnant women were the focus of a study by Pond and Kemp.[25] They compared 35 adolescent with 58 adult prenatal patients, measuring anxiety with the STAI. Although no significant differences were found between these groups, they found significant negative correlations for both state and trait anxiety during pregnancy and self-confidence for all the women.

The effects of different coping patterns on the physical health, depression, and anxiety experienced by spouse caregivers of persons with dementia were studied by Neundorfer.[44] The Brief Symptom Inventory anxiety and depression subscales were used in the assessment of 60 spouse caregivers. The patient's memory and behavior problems, caregiver's appraisal of the stressfulness of these problems, and caregiver's appraisal of their options explained 43% of the variance in both depression and anxiety.

Myocardial infarction patients were assessed in a study of heart rate variability and psychologic outcomes by Buchanan et al.[22] The psychologic outcomes included anxiety, anger, denial, and depression, with anxiety being measured by the STAI. Anxiety was higher within 4 days of hospital admission, but had significantly decreased 6 months later.

Wong and Bramwell[23] examined the relationship between uncertainty and anxiety after mastectomy for breast cancer among 25 women. Subjects completed measures of anxiety and uncertainty at 1 to 2 days before and 1 to 2 weeks after hospital discharge. Using the STAI, they found a significant positive correlation between anxiety and uncertainty at the postdischarge testing. In a 6-month study of cancer patients with advanced disease, Payne[32] sought to identify the influence of site (home or hospital) and method of palliative chemotherapy on quality of life. The operationalization of quality of life included a measure of anxiety and depression, the Hospital Anxiety and Depression Scale (HADS). Anxiety and depression accounted for 92% of the variance in quality of life.

Anxiety as a Causal Factor

Two studies in the recent literature are representative of the examination of anxiety as a causal factor. Annie and Groer studied the influence of state and trait anxiety on immunoglobulin A (IgA) concentrations in 30 women during pregnancy and at childbirth.[24] State anxiety appeared to account for some of the variance in IgA concentration at both points in time. The State subscale of the STAI was used to measure anxiety. Also using the State subscale of the STAI, Eaton and his associates explored the relationship of psychosocial variables, including anxiety, depression, family process, and health locus of control, to management and control of insulin-dependent diabetes in 127 subjects.[27] Their results showed that both anxiety and depression had weak positive correlations with blood sugar levels. Life stage had the most significant effect on management and control of diabetes.

Anxiety as the Direct Focus of an Intervention

The recent literature also includes intervention studies where anxiety is the focus of intervention. Zimmerman and her colleagues evaluated the effects of music with suggestion on the anxiety levels of patients in coronary care units.[19] Seventy-five patients were randomly assigned to one of three groups: listening to music, listening to "white noise," or having a period of uninterrupted rest. The State subscale of the STAI was administered, and blood pressure, heart rate, and digital skin temperature were measured. The authors attribute the lack of significant findings to the fact that all three groups actually experienced an intervention.

Weintraub and Hagopian examined the effect of nursing consultation sessions on anxiety, side effects experienced, and helpfulness of self-care strategies used by patients receiving radiation therapy.[18] Fifty-six subjects were randomly assigned to either the health education control or nursing consultation group. Again, the STAI was used to measure anxiety. The researchers reported that the mean state anxiety scores were consistently lower, but not statistically significant, in the nursing consultation group.

In another intervention study with cancer patients, Holland et al. conducted a multisite, randomized clinical trial of alprazolam versus progressive muscle relaxation in the treatment of anxiety and depressive symptoms.[39] Four measures of anxiety and depression, including the Affects Balance Scale and the SCL-90, were used. See the end of the chapter for a summary of this study and its findings.

Peterson conducted an anxiety intervention study with 72 patients about to undergo cardiac catheterization.[20] Subjects were randomly assigned to one of three groups: educational intervention, social intervention, or control. Anxiety was measured, using the STAI, pre- and postintervention. Both the educational and social intervention groups experienced a significant decrease in anxiety compared with the control group.

Anxiety as a Component of the Outcome of an Intervention

This last trend in the research literature is the inclusion of anxiety with a number of other related factors as the focus of an intervention. Fraser and Kerr examined the effects of back massage on the anxiety levels of elderly residents in a long-term care institution.[28] Twenty-one subjects were randomly assigned to three groups: back massage with normal conversation, conversation only, or no intervention. The STAI State subscale was the measure of anxiety, along with electromyographic recordings, systolic and diastolic blood pressure, and heart rate. There was a statistically significant difference in anxiety between the back massage group and the no-intervention group. The statistical significance of other relationships among study variables may have been affected by the sample size.

A study of the effect of timing and reinforcement of preoperative education on knowledge and recovery in patients having coronary bypass graft surgery was conducted by Cupples.[21] Forty subjects were randomized to either the preadmission and postadmission preoperative education group or the postadmission only education group. Postoperative anxiety was measured with the STAI. The Profile of Mood States measured postoperative mood. Preoperative knowledge of surgery and physiologic recovery also were monitored. Subjects in the experimental group were found to have more positive mood states than those in the control group.

Summary

The concept of anxiety has many diverse interpretations that subsequently influence the selection of a measurement instrument. Whether conceptualized as an enduring personality characteristic, a response to life events, or a psychiatric diagnosis, anxiety can be measured by one of the instruments presented in this chapter. The clear delineation of one's research question, conceptual framework, and research design will facilitate an appropriate choice. Selection of a measure that is appropriate to the target population also is important, particularly when the somatic symptoms of a preexisting physical problem can influence the validity of the measurement process. Anxiety is an important and universal experience that may influence, or be influenced by, many aspects of health and function. Trends in the recent literature demonstrate significant interest in examining this phenomenon in a variety of settings and with a variety of approaches.

Exemplar Studies

Gift, Audrey. Psychologic and physiologic aspects of acute dyspnea in asthmatics. *Nurs Res*, 1991, *40*(4):196–199.

This study compared psychologic and physiologic variables during intense dyspnea to those at times of no or low dyspnea in people with asthma. Thirty-six adults, 19 to 76 years old, were assessed upon admission to the emergency room in acute dyspnea and again when they had no or low dyspnea just prior to discharge. Psychologic and physiologic variables measured included: anxiety, overall psychologic distress, specific asthma-related distress, oxygen saturation, and airway obstruction. Clinical symptoms found to be elevated during high dyspnea were respiratory rate, pulse, wheezing, and accessory muscle use. The psychologic variables anxiety, depression, somatization, and hostility were higher during high dyspnea, and peak expiratory flow rates and oxygen saturation were significantly lower. Subscales of the Asthma Symptom Checklist, pain/fear, fatigue, dyspnea, hyperventilation/hypocapnia, congestion, and rapid breath also were higher during high dyspnea.

This study represents a comprehensive approach to the description of both psychologic and physiologic responses in an acute event, dyspnea, with a specific population, asthmatics. Two measures of anxiety, the Stait-Trait Anxiety Inventory and the anxiety dimension of the Brief Symptom Inventory, were used to measure anxiety and were found to correlate significantly, supporting their construct validity. The study clearly operationalizes the variables of interest.

Holland, J., Morrow, G., Fetting, J., Schmale, A., Derogatis, C., Berenson, S., Carpenter, P., Breitbart, W., & Feldstein, M. A randomized clinical trial of alprazolam versus progressive muscle relaxation in cancer patients with anxiety and depressive symptoms. *J Clin Oncol*, 1991, *9*(6):1004–1011.

This multi-site, randomized study compared over a 10-day period the efficacy of the anxiolytic drug alprazolam (Xanax) with the use of progressive muscle relaxation for the treatment of anxiety and depressive symptoms among 147 cancer patients. Seventy patients took alprazolam (0.5 mg three times a day), while 77 listened to an audiotape of a training session three times a day. Four measures of anxiety and depression, including the Affects Balance Scale and the SCL-90, were administered at enrollment in the study and 10 days later. Both interventions resulted in a significant decrease in observer- and patient-reported anxiety and depressed mood symptoms. Patients receiving alprazolam demonstrated a slightly more rapid decrease in anxiety and a greater reduction of depressive symptoms. As both interventions are safe, inexpensive, and effective, a decision could be made in terms of the patient's preferences for a behavioral approach or medication.

This study compared a purely physiologic intervention, medication, with a behavioral approach, progressive muscle relaxation. A multi-method approach was used in measuring anxiety and depression, including interview-observation, and self-report instruments. The findings that both interventions were successful in reducing anxiety and depression have important implications for patient care. Because either intervention is effective, patients can make a choice based on their own personal likes and dislikes.

References

1. Walker, L.G. The measurement of anxiety. *Postgrad Med J*, 1990, *66*(Suppl 2):511-517.
2. Goodwin, Donald W. *Anxiety*. New York: Oxford University Press, 1986.
3. Kellerman, H., & Burry, A. *Handbook of psychodiagnostic testing* (2nd ed.). Boston: Allyn & Bacon, 1991.
4. Derogatis, L., & Wise, T. *Anxiety and depressive disorders in the medical patient*. Washington, DC: American Psychiatric Press, 1989.
5. Spielberger, C., Gorsuch, F., & Lushene, R. *STAI manual for the S-T-A-I ("Self-evaluation Questionnaire")*. Palo Alto, CA: Consulting Psychologist Press, 1971.
6. Hoehn-Saric, R., & McLeod, D. *Biology of anxiety disorders*. Washington, DC: American Psychiatric Press, 1993.
7. Lazarus, R., & Folkman, S. *Stress, appraisal and coping*. New York: Springer, 1984.
8. Taylor, Janet. A personality scale of manifest anxiety. *J Abnorm Soc Psychol*, 1953, *48*(2):285-290.
9. Bech, P., Grosby, H., Husum, B., & Rafaelsen, S. Generalized anxiety or depression measured by the Hamilton Anxiety Scale and the Melancholia Scale in patients before and after cardiac surgery. *Psychopathology*, 1984, *17*:253-263.
10. Derogatis, L. *BSI Administration, scoring and procedures Manual II*. Towson, MD: Clinical Psychometric Research, 1992.
11. McNair, D., Lorr, M., & Droppleman, L. *EDITS manual for the profile of mood states*, San Diego: Educational and Industrial Testing Service, 1981.
12. Koeter, M., & VanDenBrink, W. The relationship between depression and anxiety: Construction of a prototypical anxiety and depression scale. *Psychol Med*, 1992, *22*:597-606.
13. Zigmond, A.S., & Swaith, R.P. The hospital anxiety and depression scale. *Acta Psychiatr Scand*, 1983, *67*:361-370.
14. Roberts, N., Vargo, B., & Ferguson, H.B. Measuring anxiety and depression in children and adolescents. *Psychiatr Clin North Am*, 1989, *12*(2):837-860.
15. Hoehn-Saric, E., Maisami, M., & Wiegand, D. Measurement of anxiety in children and adolescents using semistructured interviews. *J Am Acad Child Adolesc Psychiatr*, 1987, *26*:541-545.
16. Massie, M.J. Anxiety, panic and phobias. In J. Holland & J. Rowland (Eds.), *Handbook of psycho-oncology: Psychological issues in cancer*. New York: Oxford University Press, 1989.
17. Holland, Jimmie C. Anxiety and cancer: The patient and the family. *J Clin Psychiatr*, 1989, *50*(Suppl 11): 20-25.
18. Weintraub, F., & Hagopian, G. The effect of nursing consultation on anxiety, side effects and self-care of patients receiving radiation therapy. *Oncol Nurs Forum*, 1990, *17*(suppl 3):31-38.
19. Zimmerman, L., Pierson, M., & Marker, J. Effects of music on patient anxiety on coronary care units. *Heart Lung*, 1988, *17*(5):560-566.
20. Peterson, Marjory. Patient anxiety before cardiac catheterization: An intervention study. *Heart Lung*, 1991, *20*(6):643-647.
21. Cupples, Sandra. Effects of timing and reinforcement of preoperative education on knowledge and recovery of patients having coronary artery bypass graft surgery. *Heart Lung*, 1991, *20*(6):654-660.
22. Buchanan, L., Cowan, M., Burr, R., et al. Measurement of recovery from myocardial infarction using heart rate variability and psychological outcome. *Nurs Res*, 1993, *42*(2):74-78.
23. Wong, C., & Bramwell, L. Uncertainty and anxiety after mastectomy for breast cancer. *Cancer Nurs*, 1992, *15*(5):363-371.
24. Annie, C., & Groer, M. Childbirth stress: An immunologic study. *JOGNN*, 1991, *20*(5):391-397.
25. Pond E., & Kemp, V. A comparison between adolescent and adult women on prenatal anxiety and self-confidence. *Maternal-Child Nurs J*, 1992, *20*(1):11-20.
26. Gift, Audrey. Psychologic and physiologic aspects of acute dyspnea in asthmatics. *Nurs Res*, 1991, *40*(4):196-199.
27. Eaton, W., Mengel, M., Larson, D., et al. Psychosocial and psychopathologic influences on management and control of insulin-dependent diabetes. *Int J Psychiatr Med*, 1992, *22*(2):105-117.
28. Fraser J., & Kerr, J. Psychophysiological effects of back massage on elderly institutionalized patients. *J Adv Nurs*, 1993, *18*:238-245.
29. Zung, William. A rating instrument for anxiety disorders. *Psychosomatics*, 1971, *12*(6):371-379.
30. Tyrer, P., Owen, R.T., & Cicchetti, D.V. The brief scale for anxiety: A subdivision of the comprehensive psycho-pathological rating scale. *J of Neurosurg Psychiatr*, 1984, *47*:970-975.
31. Gottschalk, L.A., & Bechtel, R.J. The measurement of anxiety through the computer analysis of verbal samples. *Comp Psychiatr*, 1982, *23*(4):364-369.
32. Payne, S.A. A study of quality of life in cancer patients receiving palliative chemotherapy. *Soc Sci Med*, 1992, *35*(12):1505-1509.
33. Watson, M., & Greer, S. Development of a questionnaire of emotional control. *J Psychosom*, 1983, *27*(4):299-305.
34. Derogatis, L., Lipman, R., & Covi, L. SCL-90: An outpatient psychiatric rating scale—Preliminary report. *Psychopharmacol Bull*, 1973, *9*:13-23.
35. Derogatis, L. *SCL-90-R Administration, scoring and procedures manual II*. Towson, MD: Clinical Psychometric Research, 1992.
36. SCL-90-R. In J.V. Mitchell (Ed.), *The ninth mental measurements yearbook (Vol. II)*. Lincoln: University of Nebraska Press, 1985.
37. Rief, W., & Fichter, M. The Symptom Check List SCL-90-R and its ability to discriminate between dysthymia, anxiety disorders and anorexia nervosa. *Psychopathology*, 1992, *25*:128-138.
38. Derogatis, L., Morrow, G., Fetting, J., et al. The prevalence of psychiatric disorders among cancer patients. *JAMA*, 1983, *249*(6):751-757.
39. Holland, J., Morrow, G., Schmale, A., et al. A randomized clinical trial of alprazolam versus progressive muscle relaxation in cancer patients with anxiety and depressive symptoms. *J Clin Oncol*, 1991, *9*(6):1004-1011.
40. Derogatis, L., & Melisaratos, N. The brief symptom inventory: An introductory report. *Psychol Med*, 1983, *13*:595-605.

41. The Brief Symptom Inventory. In J. Conoley & J. Kramer (Eds.), *The tenth mental measurements yearbook.* Lincoln: University of Nebraska Press, 1989, pp. 111-113.

42. Stefanek, M., Derogatis, L., & Shaw, A. Psychological distress among oncology patients. *Psychosomatics,* 1987, *28*(10):537-539.

43. Zabora, J., Smith-Wilson, R., Fetting, J., & Enterline, J. An efficient method for psychosocial screening of cancer patients. *Psychosomatics,* 1990, *31*(2):192-196.

44. Neundorfer, M. Coping and health outcomes in spouse caregivers of persons with dementia. *Nurs Res,* 1991, *40*(5):260-265.

45. Goldberg, D.P., & Hillier, V.F. A scaled version of the general health questionnaire. *Psychol Med,* 1979, *9*:139-145.

46. McDowell, I., & Newell, C. *Measuring health: A guide to rating scales and questionnaires.* New York: Oxford University Press, 1987.

47. Derogatis, L. *The Affects Balance Scale.* Baltimore, MD: Clinical Psychometric Research, 1975.

48. Sangal, R., Coyle, G., & Hoehn-Saric, R. Chronic anxiety and social adjustment. *Comp Psychiatr,* 1983, *24*(1):75-78.

49. Derogatis, L., Abeloff, M., & Melisaratos, N. Psychological coping mechanisms and survival time in metastatic breast cancer. *JAMA,* 1979, *242*(4):1504-1508.

50. Cella, D., Jacobsen, P., Orav, E., et al. A brief POMS measure of distress for cancer patients, *J Chron Dis,* 1987, *40*(10):939-942.

51. Hoehn-Saric, R. Comparison of generalized anxiety disorder with panic disorder patients. *Psychopharmacol Bull,* 1982, *18*(4):104-108.

23

Measuring Depression

Jeannie V. Pasacreta

Misconceptions concerning depression exist in various populations and stem from the fact that the concept of depression has a variety of meanings and is commonly used to describe a broad spectrum of human emotions and behaviors. This spectrum can range from expected, transient, and nonclinical sadness following upsetting life events to the clinically relevant extremes of suicidality and major depressive illness. Because depression is described as a common malady among individuals with chronic illness, researchers are in an optimal position to clarify the components and consequences associated with this often elusive concept. The literature on primary depressive phenomena is large and reveals advances in the understanding of etiologic factors, classification, prevalence, course, and treatment. These strides are somewhat obscured when examining the literature on depression in medically ill patients, particularly because depression often is conceptualized differently from study to study. The ultimate goal of this chapter is to describe various models and measurement systems for delineating depression and provide some guidelines for choosing appropriate measurement strategies. The need to broaden the definition of depression beyond the discrete psychiatric varieties and to clarify outcomes associated with depression secondary to medical illness is stressed as an important means of expanding knowledge in this area.

Terms that will be used throughout this chapter include *depressive syndromes*, which refers to a specific constellation of symptoms that comprise a discrete psychiatric disorder. Types of depressive syndromes that will be referred to in this chapter include: major depression dysthymia, organic affective disorder and adjustment disorder with depressed features. *Depressive symptoms* is used to describe varying degrees of depressed feelings not necessarily associated with psychiatric illness. The clinical significance of psychiatric symptoms in most settings remains to be seen and is an important area for ongoing research.

Defining Depression

The literal meaning of *melancholia*, "black bile," vividly suggested a state of gloom and darkness with explicit biologic connotations.[1] Unfortunately, the adoption of the term depression failed to eliminate conceptual confusion. In fact this current review revealed 46 definitions and classification schemas and 133 psychometric instruments aimed at determining the presence of the phenomena. Even today, definitions of depression continue to be used loosely and interchangeably in research studies, and clinicians and researchers have still not reached agreement on the basic concepts of depression and the best methods of classification and measurement.

Despite extensive research, the mechanisms that underlie depressive phenomena (particularly those secondary to medical illness) are in general poorly understood.[2] There is growing consensus however, that depression often is the consequence of multiple biologic, psychologic, cognitive, and sociologic interacting mechanisms. As suggested by Akiskal and McKinney,[1] depressive syndromes most likely represent a "psychobiological final common pathway."[1,p285] The five theoretical frameworks that are briefly reviewed advance the understanding of depressive phenomena. Unfortunately, and as described, the theoretical frameworks often elude accurate measurement, and many studies of depression are only loosely based on a theoretical foundation.

Depression and the Psychodynamic View

The psychoanalytic approach to depression was first described by Abraham[3] and elaborated on by Freud. Freud theorized individuals to be in a perpetual state of conflict motivated by unconscious sexual and aggressive drives.[4] According to the classical Freudian view, depression represents the introjection of hostility subsequent to the loss of an ambivalently loved object.[5] Within the psychoanalytic frame, depression is described on a continuum from neurotic (mild, reactive) to classic melancholia, which is the most severe form and includes the clinical extremes of psychosis and mania. The model largely disregarded the effect of object loss on the ego and focused largely on the introjection of primal, aggressive energy, concepts that elude an operational definition and precise measurement. Despite the fact that the analytic view is one of the most widely quoted conceptualizations of depression, there is little empirical support for its propositions[1,4] and any attempts at confirming depression as the inward turning of aggressive drives have yielded conflicting results.[6]

Several investigators have viewed separation from the central figure of attachment to be primary in the genesis of depression.[7,8] Empirical support for these hypotheses has been inconsistent. Some studies suggest that depression may precede separation and be the consequence of isolative, alienating behavior.[9] Others argue that separation is not a prerequisite for depression as many depressed individuals have not experienced it.[1] Other investigators note that separation is not specific to depression as it may predispose individuals to medical disorders[10] and sociopathy.[11] The inconsistent empirical support that these theories have received speaks to the likely multifaceted nature of depression, the problems inherent in adopting a narrow view, and the importance of considering life experiences and individual meaning when exploring depressive phenomena.

Depression and the Cognitive View

Cognitive views of depression are based on the general premise that the process of acquiring knowledge and formulating beliefs is a primary determinant of mood and behavior. Cognitive approaches represent a departure from psychodynamic theories in that they emphasize the mediating role that distorted thinking plays in determining affective state.[12] Two cognitive models of depression that have received considerable attention are the cognitive schema approach proposed by Beck[12] and the learned helplessness model developed by Seligman and Maier.[13]

Beck's cognitive model describes depression as "the activation of primitive negative schemas that lead to a selective negative bias in interpreting experiences."[14,p1121] Basic principles of the theory hold that: (1) negative schemata exist outside of conscious awareness and are automatically activated by stressful events and/or neurochemical changes; (2) the negative cognitive schema interprets environmental events in a distorted and illogical fashion that is consistent with its negativity; (3) persistently negative cognition reinforces sadness and depressive behaviors and leaves the individual oblivious to positive factors; and (4) the cognitive set is but one component of depressive syndromes, yet it provides a useful model to develop intervention strategies.[12,14]

Seligman and colleagues[15] coined the term *learned helplessness* to describe a phenomenon first noticed in dogs repeatedly exposed to inescapable electric shock. A serendipitous finding emerged in that once the dogs were exposed to the shock they were unable to escape it, even when an exit was made readily available.[13] Following repeated exposure to aversive stimuli, the inability of humans to escape, even when given the opportunity has been documented.[15] Based on these observations, the learned helplessness model describes a cognitive and behavioral state characterized by an inability to engage in adaptive behaviors because of a lack of recognition that one can control unpleasant events. The theory suggests that depressed individuals generalize their failure experiences. Eventually they perceive themselves as losing control over their environment in a pervasive sense ultimately leading to the paralyzing effects of helplessness, passivity, powerlessness, and depression.

Some investigators have questioned cognitive approaches to depression by challenging the belief that cognitive and motivational problems induce depression. An alternative view is that cognitive and motivational problems merely are the consequence of depression and as such should be regarded as symptoms. Proponents of the cognitive view of depression readily acknowledge the multiplicity of factors underlying depressive disorders.[14] Akiskal and McKinney[1] suggest that "interpersonally induced states of helplessness, whether from separation, chronic aversive stimulation or loss of control over reinforcement could result in the alteration of biogenic amines."[1] Because depression is a complex, multifaceted concept, diverse explanatory frames of reference must be considered if knowledge in this area is to progress.

Depression and the Sociologic View

The ego, which is rooted in social reality, is made up of socially learned symbols and motivations. Thus, according to Becker,[16] depression is a social phenomenon. A breakdown of self-esteem (which according to the psychodynamic and cognitive view is intimately connected to loss, helplessness, and depression) may involve the loss of symbolic possessions such as status, roles, relationships, and life meaning in addition to object losses.[1] Cultural and societal factors may increase social vulnerability to depression when exposed to certain circumstances,[17] and individuals exposed to illnesses that threaten the ability to perform desirable social roles are particularly at risk.[18]

Depression and the Biologic View

The importance of genetic vulnerability has been conclusively demonstrated in bipolar illness and recurrent unipolar depressions.[1,19] Several genetically determined biochemical alterations have been implicated, particularly in the etiology of primary and severe depressive disorders. These biologic hypotheses have been based largely on psychopharmacologic inference.[1,19]

Most biochemical hypotheses have suggested alterations in two major classes of neurotransmitters, the catecholamines (i.e., norepinephrine) and the indolamines (i.e., serotonin) in the etiology of depression. Early studies suggested a decrease in brain sero-tonin or norepinephrine levels but failed to favor one class over the other.[15] The per-missive amine hypothesis of affective disorders, which has been heralded as an important development in the synthesis of biologic hypotheses of depression, suggests that a central serotonergic deficiency may represent the vulnerability to affective illness. Lowered catecholamines correspond to depression and increased catecholamines to mania. Within this view, depression and mania are viewed along a continuum, rather than being polar opposites with mania representing a more severe deviation from nor-mal mood.[20]

At this point, there are no biologic markers that characterize depression secondary to specific medical illnesses,[21] although some are treated effectively with psychophar-macologic agents that increase central levels of norepinephrine and serotonin.

Depression and the Crisis Model

In several studies that examine the occurrence of depression in medically ill patients, de-pression is equated with a crisis response. According to Caplan,[22] receiving catastrophic news about a medical diagnosis results in immediate problem-solving efforts, and yet demands on the individual exceed the ability to respond, producing both physiologic and psychologic arousal. Problem-solving ability is consequently reduced by physio-logic arousal resulting in poor attention, poor concentration, poor judgment, a sense of disorganization and erosion of self-concept. The inability to use adaptive skills results in transient dysphoria, manifested by depression and anxiety.

As a result of numerous theoretical orientations, and their lack of clear association to particular measurement strategies, numerous diagnostic and measurement systems that identify overlapping populations have been used to document depression in re-search studies. With the exception of the Beck Depression Inventory, a depression rating scale based on Beck's theoretical formulation of depression, most measurement systems are only loosely tied to a theoretical framework. Criteria-based systems are grounded in the medical model and thus loosely tied to biologic theories of depression. The link be-tween theory and the measurement of depression becomes particularly vague when mild to moderate levels of depression or those secondary to a medical condition are de-scribed. The following sections describe the primary measurement systems used to as-certain the prevalence of depression among primary psychiatric, medical patients as well as nonpatient groups. The notion that varied instruments produce varied results and issues relevant to special populations are stressed. Special attention is paid to the in-terplay between somatic and psychologic symptoms among medically ill subjects. Sug-gestions are offered for handling these issues in research studies.

Primary Measurement Systems for Delineating Depression

Two major systems are used to delineate depression among various populations, criteria-based systems, and rating scales, some specific to depression and some self report scales that measure general psychologic profiles and include depression as a separate dimen-sion. Each system, as well as some of the problems associated with each, are described.

Criteria-Based Systems

In 1972, the Feigner Criteria were published, along with a structured interview to elicit information needed to apply specific diagnostic criteria.[23] The Feigner Criteria were later modified by Spitzer, Endicott, and Robins,[24] who published specific criteria for making[25] psychiatric diagnoses called the Research Diagnostic Criteria (RDC). The RDC consists of descriptions of the clinical features of select disorders and sets forth specific inclusion and exclusion criteria. It is supplemented by a structured interview, the Schedule for Affective Disorders and Schizophrenia (SADS).[24]

Much of the literature that attempts to describe and classify depressive phenomena according to criteria-based systems originates in psychiatry. The focus, throughout much of the last century, has been to classify depressions into discrete categories based on family history, symptoms, treatment, and course. Classification schemes are based on the medical model and nosology, the grouping of symptoms into single disease states with prediction of course and response to treatment as the goal.[25] The current focus in psychiatry is to separate depressions into distinct heterogeneous categories, often with the intent of distinguishing those types that will respond to pharmacotherapy.

The second edition of the *Diagnostic and Statistical Manual of Mental Disorders* (DSM-II),[26] which was used until 1980, classified depression into two broad categories: (1) those presumed to be reactive to life events were characterized by antecedent psychosocial conditions and supposed to be psychogenic in nature (neurotic depression and psychotic depressive reaction); and (2) those not related to a precipitating life experience and presumed to be biologic or endogenous (coming from within) in nature (i.e., involutional melancholia, manic depressive illness).

The third edition of *The Diagnostic and Statistical Manual of Mental Disorders* (DSM-III)[27] heralded a major change in approach. DSM-IV,[28] (1994), is the current, criteria-based method of classifying depression and is based on the RDC approach. The RDC consists of descriptions of the clinical features of select disorders and sets forth specific inclusion and exclusion criteria. It is supplemented by a structured interview, the Schedule for Affective Disorders and Schizophrenia (SADS).[24] Similarly, DSM-IV is largely descriptive and for the most part disregards etiologic considerations. Several distinct categories of depressive phenomena are outlined in DSM-IV. Clinically significant depressions are defined in terms of a constellation of symptoms (syndrome). Depressive syndromes are classified according to course (whether a single episode or recurrent), and recurrent episodes are defined as disorders. DSM-IV distinguishes depressive phenomena into bipolar and depressive types. The essential feature of the bipolar type is the presence of manic or hypomanic episodes in an individual or close relative. Depressed mood may or may not be present. "Major depressive episode/disorder" is used to describe a syndrome characterized by depressed mood, a change from previous functional level and loss of interest or pleasure. These attributes often are accompanied by neurovegetative symptoms (i.e., insomnia, psychomotor retardation, diminished appetite), as well as suicidality, guilt, and feelings of worthlessness. A "melancholic type" of major depression is described in DSM-IV as the most severe type of depression and is believed to be particularly responsive to somatic therapy.

Dysthymia, or "depressive neurosis," is a diagnosis reserved for chronic depression that interferes with function but does not fulfill the severity criteria for major depression. Depressive symptoms must be present almost continuously for a period of 2 years or longer.

An additional DSM-IV category of depressive phenomena particularly germane to a description of depression in medically ill patients as they frequently receive this diagnosis[29] is "adjustment disorder with depressed features." This is not considered a primary mood disturbance, however, and is so general that it does not define a discrete population.[30] Thus, this diagnosis is not considered in epidemiologic studies of depression in the general population.

The development of DSM-IIIR[28A] (edition prior to DSM-IV) made a fundamental change in criteria by excluding depressive symptoms related to a physical condition. By excluding these symptoms, DSM-III-R decreased the number of symptoms patients could exhibit and still be considered depressed but did not decrease the number of symptoms necessary to meet the criteria for a depressive diagnosis. Although the purpose of this change was to make standardized criteria for psychiatric diagnosis more rigorous to enhance reliability, the change excluded a group of the medically ill from further study and thus eventual effective treatment. None of the interview schedules designed to obtain criteria-based diagnoses have been standardized on medically ill populations.[31]

Because of the difficulties diagnosing depression in the medically ill (associated with the overlap of somatic and affective symptoms), some investigators have suggested that somatic items be excluded from criteria-based systems in this population. Such modification threatens the validity of the modified system and also increases the severity of criteria for a depressive syndrome in patients with cancer.[32] To counter these problems, Endicott proposed that alternative symptoms be used to replace those most likely to be affected by the medical condition and its treatment.[32] Depending on the type of cancer and type of treatment, an investigator can decide that one symptom, for example, appetite loss, is not to be used and substitute some other common depressive symptom in its place (e.g., tearfulness or depressed appearance). If several of the associated clinical features are apt to be affected by the cancer and/or its treatment, the investigator must decide which list of alternative symptoms will be used. Endicott[32] stresses that training procedures for clinical evaluators must ensure that modified criteria be used similarly and consistently for all subjects. It is important that replacement symptoms be of equal validity and reliability to those being replaced. However, to date, such assessment has not been performed.[30]

A study of depression in cancer patients by Kathol and colleagues,[30] reports that different criteria-based diagnostic systems (specifically, DSM-III, DSM-III-R and RDC criteria) identify different patients as having major depression. In a cohort of 151 cancer patients, 57 received a diagnosis of major depression according to DSM-III; 44 according to DSM-III-R, and 37 according to RDC criteria. As mentioned, a fundamental change in criteria was made between the DSM-III and the DSM-III-R so that the latter excludes depressive symptoms related to a physical condition. Although more stringent criteria may increase diagnostic reliability, the fact that the process also may eliminate a full inquiry into the subtleties of depression among the medically ill must be addressed.

Most investigations of depression in the medically ill point to a small number of patients with major depressive syndromes or dysthymia and a much larger number with symptoms of lesser intensity. The immediate and long-term significance of depressive symptoms, because they are not of the type or intensity to be included in rigorous syndromic diagnoses, remains unclear.

Rating Scales

Rating scales have been used primarily as screening instruments or as a means of quantifying the severity of depression, particularly in intervention studies that aim at assessing treatment response. Screening is a process whereby a disorder is presumptively identified in a particular population. Screening studies have based the definition of a case of depression on the attainment of a certain score on one of many depression rating scales. For a rating scale to be used for research purposes, Nunnally recommends that a coefficient alpha be at least 0.6 or at least 0.8, if a rating scale is used as a screening instrument in the clinical setting.[33] For some rating scales, norms exist that have been established using homogeneous samples (e.g., normal controls, psychiatric inpatients, medically ill patients). Fundamentally, norms provide an interpretive point of reference and allow an individual to be assessed in terms of an existing standard.

Several issues are inherent in the use of rating scales to measure depression. Primarily, differing scale construction leads to serious difficulty when comparing studies that used different instruments.[34] It is virtually impossible to assume the measurement of like concepts when using different measures. In addition, self-report measures may produce high false-positive or false-negative diagnoses (when using criteria-based diagnoses as the standard) depending on the cutoff points used (which may differ in separate investigations, even when the same scale was used).[35] In addition, some individuals may not be willing or able to report affective symptoms during a severe depressive state.[36]

Some investigators have used depression symptom scales as sole diagnostic instruments in patients with possible depression associated with medical illness.[37] Rating scales can be self-report or observer-rated scales. The singular use of self-report instruments, to measure depression, has been questioned,[30] suggesting that the positive predictive power of various self-report instruments is limited (i.e., the probability that a patient with a scale score greater than a certain value will have a criteria-based depression). In a study regarding the predictive value of the Beck Depression Inventory (BDI),[30] 768 consecutive cancer outpatients were screened for depression. Five hundred eighty nine subjects completed the BDI, 117 of whom had scores of 10 or greater. Only 12 of those 117 patients met the criteria for major depression according to DSM-III. The prevalence rate of depression in this sample was only 2%. The authors concluded that the predictive power of the BDI among cancer patients was poor and that other screening instruments be used with caution as they inflate the prevalence of depression in patients with cancer.

As stated, most depression rating scales have corresponding cutoff points that distinguish those patients with clinical depression (scoring above cutoff point) from those without it (scoring below cutoff point). When used this way, rating scales are considered to be screening instruments. The relationship between symptom scale scores and clinical depression as it is understood in primary psychiatric patients suggests that such scales are poorly correlated.[37] The underlying assumption regarding the practice of correlating scale scores with criteria-based diagnoses to determine their validity is that criteria-based diagnoses of depression are inherently better than other methods in the medically ill. Data regarding untoward outcomes associated within depressive syndromes, as well as less severe depressive symptoms, are slowly emerging and challenge the singular use of the medical paradigm in determining the types of depression that are of clinical significance among medically ill patients. Only when the full range of depressive symptoms experienced by these populations are studied and understood will effective treatments, both pharmacologic and psychotherapeutic, be tested and developed.

Rating scales are devised as: (1) self-report scales whereby the subject fills out responses on a structured scale without assistance from an interviewer; (2) observer-assisted scales whereby the subject responds to the scale with assistance from an interviewer who may read questions from the scale; and, (3) clinical observer scales whereby ratings are based on clinical observation and interview by a trained individual. Each variety of rating scale has its advantages and disadvantages. Self-report measures, for example, may yield inaccurate information from severely depressed individuals. Subjects who are severely depressed may be unable to respond on their own because of problems with apathy, psychomotor retardation, and poor concentration, to name just a few. On the other hand, observer-rated scales may be subject to observer bias and relia-bility problems, thus stringent interviewer training is imperative. The issues mentioned stress the need to plan carefully regarding the type of instrument that will be used to measure depression in research and to anticipate potential problems and solutions be-fore they occur.

General Psychologic Profiles to Measure Depression

In several studies that examine the occurrence of depression, self-report instruments that reveal general psychologic profiles and include depression as a specific dimension or subscale are used. Examples of multidimensional inventories that have been used in this regard include the Hospital Anxiety and Depression Scale (HAD); the Hopkins Symptom Checklist-90 (SCL-90); and the Brief Symptom Inventory (BSI). Several factors account for the use of multidimensional rather than depression specific scales. Multidi-mensional scales provide information regarding other emotional states that may ac-company depression in select populations. This may be useful in descriptive studies, as well as to note the differential effects of research interventions. In addition, numerous studies equate the occurrence of depression in medically ill patients with a crisis re-sponse[38] and associate its existence with other psychologic states. An ongoing debate re-garding the ability to separate clearly symptoms of anxiety and depression has contributed to the use of scales that measure general, as opposed to specific, distress in patients with cancer. Some investigators view less severe, reactive, or situational de-pressions as indistinguishable from anxiety disorders. Historically, this viewpoint is based on the work of Lewis[39] and the observation of high overlap in the symptomatic presentation of the two classes of disorders and their similar responses to therapeutics. Several investigators, however, have reviewed evidence for both unitary and distinct positions and found that there was strong support for the contention that anxiety and depression could be distinguished as separate diagnostic entities.[40]

The Conceptualization of Depression

As Wells et al. outlined,

> In current clinical practice and research, there are two major paradigms for defining de-pression: the general phenomena of depressive symptoms; and, specific psychiatric, de-pressive disorders. While the general medical sector tends to conceptualize depression according to the former definition, much of the mental health specialty sector conceptu-alizes depression according to the latter.[41,p915]

The psychiatric specialty, with its focus on categorizing depressions into discrete groups or syndromes, has hindered inquiry into less severe depressive symptoms among the medically ill that do not meet current criteria for psychiatric disorder status. As criteria for depressive syndromes have become more stringent (as per the changes from DSM-II to DSM-III to DSM-III-R), more and more medical patients are being ex-cluded from diagnostic groups. Although this may be appropriate considering the in-trinsic differences between primary and secondary depression, the need to examine the course and consequences associated with less severe depressive symptoms among the medically ill is needed so that ultimately definitions of and treatment for the broad spec-trum of depression in this unique population can be expanded. The relevance of this view is supported by several studies that associate untoward outcomes with persistent depressive symptoms in the medically ill.

In a study by Mossey and colleagues,[42] the effects of persistent depressive symp-toms on hip fracture recovery were examined. Depressive symptoms were measured using the Center for Epidemiologic Studies-Depression (CES-D). After controlling for age, prefracture physical function, and cognitive status, which were found to be predictors of recovery, subjects consistently reporting few depressive symptoms were three times more likely than those with persistently elevated CES-D scores to achieve independence in walking; nine times more likely to return to prefracture levels in at least five of seven physical function measures; and nine times more likely to be in the highest quartile of overall physical function. These findings emphasize the significance of persistently elevated depressive symptoms in the recovery process and the importance of routine screening, evaluation, and treatment of depressed mood states.

The preceding study used CES-D scores over 16 to define elevated depressive symptoms, and although the authors did not evaluate the presence of criteria-based depressive syndromes, it can be assumed that a large percentage of them would not have met specific criteria. This assumption is based on a study by Schulberg and colleagues[43] that analyzed the efficiency of the CES-D against a criterion measure, the Diagnostic Interview Schedule (DIS), which permits clinicians to formulate psychiatric diagnoses according to DSM-III criteria. Sixty-two percent of high-scoring medical patients (from a total sample of 294) were assigned no psychiatric diagnosis by the DIS. It was suggested by the authors that considerably higher than usual cut-off scores be used to improve the efficiency of the CES-D. Although this may improve the ability of the instrument to predict psychiatric syndromes, it minimizes the clinical significance of less severe symptom profiles, as well as the importance of exploring their associated risk factors, course, outcomes, and treatment response.

Routine psychiatric evaluations of 100 adult patients undergoing allogeneic bone marrow transplantation for acute leukemia were reviewed to examine the possible relationship between psychiatric and psychosocial factors and survival time following the procedure.[44] Three variables were found to affect outcome independently: (1) illness status (first remission versus other status); (2) the presence of depressed mood; and (3) the extent of perceived social support. Patients with depressed mood ($n = 13$) as a prominent symptom at the pretransplant evaluation had significantly shorter survival following transplantation. Only one patient in the depressed group had a diagnosis of major depression. The authors admit that their sample was small and that the mechanism by which depressed mood impacts outcome remains highly speculative. The important point was that depressive symptoms of lesser magnitude than those associated with stringent psychiatric diagnoses are coupled with unfavorable outcomes in medically ill patients. Further study that expands the conceptual and operational nature of depression among the medically ill is warranted.

A recent, large-scale study specifically examined and compared outcomes associated with depressive disorders, depressive symptoms, chronic medical conditions, and no chronic conditions.[41] Data from 11,242 outpatients at three health-care sites were collected. The study associated significant morbidity with depressive symptoms and further pointed to the need to expand the study of depression among the medically ill to include depressive symptoms that do not qualify for disorder status.

Depression, Somatic Symptoms, and Functioning

The effects of medical treatments often inflict transient and/or permanent physical changes, somatic symptoms, and functional impairments in patients. It is well-known that excessive psychologic distress can exacerbate the side effects of various treatment agents.[45] Conversely, treatment side effects can dramatically impact recipient mood and affect.[46]

Because of the expected nature of somatic and affective changes secondary to many medical problems and their treatments, symptoms of depression that reach clinical significance often go unnoticed and untreated. Somatic symptoms imposed by various illnesses and treatments often coexist with somatic symptoms that are characteristic of depressive syndromes. The coexisting and competing nature of somatic and affective symptoms (treatment of physical problems often assumes priority in the medical treatment setting) has led to an underrecognition of clinically significant depression as well as to the assumption that depression is an appropriate response to a physically and emotionally disruptive chronic illness.

Although it is true that transient symptoms of depression occur with some regularity throughout the chronic illness trajectory, severe depressive symptoms or a constellation of depressive symptoms (syndrome) are not expected or typical. The frequent inability to recognize symptoms of depression that go beyond the expected often is due to the difficulty separating somatic changes due to illness from those associated with severe depression. The need to measure somatic symptoms and depression separately to ascertain an accurate prevalence of the latter is crucial. Defining symptom distress secondary to illness and treatment separate from depressive phenomena is an important step in that direction. Early attempts to measure the impact of physical symptoms experienced by medically ill patients focused on one dimension of the individual's life, physical performance. Karnofsky and Burchenal[47] developed a scale that rates physical activity from 1% to 100% in increments of 10%. The Karnofsky scale, extensively used by cooperative cancer research groups, has been shown to be correlated with tumor response and survival. The scale was originally developed in response to an urgent need for a brief measure that could demonstrate response to cancer treatment protocols. The value of instruments such as the Karnofsky scale in adequately describing the multiple dimensions of human functioning and their relationship to concepts such as affect and quality of life has been questioned.[48] Many prevalence studies of depression secondary to medical illness used Kornofsky measures alone. Their findings in regard to the highly interrelated nature of somatic symptoms and affect represent a relatively limited view. According to some researchers, the variable with the strongest relationship to clinical depression is physical performance as measured by the Karnofsky scale.[21] Bukberg and colleagues[21] reported that of the patients who scored 40 or less on the Karnofsky scale (the most physically disabled), 77% met the criteria for clinical depression. Only 23% of those with scores above 60 (better physical function) had clinical depression. Although somatic items were excluded from depression criteria to account for the fact that physical symptoms of depression often overlap with symptoms of illness and treatment, use of the Karnofsky measure alone sheds little light on factors that can enhance a depressive response. These findings merely illustrate the extreme difficulty in assigning symptoms to either a medical or a psychologic origin. A more comprehensive measure of somatic symptoms and functional status outcomes should expand our understanding of the dynamic balance between somatization, affect, and functional outcomes and help to clarify factors associated with and consequential to degrees of depressive phenomena.

Sadness is an expected emotional reaction to the diagnosis of a chronic illness at key points along the illness trajectory.[40] It is important, but often difficult, to distinguish between "normal" degrees of sadness and "abnormal" levels of depression. One of the major problems in making this distinction stems from an inability to separate neurovegetative symptoms of depression from the somatic symptoms characteristic of a particular illness and treatment. Some studies of depression among the medically ill conclude that depression is best evaluated by the severity of dysphoric mood, the degree of feelings of hopelessness, guilt, and worthlessness, and the presence of suicidal thoughts.[21,49] Theoretically, excluding somatic items from an evaluation for depression in cancer patients sounds reasonable. In practice, however, the ability to separate affect and soma is extremely difficult. In addition, some investigators question the necessity of removing somatic items,[30] stating that doing so may threaten an established instrument's validity. When criteria developed by Endicott[32] were used to diagnose depression in patients with cancer (because the physical conditions and resultant symptoms were considered to be an interfering variable), the number identified as depressed was about the same as the number diagnosed by the older DSM-III criteria. Only two patients were not concordant. According to Kathol and colleagues,[30] these findings suggest that, "although somatic symptoms are less satisfactory as predictors of the syndrome of major depression, in fact when coupled with the psychologic complaints found in DSM-III, most of the same patients will meet the criteria for depression whether somatic symptoms are replaced by psychologic symptoms or not.[11,p447] According to this view, somatic symptoms may not confound depression among cancer patients provided that a sufficient number of psychologic symptoms are present.

The addition of a comprehensive measure of symptom distress to a study of depressive phenomena in medically ill patients should enhance our understanding of the relationships among somatic symptoms associated with illness, treatment, and depression. Efforts in this domain could help to determine the somatic aspects of illness and treatment that are most strongly associated with the development of depression and may clarify discrepancies regarding the prevalence of depression among the medically ill.

Organic Mental Symptoms and Depression

Organic mental impairment can have a direct causal relationship to depression in some patients. Certain drugs, including chemotherapy, steroids, and commonly prescribed medications, such as those for anxiety and pain, can produce depression in some individuals.[50] Pancreatic and neurologic cancers, cerebral metastasis, uncontrolled pain, and certain metabolic, nutritional, and endocrine derangements also are associated with a depressionogenic effect.[50] These problems present special challenges to the study of depression among the medically ill and highlight the need to screen for organic impairment with a well-established, valid, and reliable instrument.

When to Measure Depression

Given that a multisymptom crisis response occurs close to the time of diagnosis among the medically ill, it seems reasonable that investigators allow adequate time for patients to adjust to their situation before examining the nature of ongoing or residual depressive phenomena. Studies that do not consider this issue leave the differentiation between a transient crisis reaction and ongoing depression unclear. Because depression is characterized by change, a longitudinal design may best shed light on the course of depression over time.

Overview of Selected Instruments to Measure Depression

Ten instruments representing each of the measurement systems described earlier are presented in a concise format in Appendix 23A. The chosen instruments have been widely used, have had their psychometric properties assessed in depth, and can be used with a variety of populations.

Summary

Despair, hopelessness, lack of compliance with medical and psychiatric treatment, social isolation, and even premature death are but a few of the consequences frequently associated with depression. Despite significant strides in the understanding and treatment of certain types of depression, our understanding, particularly of less severe, secondary depression has been obscured by methodologic problems and inconsistencies. Although it has been difficult to bridge the gap between depressive disorders and less severe depressive symptoms within our current state of knowledge, recommendations made in this chapter are important steps in clarifying the nature of depressive phenomena. The following key points are important to help us understand depressive phenomena better:

- Rates of depression should be placed within the context of established norms for similar populations.
- Clinical interviews or observer-rated scales should be used in addition to the use of self-report measures to minimize the chance that severe depression will interfere with accurate reporting.
- For medically ill samples, physical symptom distress should be measured separately from depressive phenomena so that conceptual clarity can be maximized.
- Removal of somatic items from depression scales may not improve their sensitivity among the medically ill and can threaten the validity of established instruments.
- Outcome variables associated with various types and degrees of depressive phenomena should be described.
- Patients should be screened for organic mental impairment.
- Because to its changing nature, depression should be measured longitudinally.
- For medically ill samples, instruments with fewer somatic items should be used.
- The use of multiple measures of depression can clarify the conceptual nature of the phenomena among select populations.
- A program of research should utilize consistent measures of depression across studies to foster meaningful comparisons.

All too often, psychologic services for depressed patients are thought to be dispensable. They are viewed as expensive and without tangible need or benefit. Documentation regarding the nature of depression, its response to systematically tested interventions, and the cost of depression in terms of exaggerating the impact of chronic illness, increasing days in bed, and time off work are just beginning to emerge and deserve ongoing, careful investigation. Only when meticulous attention is paid to the theoretical, methodologic, and measurement issues addressed in this chapter will the nature and consequences associated with depressive phenomena be realized and the development of effective treatments viewed as a research and clinical priority.

Exemplar Study

Wells, K.B., Stewart, A., Hays, R.D., Burnam, N.A., Rogers, W., Daniels, M., Greenfield, S., & Ware, J. The functioning and well being of depressed patients: Results from the medical outcomes study. *JAMA*, 1989, 262:914-919.

A large-scale study specifically examined and compared outcomes associated with depressive disorders, depressive symptoms, chronic medical conditions, and no chronic conditions.[41] Data from 11,242 outpatients at three health-care sites were collected. The study associated significant morbidity with depressive symptoms and further pointed to the need to expand the study of depression among the medically ill to include depressive symptoms that do not qualify for disorder status. According to the authors:

Patients with either current depressive disorder or depressive symptoms in the absence of disorder tended to have worse physical, social and role functioning, worse perceived current health status and greater bodily pain than patients with no chronic conditions. The poor functioning uniquely associated with depressive symptoms with or without depressive disorder was comparable to or worse than that uniquely associated with eight major chronic medical conditions. For example, the unique association of days in bed with depressive symptoms was significantly greater than the comparable association with hypertension, diabetes and arthritis. Depression and chronic medical conditions had unique and additive effects on patient functioning.[41,p914]

This research emphasizes the need to measure depression with instruments that broaden the conceptual perspective beyond criteria-based psychiatric depression and to describe associations and outcomes related to depressive symptoms and syndromes among research samples. The ultimate utility of these issues in terms of patient well-being, quality of life, and health-care expenditures is not currently within grasp and will not be fully appreciated until the knowledge base in this area is expanded and more thoroughly understood.

References

1. Akiskal, H.S., & McKinney, W.T. Overview of recent research in depression: Integration of ten conceptual models into a comprehensive clinical frame. *Arch Gen Psychiatr*, 1975, *32*:285-305.
2. Boyd, J.H., & Weissman, M. Epidemiology of affective disorders, a reexamination and future directions. *Arch Gen Psychiatr*, 1981, *38*:1039-46.
3. Abraham, K. Notes on the psychoanalytic investigation and treatment of manic depressive insanity and allied conditions. In *Selected papers on psychoanalysis*. New York: Basic Books, pp. 152-172. (Original work published in 1927.)
4. Hjelle, L.A., & Zeigler, D.J. Sigmund Freud: A psychoanalytic theory of personality. In L.A. Hjelle & D.A. Zeigler (Eds.), *Personality theories: Basic assumptions, research and applications* New York: McGraw-Hill, 1976.
5. Freud, A. Certain types and stages of social maladjustment. In K.R. Eissler (Ed.), *Searchlights on delinquency*. New York: International University Press, 1949.
6. Fava, G.A., Kellner, R., Munari, F., et al. Losses, hostility and depression. *J Nerv Ment Dis*, 1982, *170*:474-478.
7. Bowlby, J. Grief and mourning in infancy and early childhood. *Psychoanal Study Child*, 1960, *15*:9-52.
8. Kaufman, I., & Rosenblum, L. Imipramine effects upon hostility in depression. *J Nerv Ment Dis*, 1970, *150*:127-132.
9. Cardoret, R., Winokur, G., & Dorzab, J. Depressive disease: Life events and onset of illness. *Arch Gen Psychiatr*, 1972, *26*:133-136.
10. Schmale, A. Relationship of separation and depression to disease. *Psychosom Med*, 1958, *20*:259-277.
11. Heinicke, C. Parental deprivation in early childhood. In S.J. Senay (Ed.), *Separation and depression: Clinical and research aspects*. Washington, DC: American Association for the Advancement of Science, 1973.
12. Beck, A.T. Thinking and depression, I. Idiosyncratic content and cognitive distortions. *Arch Gen Psychiatr*, 1963, *9*:36-45.
13. Seligman, M., & Maier, S. Failure to escape traumatic shock. *J Exp Psychol*, 1967, *74*:1-9.
14. Wright, A.T., & Beck, J.H. Cognitive therapy of depression: Theory and practice. *Hospital Comm Psychiatr*, 1983, *34*:1119-1126.
15. Hiroto, D.S., & Seligman, M.E. Generality of learned helplessness in man. *J Person Social Psychol*, 1975, *31*:311-327.
16. Becker, E. *The revolution in psychiatry*. London: Free Press, Collier Macmillan, 1964.
17. Molina, J.A. Understanding the biopsychosocial model. *Int J Psychiatr Med*, 1983, *13*:29-36.
18. Lipowski, Z.J. Psychosocial aspects of disease. *Ann Int Med*, 1969, *71*:1197-1206.
19. Sachar, E.J., & Baron, M. The biology of affective disorders. *Ann Rev Neurosci*, 1979, *2*:505-518.
20. Prange, A., Wilson, I., & Lynn, C.W. L-tryptophan in mania: Contribution to a permissive hypothesis of affective disorders. *Arch Gen Psychiatr*, 1974, *30*:56-62.
21. Bukberg, J., Penman, D., & Holland, J.C. Depression in hospitalized cancer patients. *Psychosom Med*, 1984, *46*:199-212.
22. Caplan, G. Mastery of stress: Psychosocial aspects. *Am J Psychiatr*, 1981, *138*:413-420.
23. Feighner, J.P., Robins, E., & Guze, S.B. Diagnostic criteria for use in psychiatric research. *Arch Gen Psychiatr*, 1972, *26*:57-63.
24. Spitzer, R.L., Endicott, J., & Robins, L.N. *Schedule for Affective Disorders and Schizophrenia*. New York: Biometrics Research Division, Evaluation Section: New York Psychiatric Institute, 1978.
25. Feinstein, A.R. A critical overview of diagnosis in psychiatry. In V.M. Rakoff, H.C. Stancer, & H.B. Kedward (Eds.), *Psychiatric diagnosis*. New York: Brunner-Mazel, 1977, pp. 189-206.
26. American Psychiatric Association. *Diagnostic and statistical manual of mental disorders (DSM-II)* (2nd ed.). Washington, DC: American Psychiatric Association, 1968.
27. American Psychiatric Association. *Diagnostic and statistical manual of mental disorders (DSM-III)* (3rd ed.). Washington, DC: American Psychiatric Association, 1980.
28. American Psychiatric Association, *Diagnostic and statistical manual of mental disorders (DSM-IV)* (4th ed.). Washington, DC: American Psychiatric Association, 1994.
28A. American Psychiatric Association. *Diagnostic and statistical manual of mental disorders (DSM-III-R)* (3rd ed., rev.). Washington, DC: American Psychiatric Association, 1987.

29. Massie, M.J. Depression. In J.C. Holland & J.H. Rowland (Eds.), *Handbook of psychooncology: Psychological care of the patient with cancer*. New York: Oxford University Press, 1989, pp. 75-100.

30. Kathol, R.G., Noyes, R., Williams, J., et al. Diagnosing depression in patients with medical illness. *Psychosomatics*, 1990, *31*:436-449.

31. Rodin, G., & Voshart, K. Depression in the medically ill: An overview. *Am J Psychiatr*, 1986, *14*:696-705.

32. Endicott, J. Measurement of depression in patients with cancer. Proceedings of the working conference on methodology in behavioral and psychosocial cancer research. *Cancer*, 1984, *53*(suppl):2243-2248.

33. Nunnally, J.C. *Psychometric theory*. New York: McGraw-Hill, 1978.

34. Snaith, R.P. The concepts of mild depression. *Br J Psychiatr*, 1987, *150*:387-393.

35. Meyers, J.K., & Weissman, M. Use of a self report symptom scale to detect depression in a community sample. *Am J Psychiatr*, 1980, *137*:1081-1084.

36. Prusoff, B.A., & Klerman, G.L. Differentiating depressed from anxious neurotic outpatients. *Arch Gen Psychiatr*, 1974, *30*:302-308.

37. Cavanaugh, S., Clark, D., & Gibbons, R.D. Diagnosing depression in the hospitalized medically ill. *Psychosomatics*, 1983, *24*:809-815.

38. Holland, J.C. Clinical course of cancer. In J.C. Holland & J.H. Rowland (Eds.), *Handbook of psychooncology: Psychological care of the patient with cancer*. New York: Oxford University Press, 1989, pp. 75-100.

39. Lewis, A.J. Psychological medicine In R.B. Scott (Ed.), *Price's textbook of the practice of medicine*. Section 18. London: Oxford University Press, 1966.

40. McNair, D.M., & Fisher, S. Separating anxiety from depression In M.A. Lipton, A. DiMascio, & K.F. Killiam (Eds.), *Psychopharmacology: A generation in progress*, 1978.

41. Wells, K.B., Stewart, A., Hays, R.D., et al. The functioning and well being of depressed patients: Results from the medical outcomes study. *JAMA*, 1989, *262*:914-919.

42. Mossey, J.M., Knott, K., & Craik, L. The effects of persistent depressive symptoms on hip fracture recovery. *J Gerontol*, 1990, *45*:163-168.

43. Schulberg, H.C., Saul, M., McClelland, M.A., et al. Assessing depression in primary medical and psychiatric practices. *Arch Gen Psychiatr*, 1985, *42*:1164-1170.

44. Colon, E., Callies, A.L., Popkin, M., & McGlave, P.B. Depressed mood and other variables related to bone marrow transplantation survival in acute leukemia. *Psychosomatics*, 1991, *32*:420-425.

45. Andrykowski, M.A., Redd, W.II., & Hatfield, A.K. The development of anticipatory nausea: A prospective analysis. *J Consult Clin Psychol*, 1985, *4*:447-454.

46. Burish, T.G., & Lyles, J.N., Effectiveness of relaxation training in reducing adverse reactions to cancer chemotherapy. *J Behav Med*, 1981, *4*:65-78.

47. Karnofsky, D.A., & Burchenal, J.H. The clinical evaluation of chemotherapeutic agents in cancer. In C.M. Macleod (Ed.), *Evaluation of chemotherapeutic agents*. New York: Columbia University Press, 1949.

48. Frank-Stromborg, M. Single instruments for measuring quality of life. In M. Frank-Stromborg (Ed.), *Instruments for clinical nursing research* (1st ed.). Norwalk, CT: Appleton & Lange, 1988, pp. 79-106.

49. Lansky, S.B., List, M.A., Hermann, C.A., et al. Absence of major depressive disorder in female cancer patients. *J Clin Oncol*, 1985, *3*:1553-1558.

50. Breitbart, W., & Holland, J.C. Psychiatric complications of cancer. *Curr Ther Hematol Oncol*, 1988, *3*:268-274.

51. Spitzer, R.L., Williams, J.B.W., Gibbon, M., & First, M.B. The structured clinical interview for DSM-III-R (SCID) I: History, rationale and description. *Arch Gen Psychiatr*, 1992, *49*:624-629.

52. Williams, J.B.W., Gibbon, M., First, M.B., et al. The structured clinical interview for DSM-III-R (SCID) II: Multi site test-retest reliability. *Arch Gen Psychiatr*, 1992, *49*:630-636.

53. Helzer, J.E., Robins, L.N., McEvoy, L.T., et al. A comparison of clinical and Diagnostic Interview Schedule diagnoses. *Arch Gen Psychiatr*, 1985, *42*:667-676.

54. Koenig, R., Goli, V., & Shelp, F. Major depression and the diagnostic interview schedule: Validation in medically ill patients. *Int J Psychiatr Med*, 1989, *19*:121-132.

55. Wells, K.B., Burnam, M.A., Leake, B., & Robins, L.N. Agreement between face-to-face and telephone administered versions of the depression section of the Diagnostic Interview Schedule. *J Psychiatr Res*, 1988, *22*:207-220

56. Buka, S., McEvoy, L.T., Robins, L.N., & Marcus, S.C. *Data entry, cleaning and scoring program (Version 1.0) for the Diagnostic Interview Schedule Version III Revised*. St. Louis, MO, Washington University, 1989.

57. Beck, A.T., & Beamsderfer, A. Assessment of depression: The depression inventory. In *Modern problems in pharmacopsychiatry* (vol. 7). Basel: Basel & Karger, 1974.

58. Beck, A.T., Ward, C., & Mendelson, D. An inventory for measuring depression. *Arch Gen Psychiatr*, 1961, *4*:53-63.

59. Radloff, L.S. The CES-D Scale: A self-report depression scale for researching the general population. *Appl Psychol Meas*, 1977, *1*:385-401.

60. Roberts, R.E. Reliability of the CES-D scale in different ethnic contexts. *Psychiatr Res*, 1980, *2*:125-134.

61. Derogatis, L.R. *SCL-90 Administration, scoring and procedures manual* (2nd ed.). Baltimore, Procedures Psychometric Research, 1983.

62. The SCL-90-R, BSI and matching clinical rating scales. In M. Maruish (Ed.), *Psychological testing, planning and outcome assessment*. New York: Lawrence Erlbaum, 1993.

63. Derogatis, L.R., & Spencer, P.M. *The Brief Symptom Inventory (BSI): Administration, scoring and procedures manual-I*. Baltimore, MD: Johns Hopkins University School of Medicine, 1982.

64. Derogatis, L., & Melisaratos, N. The Brief Symptom Inventory: An introductory report. *Psychol Med*, 1983, *13*:595-605.

65. Yesavage, J.A., Brink, T.L., Rose, T.L., et al. Development and validation of a geriatric depression screening scale: A preliminary report. *J Psychiatr Res*, 1982-83, *17*:37-49.

66. Koenig, H.G., Meador, K.G., Cohen, H.J., & Blazer, D.G. Self-rated depression scales and screening for major depression in the older hospitalized patients with medical illness. *J Am Geriatr Soc*, 1988, *36*:699-706.

67. Hamilton, M.A. A rating scale for depression. *J Neurol Neurosurg Psychiatr*, 1960, *23*:56-62.

68. Williams, J.B.W. A structured interview guide for the Hamilton Depression Rating Scale. *Arch Gen Psychiatr*, 1988, *45*:742-747.

69. Carroll, B.J., Fielding, J.M., & Blashki, T.G. Depression rating scales: A critical review. *Arch Gen Psychiatr*, 1973, *28*:361-366.

70. Potts, M.K., Daniels, M., Burnam, A., & Wells, K.B. A structured version of the Hamilton Depression Rating Scale: Evidence of reliability and ease of administration. *Psychiatr Res*, 1990, *24*:335-350.

71. Simon, G.E., Revicki, D., & VonKorff, M. Telephone assessment of depression severity. *J Psychiatr Res*, 1993, *27*:247-252.

72. Zigmond, A.S., & Snaith, R.P. The hospital anxiety and depression scale. *Acta Psychiatr Scand*, June 1983, *67*:361-370.

73. Klein, D.G. Endogenomorphic depression. *Arch Gen Psychiatr*, 1974, *31*:447-454.

74. Bramley, P.N., Easton, A.M.E., & Morley, S. The differentiation of anxiety and depression by rating scales. *Acta Psychiatr Scand*, 1988, *77*:136-139.

75. Aylard, P.R., Gooding, G.H., & McKenna, P.J. A validation study of three anxiety and depression self assessment scales. *J Psychosom Res*, 1987, *31*:261-268.

76. Barczak, P., Kane, N., & Andrews, S. Patterns of psychiatric morbidity in a genitourinary clinic: A validation of the Hospital Anxiety and Depression Scale. *Br J Psychiatr*, 1988, *152*:698-700.

77. Moorey, S., Greer, S., Watson, M., et al. The factor structure and factor stability of the Hospital Anxiety and Depression Scale in patients with cancer. *Br J Psychiatr*, 1991, *158*:255-259.

78. Zung, W.W.K. A self-rating depression scale. *Arch Gen Psychiatr*, 1965, *112*:63-70.

79. Zung, W.W.K., Broadhead, W.E., & Roth, M.E. Prevalence of depressive symptoms in primary care. *J Fam Pract*, 37:337-344.

80. Zung, W.W.K., Magruder, H.K., Valez, R., & Alling, W. The comorbidity of anxiety and depression in general medical patients: A longitudinal study. *J Clin Psychiatr*, 1990, *51*(suppl 6):77-80.

Appendix
23A. Selected Instruments to Measure Depression

Instrument	Description	Psychometric Indices
Structured Clinical Interview for DSM-III-R (SCID) (51,52)	Semistructured interview for making major psychiatric diagnoses according to DSM-III-R Administered by a trained psychiatric clinician Includes introductory overview and 9 modules Modular approach allows use in specific diagnostic areas of interest Uses decision tree to test diagnostic hypotheses Questions grouped by diagnostic criteria required to meet the specific diagnoses Ratings for diagnostic criteria: (1) symptom absent; (2) subthreshold condition; (3) symptom present; (4) inadequate data for a rating 2 editions: SCID-P: adults identified as psychiatric patients; SCID-NP: not identified as psychiatric patients	Test-retest reliabilities performed (sample = 4 patient sites, 2 nonpatient sites; 592 subjects) Agreement between interviewers: patient sample: $k = 0.65$ (current lifetime diagnoses of major depression); nonpatient sample: $k = 0.42$ (major depression) Raises questions regarding source of diagnostic disagreement
Diagnostic Interview Schedule (DIS) (53-56)	Criteria-based system designed to make DSM-III diagnoses Can be used to evaluate the presence of depressive disorders, including depression and dysthymia Highly structured, comprehensive interview Clinically significant symptoms unexplained by physical causes coded on a structured form Nonpsychiatric person can be trained as interviewer Data can be scored to obtain current and lifetime diagnoses of major depression and dysthymia (56)	Validated for use in medically ill patients (54) Face-to-face and telephone-administered versions of depression section of the DIS are equivalent (55)
Beck Depression Inventory (BDI) (56,57)	Based on cognitive model of depression as "activation of primitive negative schemas that lead to a selective negative bias in interpreting experiences" (12) Unidimensional, self-report scale designed to measure the behavioral manifestations and depth of depression Scale statements read to patients who select most appropriate choice (really an interviewer-adjusted scale) 21 "symptom-attitude categories," each representing a characteristic manifestation of depression 4-point discrete scale for responses	Factor analysis: 3 highly correlated factors: (1) negative attitude toward self; (2) performance impairment; (3) somatic disturbance Internal consistency: 0.86 Test-retest reliability: 0.48–0.86 Concurrent validity established with other widely used measures of depression: Hamilton (0.73); Zung (0.76); MMPI depression subscale (0.76) Instrument open to observer bias BDI used to study medical inpatients, depressed psychiatry patients, and normal subjects (37)

23A. Selected Instruments to Measure Depression (*cont.*)

Instrument	Description	Psychometric Indices
BDI (*cont.*)	Individual items summed for total depression score (0–63): 0–9: normal range; 10–15: mild depression; 16–19: mild to moderate depression; 20–29: moderate to severe depression; 30–63: severe depression Widely used with psychiatric patients as a measure of symptom severity (depressed mood) and as a screening tool in nonpsychiatric populations	Latent trait model of analysis BDI measures one underlying general syndrome of depression 6 cognitive BDI items able to discriminate severity of depression in each subject group Dissatisfaction and social interest were items that discriminate best; these were related to the subject's pleasure capacity Crying (single item) discriminated well for depression among medical patients only
Center for Epidemiological Studies of Depression Scale (CES-D) (58,60)	Developed as a brief, inexpensive measure of depression to use in community surveys (large epidemiologic studies) Consists of 20 items, derived from other depression scales 6 major symptom areas: (1) depressed mood; (2) guilt/worthlessness; (3) helplessness/hopelessness; (4) psychomotor retardation; (5) loss of appetite; (6) sleep disturbance Scoring: responses 0–3 except for 4 items that are reverse-scored Higher scores mean more impairment Total scores range from 0 to 60 In some studies, patients with scores > 15 experience major depressive or dysthymic disorders (43)	Reliability tested (sample: clinic populations, and probability samples of households in 3 communities across the U.S.) High internal consistency Acceptable test–retest stability Good construct validity Some criterion validity (clinic samples)
Symptom Checklist-90 (SCL-90) (61-62)	90-item self-report symptom inventory designed to assess psychologic status of individuals, including medical patients Measures multidimensional psychologic distress, including 9 primary symptom dimensions: (1) somatization; (2) obsessive-compulsive; (3) interpersonal sensitivity; (4) depression; (5) anxiety; (6) hostility; (7) phobic anxiety; (8) paranoid ideation; (9) psychoticism 3 global indices measured, giving as a single value, the depth of symptomatic distress: (1) General Severity Index (GSI); (2) Positive Symptom Distress Index (PSDI); (3) Positive Symptom Total (PST)	Internal consistency (Cronbach's alpha): 0.79–0.90 Test–retest reliability (stability) coefficient: 0.68–0.83 Factor analysis: supported 7–9 dimensions
Brief Symptom Inventory (BSI) (62-64)	53-item, self-report symptom inventory assessing psychologic status of individual, including medical patients Short-version of SLC-90, measuring multidimensional psychologic distress	Internal consistency (Cronbach's alpha): 0.68–0.91 Stability (global indices): PST: 0.80; PSDI: 0.87; GSI: 0.90 Validity: correlated positively with MMPI, >0.30 Factor analysis: empirical support for 7–9 dimensions

Instrument	Description	Psychometric properties
	9 primary symptom dimensions are same as for the SLC-90 Depression dimension reflects broad range of signs/symptoms of clinical depression 3 global indices: (1) PSDI: Positive Symptom Distress Index; (2) PST: Positive Symptom Total; (3) GSI (General Severity Index), the single best indicator of current distress level(s) (GSI combines and the information on the numbers of symptoms intensity of perceived distress)	
Geriatric Depression Scale (GDS) (65,66)	30-item self-report questionnaire assessing symptoms of depression in the elderly Contains yes–no categories, takes 5 minutes to complete Scores range 0 to 30, higher scores mean greater depression Advantages: (1) binary response options easily understood by elders; (2) does not contain potentially confounding somatic items; (3) completion time is 5 minutes; (4) contains more criteria characteristic of late life depression than other scales; (5) one of few scales validated in older hospitalized population	Sensitive to depression in elders suffering from mild to moderate dementia and physical illness Reliability estimates: good internal consistency (Cronbach's alpha): 0.94 Test–retest: 0.86 Screening instrument: (cutoff score of 11): sensitivity: 92% (distinguishes subjects with and without depression); specificity: 89% (accuracy in selecting individuals with depressive disorders); positive predictive power: 56%; negative predictive power: 99%
Hamilton Depression Scale (HDRS) (67-71)	Most widely used scale in depression research as measures change over time in severity of depression Total score based on 17 of its 21 items, but some investigators use all 21 items Face-to-face clinical interview Depression viewed as unitary concept Relies heavily on the expertise of an interviewer with extensive psychiatric background so use limited Revised version (14 or 17 items): interviewers without psychiatric background can be trained to use the schedule; telephone or face-to-face interviews yield similar results; heavily weighted with somatic items	High overall scale reliability Concurrent, discriminant, and construct validity established Limitations: interrater reliability on individual items criticized (–0.02 to 0.76); interpretative differences Clinicians instructed to consider intensity and frequency of symptoms when assigning values on an anchored rating scale, but there are no defined response categories Questions directed at a timeframe of a few days to a week 3 scale items (insight, psychomotor agitation, psychomotor retardation) demonstrate very poor test–retest correlations Structured interview developed to overcome limitations removed 3 poorly performing items; alpha reliability for 17-item version: 0.82; test–retest reliability for 14-item version: 0.67
Hospital Anxiety and Depression Scale (HADS) (72-77)	Brief, self-administered measure of anxiety and depression in patients with medical illness: screens for significant depression; measures/monitors severity of depression over time Focuses on psychologic rather than somatic manifestations Contains 14 items, 7 each for anxiety and depression	Concurrent validity established in heterogenous populations (97-99) Validation studies demonstrated HADS functions as 2 scales, measuring 2 distinct psychologic states Factor analysis (100) (sample 568 cancer patients): 2 distinct but correlated factors (2 subscales)

23A. Selected Instruments to Measure Depression (*cont.*)

Instrument	Description	Psychometric Indices
HADS (*cont.*)	Depression subscale emphasizes anhedonia, which may be amenable to antidepressants Overall severity of depression rated on a 4-point (0 to 3) scale; range of scores on depression subscale 0 to 21; score of 8 to 10 indicates probable presence of clinically significant depression	Internal consistency (coefficient alpha): anxiety (0.93); depression (0.90) Limitations: brevity may exclude important aspects of each subscale
Zung Self-Rating Depression Scale (SRS) (69,78-80)	Widely used, 20-item self-report scale (unassisted) Screening instrument for major depressive disorders and measure of severity of depressive symptoms 10 items positively worded, 10 negatively worded Subjects indicate frequency with which they experience a symptom or feeling described Scale includes affective, behavioral, somatic features	Comparison of scores to DSM-III-R criteria for major depression (80): sensitivity of 97%; specificity of 63%; positive predictive value of 77%; negative predictive value of 95% Limitations: subjects may require assistance, increased length of time to complete tool

Numbers in parentheses correspond to studies cited in the References.

III

Instruments for Assessing Health-Promotion Activities

24

Measuring Healthy Lifestyle

Ann Malone Berger and Susan Noble Walker

Since the mid-1970s, increasing interest in the relationship between lifestyle behavior and health has been evident in nursing and a variety of other disciplines. Researchers have examined the patterns of healthy lifestyle and the stages and processes of lifestyle behavior change to further understanding of health-related behaviors. Since the publication of the Canadian LaLonde[1] report in 1974, national and international public health initiatives have emphasized disease prevention and health promotion and focused on lifestyle behaviors and individuals' responsibility to influence their own health. In most industrialized nations today, the leading causes of illness and death have shifted from communicable diseases to those chronic diseases strongly linked with personal lifestyle.

In the 1979 *Surgeon General's Report on Health Promotion and Disease Prevention*,[2] it was estimated that at least 50% of all deaths in the United States each year were due to unhealthy lifestyles. Following the release of that report, an agenda of national health objectives to be achieved by 1990 was developed. It emphasized lifestyle modification as one major strategy to enhance health and prevent illness.[3] Although the objectives clearly focused more heavily on disease prevention than on health enhancement, the idea of health as a positive concept was introduced. Throughout the 1980s, data systems were established and expanded to track progress toward meeting the objectives, and nearly half were wholly or partially accomplished by 1990.[4] Much of the major decline in death rates from heart disease, stroke, and unintentional injuries was attributed to reduction in risk factors associated with lifestyle behaviors, such as cigarette smoking, alcohol consumption, dietary fat intake, and sedentary lifestyle.

The current U.S. public health initiative, *Healthy People 2000*,[5] challenges the nation to move beyond measuring the health of the population by death rates to defining good health by reduction of unnecessary suffering, illness, and disability and by improvement in quality of life. The report suggests that personal responsibility is the key to good health and sets forth objectives for the year 2000 in three broad categories: health promotion, health protection, and preventive services. The health-promotion objectives concern "individual lifestyle—personal choices made in a social context—that can have a powerful influence over one's health prospects."[5,p6] If the vision set forth in *Healthy*

People 2000 is to be achieved, a clear understanding of the nature of a healthy lifestyle and of why and how individuals acquire and maintain healthy lifestyle behavior patterns is essential.

The Concept of Healthy Lifestyle

Although the term *healthy lifestyle* is used frequently in everyday conversation and in the public media, its use in scientific discourse has been far from consistent. It has been described in the literature in various ways; sometimes narrowly as simply the avoidance of bad health habits, and sometimes broadly as all behaviors that have an impact on health status. It is central to the *American Journal of Health Promotion*'s definition of health promotion as "the science and art of helping people to change their lifestyle to move toward a state of optimal health."[6,p4] Issues surrounding the conceptualization of healthy lifestyle and the related concepts of health and health promotion have been addressed thoughtfully and quite comprehensively by several nursing authors[7-10] who have recognized the considerable ambiguity that currently exists. Healthy lifestyle has been conceptualized within the broader contexts of lifestyle and of health behavior. Both contexts provide important information contributing to the definition of the concept of healthy lifestyle.

Healthy Lifestyle as a Component of Lifestyle

The themes of personal responsibility and individual choice of behavior patterns are evident in definitions of both global and healthy lifestyle. For their study of the influence of selected lifestyle or personal practices on physical health, Wiley and Camacho defined lifestyle as "discretionary activities which are a regular part of an individual's daily pattern of living."[11,p1] Ardell[12] advocated a wellness lifestyle to enable individuals to realize their highest potential for well-being. He described lifestyle as "the aggregation of all individual decisions affecting health status," incorporating "all those behaviors over which we have control, including those actions which affect our health risks."[12,p19]

Many definitions also recognize that lifestyle choices take place in an environmental context. Bruhn[13] described lifestyle as: (1) a person's way of life, with some aspects chosen and others determined by socioenvironmental factors; (2) long-term patterns encompassing behaviors and attitudes as well as a philosophy or outlook on life; and (3) components that are acquired and modified throughout life. He viewed health behaviors as an integral part of lifestyle and outlined characteristics that might comprise illness and wellness lifestyles. Abel addressed the need for a definition that could be operationalized in empirical research, and suggested that "health lifestyles comprise patterns of health-related behavior, values, and attitudes adapted [sic] by groups of individuals in response to their social, cultural and economic environment."[14,p901] Milio characterized lifestyles as "patterns of choices [concerning personal behavior] made from the alternatives that are available to people according to their socioeconomic circumstances and to the ease with which they are able to choose certain ones over others."[15,p76] Pender suggested that health as a positive life process may be experienced and expressed through lifestyle patterns, "person/environment interactional patterns that become increasingly complex throughout the lifespan."[16,p117] She proposed five dimensions of lifestyle patterns through which health may be expressed—affect, attitudes, activity, aspirations, and accomplishments—and noted that some can be directly observed whereas others must be self-reported.

Healthy Lifestyle as a Component of Health Behavior

The term *health behavior* first appeared in the literature when Kasl and Cobb differentiated sick role behavior and illness behavior from health behavior.[17] They defined health behavior as "any activity undertaken by a person believing himself to be healthy, for the purpose of preventing disease or detecting it in an asymptomatic stage."[17,p246] Since that time, the term has been used in a variety of ways and applied in a variety of populations. Although some authors, like Kasl and Cobb, restrict the definition of health behavior to action or activity, others expand the definition to encompass various cognitive elements of behavior. Gochman provides a broadly constructed definition of health behavior as "personal attributes such as beliefs, expectations, motives, values, perceptions, and other cognitive elements; personality characteristics, including affective and emotional states and traits; and overt behavior patterns, actions and habits that relate to health maintenance, to health restoration and to health improvement."[18,p3] He notes that such a definition includes mental events and feeling states that must be measured indirectly, as well as overt actions that can be observed directly. Although health behavior was initially conceptualized as applicable only to those who were healthy,[17] its relevance for those with chronic illness has since been recognized. Miller[19] includes the pursuit of a healthy lifestyle as a goal for persons with diabetes and other chronic illnesses, and others[20-22] advocate the value of health-promoting behaviors for those with cancer.

Laffrey, Loveland-Cherry, and Winkler[23] summarized the definitions of health behavior found in the nursing and public health literature as including the use of health-care services, compliance with medically prescribed regimens, routine activities of one's life, actions taken to prevent illness, and actions taken to achieve a higher level of well-being. They associated these diverse definitions of health behavior with two major paradigms that reflect different views of health: the pathogenic or disease paradigm, in which health behavior is conceptualized as preventing or detecting disease, and the health paradigm, in which health behavior is conceptualized as promoting higher levels of health or wellness. In the disease paradigm, health behavior is variously labeled as illness-preventing, risk-reducing, or health-protecting. The original definition by Kasl and Cobb[17] reflects this preventive orientation. An extensive body of evidence linking certain lifestyle behaviors (such as cigarette smoking, physical inactivity, and alcohol consumption) to disease and death has accumulated since the 1960s.[24,25] Preventive health behaviors may be isolated acts, such as obtaining an influenza vaccination, or may be components of a person's lifestyle, such as performing monthly breast self-examination or regularly wearing seat belts.

Within the health paradigm, health behavior is labeled as health-promoting or wellness-enhancing. Although a preventive orientation dominates much of the literature on health behavior, a promotive orientation is increasingly prominent. It is strongly evident in the salutogenic framework for health proposed by Antonovsky,[26] in the high-level wellness literature,[27,28] and in the work within nursing of Laffrey[29] and Pender.[30] As an expression of the actualizing tendency, health-promoting behaviors are pursued because they are satisfying and enjoyable rather than to avoid disease or premature death.[12,30] Walker et al. defined health-promoting lifestyle behavior as "a multidimensional pattern of self-initiated actions and perceptions that serve to maintain or enhance the level of wellness, self-actualization, and fulfillment of the individual."[31,p77] The Alameda County Study of Health and Ways of Living, begun in 1965 at the Human Population Laboratory, provided perhaps the first definitive link between lifestyle behaviors and positive health consequences (defined as physical, mental, and social well-being). That work was important because it suggested that "certain behaviors have generalized health, rather than just specific disease, consequences."[32,p54] Support for the association of health behaviors with high-level wellness, a wholistically oriented outcome, is more theoretical than empirical at this time. As health disciplines embrace wellness and quality of life as outcomes valued as highly as declines in morbidity and mortality rates, more research undoubtedly will address such connections. Health-promoting behaviors "almost without exception are continuing activities that must be an integral part of an individual's lifestyle."[30,p59]

Dimensions of Healthy Lifestyle

The concepts of health promotion and healthy lifestyle are still relatively new in the scientific arena, including that of nursing science. A literature review identified only one nursing research report concerned with preventive health behavior or health-promotion behavior published between 1958 and 1980, and thirty between 1980 and 1992.[12] There has been much discussion among nurse researchers as to whether (1) health-promoting behavior should be differentiated from illness-preventing behavior; (2) preventive behavior might be subsumed as a category of promotive behavior; (3) illness-preventing, health-maintaining, and health-promoting behaviors might be placed on a continuum of promotiveness; or (4) health-protecting and health-promoting behaviors might be viewed as two complementary components of a healthy lifestyle.[7,9,23,29,30,33] It is recognized that particular lifestyle behaviors (e.g., exercise) may be undertaken by some individuals to prevent cardiovascular disease, by others to promote a feeling of well-being, and by still others for reasons such as socialization that are unrelated to health. For some research purposes the nature of motivation for healthy lifestyle behaviors will be important, whereas for others it will not. The state of the science is such that many questions remain concerning the dimensionality of healthy lifestyles. Categories of preventive and promotive behaviors mentioned in the literature as components of healthy lifestyles can be summarized as:

Self-responsibility for health	Stress management
Exercise	Accident or injury prevention
Nutrition	Smoking avoidance or cessation
Interpersonal relationships/support	Spiritual growth, fulfillment of potential, or
Safe use of medications and alcohol	self-actualization

Continued identification of the dimensions of healthy lifestyle is important to further the development of instruments as well as knowledge in this area.

Summary

Some defining characteristics of a healthy lifestyle emerge repeatedly, although not unanimously, from the literature. Healthy lifestyle includes complex multidimensional patterns of behavior that have cognitive, affective, or emotional, and action or activity elements. Healthy lifestyle behavior is self-initiated, voluntary, and individually chosen from available options and influenced by socioenvironmental and other contextual factors. It is a continuing and consistent long-term, but modifiable, pattern of behavior integrated into daily living as a way of life. Healthy lifestyle serves to prevent illness and maintain or enhance wellness, whether engaged in for health consequences or not, and regardless of the individual's current state of health.

Issues in Instrument Selection

Relatively few instruments measure healthy lifestyle behaviors. Early tools were developed as Health Risk Appraisals (HRAs) and focused on risk reduction through adoption of preventive behaviors specific to particular diseases (i.e., smoking and lung cancer).

More recent instruments measure both risk potential and health-promoting lifestyle behaviors, or health-promoting lifestyle alone.

When selecting an instrument, it is important to consider the lifestyle dimensions assessed, relevance for the population being studied, length, method of administration and reporting results, cost for use, and, for intervention research, availability of supplemental educational materials. The researcher should look for evidence of reliability and validity, including the populations in which they were evaluated and the instrument's ability to discriminate among distinct groups.[14] Caution must be taken that a tool developed for one population is not automatically transferred to a second with different characteristics, such as race, culture, or age. With HRAs, it is important to consider whether the tool identifies individual characteristics that affect life expectancy based on current scientific knowledge.[34]

It is recognized that, although some healthy lifestyle behaviors may be observed directly, self-report is necessary for comprehensive measurement of the concept. Kirscht[35] points out that self-report is needed because many behaviors cannot be observed at all or can't be observed over enough occasions to provide reliable data. The accuracy of self-report is generally good, but may be threatened by inaccurate recall or by intentional false responses due to sensitive issues or perceived social desirability. Information on health issues obtained by telephone interviews has been shown to be as reliable and valid as information obtained face-to-face or by mail interview.[36] A few self-reported behaviors, such as smoking and drug use, can be validated with biologic measures. Reliability and validity can be enhanced by the specificity of measurement tools and by multiple modes of assessment of the same behavior when feasible.[35,37]

A major issue in selecting instrumentation is that if lifestyle represents patterns of coherent behaviors, then measurement must go beyond single health behaviors to clusters of behaviors that show linkages. Clusters of behaviors have been demonstrated in several studies, with correlations among preventive health behaviors varying across studies but generally of low to moderate magnitude.[35,38] Higher correlations have been shown among promotive health behaviors.[31] There clearly is not yet sufficient internal consistency of items or statistical association among a comprehensive set of preventive and promotive healthy lifestyle behaviors to permit measurement by any single scale.

Instruments designed to measure healthy lifestyle operationalize the concept in a variety of ways, some narrower and some broader. Instruments included in this chapter provide more comprehensive measurement of either or both of the health-protecting and health-promoting behavioral components of a healthy lifestyle, rather than measurement of single behaviors or behavioral sets (such as nutrition or smoking). They are arranged in sequence from those that emphasize preventive behaviors to those that emphasize promotive behaviors.

Health Risk Appraisal

Although many HRAs are available, most are derived from the original Centers for Disease Control and Prevention (CDC) version developed by the U.S. government in the late 1970s or from the Carter Center revision in 1988. HRA was developed primarily to assist health professionals in practice settings to educate and counsel patients to modify hazardous behaviors. HRA also has been used as a screening tool, a research tool, and a baseline or outcome measure to evaluate health-promotion programs.

Health risk appraisal is a personalized estimation of one's risk for dying or major illness in the next 10 years from each of the most frequent causes of death. Risks are calculated by a computer program that compares the individual's characteristics to national mortality statistics using equations developed by epidemiologists and updated on a routine basis. These risks are communicated to the client through a personalized or group report, as illustrated in Figure 24.1. The report accounts for both controllable and uncontrollable risk factors, but emphasizes that the individual should focus on modifiable risk factors. Although the HRA estimates the probability of specified outcomes among groups of persons with similar characteristics, it cannot predict the precise outcome for each individual.

In HRAs risk is expressed in terms of both risk age and health score. The ideal score is a risk age lower than real age or a health score of 100 points. Risk age is calculated first on the basis of current risk factors and a second time as if the risk factors were reduced as much as possible by adopting healthier lifestyle behaviors. The second "target" risk age shows the potential health benefit to the individual of improving lifestyle through the elimination of risky behaviors. Estimates of risks are imperfect because of individual variance in susceptibility to disease. Risk age provides useful feedback to stimulate individual behavior change, but the health score appears most suitable in research, particularly when it involves inferential statistical analysis. Health scores range from 0 to 100 (maximum incorporation of risk-reducing behaviors into one's lifestyle).[39] Gustafson[40] states that the effectiveness of the HRA should be measured by how it influences individuals to make recommended behavior changes to improve their health score.

The HRA has a high degree of face validity, and its use as an awareness and educational tool in health-promotion programs is strongly supported in the literature. Estab-

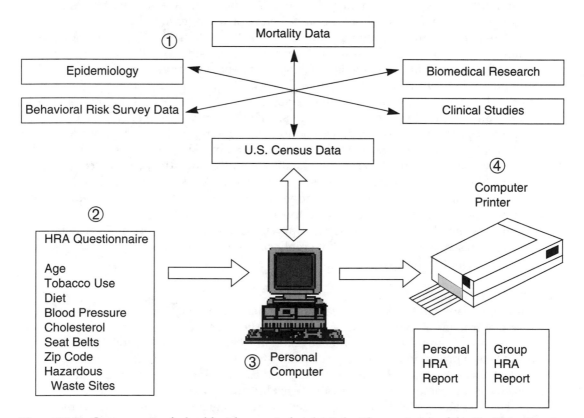

Figure 24.1 Components of a health risk appraisal. Adapted with permission of the Healthier People Network, Inc., Decatur, GA.

lishing the reliability, validity, and effectiveness of HRAs is critical to future use and development of this technology for research purposes. When it is used to predict risk or evaluate a program, questions remain unanswered. In the most rigorous scientific sense, reliability and validity are minimally acceptable because many health risk factors have yet to be determined.[41] Test–retest reliability coefficients have ranged from 0.99 on many items to considerably lower levels (0.23–0.65) for self-reported blood pressure, cholesterol levels, and dietary patterns.[41] Item reliability is enhanced when clinical screening includes the actual measurement of blood pressure, cholesterol, and body weight and height at the time of HRA administration.[42]

To be scientifically credible, the HRA must identify high-risk individuals. The validity of risk estimates depends on the ratio of known to unknown plus chance etiologic factors related to the leading causes of death. Validity is based on the accuracy of the algorithms derived from death certificate data, epidemiologic and clinical data, and respondents' self-reports of risk factors. Results are limited by the availability and accuracy of statistics used to estimate risks and by the method used to handle missing data.[43,44] When comparing the CDC version with the Carter Center version, Gazmararian[44] found that, although the CDC version was a more accurate predictor of 10-year mortality, the predictive validity of each version was sufficient to warrant their continued use.

Despite steady growth in the 1990s since their widespread distribution, there are many areas in HRAs can be further developed. No risk indicators are available yet for many common and serious health problems and only healthy people receive reliable risk estimates from the HRAs, as they are not designed to be used with people already diagnosed with chronic diseases. In summary, HRA technology has demonstrated adequate reliability, validity, and effectiveness to encourage continued development for use in research.

HRA-CDC-Carter Center

The Carter Center of Emory University was founded in 1982 by former President Jimmy Carter. The Carter Center's HRA program was the result of a joint venture between the CDC and the private sector to update the CDC-HRA instrument, which was first available in 1980. *Healthier People* Version 4.0 is a microcomputer-based HRA developed and published in 1991 by the Carter Center. A set of 43 questions cover topics such as demographics, blood pressure, cholesterol, driving, smoking, alcohol use, and gender-specific health issues. An example of an item is: "On the average, how close to the speed limit do you usually drive?" Most questions require a fill-in-the-blank response and can be completed in minutes. After completion and computer analysis based on the latest mortality data, the two-page report to the participant highlights health risks affecting life expectancy and pinpoints risks that the individual can control. The report also provides information and general recommendations about preventive services. The *Healthier People* report should always be interpreted to the client by a qualified health professional. A group report also is available to assess the health status of an employee group as a basis for establishing priorities for an organization's health-promotion program efforts.

In addition to the software program, a camera-ready copy of the four-page questionnaire and a 532-page manual are provided. The manual outlines the computer program's structure and risk calculations and includes step-by-step operating instructions. The Carter Center discontinued its involvement in updating the HRA in 1991. The Healthier People Network is a nonprofit organization that continues the work of the CDC and the Carter Center. The Network's goals are to update the HRAs in a timely manner as scientific knowledge changes and to disseminate them to health-promotion professionals so they can inform the public of their health risks. *Healthier People* Version 4.1 was released in 1995.

The UM-HRA

The University of Minnesota-HRA Version 3.0, released in 1993, is based on the health risk statistics from the CDC and the Carter Center. It includes items from the original CDC version plus questions on risk behaviors for AIDS. This program takes 8 to 12 minutes to complete. The computer printout provides immediate feedback about an individual's risk for 10 leading causes of death, good health habits, and risk age. It also suggests interventions to decrease the risk age and lists an achievable risk age based on the elimination of one or more changeable risk factors.[45] A Spanish-language version is available.

The HRA-U.S. Army

This tool is a modification of the HRA-CDC version with specialized content for U.S. Army military personnel. It has been customized by the addition of questions concerning military branch, service and rank (6 items); psychologic status (10–12 items); alcoholic use/abuse (2 items); testicular self-exam (1 item); nutrition (3 items); exercise pattern (1 item); and suicide (2 items). The HRA-U.S. Army has 29 items with base predictions and equations borrowed from the CDC version. The additional items listed are not yet included in the algorithms, but they provide a means to collect information about lifestyle behaviors such as stress management, exercise and nutrition, where scientific knowledge is now advancing. Version 5.0 includes a component focusing on morbidity and functional status for use with older adults.

Other Instruments

Youth Risk Behavior Survey (YRBS)

The Youth Risk Behavior Survey is a survey instrument developed by the Centers for Disease Control and Prevention (CDC) for use within the Youth Risk Behavior Surveillance System (YRBSS).[46] The YRBSS is a school-based epidemiological surveillance system designed to monitor progress toward 26 of the national health objectives for the Year 2000[5] and to provide comparable national, state, and local data across six categories of behavior. The Division of Adolescent and School Health (DASH) in the CDC conducts a biennial survey to measure the prevalence of the identified priority health risk behaviors among a national probability sample of students in grades 9–12. The CDC also provides fiscal and technical assistance to state and local education departments who wish to use the YRBS to assess the prevalence of these health risk behaviors among youth in their locales.

The YRBS focuses on those behaviors established during youth that result in the most significant mortality, morbidity, and social problems during both youth and adulthood. Those six priority areas of health risk behavior include: (1) behaviors that result in intentional and unintentional injuries; (2) alcohol and other drug use; (3) tobacco use; (4) sexual behaviors that result in HIV infection, other sexually transmitted diseases, and unintended pregnancies; (5) dietary behaviors; and (6) physical activity. The YRBS is a self-administered 75-item multiple-choice questionnaire with a standard scannable "bubble sheet" that can be used to record responses. It has a 7th-grade reading level and was designed for use with adolescents during a typical 45-minute school class period. It includes five demographic items and 70 behavioral items; varied response options include yes–no, age when a behavior was started, and frequency of behaviors within the past 30 days or the past 12 months. An example of an item is: "How old were you when you had your first drink of alcohol other than a few sips?" (never, less than 9, 9 or 10, 11 or 12, 13 or 14, 15 or 16, 17 or more years old).

Results are reported for aggregates rather than individuals. The process of development of the YRBS produced content validity through the use of panels of experts who delineated priority behaviors consistent with national health objectives and devised questions to measure those behaviors. No empirical evidence of validity or reliability is available. However, development included four waves of field testing with national, state, and local samples of high school students that strengthened the tool through various revisions of wording, response categories, and recall periods before its release in 1990. The CDC currently is modifying the questionnaire for college populations and plans to conduct national college surveys.

Index of Health Practices

The Index of Health Practices was developed as one component of a more extensive questionnaire used within the Human Population Laboratory Studies in Alameda County, California, in the 1960s,[24] and is the first measure of health behaviors to be used as a public health screening instrument. The index contains seven items pertaining to habits of sleep, eating, exercise, alcohol consumption, and smoking. The items were developed from a literature review; however, little empirical evidence to support the selected items was available at the time. The index was designed to measure health habits in a study examining the relationship between "good" health habits and physical health status. Based on data from that survey of 6,928 adults, the researchers reported that responses to the items were highly reliable. Although the small number of items gives rise to concerns about the instrument's sampling validity as a comprehensive measure of healthy lifestyle, the criterion-oriented validity for this tool appears to be excellent. Health practices measured by this index have been correlated with physical health status and with mortality. The tool's restricted number of items and lack of detail concerning the assessed health habits limit its usefulness.

Lifestyle Assessment Questionnaire (LAQ)

The Lifestyle Assessment Questionnaire (LAQ), developed in 1976 by the National Wellness Institute, has been a popular and useful lifestyle assessment instrument for research. Wellness is described by the developer of this instrument as a continuous, active process rather than as a single goal or achievement. The process involves becoming aware of the different areas in one's life, identifying the areas that need improvement, and then making choices that will help to attain a higher level of health and well-being. The methodology used to develop the tool is not presented by the authors. The extensive appraisal instrument consists of a 270-item questionnaire that not only assesses adult lifestyle behavior and major health risks, but also provides suggestions for lifestyle improvement and a guide to effective behavior change. The LAQ report provides the individual with (1) a TestWell® Wellness Inventory (assessment of lifestyle behaviors); (2) an HRA (appraised and achievable health age); (3) a behavioral change facilitation guide (steps to make a positive change in lifestyle); and (4) a personal growth resources list (bibliography of resources). Divided into six dimensions of wellness, the tool includes: physical, emotional, occupational, intellectual, spiritual, and social areas in 11 assessment categories. An example of an item is: "I examine my breasts or testes on a monthly basis."

Each item is scored on a scale ranging from 1 (almost never) to 5 (almost always). Item scores are summed to obtain a subscale score for each section, and subscale scores then are summed to obtain a total score. Subscale scores can be used to determine specific areas for wellness instructions. The questionnaire is available in both paper-and-pencil and computer versions. The instrument's strengths include use of the latest statistics from the CDC, availability of reliability and validity estimates, and access to technical support for the user. Users can purchase the software program or submit completed paper version questionnaires to the National Wellness Institute Processing Center for scoring and feedback. Test–retest reliability coefficients range from 0.57 to 0.87 for the subscales with a coefficient of 0.76 for the total scale. Content validity has been established, and low to moderate intercorrelations have been found among the LAQ wellness subscales. A college version is available for use with young adults. The instrument has been used at health fairs, employee wellness education offerings, in wellness consulting, and for classroom instruction on health promotion.

Wellness Index and Wellness Inventory

Wellness Associates is a nonprofit educational organization that is the successor to the Wellness Resource Center founded by Dr. John W. Travis in 1975. In the *Wellness Workbook*, Travis and Ryan[28] describe a model of wellness that views the individual and environment as interacting in a Wellness Energy System, with system output consisting of 12 dimensions of wellness: self-responsibility and love; breathing; sensing; eating; moving; feeling; thinking; playing and working; communicating; sex; finding meaning; and transcending. These dimensions are depicted on 12 sections of a Wellness Wheel that reflects how well an individual's energy is balanced. Dimension scores to be recorded on the Wellness Wheel can be obtained from a full-length Wellness Index or an abbreviated Wellness Inventory.

The Wellness Index is a 378-item self-scoring questionnaire for adults that is included in the *Wellness Workbook*.[28] The number of items in each of the 12 sections varies from 19 in the wellness and thinking section to 71 in the wellness, self-responsibility, and love section. Responses are recorded on a 5-point scale ranging from 0 (no, never, or hardly ever) to 4 (yes, always, or usually). The Wellness Inventory (3rd edition) is a 120-item abridged form of the questionnaire that contains 10 items in each of the 12 sections and is available both in a 12-page pamphlet and in an interactive computer (IBM) version. The response format also is abridged to 3-point scale ranging from 0 (no, rarely) to 2 (yes, usually). Items on the Wellness Index and Wellness Inventory are described as wellness attributes that reflect both awareness and action based on awareness. An example of an item is: "I meditate or relax myself for at least 15 (to 20) minutes each day." Both questionnaires can be self-scored, and scores for each of the 12 wellness dimensions transferred onto the Wellness Wheel to assess balance. The interactive computer version of the Wellness Inventory displays both the individual's score and level of satisfaction with answers in each section. The experience of completing either of these tools is designed to educate more than to test the individual. These questions are recommended for initial wellness assessment sessions to increase clients' awareness of healthy lifestyle and assist in developing priorities and plans for lifestyle change. They have not been subjected to psychometric evaluation for use in research. The authors do not present their methodology for item or scale development and state that "much wellness information is subjective and 'unprovable' by current scientific methods."[28,pxxviii] No information about reliability or validity is available.

Personal Lifestyle Questionnaire (PLQ)

The Personal Lifestyle Questionnaire (PLQ) was developed by Muhlenkamp and Brown[47-49] to measure the extent of individuals' participation in health-related or health-promotion activities; these terms are not conceptually defined. The 24-item instrument includes three to five items in each of six categories of health practices: exercise; substance use; nutrition; relaxation; safety; and general health promotion. Items are scored on a 4-point Likert scale ranging from 1 (never) to 4 (almost always). An example of an item is: "See a health-care provider for a check-up at least yearly." A subscale score may be obtained for each of the six categories; a total score, called Lifestyle, is computed by adding the scores obtained on the six subscales. The authors indicated that they have more confidence in the use of the total score than in the subscale scores,[47] and validity and reliability data support that conclusion.[47,48]

Development of the item pool for the PLQ is not described. Construct validity was assessed by means of a factor analysis of the responses of 380 subjects to determine the validity of the six theorized categories. Seven factors emerged, five of which were almost identical to the original subscales. Intercorrelations between subscale scores ranged from 0.003 to 0.42.[47] Only 0.002% of the variance on the PLQ total score was attributed to social desirability in a sample of 175 nursing clinic clients.[48] Convergent validity of the scale was assessed by administering it with the National Wellness Institute's Lifestyle Assessment Questionnaire; correlation coefficients of 0.83 and 0.72 were obtained in two separate samples. Concurrent validity was assessed in a sample of 127 individuals by correlating the PLQ score with an HRA-modifiable risk score (risk that can be lowered by changing health behaviors), with a result of $r = -0.25$.[47] Internal consistency of the total scale was acceptable, with alpha coefficients of 0.74 and 0.76 in samples of 133 and 383 subjects. Subscale coefficients ranged from 0.24 to 0.75, so that some would not be acceptable for use in inferential research. The PLQ's test–retest reliability coefficient was 0.78 over a 4-week period and 0.88 over a 3-week period with small samples.[47,48] The PLQ may be a useful short instrument to measure a combination of preventive and promotive health practices among adults when restricted to use of the total score.

Health-Promoting Lifestyle Profile (HPLP)

The Health-Promoting Lifestyle Profile (HPLP) was developed by Walker et al.[31] for use in testing the Health Promotion Model, has been widely used. It measures health-promoting lifestyle, conceptualized as a "multidimensional pattern of self-initiated actions and perceptions that serve to maintain or enhance the level of wellness, self-actualization, and fulfillment of the individual."[31,p77] The item pool for the original HPLP was developed from a 100-item yes–no checklist designed as a clinical nursing tool. Items concerned with prevention or detection of specific diseases were deleted because they lacked concept validity. Empirical validation that included item analysis, factor analysis and reliability estimates resulted in the elimination of all items concerned with undesirable health behaviors (e.g., smoking and excessive alcohol consumption).

Factor analysis isolated six dimensions used as subscales and second-order factor analysis yielded a single factor, interpreted as health-promoting lifestyle, the multidimensional construct measured by the instrument. Subsequently, the HPLP has been used with numerous healthy populations representing the full adult age range[50] and with a few clinical populations, including those with heart disease, cancer, and multiple sclerosis. A Spanish-language version of the tool became available in 1990. It was found to be culturally relevant, reliable (total alpha 0.93, subscale alphas 0.70–0.87), and valid as evidenced by factor analysis that explained 45.9% of the variance in the measure.[51]

A revised and updated version, the Health-Promoting Lifestyle Profile II (HPLPII), was released in 1995.[52] This 52-item instrument summated behavior-rating scale uses a 4-point ordinal response format to measure the frequency of self-reported health-promoting behaviors. Responses range from 1 (never) to 4 (routinely). The HPLPII consists of a total scale and six subscales (8 to 9 items each) that measure the dimensions of health-promoting lifestyle: health responsibility; physical activity; nutrition; interpersonal relations; spiritual growth; and stress management. An example of an item is: "Eat 3–5 servings of vegetables each day." A score for overall health-promoting lifestyle is obtained by calculating a mean of the individual's response to all 52 items; six subscale scores are the means of response to subscale items. The use of mean scores retains the 1- to-4 measurement of item responses and allows meaningful comparisons of scores across subscales.

Psychometric evaluation of the HPLPII was undertaken in a community sample of 712 adults.[52] Construct validity was examined with traditional factor analysis employing principal axis extraction followed by oblique rotation. A six-factor solution resulted in the Spiritual Growth and Interpersonal Relations subscale items loading together, the other four subscale items loading cleanly on separate factors at levels of 0.43 or greater, and a nuisance factor with no significant loadings. Spiritual Growth and Interpersonal Relations were recognized as closely aligned concepts, both involving a sense of connectedness and belonging. A seven-factor solution included six factors that were interpretable as hypothesized and the nuisance factor. Confirmatory factor analysis using LISREL was used to evaluate the hypothesized six-dimensional structure of health-promoting lifestyle, with the subscales permitted to correlate with each other. Fit indices indicated that the model fit the data well (GFI 0.980; AGFI 0.940; RMSR 0.034). Convergent validity was assessed by comparing it to the Personal Lifestyle Questionnaire; the correlation of the HPLPII and the PLQ total scores among a subset of 80 adults was 0.678. In addition, social desirability explained only 1.4% of the variance in responses on the HPLPII among a subset of 80 adults. Concurrent criterion-related validity was evidenced by the relationship of health-promoting lifestyle to the outcomes of perceived health status and quality of life. The correlation of the HPLPII with the Medical Outcomes Study Short-Form General Health Survey general health perception scale was 0.269 in a subset of 158 adults, and with the Quality of Life Index, was 0.464 in a subset of 49 adults. The total scale was found to have high internal consistency with an alpha coefficient of 0.943, and the subscales to have acceptable internal consistency with alpha coefficients ranging from 0.793 for Stress Management to 0.872 for Interpersonal Relations among a sample of 712. Test–retest stability among 26 undergraduate nursing students at a 3-week interval was reported as $r = 0.892$. The HPLPII is copyrighted.

Health Diary

The Health Diary was developed by Frank-Stromborg[20,p38] to measure health-promoting behaviors in ambulatory adult cancer patients. Health-promoting behaviors were defined as "those actions that are directed toward sustaining or increasing the levels of well-being, self-actualization, and fulfillment of an individual." The Health Diary is based on the six dimensions of health-promoting lifestyle measured by the subscales of the Health-Promoting Lifestyle Profile.[31] The Health Diary is a 12-item personal record of health perceptions and health-promoting activities. It is completed daily by cancer patients for 4 weeks. Each week a separate instrument is mailed postage-paid from the subject to the investigator. Four of the 12 items have a 7-point Likert format; eight openended questions allow individuals to document the methods they have used to make themselves feel better. An example of an open-ended item is: "What specifically did you do today that you feel helped your physical health or decreased a physical problem you were having?" (For instance, reporting any unusual symptoms to your doctor or nurse). The Health Diary is primarily qualitative in nature, and content analysis is used for data analysis. Kosa, Alpert, and Haggerty[53] reported several advantages to the diary method: high levels of reporting; sensitivity to detail; reduction in memory recall bias and error; and the ability to reflect accurately daily health perceptions and health behaviors. Assessments of reliability and validity of the data obtained with the diary were not reported.[20] Since the items are not specific to the experience of individuals with cancer, the diary potentially could be used with various other clinical populations.

Summary

In the 1970s HRAs were developed by epidemiologists to assess lifestyle behaviors associated with an increased risk of preventable death. During the 1980s, an emerging emphasis on health promotion was accompanied by the development of a few instruments to measure lifestyle behaviors believed to be associated with health and wellness. Most instruments presented in this chapter have established reliability and validity. Most are designed for use with adults and late adolescents. The development of additional instruments to measure the healthy lifestyle behaviors of children and adolescents is needed to further understanding of behavior patterns during these critical developmental periods.

Healthy lifestyle behavior is an emerging area of interdisciplinary interest. Research has focused largely on descriptive studies and the testing of conceptual frameworks and is just beginning to include intervention studies. Findings from a few studies point to the existence of discrete clusters of behavior in various samples.[7,38,48,50,54] Many investigations examine only a few preventive and/or promotive behaviors, and little is currently known about how the full range of healthy lifestyle behaviors relate to one another. More work is needed to further understanding of the nature of clusters and patterns of behavior in different samples. The development of childhood health beliefs and behaviors and of family patterns of behavior also are important areas for investigation.

Researchers have proposed a variety of paradigms to explain why people engage in healthy lifestyle behavior; these include the Health Belief Model,[55] the Health Promotion Model,[30] the Theory of Reasoned Action,[56] the Resource Model of Preventive Health Behavior,[8] and others that focus on the determinants of individual behavior. Research is just beginning to build a knowledge base concerning the linkages between demographic, cognitive/perceptual and socioenvironmental factors, and patterns of healthy lifestyle in individuals and populations. Several literature reviews have summarized the findings published to date.[30,33,35,57,58] In addition, much yet unpublished doctoral dissertation research has focused on healthy lifestyle. It remains to be seen whether the 1990s will fulfill their promise of focusing on health promotion to reduce chronic disease, control health-care expenditures and improve the well-being of Americans.

Exemplar Study

Frank-Stromborg, M., Pender, N., Walker, S., & Sechrist, K. Determinants of health-promoting lifestyle in ambulatory cancer patients. *Soc Sci Med*, 1990, 31(10):1159-1168.

This study sought to determine the degree to which cognitive-perceptual and modifying variables identified in the Health Promotion Model[30] explained the occurrence of health-promoting behaviors in a sample of 385 adults undergoing cancer treatment. A secondary purpose was to determine the potential for illness-specific cognitive-perceptual and modifying variables to explain further the occurrence of health-promoting behaviors in adults with cancer. Multiple regression analyses revealed that 23.5% of the variance in health-promoting lifestyle was explained by three cognitive-perceptual variables from the model (definition of health, perceived health status, and perceived control of health) and four modifying variables (education, income, age, and employment). When illness-specific variables were added to the analysis, initial reaction to the diagnosis of cancer was found to be a significant contributor to the regression. The study results support the importance of both general health-related and cancer-specific cognitive-perceptual factors in explaining the occurrence of health-enhancing behaviors among ambulatory cancer patients. Researchers concluded that these factors may therefore be suitable targets for interventions to encourage the adoption of healthy lifestyles. This study is exemplary in that it uses a conceptual model to frame the study, increases understanding of health-promoting lifestyles in adults with cancer, and establishes a rationale for future theory testing and research in clinical populations.

References

1. LaLonde, M. *A new perspective on the health of Canadians*. Ottawa: Government of Canada, 1974.
2. U.S. Department of Health Education and Welfare. *Healthy people: The Surgeon General's Report on Health Promotion and Disease Prevention*. Washington, DC: U.S. Government Printing Office, 1979.
3. U.S. Department of Health and Human Services. Public Health Service. *Promoting health: Preventing disease: Objectives for the nation*. Rockville, MD: U.S. Department of Health and Human Services, 1980.
4. National Center for Health Statistics. *Health, United States, 1989 and prevention profile*. Hyattsville, MD: U.S. Department of Health and Human Services, 1990.
5. U.S. Department of Health and Human Services. *Healthy People 2000: National health promotion and disease prevention objectives*. Washington, DC: U. S. Government Printing Office, 1991.
6. O'Donnell, M.P. Definition of health promotion. *Am J Health Prom*, 1986, 1:4-5.
7. Brubaker, B.H. Health promotion: A linguistic analysis. *Adv Nurs Sci*, 1983, 5(3):1-14.
8. Kulbok, P.A. Social resources, health resources, and preventive health behavior: Patterns and predictors. *Public Health Nurs*, 1985, 2(2):67-81.
9. Pender, N. Health and health promotion: Conceptual dilemmas. In M. Duffy & N. Pender (Eds.), *Conceptual issues in health promotion*. Indianapolis, IN: Sigma Theta Tau, 1987, pp. 7-23.
10. Pender, N.J., Barkauskas, V.H., Hayman, L., Rice, V.H., & Anderson, E.T. Health promotion and disease prevention: Toward excellence in nursing practice and education. *Nurs Outlook*, 1992, 40(3):106-112.
11. Wiley, J. & Camacho, T. Life-style and future health: Evidence from the Alameda County study. *Prev Med*, 1980, 9:1-21.
12. Ardell, D.B. The nature and implications of high level wellness, or why "normal health" is a rather sorry state of existence. *Health Values Achiev High Lev Wellness*, 1979, 3(1):16-24.
13. Bruhn, J.G. Life-style and health behavior. In D.S. Gochman (Ed.), *Health behavior: Emerging research perspectives*. New York: Plenum, 1988.
14. Abel, T. Measuring health lifestyles in a comparative analysis: Theoretical issues and empirical findings. *Soc Sci Med*, 1991, 32(8):899-908.
15. Milio, N. *Promoting health through public policy*. Philadelphia: Davis, 1981.

16. Pender, N.J. Expressing health through lifestyle patterns. *Nurs Sci Q*, 1990, 3(3):115-122.
17. Kasl, S., & Cobb, S. Health behavior, illness behavior. *Arch Environ Health*, 1966, 12:246.
18. Gochman, D.S. Health behavior: Plural perspectives. In D.S. Gochman (Ed.), *Health behavior, emerging research perspectives*. New York: Plenum, 1988.
19. Miller, J.F. Categories of self-care needs of ambulatory patients with diabetes. *J Adv Nurs*, 1982, 7(1):25.
20. Frank-Stromborg, M. Health promotion behaviors in ambulatory cancer patients: Fact or fiction? *Oncol Nurs Forum*, 1986, 13(4):37-43.
21. Frank-Stromborg, M., Pender, N.J., Walker, S.N., & Sechrist, K.R. Determinants of health-promoting lifestyle in ambulatory cancer patients. *Soc Sci Med*, 1990, 31(10):1159-1168.
22. MacVicar, M., Winningham, M., & Nickel, J. Effects of aerobic interval training on cancer patients' functional capacity. *Nurs Res*, 1989, 38(6):348-351.
23. Laffrey, S.C., Loveland-Cherry, C.J., & Winkler, S.J. Health behavior: Evolution of two paradigms. *Public Health Nurs*, 1986, 3(2):92-100.
24. Belloc, N.B., & Breslow, L. Relationship of physical health status and health practices. *Prev Med*, 1972, 1(3):409-421.
25. U.S. Preventive Services Task Force. *Guide to clinical preventive services*. Baltimore, MD: Williams & Wilkins, 1989.
26. Antonovsky, A. *Unraveling the mystery of health*. San Francisco: Jossey-Bass, 1987.
27. Ardell, D.B. *High level wellness*. Berkeley, CA: Ten Speed Press, 1986.
28. Travis, J.W. & Ryan, R.S. *Wellness workbook for health professionals* (2nd ed., rev.). Berkeley, CA: Ten Speed Press, 1988.
29. Laffrey, S.C. An exploration of adult health behaviors. *West J Nurs Res*, 1990, 12(4):434-447.
30. Pender, N. *Health promotion in nursing practice* (3rd ed.). Stamford, CT: Appleton & Lange, 1996.
31. Walker, S.N., Sechrist, K.R., & Pender, N.J. Health-promoting lifestyle profile: Development and psychometric characteristics. *Nurs Res*, 1987, 36(2):76-81.
32. Berkman, L., & Breslow, L. *Health and ways of living*. New York: Oxford University Press, 1983.
33. Kulbok, P.A., & Baldwin, J.H. From preventive health behavior to health promotion: Advancing a positive construct of health. *Adv Nurs Sci*, 1992, 14(4):50-64.

34. Acquista, V.W., Wachtel, T.J., Gomes, C.I., Salzillo, M., & Stockman, M. Home-based health risk appraisal and screening program. *J Comm Health*, 1988, 13(1):43-52.

35. Kirscht, J.P. Preventive health behavior: A review of research and issues. *Health Psychol*, 1983, 2(3):277-301.

36. Frey, J.H. *Survey research by telephone*. Beverly Hills, CA: Sage, 1983.

37. Kirscht, J. Process and measurement issues in health risk appraisal. *Am J Public Health*, 1989, 79(12):1598-1599.

38. Rakowski, W., Julius, M., Hickey, T., & Halter, J. Correlates of preventive health behavior in late life. *Res Aging*, 1987, 9(3):331-355.

39. Killeen, M.L. What is the health risk appraisal telling us? *West J Nurs Res*, 1989, 11(5):614-620.

40. Gustafson, D.H. Health risk appraisal: Its role in health services research. *Health Serv Res*, 1987, 22(4):453-465.

41. Edington, D.W., & Yen, L. Reliability, validity, and effectiveness of health risk appraisals. *Directory Health Risk Appraisals*, 1992, 1(1):27-38.

42. Berlin, J., Thorington, B., McKinlay, J., & McKinlay, S. The accuracy of substitution rules for health risk appraisals. *Am J Health Prom*, 1990, 4(3):214-219.

43. DeFriese, G.H., & Fielding, J.E. Health risk appraisal in the 1990s: Opportunities, challenges, and expectations. *Ann Rev Public Health*, 1990, 11:401-418.

44. Gazmararian, J., Foxman, B., Yen, L., Morgenstern, H., & Edington, D.W. Comparing the predictive accuracy of health risk appraisal: The Centers for Disease Control versus Carter Center program. *Am J Health Prom*, 1991, 81(10):1296-1301.

45. Ellis, L.B., Joo, H., & Gross, C.R. Use of a computer-based health risk appraisal by older adults. *J Fam Pract*, 1991, 33(4):390-394.

46. Measuring the health behavior of adolescents: The Youth Risk Behavior Surveillance System and recent reports on high-risk adolescents. *Public Health Reports*, 1993, 108(suppl 1):1-96.

47. Muhlenkamp, A.F., & Brown, N.J. The development of an instrument to measure health practices. Paper presented at the American Nurses' Association Council of Nurse Researchers Conference, Minneapolis, MN, 1983.

48. Muhlenkamp, A.F., Brown, N.J., & Sands, D. Determinants of health promotion activities in nursing clinic clients. *Nurs Res*, 1985, 34(6):327-332.

49. Brown, N.J., Muhlenkamp, A., Fox, L., & Osborn, M. The relationship among health beliefs, health values, and health promotion activity. *West J Nurs Res*, 1983, 5(2):155-163.

50. Walker, S.N., Volkan, K., Sechrist, K.R., & Pender, N.J. Health-promoting life styles of older adults: Comparisons with young and middle-aged adults, correlates and patterns. *Adv Nurs Sci*, 1988, 11(1):76-90.

51. Walker, S.N., Kerr, M.J., Pender, N.J., & Sechrist, K.R. A Spanish language version of the Health-Promoting Lifestyle Profile. *Nurs Res*, 1990, 39(5):268-273.

52. Walker, S.N., & Hill-Polerecky, D.M. (1995). Psychometric evaluation of the revised Health-Promoting Lifestyle Profile. Paper presented at the 123rd Annual Meeting of the American Public Health Association, San Diego, CA, October 29–November 2.

53. Kosa, J., Alpert, J., & Haggerty, R. On the reliability of family health information: A comparative study of mother's reports on illness and related behavior. *Soc Sci Med*, 1967, 1(2):165-181.

54. Langlie, J.K. Interrelationships among preventive health behaviors: A test of competing hypotheses. *Public Health Rep*, 1979, 94(3):216-225.

55. Rosenstock, I. Historical origins of the health belief model. *Health Educ Monographs*, 1974, 2(4):328-335.

56. Fishbein, M., & Ajzen, I. *Beliefs, attitudes, intention, and behavior: An introduction to theory and research*. Reading, MA: Addison-Wesley, 1975.

57. Gillis, A.J. Determinants of a health-promoting lifestyle: An integrative review. *J Adv Nurs*, 1993, 18:345-353.

58. Palank, C.J. Determinants of health-promotive behavior: A review of current research. *Nurs Clin North Am*, 1991, 26(4):815-831.

25

Measuring Self-Care Activities

Marilyn J. Dodd

Many individuals and families have performed self-care in the past. Today many more health-care consumers are taking increased interest in their health and assume greater responsibility for their own care. Three main reasons can be identified and explained for this resurgence of interest. The first concerns dissatisfaction with current cost control systems and measures, maldistribution of physicians and medical facilities, and iatrogenic outcomes. The second is the shift from acute to chronic health problems. The third is the gradual change in value and belief systems in which clients desire more control over themselves, their environment, and their social systems, including health-care systems.[1,2,3]

Since the 1960s, health-care professionals have incorporated self-care philosophy into their practice. However, in this era of dwindling community health resources and diagnostic-related groups (DRGs), the concept of self-care has taken on a new central and critical importance in the attainment of quality health-promotion and illness-related care. Now people (healthy individuals, patients, and families) simply must manage more by themselves. The mandate for health-care professionals to provide health information and teach skills to everyone is clear.

The concept of self-care has a wide range of meaning given the various perspectives from which self-care is viewed in the health-care system and by professional practitioners. These views range from a conservative ideology,[4,5] with emphasis on minimal dependence on the current health-care system, to a less conservative view,[6] in which the health-care professional, for example, the nurse, plays a significant role not only in assisting the patient in acquiring self-care skills but also in managing the patient's self-care.

Levin defines self-care as "a process whereby a lay person can function effectively on his/her own behalf in health promotion and prevention and in disease detection and treatment at the level of the primary health resource in the health care system."[4,p170] It is important to note that Levin's definition implies that self-care is part of the health-care system, that is, that the patient is presumed to have access to the technology and skills of the health-care system.

At an international symposium on self-care, Frye,[5] a leading British proponent of self-care identified the following self-care roles: health maintenance, disease prevention, self-diagnosis, self-medication and self-treatment, and participation by the patient in professional care. Frye went on to define self-care as:

> a voluntary, self-limiting, non-organized, universal, varying complex of behaviors evolved through a mixture of socializing and cognitive experiences . . . an indigenous phenomenon, wholly outside the framework of professional health resources, although obviously influenced by the nature of social institutions of care and the context of economic, social and political structures.[5,p10]

Norris, somewhat on the liberal side of the continuum, defines self-care as "those processes that permit people and families to take initiative, to take responsibility, and to function effectively in developing their own potential for health."[2,p486]

In Orem's Self-Care Deficit Nursing Theory, the concept of self-care is central and is defined as "the practice of activities that individuals initiate and perform on their own behalf in maintaining life, health, and well-being."[6,p117] She clearly emphasizes the significant role of the nurse in assisting patients to meet their self-care demands when actual or potential deficits exist.

The meaning of self-care as described by some of its proponents is presented here in an attempt to identify similarities in ideology as well as to create an awareness that significant differences exist. Similarities identified include the performance of activities for oneself in relation to matters that affect health. There is recognition that this performance requires both knowledge and skills, ranging from simple to complex, on the part of the one providing self-care. Access to medical technology is considered a part of self-care. Another common belief is the need for client input in setting client goals and program planning and evaluation. A major difference is the extent to which the client performs self-care activities independently of the health-care system and its professionals. Inherent in this difference are issues of control and the extent to which the patient should have unsupervised access to medical technology. The researcher desiring to measure self-care needs to consider these varying definitions and select an instrument congruent with the purposes of determining self-care.

What emerges from a review of the literature on self-care is the individual's readiness to learn about a health- or disease-related situation,[7] knowledge of what to do,[8] beliefs in ability,[9,10] and possession of the functional ability to perform self-care activities.[11,12] Suggestions on how to assess the individual's readiness to learn, instruments to determine knowledge about the situation, and the psychophysiologic capabilities to initiate self-care are not within the scope of this chapter. These concepts are found elsewhere in this text. The focus of the chapter is a review of tools to measure actual self-care activities.

Orem's conceptualization of self-care as consisting of three categories is useful in organizing this review.[6] According to Orem, self-care is undertaken to meet three types of self-care requisites: (1) universal; (2) developmental; and (3) health-deviation. Universal self-care requisites focus on life processes and the maintenance of human structure and function, such as, sufficient air, water, and food. Developmental self-care requisites focus on human developmental processes and events during various stages of the life cycle and on events that may adversely affect development. Health-deviation self-care requisites arise from disabilities, deviations, or defects in human structure and function and from medical diagnosis and treatment of disease conditions. The greatest preponderance of self-care research and many of the methodologic issues that the researcher must consider have involved health-deviation self-care.

Health-Deviation Self-Care Requisite

Several methodologic problems have plagued research in health-deviation self-care and thwarted the development of the concept. First, the conceptualization in these studies often is nonexistent or inadequately developed, and the operational definition of self-care rarely is given. Second, the measure of self-care activities is limited to only a few interview or questionnaire items[8,13] embedded in an instrument that also assesses patients' attitudes, values, knowledge, disease and treatment parameters, and functional (psychomotor) abilities. Third, the interview or questionnaire items[14] and patients' self-reports[15] are not described clearly, and their psychometric properties (reliability and validity data) frequently are not reported. Finally, in some studies, self-care activity items can be identified in instruments that have not been developed for the specific measurement of self-care per se.[15]

These methodologic issues are especially grave given the flood of intervention studies designed to enhance self-care activities in arthritic,[8] elderly,[12] hypertensive,[16] cerebral vascular accident,[17] neurologically impaired (e.g., quadriplegic and paraplegic),[18] chronic obstructive pulmonary disease,[19] obese,[20] dental,[21] cancer,[22-24] and ambulatory[25] patients. The vast majority of these experimental studies have focused on disease outcomes, that is, normal glucose, blood pressure, or cholesterol levels, and have failed to assess systematically the self-care activities patients perform to obtain the desired disease and treatment outcomes. Two important instruments are comprehensively discussed,[26-33] and others are shown in Appendix 25A.[34-51]

Self-Care Behavior Log

The Self-Care Behavior Log was developed by Dodd to measure the self-care activities of cancer patients experiencing side effects of radiation therapy[26,27] and chemotherapy.[28] In an earlier study,[29] in which Dodd developed and tested the Self-Care Behavior Questionnaire, the patients were asked to recall in an interview what self-care activities they had performed. Concerned with the lack of accuracy of the patients' memory, Dodd devised an adaptation of this questionnaire, the Self-Care Behavior Log, in which the patient records the experienced side effects of either radiation therapy or chemotherapy as they occur.

For each side effect experienced, the patient indicates the date of onset of the side effect and, on two 5-point Likert scales, how severe and how distressing the side effect is. The patient also records the activities performed to alleviate the side effect and the date on which the activities occur. The patient's perception of the effectiveness of each self-care behavior is obtained on a third 5-point Likert scale. Finally, the patient records the source of information for each self-care behavior. The patient maintains his or her log for the duration of the study period and is instructed to bring it in for the nurse to review every cycle of chemotherapy or every 2 weeks with radiation therapy. Four ratios have been established to score the quantitative variable of self-care behavior. Details of these scoring ratios are available in another report.[26]

A preventive self-care dimension also is included in the Self-Care Behavior Log.[30] Patients are asked to record the potential side effects that can occur with their chemotherapy, to think about what self-care activity can be taken to prevent the side effect from occurring, and the date the activity takes place. They are asked to record the source of the idea for the activity. The scoring method for the preventive self-care activity has been limited to frequency counts because of the lack of patient recall of potential side effects and preventive self-care activities for the potential side effects.[30]

Reliability and validity data have been documented for the original Self-Care

Behavior Questionnaire from which the Self-Care Behavior Log was derived.[23,26] Concurrent validity is evidenced in significant negative correlations with the self-care behavior scores and severity of symptoms, increased age, and lower performance scores.[31]

The investigator has identified two methodological issues concerning the use of the log. First, dates are requested on the log for the occurrence of a side effect and the performance of a self-care behavior. The intent of these items was to determine the delay that occurred between the side effect being experienced and the performance of an activity and to determine in what sequence self-care behaviors occurred. Because of missing data, this intent was never fulfilled. Another related issue is that in the earlier smaller self-care studies the patients performed fewer study-related activities and their reporting in the logs was more complete. In later randomized clinical trials the patient is more of an active participant in the intervention protocol, that is, has more activities to do, and completing the log has become problematic for a large number of patients. The log has again been modified and is now collapsed to a 5" x 7" checklist where the patient records when she or he has completed the oral protocol for the prevention and treatment of chemotherapy-induced oral mucositis.[32]

The utility of this log for other patient populations is clear. Self-report of signs and symptoms of diseases other than cancer or other treatment side effects could be incorporated easily into the Self-Care Behavior Log.

Self-Care Diary (SCD)

The Self-Care Diary was developed by Nail and her colleagues[33] to measure the incidence and severity of selected side effects of cancer treatment and the use and efficacy of self-care activities used to manage those side effects. The patient is instructed as to when (date) to complete the diary and what time frame to consider (i.e., "since your treatment" or "in the past three days"). For each of the sixteen side effects, the patients indicates whether or not she or he experienced the side effect in the time frame given. If the patient responds negatively, she or he is directed to the next side effect item. If the patient responds affirmatively, she or he is asked to rate the severity of the side effect (not at all, a little, moderately, quite a lot, or extremely), indicate which of the listed self-care activities she or he used to manage the side effect, and to indicate how effective the activities were on a 6-point scale with descriptors. The number of self-care activities listed for specific side effects varies from 3 to 17, and there is space to write in self-care activities not included in the list. A place also is provided to list a side effect not included in the instrument and list the self-care activities used to manage it. Patients complete the diary at home and return it to the investigators in a stamped, self-addressed envelope.

The scoring of the SCD is descriptive, and the incidence and severity of side effects are obtained by summing and averaging. Similarly, the number of self-care activities and their efficacy can be summed and averaged. Individual side effects and self-care activities also can be derived depending on the purpose of investigators.

Reliability and validity data are available for the SCD. The overall side effect severity scores at day two and day five were correlated at $r = 0.80$, demonstrating an acceptable level of test–retest reliability.[33] The list of side effects and self-care activities was derived from literature concerning patients' experiences with chemotherapy. Further content validity was provided by two patients who were undergoing treatment and three experienced oncology clinical nurse specialists. Nail and her colleagues describe two scoring issues related to the SCD.[33] First, many patients in their study used multiple combinations of self-care activities, but the methodology employed in this study did not lend itself to measuring the efficacy of combinations of self-care activities. Second, the evaluation of the efficacy of single self-care activity is limited to the fact that combinations are used and no data were collected on the sequence of initiation of self-care activities. As the combinations are used and no data were collected on the sequence of initiation of self-care activities, and the order in which the self-care activities are performed is unknown, a patient who moves from using an effective self-care activity to using an ineffective activity will receive the same score as a patient taking the opposite path.

The SCD was designed to be used with cancer patients receiving chemotherapy. The investigators describe their sample as predominantly Caucasian, married, middle-aged women with a diagnosis of breast cancer.

Universal Self-Care Requisite

The definition of the universal self-care requisite includes the life processes and the maintenance of human structure and function, such as sufficient air, water, and food. In this chapter both prevention and screening activities are incorporated in this definition. These preventive and screening activities include breast self-examination, smoking behaviors, and frequency of annual checkup. Many of the methodologic issues of the research with health-deviation self-care are evident in studies of universal self-care. For example, a conceptual framework for the study and the definition of self-care often are not given; measurement of universal self-care activities includes only a few interview or questionnaire items within an instrument, and the interview items or self-reports are inadequately described.

Several instruments have been developed to measure self-care agency, a central construct of Orem's self-care theory.[51,52] Orem's definition of self-care agency is both the capability to act on behalf of oneself as agent of the action and the operability of the construct that prompts one toward action on behalf of self.[6] The instruments focus on the delineation of subconstructs that contribute to a person's exercise of self-care agency, *not* on actual self-care activities. Reporting on these instruments is beyond the scope of this chapter.

Universal Self-Care Instruments

In Chapter 24, Measuring Healthy Lifestyle, by Berger and Walker, a number of instruments for health-promotion self-care are described. Given the emphasis of Chapter 24, only one instrument of particular interest is described here.

Self-Care Health Diary

The Self-Care Health Diary was developed by Freer[53] to measure any health upsets and activities to manage these upsets. The investigator contends that the health upsets are transient problems, and just as health is not the absence of symptoms, the presence of health problems does not indicate illness.[53,p860] The conceptual model used to develop and test the Self-Care Health Diary is not provided. Self-care is defined as including self-medication, self-referral, and resting. The diary consists of a structured sheet of questions that are answered each evening by the participants. Examples of these questions are: "What kind of a day has it been for you?" (responses are made on a 7-point Likert scale from 1 for poor to 7 for good); or "If you recorded any problems yesterday, which, if any, persist today?" (open-ended response).

The diary questions were tested, and some were modified through a series of pilot studies.[53] Subjects are instructed to record health upsets no matter how trivial or transient. By design, the study was restricted to those aspects of self-care practiced in response to perceived upsets in health and recorded as answers to the relevant questions in the diary. This excluded any preventive health measures. The frequency of reported health upsets and activities (medical and nonmedical self-care responses) to manage these upsets is the scoring method. The diary questions yield both quantitative and qualitative data.

Reliability data are not presented. However, Freer contends that the diary questions are valid in that the participants' reported morbidity and self-referral patterns were very similar to published results from a British diary study that included a comparable sample. Furthermore, the amount and type of self-medication agree with the extensive literature on the subject.[53]

Considering the lack of specificity for any health upset, the Self-Care Health Diary could be used with many different populations across a variety of settings. The advantages and disadvantages associated with the diary when used as a research instrument in health-related situations has been described by Richardson.[54]

Developmental Self-Care Requisite

The definition of developmental self-care requisite includes human developmental processes and events during various stages of the life cycle and events that may adversely affect development. This area of self-care has received the least amount of attention by researchers. In a dissertation, Denyes[55] developed a self-care agency instrument in a sample of healthy adolescents. However, this research did not focus on measuring self-care activities in adolescence as a developmental phase with certain tasks of self-care to be performed and therefore is not included in this chapter.

Summary

Self-care as a concept for clinical practice is flourishing. However, the empiric development and testing of self-care theory lag seriously behind, in part because of the atheoretical use of self-care tools to measure this important concept. Greater effort is needed in this area, especially in developmental, family, and community self-care instruments.

Exemplar Study

Nail, L.M., Jones, L.S., Green, D., Schupper, D.L., & Jensen, R. Use and perceived efficacy of self-care activities in patients receiving chemotherapy. *Oncol Nurs Forum*, 1991, *18*(5):883-887.

This study exemplifies the evolution in the measurement of self-care. Nail and her colleagues have improved on earlier instruments that measured self-care by listing the 16 possible side effects of chemotherapy and their related self-care activities. Their modification has made it easier for participants to answer by checking a response, rather than the earlier "fill-in-the-response" format. The design is descriptive with repeated measures of side effects and self-care activities. The methods are carefully detailed. The Self-Care Diary retained the incidence and severity of side effects and the efficacy of self-care activities included in earlier instruments that measured self-care. The investigators have demonstrated good psychometric characteristics for the Self-Care Diary, with test–retest reliability and two forms of content validity. More frequent self-care activities were performed by participants for the side effects of fatigue, sleep difficulty, nausea, decreased appetite, and changes in food taste and smell. The efficacy of the self-care activities were rated by participants as moderate to moderately high in relief of the side effects. The issue of evaluation of the efficacy of single self-care activities when participants use combinations of self-care activities to manage a side effect remains unresolved.

References

1. Green, L.W., Weelin, S.H., Schauffler, H.H., et al. Research and demonstration issues in self-care: Measuring the decline of medicocentrism. *Health Educ Monogr*, 1977, 5(2):161-189.
2. Norris, C. Self-care. *Am J Nurs*, 1979, 79(3):486.
3. McCorkle, R. Nurses as advocates for self-care. *Cancer Nurs*, 1983, 6(1):17.
4. Levin, L. Patient education and self-care: How do they differ? *Nurs Outlook*, 1978, 26:170-175.
5. Frye, J. Self-Care: Its place in the total health care system, a report by an independent working party. London, England, 1973.
6. Orem, D. *Nursing: Concepts of practice*. St. Louis, MO: Mosby Year Book, 1991.
7. Steiger, N.J., & Lipson, J.G. *Self-care nursing*. Bowie, MD: Brady, 1985.
8. Lorig, K., Laurin, J., & Gines, G.E.S. Arthritis self-management. *Nurs Clin North Am*, 1984, 19(4):637-645.
9. Hurley, A.C. Measuring self-care ability in patients with diabetes: The Insulin Management Diabetes Self-Efficacy Scale. In O. Strickland & C.F. Waltz (Eds.), *Measurement of nursing outcomes: Vol 4. Measuring client self-care and coping skills*. New York: Springer, 1990, pp. 28-44.
10. Gortner, S., & Jenkins, L. Self-Efficacy and activity level following cardiac surgery. *J Adv Nurs*, 1990, 15:1132-1138.
11. Rameizl, P. CADET, a self-care assessment tool. *Geriatric Nurs*, 1984, 7(1):43.
12. Karl, C.A. The effect of an exercise program on self-care activities for the institutionalized elderly. *J Gerontol Nurs*, 1982, 8(5):282-285.
13. Kubricht, D.W. Therapeutic self-care demands expressed by outpatients receiving external radiation therapy. *Cancer Nurs*, 1984, 7(1):43-52.
14. Dropkin, M.J. Compliance in postoperative head and neck patients. *Cancer Nurs*, 1979, 2(5):379-384.
15. Avery, C.H., March, J., & Brook, R.H. An assessment of the adequacy of self-care by adult asthmatics. *J Comm Health*, 1980, 5(3):167-180.
16. Stahl, S.M., Kelley, C.R., Neil, P.J., et al. Effects of home blood pressure measurement on long-term BP control. *Am J Public Health*, 1984, 74(7):704-709.
17. Anna, D.J., Hohon, S.A., Ord, L., & Wells, S.R. Implementing Orem's conceptual framework. *J Nurs Admin*, 1978, 8(11):entire issue.
18. Shillam, L.L., Geeman, C., & Loshin, P.M. Effect of occupational therapy intervention on bathing independence of disabled persons. *Am J Occup Ther*, 1983, 37(11):744-748.
19. Brough, F.K., Schmidt, C.D., Rasmussen, T., & Boyer, M. Comparison of two teaching methods for self-care training for patients with chronic obstructive pulmonary disease. *Patient Couns Health Educ*, 1982, 4(2):111.
20. Behn, S., & Lane, D.S. A self-teaching weight-control manual: Method for increasing compliance and reducing obesity. *Patient Educ Couns*, 1983, 5(2):63.
21. Weinstein, P., Fiset, L.O., & Lancanter, B. Assessment of a behavioral approach in long-term plague control using a multiple baseline design: The need for relapse research. *Patient Educ Couns*, 1984, 5(3):135.
22. Dodd, M.J. Self-care for side effects of cancer chemotherapy: An assessment of nursing interventions. *Cancer Nurs*, 1983, 6(1):63-67.
23. Dodd, M.J. Measuring informational intervention for chemotherapy knowledge and self-care behavior. *Res Nurs Health*, 1984, 7(1):43-50.
24. Dodd, M. Efficacy of proactive information on self-care in chemotherapy patients. *Patient Educ Couns*, 1988, 11:215-225.
25. Vickery, D.M., Kalmer, H., Lowry, D., et al. Effects of a self-care education program on medical visits. *JAMA*, 1983, 250(21):2952-2956.
26. Dodd, M.J. Assessing patient self-care for side effects of cancer chemotherapy. Part 1. *Cancer Nurs*, 1982, 5(6):447-451.
27. Dodd, M.J. Patterns of self-care in cancer patients receiving radiation therapy. *Oncol Nurs Forum*, 1984, 10(3):23-27.
28. Dodd, M.J. Efficacy of proactive information on self-care in radiation therapy patients. *Heart Lung*, 1987, 16(5):538-544.
29. Dodd, M.J. Patterns of self-care in patients with breast cancer. *West J Nurs Res*, 1988, 10(1):7-24.
30. Dodd, M.J. Self-care for patients with breast cancer to prevent side effects of chemotherapy. *Public Health Nurs*, 1984, 1(4):202-209.
31. Musci, E., & Dodd, M.J. Predicting self-care with patients and family members' affective states and family functioning. *Oncol Nurs Forum*, 1990, 17(3):394-400.
32. Dodd, M.J., Larson, P., Miaskowski, C., et al., *Self-care intervention to decrease mucositis morbidity*. (R01 CA55555 funded by NCI, 1992-1995.) San Francisco: University of California, 1992-1995.
33. Nail, L.M., Jones, L.S., Greene, D., et al. Use and perceived efficacy of self-care activities in patients receiving chemotherapy. *Oncol Nurs Forum*, 1991, 18(5):883-887.
34. Klein, R.N., & Bell, B. Self-care skills: Behavioral measurement with Klein-Bell ADL scale. *Arch Phys Med Rehabil*, 1982, 63(7):335-338.
35. Chen, M.J., Henderson, A., & Cermak, S.A. Patterns of visual spatial inattention and their functional significance in stroke patients. *Arch Phys Med Rehab*, 1993, 74(4):355-360.
36. Bolding, D.J., & Llorens, L.A. The effects of habilitative hospital admission on self-care, self-esteem, and frequency of physical care. *Am J Occup Ther*, 1991, 45(9):796-800.
37. Stetz, K.M., & Dodd, M.J. Behavior checklist for the self-efficacy scale *Final report of coping and self-care of cancer families: Nurse Prospectus* (R01-CA01441 funded by National Center for Nursing Research, Bethesda, MD., 1986-1990.) San Francisco: University of California, 1991.
38. Dodd, M.J., & Dibble, S.L. Predictors of self-care: A test of Orem's Model. *Oncol Nurs Forum*, 1993, 20(6):895-901.
39. Hagopian, G. The measurement of self-care strategies of patients in radiation therapy. In O. Strickland & C.F. Waltz (Eds.), *Measurement of nursing outcomes: Vol. 4. Measuring client self-care and coping skills*. New York: Springer, 1990, pp. 45-57.

40. Weintraub, F.N., & Hagopian, G.A. The effect of nursing consultation on anxiety, side effects, and self-care of patients receiving radiation therapy. *Oncol Nurs Forum*, 1990, *17*(3):31-38.

41. Stephens, M.A.P., Norris-Baker, C., & Willems, E.P. Patient behavior monitoring through self-reports. *Arch Phys Med Rehabil*, 1983, *64*(4):167.

42. Freeman, E.M. *Self-care agency in gay men with HIV infection.* Unpublished doctoral dissertation. San Francisco: University of California, 1992.

43. Saunders, J. *Nursing Self-Care and HIV Disease.* (KO8 NR00033 funded by National Institute for Nursing Research, Bethesda, MD., 1990-1995.) Duarte, CA: City of Hope, 1990-1995.

44. Valente, S.M., Saunders, J., & Uman, G. Self-care, psychological distress, and HIV disease. *JANAC*, *4*(4):15-64.

45. Smith, R.A., Aldag, J.C., & Gerstner, J.B. *Self-care and control: A multifaceted approach.* (R01 CA48280, funded by NCI, 1990–1993.) Bloomington: Indiana University, Walther Cancer, Institute, 1990-1993.

46. Hinds, P., Quargnenti, A., Meyer, W., et al. *Self-care outcomes in adolescents with cancer during the first six months of treatment.* (R01 CA48432 funded by the NCI, 1990-1994.)

47. Hinds, P., & Martin, J. Hopefulness and the self-sustaining process in adolescents with cancer. *Nurs Res*, 1988, *37*(6):336-340.

48. Jones, L.C. Measuring guarding: A self-care management process used by individuals with chronic illness. In O. Strickland & C.F. Waltz (Eds.), *Measurement of nursing outcomes: Vol. 4. Measuring client self-care and coping skills.* New York: Springer, 1990, pp. 58-75.

49. Jones, L.C., & Preuett, S. Self-care activities and processes used by hemodialysis patients. *Am Nephrol Nurs Assoc J*, 1986, *13*:73-79.

51. Hanson, B., & Bickel, L. Development and testing of the questionnaire on perception of self-care agency. In J. Riehl-Sisca (Ed.), *The science and art of self-care.* Norwalk, CT: Appleton-Century-Crofts, 1985.

52. Geden, E., & Taylor, S. Construct and empirical validity of the self-as-carer inventory. *Nurs Res*, 1991, *40*(1):47-50.

53. Freer, C.B. Self-care: A health diary study. *Med Care*, 1980, *18*(8):853-861.

54. Richardson, A. The health diary: An examination of its use as a data collection method. *J Adv Nurs*, 1994, *19*:782-791.

55. Denyes, M.J. Development of an instrument to measure self-care agency in adolescents. University of Michigan, *Dissertation Abstracts International*, 1980, *41*(5):1716B.

Appendix

25A. Additional Measures of Self-Care

Instrument	Description	Psychometric Indices
Klein-Bell Activities of Daily Living (ADL) Scale Developed by Klein and Bell (34)	Measure of performance of self-care in ADL 170 behavioral items expressed in terms that apply to all people (e.g., "achieving bathing position") Categories include: bathing/hygiene; mobility; elimination; eating; emergency telephone use Based on belief that important activities are currently observed through any thorough ADL evaluation Scoring takes 15 minutes for initial evaluation, less for subsequent ones Scored as either "achieved" (performed without verbal or physical assistance from another) or "failed" (assistance is needed) Item weighted by difficulty (0 failed, 1,2,3 most difficult) Total points in each category summed to give an overall ADL independence score Accurate measurement tool, with many research and clinical applications (34): documenting patient's progress; communicating objective results to patient, family, medical insurers; overall program evaluation; bathing section used to demonstrate whether or not occupational therapy increases independence in bathing for disabled people Advantages: precision in breaking function into component parts to allow an accurate evaluation	Interrater reliability (20 patients were independently rated by 2 occupational therapists and 2 rehabilitation nurses, using 3 pairs of OTs and 3 pairs of nurses): 92% agreement between raters (raters not extensively trained in the use of the scale; raters simply introduced to it and asked to complete the items) Validity: 14 patients with disabling conditions, who had initially been rated on the scale at discharge, were contacted 5–10 months following discharge using a structured telephone interview to elicit number of hours per week of assistance in ADL received: significant negative correlation coefficient found between ADL scale scores at discharge and the number of hours per week of assistance received 5–10 months after discharge ($r = -0.86$, $p < 0.01$); thus, people with low ADL scores at discharge can be predicted to require assistance Used in diverse populations, such as stroke patients (35), children with spina bifida, and children with arthritis (36)
Self-Care Behavior Checklist (SCB Checklist for the Self-Efficacy Scale) Developed by Stetz and Dodd (37)	Measure of self-care behaviors of cancer patients experiencing 5 common side effects of chemotherapy (nausea/vomiting, oral mucositis, fatigue, pain, hair loss) Self-care behaviors derived from Dodd's earlier self-care studies (22,23,28,29) 40-item checklist eliciting whether subject has experienced any of 5 target side effects: if "yes," subject asked if self-care measures specific to the side-effect were performed Subscale self-care behaviors: nausea/vomiting (9 items), mucositis (8), fatigue (6), pain (10), hair loss (7) If self-care behavior not performed, subject asked "why not?" Scoring: subscale and total scores derived by summing "yes" responses; "why not" responses received content analysis	Content validity established Predictive validity established (38) Methodologic issue: completion of "why not?" item: some patients are disinclined to complete Limitations: SCB checklist targets only 5 side effects of chemotherapy
Radiation Side Effects Profile (RSEP) Developed by Hagopian (39)	Measures radiation side effects experienced and self-care strategies used to manage them Orem's Self-Care Deficit Theory provided conceptual model (6) 5 sections: subjects asked to: (1) Check off side effects experienced from	Test–retest reliability (4-week interval) using Pearson's product–moment correlation Severity Index, $r = 0.59$–0.83 Helpfulness Index, $r = 0.46$–0.56

Instrument	Description	Reliability/Validity
	a list of 11 common side effects and to write in another if not listed; (2) rate the severity of side effect on 4-point scale (0 none to 3 very bad); (3) list self-care activities used to relieve side effects; (4) rate effectiveness of self-care behavior(s) on 4-point scale; (5) indicate source of information for symptom management. Reading level is 4th grade. Scoring: severity index: summed scores on first 4-point scale; helpfulness index: summed scores on 2nd 4-point scale	All correlations significant, beyond 0.001 level. Side effects are cumulative, increasing in severity with continued treatments so daily treatment is source of interference with results of repeated tool administration. Content validity established (index 0.84). Construct validity established. Comments: very low Helpfulness Index indicates patients did not obtain much relief and underscores need for more effective interventions (40)
Self-Observation and Report Technique (SORT) Developed by Stephens et al. (41)	Measures everyday behaviors of patients with recent spinal injuries: behavioral unit defined as something overtly done by, or to the patient, spans at least 5 minutes, and is a discrete molar event; subject observes and reports own behavior after being taught specific guidelines. 25 categories of behavior, 5 categories of location (where behaviors occur), 5 categories of aid. Differs from other instruments in that it (1) records behavior wherever and whenever it occurs; and (2) provides direct behavioral assessments by recording discrete units of behavior as or soon after it occurs	Accuracy of self-reporting tested with moderate to high levels of agreement. Structural agreement of reports (self and observer): 77.1–94.9%. Frequency of occurrence agreement: 86.3%–99.7%. Major advantages of self-report: can use in many settings, flexibility (41)
HIV-Related Self-Care Behavior Checklist Developed by Freeman (42)	Measured self-care operations (activities) of 301 gay men who were HIV-positive (<200 T-helper cells). 15 items represent possible self-care behaviors for HIV-infected persons. Subject asked to rate the frequency of self-care behaviors on a 6-point Likert scale (1 never, 5 at least once a day, 6 not applicable). Total score obtained by summing the items	Content validity of items established. Cronbach's alpha for items: 0.57–0.63, improved to 0.59 with removal of lowest alpha scoring items. Principal components analysis for 3 factors (maintaining wellness, taking medications and vitamins, modifying self-care practices). Utility limited to HIV-infected population
Self-Care Activity Report Scale (SCARS) Developed by Saunders et al. (43,44)	Measures changes in self-care in relation to a specific situation or important event (e.g., becoming HIV-positive, motor vehicle accident, change in beliefs). 4 parts: (I) description of important event; (II) 31 items, changes in usual activities; (III) 23 symptoms listed; subject checks appropriate symptoms experienced, what was done to manage them, and effectiveness of intervention; (IV) list of support groups; subject to check one(s) attended and rate helpfulness	Scores include total changes in self-care. Consistency reliability: Cronbach's alpha (tested in HIV group): total change score: 0.88; positive change score: 0.82; negative change score: 0.67. Factor analysis for 2 factors: (I) promoting health (alpha 0.85); (II) overcoming health barriers and risks (alpha 0.76). Test–retest reliability (Pearson's correlation): 0.90. Must modify for other study populations
Yesterday's Daily Health Diary Developed by Smith et al. (45)	Used to assess health-related dimensions with cancer patients receiving chemotherapy. 4 sections: the subject is asked to: (I) rate activity physical, and emotional status (4 items) compared to when feels well, on a 10-point numeric rating	Reliability: stability of significant correlations shown among study variables over repeated cycles of chemotherapy. Concurrent validity established

25A. Additional Measures of Self-Care (*cont.*)

Instrument	Description	Psychometric Indices
Yesterday's Daily Health Diary (*cont.*)	scale with descriptive anchors; (II) indicate number of persons contacted during previous day, and whether received chemo the previous day; (III) check symptoms experienced previous day and rate severity on a 10-point scale; (IV) report all self-care actions to manage or prevent symptoms, and rate symptom severity after action on a 11-point scale Subject completes diary at a regular time each morning for previous day Scoring: descriptive or summation of responses (II,III,IV)	Limitations: how to examine data over time; compliance problems; difficulty reading small print in the diary
Self-Care Coping Interview Guide Developed by Hinds et al. (46,47)	Used to measure self-care coping in adolescents newly diagnosed with certain cancers 2 forms, one to assess adolescents after completing an intervention program on self-care coping strategies, and the other for the control group, administered at 5–7 weeks, 12 weeks, and 6 months 6 questions elicit what adolescents do or think about to cope emotionally and mentally with cancer; which self-care measures are most effective; what or who enables them to help themselves; and what makes it hard to practice self-care coping Finally, subject asked to indicate how often a particular coping strategy is is attempted on a 5-point scale with descriptive anchors Language geared toward adolescents	Scoring: content analyses for types of coping strategies and frequencies of use; analyze responses on 5-point scale for frequency of effort Clear differences in responses between control and experimental group Reliability and validity data being established Measurement issues: yields more detailed data if administered by an investigator rather than the subject
Self-Care Management Process-Guarding (SCMP-G) Developed by Jones (48)	Measure of self-management process that individuals use to manage chronic illness self-care Derived from earlier work (49) and defines SCMP as adaptive, behavioral, psychologic, and cognitive mechanisms used in illness self-care actions (50); guarding is a SCMP process providing "vigilance over self, illness. . . . and important relationships" (51) 2 subscales of guarding: (A) self guarding: protect oneself, exert controls over treatment plan, other actions, has 20 items; (B) social guarding: includes "attempts by individuals to protect their social network person from negative aspects of the illness, has 15 items. Each subscale has 4 critical guarding elements (vulnerability, controllability, self-absorption, sense of obligation); 5-point scale used for responses (5 strongly agree, 1 strongly disagree) Scoring: 4 reverse-scoring items indicate lack of guarding; scores range from 20 to 80 (self-subscale) and 15 to 60 (social subscale); higher score indicates use of guarding	Content validity established; item-to-scale congruence: 0.92 Internal consistency (56 chronically ill adults): alpha coefficients: 0.75; and 0.78 for both subscales Factor analyses currently being performed

Numbers in parentheses correspond to studies cited in the References.

388

26

Instruments for Measuring Breast Self-Examination

Victoria Champion

Breast cancer is the most common cancer in U.S. women and the incidence is steadily increasing. Estimates are that 180,200 breast cancer cases will be discovered in 1997 with an expected 43,900 deaths.[1] Most effective in combating mortality is early diagnosis by appropriate screening. The American Cancer Society recommends the constellation of routine mammography screening, clinical breast exam, and breast self-examination (BSE) for early detection. Although breast cancer screening has the potential to dramatically lower disease mortality, compliance with screening practices has been poor. Breast self-examination, the focus of this chapter, has been reported to be very poor when considering both frequency and proficiency.[2-4] These facts have led to many research studies on BSE, both descriptive and intervention, which have required the development of attitudinal or belief scales, knowledge scales, and self-report or observational instruments to measure BSE behavior. Additional research is needed to find the most cost-effective methods to increase both BSE frequency and proficiency, which will require meticulous attention to the instruments used to measure variables.

The focus of this chapter will be on describing instruments to measure BSE-related beliefs, knowledge, and behavior. First, information about the efficacy of BSE and past research are reviewed. Then, a review of instruments to measure BSE beliefs and knowledge is presented. BSE belief scales primarily have been developed using the Health Belief Model (HBM) and the Theory of Reasoned Action. Finally, instruments to measure BSE behaviors are described.

Prior to the advent of readily available mammography, BSE, in conjunction with yearly clinical breast examination (CBE), were the only methods of detecting breast cancers at a stage in which cure might be possible. As health professionals attempted to increase the frequency and proficiency of BSE for all women, this behavior became the focus of many research studies.

Although mammography currently is the method of choice for early breast cancer detection, several factors indicate that BSE will continue to play a role in this effort. Both the American Cancer Society and the National Cancer Institute recommend that mammography be supplemented by yearly CBE and monthly BSE. Approximately 17% of lumps in the breast cancer detection project (BCDP)[5] were detected by women between annual exams. A new analysis[5] suggests mortality benefit for BSE even when mammography and CBE are completed. Based on mathematical models, it was proposed that the high survival rate for women with interval tumors in the BCDP data set may be due to the fact that 85% of the women practiced regular BSE. One study[6] found that even when women were screened every year with high-quality mammography and CBE, 13% of cancers surfaced between screenings.

Currently prospective mortality studies for BSE are under way, and preliminary results favor BSE groups for detection of cancer in an early stage of disease.[7,8] Retrospective studies have linked BSE to detection at an earlier stage, smaller tumor size, and/or decreased nodal involvement.[9-13] Three studies have supported a relationship between BSE and survival, and a metaanalysis of past reports found a significant effect for BSE.[10,14-16] A prospective trial in the United Kingdom found significantly better actuarial survival among members of a group who attended BSE instruction classes than among those in a control group.[17] Although several studies have found no effect for BSE, design problems have been cited.[18-20] A recent study found no difference in prior BSE frequency between patients with late-stage breast cancer and case control subjects, but found 35% less mortality in advanced-stage breast cancer when women who were proficient for BSE were analyzed separately.[4] Mamon and Zapka[21] found that verbal reports of BSE proficiency were correlated with BSE performance ($r = 0.62$). A second finding, however, was that BSE frequency was not correlated with proficiency. These studies suggest the importance of measuring proficiency as well as frequency when analyzing the effect of BSE on mortality.

Research

Breast self-examination research primarily has focused on identifying beliefs and knowledge that may be significantly related to frequency and/or proficiency. Only a few descriptive studies have looked at the actual ability to detect lumps in a simulated breast.[22] Many studies have found BSE practice to be significantly related to perceived susceptibility, benefits and/or barriers, health motivation, perceived control, self-efficacy, and/or knowledge.[23-28] The preponderance of evidence suggests that susceptibility, benefits, barriers, self-efficacy, and knowledge are the variables most significantly related to self-reported BSE behavior.

In addition to descriptive studies, many approaches have been used to test the effect of interventions on increasing BSE frequency, proficiency, and, in a few cases, nodule detection. These approaches range from merely handing out pamphlets to prospective, randomized trials incorporating both procedural and belief interventions. Several studies incorporated attitudinal messages into their interventions, with significant results.[29-32] Although research on BSE has been prolific, many studies provide limited information about instrument validity and reliability. The remainder of this chapter will describe instruments to measure variables important in BSE research: beliefs, knowledge and behavior.

Instruments

Instruments to measure constructs related to BSE or the actual practice of BSE fall into three major categories. First, are the instruments that measure beliefs related to BSE practice, mostly based on Health Belief Model (HBM) constructs; second, instruments measuring knowledge related to both BSE and breast cancer; and third, instruments measuring both frequency and proficiency in BSE practice. The instruments reported here attend to issues of validity and reliability and have been used in primary research or by other researchers. The first set of instruments described relates to health beliefs or knowledge about breast cancer and BSE. The second group of instruments frequency and proficiency measurements.

Belief Instruments

Stillman Knowledge and Belief Scale

Stillman[33] developed one of the first questionnaires to measure perceived susceptibility to breast cancer and perceived benefits of BSE. She used HBM constructs to define susceptibility as the subjective risk of contracting a condition, in this case breast cancer. Perceived benefits were defined as the perceived effectiveness of BSE in reducing the threat of breast cancer. A series of nine items was initially designed, with four items measuring susceptibility and five items measuring benefits. The scale to measure susceptibility and benefits is reported later in this chapter as part of a study that links health beliefs about breast cancer and BSE to actual behavior. Items were scaled from "strongly disagree" to "strongly agree." The knowledge component included four items related to factual knowledge about breast cancer. Measures were tested with a convenience sample of 122 women. Content validity was established by submitting the questionnaire to five graduate students, who reviewed the instrument for clarity, readability, and understanding, as well as congruence with definitions for susceptibility and benefits. One hundred percent agreement was required from the content experts. The questionnaire also was submitted to two nonmedical personnel to determine readability and understandability. Reliability and validity information was limited, but many subsequent researchers used items from this tool as a basis for further studies. Examples of items for each construct follow.

> Knowledge. "Most lumps discovered turn out to be cancer."
> Susceptibility. "My health is too good to even consider thinking that I might get breast cancer."
> Benefit. "If more women examined their breasts regularly, there would be fewer deaths from breast cancer."

Champion Health Belief Model Scales

One of the earliest reports of scale development using HBM constructs for the behavior of BSE appeared in 1984.[34] In this initial report, conceptual definitions for each of the variables were developed based on extensive literature reviews. Initially, 20 to 24 items were written for each concept, with statements reflecting construct attributes. Content validity was tested by submitting items to judges who were familiar with the HBM. A 75% agreement among judges was required for item retention. Items were scaled on a 5-point Likert scale with responses varying from "strongly agree" to "strongly disagree." Internal consistency reliabilities from 0.61 to 0.78 were reported, as well as test–retest reliabilities from 0.47 to 0.86. The scale for susceptibility contained 6 items; seriousness 12; benefits 8; barriers 8; and health motivation 8. Construct validity was assessed by exploratory factor analysis and multiple regression. The scales for susceptibility, seriousness, benefits, barriers, and health motivation were considered valid and reliable in measuring BSE beliefs.

Scale revision was completed in 1993[35] with the addition of a confidence scale measuring perceived ability to complete breast self-examination. The conceptual definitions were modified as follows:

> Susceptibility. Perceived personal risk of contracting breast cancer
> Seriousness. Perceived degree of personal threat related to breast cancer
> Benefits. Perceived benefits of BSE for the individual

Barriers. Perceived negative components of BSE for the individual
General health motivation. Beliefs and behavior related to state of general concern about health
Confidence. Perceived ability to detect abnormal lumps while completing BSE

After initial revision, scales were reviewed by a panel of three experts, one of whom was involved with the original development of the HBM.

Instruments were tested for validity and reliability using a random sample of 581 women. Data were collected through a self-administered mailed questionnaire and 2 to 8 weeks later using the same questionnaire during an in-home interview. Reliability and validity were again addressed. The internal consistency correlation coefficients represented improvement over the previously reported scales. Test–retest reliabilities ranged from 0.45 to 0.70, again evidencing only moderate test–retest reliability. Construct validity was assessed using exploratory factor analysis, with resulting deletion of four items. All remaining items loaded at 0.45 or above on the respective factors. Predictive validity was established by looking at the relationship between the respective HBM scales and BSE behavior. Predictive validity was demonstrated by the significant correlation of all scales with the BSE behavior. The current revision resulted in a substantial improvement for the susceptibility, seriousness, benefits, barriers, and health motivation scales over what was previously reported. In addition, the confidence scale demonstrated satisfactory validity and reliability. An example of an item from each scale follows:

Susceptibility. "It is extremely likely that I will get breast cancer."
Seriousness. "Breast cancer is an extremely serious disease."
Benefits. "When I do breast self-examination, I don't worry as much about cancer."
Barriers. "Breast self-examination would be embarrassing to me."
Health motivation. "I try to discover health problems early."

Beliefs and Attitudes Scale for BSE

Lauver and Angerame[36] developed a BSE belief and attitude scale using the literature and previously constructed items. Content validity was assessed by 20 nurses who included university faculty in women's health care, clinicians, and postdoctoral fellows. The nurses reviewed items for adequacy of beliefs and attitudes about BSE. A total of 95% of the nurses judged items to be relevant, 85% judged representation of attitudes about BSE to be adequate, and 85% judged an even distribution of items across content areas. A 5-point response set ranged from "strongly agree" to "strongly disagree." Several constructs were measured: general efficacy of BSE, specific efficacy of BSE, confidence in doing BSE, and attitudinal items addressing remembering, interference, comfort, fear, and pain. A total of 64 women were recruited for teaching sessions from employees in an industrial occupational setting. Cronbach alpha for the subscales ranged from 0.65 to 0.89. BSE frequency scores were compared using Spearman ranked-correlation coefficients. Competence, remembering, and comfort scales had moderately strong positive relationships with frequency (0.35 to 0.58), and the interference scale had a negative correlation of −0.44. Correlations between efficacy and frequency were not significant. Fear and pain subscales had weak and nonsignificant relations. Examples of items from each scale follow:

General self-efficacy. "BSE is an effective way to find changes in breasts."
Specific efficacy of BSE for self. "If I did BSE, I could protect my future health."
Perceived competence. "I may find a lump before it is discovered at a regular exam."
Remembering. "I am reminded to do BSE by things seen or heard."
Interference. "To do BSE I have to give up quite a bit."
Comfort. "I am comfortable with touching breasts."

The authors suggest further replication given the small sample size.

General Attitude and Social Norm Scale

The Theory of Planned Behavior has been operationalized in the context of BSE to develop the General Attitude and Social Norm Scale.[37] In developing this scale, both beliefs and social influences on BSE behavior and experience were elicited. Women first were asked to identify individuals or groups who approved of their monthly BSE or who might influence this behavior. Salient beliefs regarding advantages and disadvantages associated with BSE were elicited. Content analyses and instrument construction followed. Attitudinal and normative scales were developed based on the Theory of Reasoned Action. The approach to measuring beliefs is somewhat different than that specified by the HBM. Belief and evaluation items are combined to form an attitude scale. For instance, salient beliefs were identified by in-depth interviews with a subsample of 29 women from an HMO. Qualitative data were used to define belief statements about BSE performance, cancer and cancer treatment, social influences, and experience. Salient beliefs were obtained by asking women to list advantages and disadvantages associated with the performance of BSE. Belief statements with matching evaluation items were developed. The most frequent qualitative responses were used in the pilot instrument as belief items and normative beliefs. For each belief, a corresponding evaluation item was considered. For each normative belief, a motivation-to-comply item was developed. Belief and evaluation items, as well as normative belief and motivation-to-comply items, were multiplied and summed. For instance, a belief item would be: "My performing BSE would allow me to detect BSE in an early stage." This would be answered on a 7-point Likert scale from "strongly disagree" to "strongly agree." An evaluation item matching the belief item would be: "Detecting breast cancer at an early stage would be. . . ." The evaluation of this item would use a 7-point scale from "extremely bad" to "extremely good." The belief and evaluation components are multiplied, and products are summed for a total score.

Normative belief and motivation-to-comply items were developed in a similar manner: "Do you think your sister feels you should perform BSE on a monthly basis?" (normative belief). Responses were scored as 1 "I don't have any sisters"; 2 "I don't know"; 3 "Definitely not"; 4 "Probably not"; 5 "She is neutral"; 6 "Probably yes"; 7 "Definitely yes." A motivation item could be: "How much do you try to do what you feel your sister thinks you should do?" Responses were scored from: 1 "I don't have a sister"; 2 "Not at all"; 3 "Slightly"; 4 "Moderate amount"; 5 "Great deal"; 6 "I don't know."

The pilot instrument was administered to three groups of women and modified after each data collection. Items with small variance were deleted and a 69-item attitude scale, and a Cronbach alpha of 0.70 resulted. A nine-item social norm scale had an internal consistency reliability of 0.86.

Attitude, Knowledge, and Proficiency Scales

Alagna and Reddy[38] developed scales to measure the HBM constructs of susceptibility, severity, self-confidence, and barriers as related to BSE. Susceptibility items include how often a person thinks about breast cancer, how often she discusses breast cancer with friends or relatives, and how likely she believes she is to get breast cancer. Items were reported to correlate at 0.65. Severity questions referred to chances of survival or the effectiveness of treating breast cancer and correlated at 0.85. Self-confidence items included strength of belief that lesions could be detected by BSE and confidence about knowing BSE. Items for this scale correlated at 0.76. Barriers included items related to fear and embarrassment and were not correlated.

Observers recorded each subject's BSE performance for a BSE proficiency measure. Items investigated included: one or two hands used, the parts of the hand used, systematic examination, motion used when examining, and full or partial examination of breasts. Behaviors were scored as correct or not correct. Overall proficiency was an unweighted sum of the number of correct detections. In addition, lesion detection was recorded. Seventy-three women attending a health fair completed the questionnaire. Self-confidence correlated with proficient BSE. Further markers of validity and reliability were not reported.

Cromer Health Belief Model Scale

The HBM constructs of susceptibility, seriousness, barriers, benefits, control, and general health motivation were operationalized to test beliefs of postmenarcheal students in grades 10 to 12 in a public high school.[39] Items were initially developed by a Q-sort methodology and presented to adolescents using stacks of cards. Relevant statements were listed in questionnaire format using a 5-point Likert response scale. Sample items are:

Threat. "Breast cancer is a serious problem."
Benefit. "Breast cancer found early is more likely to be cured."
Barrier. "Examining my breast is a real hassle."

In addition, items for control and general health motivation were developed. Although analyses were not done on reliability, the authors did compare differences between compliers and noncompliers on susceptibility, seriousness, control over health, benefits of compliance, barriers to compliance, and health motivation. A significant difference was found between compliers and noncompliers for the control scale only.

Behavior Scales

In addition to the belief scales, several researchers have developed proficiency scales to measure actual BSE behavior. Embedded within several of these instruments are scales to measure knowledge and beliefs. Instruments that address some aspect of proficiency are described next.

Proficiency

To evaluate an intervention protocol, attempts to determine the validity of BSE evaluation tools were undertaken by a group of researchers at the Fred Hutchins Cancer Research Center.[29] Observer assessment of BSE practice included five items: (1) covered 8 or more areas of the breast; (2) used finger pads; (3) used firm pressure; (4) used massage and search pattern; (5) used mirror plus supine position. When the five unweighted points were scored, 44.6% of women scored five points or more and were rated as having excellent BSE technique. Calculation of the observation score allowed differentiation of regular practitioners from those who were not regular practitioners (chi square = 15.2, $p \leq 0.004$). In addition, women were asked to palpate three models that had a total of 15 lumps of varying sizes embedded within them. BSE technique was associated with ability to detect lumps ($p \leq 0.006$). For each two-step increase in the technique scale, one additional lump was detected. Difference in lumps detected between pre- and postinstruction was significant ($p \leq 0.002$). Irregular BSE practitioners did not increase posttraining scores. Registered nurses supported using at least five observation steps in determining BSE practice.

Toronto Breast Self-Examination Instrument (TBSEI)

A self-administered survey for BSE proficiency was developed in Toronto[40] and included three subscales: (1) frequency and proficiency (proficiency); (2) susceptibility and reasons for practice (motivation); and (3) knowledge. The instrument also included sociodemographic and health history items, which will not be reported. Sixteen items were developed for perceived susceptibility and reasons for practice. Eleven items were developed for frequency and proficiency of practice and 20 items for knowledge of breast cancer and breast self-examination. Face and content validity were established by submitting items to 24 experts in the field of breast cancer and BSE. Content experts were asked to examine the items for exhaustiveness of content. Experts also were asked to evaluate the scales for practical and technical utility, including ease of use and precision of directions. Items were sorted on a 5-point Likert scale, and space for comments was allowed. Response categories ranged from "very clear/very relevant" to "very unclear/very nonrelevant." Acceptable variance of a 5-point scale was set at 0.06 or lower. A mean of 4.5 was set as an acceptable level. Twenty items were initially eliminated, two items added, and seventeen items reworded. Experts were asked to complete knowledge items anonymously. Eighty percent was set as an acceptable level for retention of an item. Five knowledge items were deleted because fewer than 80% of the respondents agreed on a correct answer. Out of 24 experts, 18 responded to the questionnaire.

For the motivation scale, the neutral category was scored as zero. Authors believed that no opinion about motivational factors indicated lack of motivation. Knowledge was scored on a 3-point scale ranging from 0 to 2 that indicated the categories of agree, neutral, and disagree with each item.

Validity was assessed by looking at item standard deviations and judged to be reasonable for the motivation, knowledge, and proficiency scales. In addition, differences between women who practiced BSE and those who did not were significant for the knowledge scale, indicating that nonpractitioners had less knowledge of breast cancer and breast self-examination than practitioners. Correlations among the scales were low, indicating their quasi-independence.

Internal consistency coefficients were calculated using Cronbach's alpha. The alpha for proficiency was 0.91, for motivation 0.69, and for knowledge 0.85. Scales were tested with systematic removal of items using the criterion of change in the Cronbach alpha. Test–retest reliability was calculated with an additional sample of 48 women who completed the survey on two separate occasions. The interval between test and retest was 2 weeks, and the coefficient for retest reliability was 0.89.

A convenience sample of nine family physicians at a university teaching hospital reviewed the final items. Items that had a consensus of 8 out of 9 were kept. Following this initial validity assessment, the proficiency scale retained 11 items, the motivation scale 16 items, and the knowledge scale 20 items.

A sample of 729 volunteers was selected from ambulatory patients, communities, universities, and non-health-related industries. Validity and reliability were calculated from the data. Sample items are:

Proficiency. "How often in the past 12 months have you done breast self-examination?" "How confident are you that you would notice a lump by BSE?"
Knowledge. "Before menopause, the best time for BSE is during menstruation." "Women with a high-fat diet have a higher chance of breast cancer."
Motivation scale. "I do not have time for BSE." "It is not important to do BSE because I am too young."

The authors suggest that the total BSE inventory will be useful as a standardized self-administered inventory to measure BSE practice, motivation, and knowledge. The authors recommend validating the proficiency scale with alternate assessments of performance.

Coleman BSE Proficiency Tool

Coleman[41] developed a scoring system to measure the eight components of BSE proficiency as specified by a BSE training technology called MammaCare. These eight components related to: (1) area; (2) pressure type; (3) motion; (4) part (fingers or hands);

(5) pattern; (6) number of fingers; (7) number of motions; and (8) duration. Using these components, a scoring system was developed and validated. A paired-comparisons procedure was used to provide each component a BSE weight. The weights were then combined to produce a value on an interval scale. A paired-comparisons survey instrument presenting each of the eight components in all[28] possible combinations was constructed.

Experts in teaching the MammaCare method of BSE completed the tool by checking which of the pairs were most important for correct BSE technique. All of the health professionals involved in this assessment had been trained in the MammaCare method of teaching BSE, and three of the expert judges were instrumental in developing the MammaCare method. Weights for each of the items were calculated by dividing the total number of responses (28 choices times 20 experts) that each component received by the overall total responses. Raw scores for each of the steps were calculated. For instance, the area score was the total percentage of breast area actually palpated divided by the number of square inches of breast surface present. Duration was the actual time of examination in minutes converted to a maximum of 1. Each subject's pressure was divided by 6 and a value of 1 given if light, medium, and deep pressures were used and less than 1 given for the other choices according to rank. The other five components (motion, number of motions, pattern, part of fingers, and number of fingers) were given a score of 0 or 1, 1 being the preferred choice. Raw scores were then multiplied by the weighted scores and all scores summed for a performance score to produce a set of weights with the following values: area, 0.216; duration, 0.06; motion, 0.14; part, 0.13; pattern, 0.1225; number of fingers, 0.075; number of motions, 0.0725; pressure type, 0.185.

To validate the scoring system, both pre- and post-tests were completed by women who were taught BSE individually using self-modeling and by women taught BSE in a group using a breast model. Instructors were trained in teaching the MammaCare method of BSE.[41] Observer scores were trained to 95% agreement on the number of palpations and 95% agreement on the number of squares examined by the standard observer. A total of 79 noninstitutionalized women 50 years of age or older were included in this study. Mean performance scores for each group on the first and second post-test showed improvement after teaching over pretest values. Pre- and post-test values demonstrated discrimination. Implications for this measure of proficiency included using all components on a checklist to evaluate persons in a clinical area. Recommendations for a checklist using components as in the overall area were suggested. Necessary components for the checklist would be: (1) correct position; (2) examination of all areas; (3) adequate pressure; (4) use of a circular motion with the application of each type of pressure; (5) use of the pads of the three middle fingers; (6) use of a vertical strip pattern; (7) squeezing the nipple to check for discharge; and (8) examining the breast for symmetrical dimpling or retraction. Using a weighted scale might be appropriate in research settings when an accurate picture of proficiency is needed.

Atkins BSE Proficiency Measure

A study by Atkins et al.[42] assesses the relative effectiveness of different search patterns on area of breast covered and number of lumps detected. To assess area covered, a videotape of each subject's BSE was recorded after a training session. A slide and matching schematic score sheet with a breast board divided into numbered 3-cm squares was provided to compare with the BSE tape. Each square that was palpated with distal finger pads of the first three fingers was counted. Percentage of coverage was calculated by dividing the number of squares palpated by the total number of squares represented in the area. The mean interrater reliability was 0.82. In addition, a measure of lump detection representing the total number of actual lumps detected in two silicon breast models was used, with the score ranging from 0 to 10. A false-positive score also was calculated representing the total number of false-positive lumps identified in two silicon breast models. Duration scores were obtained by recording duration of the exam on both the breast board and the model.

These methods of measuring area covered and number of lumps detected were used to assess differences in search patterns comparing concentric circle, radial spoke, and vertical strip patterns. Results indicated that these methods of scoring differentiated the vertical strip pattern in terms of breast area covered.

Champion BSE Performance Scale

Methods for measuring frequency and proficiency also have been developed by Champion.[35] First, frequency by self-report was assessed. Women were asked the number of times they had completed BSE in the last 12 months and about their technique (proficiency) using BSE behavior scales. Items assessed included positioning of hands, areas of breast covered, systematic examination, and length of examination. Items were scored so that increasing magnitude of the ordinal-scale response indicated more proficient practice. A Cronbach alpha internal consistency of 0.73 and test–retest correlation of 0.74 were computed.[35,43]

An observed proficiency score also was developed. An observer checklist contained 10 procedural components deemed important for BSE that corresponded to items in the self-report measurement scale. Items included those listed in the self-report instrument. Participants were given two points for each of the steps that were adequately completed, except for the last two items that indicated both position and examination of total breast, for which four points were given. A total of 24 points was possible on the proficiency checklist. An interobserver reliability of 0.90 was obtained.

A final measure of BSE frequency and proficiency was developed using self-report logs. A log kept by the participant indicating whether BSE was completed and checking what steps were completed was given to women involved in an intervention study. Each log allowed recording BSE for 12 months. Participants were given a point for each month they examined their breasts and a point for each item on the proficiency scale. A total of eight items were included: (1) examining the breast in the shower; (2) duration of examination; (3) examining right and left breast while lying on a pillow; (4) looking in the mirror with hands at the side; (5) looking in the mirror with hands over head; (6) using the pads of the fingers to examine; (7) squeezing the nipple; and (8) using a systematic pattern. A range of 0 to 96 points was possible for the total year.[43]

Jones Proficiency Scale

Jones et al.[44] measured BSE proficiency by having 11 components of BSE rated by trained observers. Components of BSE that were monitored included: duration; number of steps; number of spots (area) covered; use of 3 middle fingers; use of pads of fingers; using 3 circles at each spot; squeezing nipple; percentage of area covered; vertical strip pattern; use of opposite hand; and positioning of hand behind head. Subjects include 54 undergraduate women who were trained and assigned to tape or no-tape groups. A stop watch was used to measure duration. Strips were measured by the number of vertical movements up and down the body between the collarbone and bra line. Spots included the number of discrete points at which the fingers come into contact with the skin. Three fingers at each spot was assessed as adequate. Finger pads were to be positioned at a 45-degree angle or less. Area covered was measured by a transparency grid of 0.5" squares secured to the front of a 9" television screen. The total area that could be palpated was outlined and all squares where the fingers touched were marked on the grid with a pen.

BSE frequency was measured with seven BSE monitoring sheets, on which participants were to indicate the date on which BSE was performed. Interrater reliability for the proficiency variables was calculated using Pearson's coefficients. One item, pads of the fingers, was found to be unreliable ($r = 0.10$). Other correlations ranged from 0.81 to 0.99. Items for hands behind head and squeezing nipple were found to be 100% reliable.

Comparisons on BSE proficiency were made between members of a group who received a tape at the end of the training session and those who did not. Significant differences in the expected direction were found on number of strips covered ($t = 2.76$), percentage of area covered ($t = 2.15$), use of vertical search patterns ($t = 2.67$), and use of the contralateral hand ($t = 2.22$).

Summary

Breast self-examination was one of the earliest screening techniques for the early detection of breast cancer. Although mammography now is the major screening focus, tumors not identified by mammography, as well as interval tumors, may be found by BSE. Early work has suggested that belief variables specified by the Health Belief Model are important in predicting BSE behavior. Measurement efforts for BSE have focused on the development of belief scales, knowledge scales, and self-report behavior scales. Research efforts have been hampered by inconsistent use of valid or reliable scales for measurement of beliefs, knowledge, and BSE behavior. Instruments with reported reliability and validity now are available to measure BSE beliefs and BSE proficiency. Selection of instruments will depend on the particular research or clinical application.

Exemplar Studies

Champion, V. Instrument refinement for breast cancer screening behaviors. *Nurs Res*, 1993, *42*(3):139-143.

This study exemplifies the measurement of scales related to the behavior of BSE. The instruments are refinements of previously existing scales that had been extensively tested for validity and reliability. The methods to refine the previous scales are rigorous and well explained. The new instruments expand our ability to measure constructs that are related to BSE behavior.

Coleman, E., & Pennypacker, H. Measuring breast self-examination proficiency. *Cancer Nurs*, 1991, *14*(4):211-217.

This study exemplifies the measurement of BSE behavior. The method of paired comparisons was used to develop an interval-level scale using eight BSE components. Extensive validity testing verified the usefulness of this instrument for measuring proficient BSE behavior. The authors recommend a simpler version for use in a clinical setting that would include: (1) correct position; (2) examination of all areas; (3) adequate pressure; (4) use of a circular motion with the application of each type of pressure; (5) use of the pads of the three middle fingers; (6) use of a vertical strip pattern; (7) squeezing the nipple to check for discharge; and (8) examining the breast for symmetrical dimpling or retraction.

References

1. Parker, S.L., Tong, T., Bolden, S., & Wingo, P. Cancer statistics, 1997. *CA Cancer J Clin*, 1997, *47*(1):5-27.
2. Champion, V.L. Breast self-examination in women 35 and older: A prospective study. *J Behav Med*, 1990, *13*(6):523-538.
3. Gallup Organization. Women's attitudes regarding breast cancer. Princeton, NJ: *Gallup Organization*, 1988.
4. Newcomb, P.A., Weiss, N.S., Storer, B.E., et al. Breast self-examination in relation to the occurrence of advanced breast cancer. *J Nat Cancer Inst*, 1991, *83*(4): 260-265.
5. Shwartz, M. Validation of a model of breast cancer screening: An outlier suggests the value of breast self-examination. *Med Decision Making*, 1992, *12*(3):222-228.
6. Seidman, H., Gelb, S.K., Silverberg, E., & Lubera, J.A. Survival experience in the breast cancer detection demonstration project. *CA Cancer J Clin*, 1987, *37*(5):258-290.
7. Koroltchouk, V., Stanley, K., & Sternsward, J. The control of breast cancer. A World Health Organization perspective. *Cancer*, 1990, *65*(12):2803-2810.
8. Semiglazov, V.F., & Moiseenko, M.V. Breast self-examination for the early detection of breast cancer: A USSR/WHO controlled trial in Leningrad. *Bull WHO*, 1987, *65*(3):391-396.
9. Feldman, J.G., Carter, A.C., Nicastri, A.D., & Hosat, S.T. Breast self-examination, relationship to stage of breast cancer at diagnosis. *Cancer*, 1981, *47*(11):2740-2745.
10. Foster, R.S., & Costanza, M.C. Breast self-examination practices and breast cancer survival. *Cancer*, 1984, *53*(4):999.
11. Greenwald, P., Nasca, P., Lawrence, E., et al. Estimated effect of breast self-examination and routine physician examination on breast-cancer mortality. *N Eng J Med*, 1978, *299*(6):271-273.
12. Huguley, C., & Brown, R. The value of breast self-examination. *Cancer*, 1981, *47*(5):989-995.
13. Mant, D., Vessey, M.P., Neil, A., et al. Breast self examination and breast cancer stage at diagnosis. *Br J Cancer*, 1987, *55*(2):207-211.
14. Hill, D., White, V., Jolley, D., & Mapperson, K. Self examination of the breast: Is it beneficial? *Br Med J*, 1988, *297*(6647):271-274.
15. Huguley, C.M., Brown, R.L., Greenberg, R.S., & Clark, W.S. Breast self-examination and survival from breast cancer. *Cancer*, 1988, *62*(7):1389-1396.
16. Kuroishi, T., Tominaga, S., Ota, J., et al. The effect of breast self-examination on early detection and survival. *Jpn J Cancer Res*, 1992, *83*(4):344-350.
17. Locker, A.P., Casildine, J., Mitchell, A.K., et al. Results from a seven-year programme of breast self-examination in 89,010 women. *Br J Cancer*, 1989, *60*(3):401-405.
18. Philip, J., Harris, G., Flaherty, C., & Joslin, C.A.F. Clinical measures to assess the practice and efficiency of breast self-examination. *Cancer*, 1986, *58*(4):973-977.
19. Senie, R.T., Rosen, P.P., Lesser, M.L., & Kinne, D.W. Breast self-examination and medical examination related to breast cancer stage. *Am J Public Health*, 1981, *71*(6):583-590.
20. Smith, E.M., & Burns, T.L. The effects of breast self-examination in a population-based cancer registry. *Cancer*, 1985, *55*(2):432-437.
21. Mamon, J., & Zapka, J.G. Determining validity of measuring the quality of breast self- examination. *Eval Health Prof*, 1985, *8*(1):55-59.
22. Fletcher, S.W., O'Malley, M.S., Earp, J.A.L., et al. How best to teach women breast self-examination. A randomized controlled trial. *Ann Int Med*, 1990, *112*(10):772-779.
23. Calnan, M., & Rutter, D.R. Do health beliefs predict health behaviour? An analysis of breast self-examination. *Soc Sci Med*, 1988, *24*(6):663-665.
24. Champion, V.L. Attitudinal variables related to intention, frequency and proficiency of breast self-examination in women 35 and over. *Res Nurs Health*, 1988, *11*(5):283-291.
25. Chrvala, C.A. Breast cancer risk status as a predictor for breast cancer screening behaviors. In P.F. Engstrom & B. Rimer (Eds.) *Advances in cancer control: Screening and prevention research*. New York: Wiley-Liss, 1990, p. 239.
26. Fletcher, S.W., Morgan, T.M., O'Malley, M.S., et al. Is breast self-examination predicted by knowledge, attitudes, beliefs, or sociodemographic characteristics? *Am J Prev Med*, 1989, *5*(4):207-215.
27. Grady, K.L., Kegeles, S.S., Lund, A.K., et al. Who volunteers for a breast self-examination program? Evaluating the bases for self-selection. *Health Educ Q*, 1983, *10*(2):79-94.
28. Shepperd, S.L., Solomon, L.J., Atkins, E., et al. Determinants of breast self-examination among women of lower income and lower education. *J Behav Med*, 1990, *13*(4):359-371.
29. Mahloch, J., Paskett, E., Henderson, M., et al. An evaluation of BSE frequency and quality and their relationship to breast lump detection. In P.F. Engstrom & B. Rimer (Eds.) *Advances in cancer control: Screening and prevention research*. New York: Wiley-Liss, 1990, p. 269.
30. Nettles-Carlson, B., Field, M.L., Friedman, B.J., & Smith, L.S. Effectiveness of teaching breast self-examination during office visits. *Res Nurs Health*, 1988, *11*(1):41-50.
31. Paskett, E.D., White, E., Urban, N., et al. Implementation and evaluation of a worksite breast self-examination training program. In P.F. Engstrom & B. Rimer (Eds.) *Advances in cancer control: Screening and prevention research*. New York: Wiley-Liss, 1990, p. 281.
32. Worden, J.K., Solomon, L.J., Flynn, B.S., et al. A community-wide program in breast self-examination training and maintenance. *Prev Med*, 1990, *19*(3):254-269.
33. Stillman, M.J. Women's health beliefs about breast cancer and breast self- examination. *Nurs Res*, 1977, *26*(2):121-127.
34. Champion, V.L. Instrument development for health belief model constructs. *Adv Nurs Sci*, 1984, *6*(3):73-85.
35. Champion, V.L. Instrument refinement for breast cancer screening behaviors. *Nurs Res*, 1993, *42*(3):139-143.

36. Lauver, D., & Angerame, M. Development of a questionnaire to measure beliefs and attitudes about breast self-examination. *Cancer Nurs*, 1988, *11*(1): 51-57.

37. Young, H.M., Lierman, L.C., Powell-Cope, G., et al. Operationalizing the theory of planned behavior. *Res Nurs Health*, 1991, *14*(2):137-144.

38. Alagna, S.W., & Reddy, D.M. Predictors of proficient technique and successful lesion detection in breast self-examination. *Health Psychol*, 1984, *3*(2):113-127.

39. Cromer, B.A., Frankel, M.E., Hayes, J., & Brown, R.T. Compliance with breast self-examination instruction in high school students. *Clin Pediatr*, 1992, *31*(4):215-220.

40. Ferris, L., Shamian, J., & Tudiver, F. The Toronto Breast Self-Examination Instrument (TBSEI): Its development and reliability and validity data. *J Clin Epidemiol*, 1991, *44*:1309-1315.

41. Coleman, E.A. Practice and effectiveness of breast self-examination: A selective review of the literature (1977-1989). *J Cancer Educ*, 1991, *6*(2):83-92.

42. Atkins, E., Solomon, L.J., Worden, J.K., & Foster, R.S., Jr. Relative effectiveness of methods of breast self-examination. *J Behav Med*, 1991, *14*(4):357-367.

43. Champion, V.L., & Scott, C. Effects of a procedural/belief intervention on breast self-examination performance. *Res Nurs Health*, 1993, *16*:163-167.

44. Jones, J.A., Eckhardt, L.E., Mayer, J.A., et al. The effects of an instructional audiotape on breast self-examination proficiency. *J Behav Med*, 1993, *16*(2): 225-235.

27

Measuring Information-Seeking Behaviors and Decision-Making Preferences

Caroline Bagley-Burnett and Bettyann Heppler

Information is a key to understanding the problems, challenges, and frustrations with which an individual is faced throughout his or her lifespan. Individuals often have to seek out new information to promote health, prevent illness, or make treatment decisions. Information is essential in decision making and is considered by many to be a means of coping with and reducing stress and maintaining control.[1-8] For these reasons, it is important for health-care providers (1) to understand the concept of information seeking; (2) to possess a knowledge of the behaviors exhibited by patients seeking information; (3) to develop the skills necessary to assess the amount and type of information desired by patients; (4) to recognize the contextual and situational variables that influence a patient's desire for information and; (5) to recognize situations in which a patient desires to or not to participate in decision making.

The purposes of this chapter are to present relevant background on the concept of information-seeking and decision-making preferences as found in both consumer and health care literature, to describe the development of instruments used to measure aspects of information seeking and decision making, to evaluate the utility of these instruments for their ability to fulfill their designed purpose, to summarize pertinent research findings that have used selected instruments, and to discuss the contribution of the work toward enhancing health-care professional's understanding of the information-seeking behaviors and decision-making preferences of patients.

Consumer Information-Seeking Behavior

A review of the consumer and health-care literature from 1975 to the present reveals that the concept of information seeking is both complex and poorly understood. Research in this area can be found in the consumer literature as early as the 1920s. Early studies that focused on consumer prepurchase information-seeking activities were one component of marketing theory. The literature is sparse until the 1960s when studies that address the prepurchase activities of consumers surface.[9,10]

Since then, interest in consumer prepurchase behavior has increased significantly. There are several reasons for this increase. Manufacturers, retailers, and advertisers benefit from data on consumer prepurchase behavior. These data enable them better to target the interests of consumers and result in increased product sales. The consumers' and women's movements have highlighted individuals' rights to information, resulting in an increased demand to be informed. Researcher interest in what motivates people to seek information and make health-care decisions has increased. Legislators, health-care professionals, and policymakers have shown increased interest in information-seeking behavior. At the national and state levels, laws have been enacted that mandate informed consent, adequate disclosure concerning treatment alternatives for diseases such as breast cancer, and the inclusion of patient package inserts for such drugs as oral contraceptives and estrogens. A few health insurance companies reimburse for health education and may prorate insurance rates accordingly. Organizations, such as the American Cancer Society, the National Cancer Institute, and many drug companies, have developed their own information sources for use by consumers. Changes in the economic climate, including income and employment levels, periods of high inflation, skyrocketing medical costs, reduced provider payments, and cutbacks in federal funding all have contributed to an increased preference for more information. Finally, health-care reform will undoubtedly influence the way in which consumers seek information and make health-care decisions. It is not clear at this juncture what the outcome(s) of this reform will be. However, one might suggest that consumers' role in their health-care decisions will increase.

The changes outlined have provided consumers improved access to more complete and often complex information. Physicians and nurses are more likely to offer explanations about diagnoses, treatments, side effects, and expected outcomes. This access to and improved availability of information may enable consumers to participate in independent health-care decisions, to ask more questions, and to seek information from several sources. Sources of information may include physicians, nurses, pharmacists, such media as television, radio, newspaper, and magazines, and to a lesser degree family and friends.[11]

Discrepancy still exists between what consumers say they want to know and how much information physicians believe their patients want to know. Faden et al.[12] reported that physicians consistently underestimate the amount of information people want about treatments and their side effects. Studies performed with patients receiving patient package inserts show similar results.[11] Research has focused on distinguishing between the amount of information patients say they want and whether, once they have received that information, they choose to use it in health-care decision making.

Studies suggest that, although individuals report a desire for information, they frequently prefer not to participate in actual treatment decisions.[13-17] Caution must be exercised in generalizing these findings or in assuming that "more information is better," "all people desire complete information," "patients want to participate in health-care decisions," and "more information reduces stress and enhances the ability to cope with this stress." Many of these assumptions may be true, but research is needed that focuses on how much information a person wants, variables that may influence the amount of information desired, and whether a person wants to make the decisions and in what situations. Studies must clarify the relationship of such variables as age, sex, race, and psychosocial, cultural, economic, and educational backgrounds to desire for information and participation in decision making. Other factors that influence information-seeking and decision-making preferences, such as previous illness, severity of illness, and personal and significant others' experiences with the health-care system, need to be explored.

The problem today, then, is not so much the availability of information as the identification of the type of information a person wants, a recognition of how much and under what circumstances information is needed, a determination of the circumstances in which the individual wishes to use the information and of extent of participation desired, and a clarification of the relationship between sociodemographic variables and the process.

As a result of the research conducted on consumer prepurchase information-seeking behavior, a body of knowledge has accumulated that has conceptual relevance to research conducted in the health-care field. For example, Payne[18] and Englander and Tyszka[19] have used an information display board method. This method consists of an information display matrix that has rows listing alternatives and columns describing the attributes of each alternative.[19] They found that people proceeded in either an intradimensional or interdimensional manner; that is, when faced with several alternatives and the choice of characteristics within each alternative, the person might choose to exhaust all characteristics with one alternative (intradimensional) or might choose to explore all the alternatives (interdimensional) before investigating characteristics within each alternative. Unfortunately, the authors did not identify individual characteristics of people or contextual variables that might predict the type of approach chosen. They did find that, when faced with many alternatives, people tend to limit the intradimensional search component, thus sacrificing some depth of knowledge about an alternative, to seek more limited information on the large number of alternatives. Conversely, when faced with only two alternatives, people tended to extend the depth of search. When faced with many alternatives, people attempted to eliminate or collapse the categories to decrease the total number of options to be evaluated. The apparent purpose is to decrease both the complexity of the task and the strain or tension experienced in the evaluation process.

Fast and colleagues[20] investigated the effects of consumer education on search. They described a theoretical model that posited a relationship between consumer education and type of information source used during search. The dependent variable was time allotted to search from four information sources, advertising, sellers, friends, acquaintances, and independent product test reports (such as those found in *Canadian Consumer*, *Consumer Reports*, *Consumers' Research*, and *Protect Yourself* magazines). The independent variables in the model include consumer education (e.g., high school, community or general continuing education programs), wage rate, age, educational level, prior experience, perceived risk, and urgency of purchase. The following findings have particular application to information seeking and decision making in health care.

Friends or relatives were the only search source used in situations that were perceived as high urgency or where there was previous product ownership. In some situations the authors found that prior experience was negatively associated with search. High school continuing education, community workshops, and general public continuing education were not significantly related to information sources chosen for search. There was a significant relationship between reading consumer literature and using product test reports during search. Written product information was preferred over formal classroom presentations.

Although the findings of this study relate to search behavior associated with purchase of major household appliances, the authors define these goods as "high-involvement" items. That is, the items are high cost, involve complex technology, and are potentially uncertain and risky purchases. Framed in this manner, one may assert that findings from this study have direct relevance to information search and decision making in health care. Health-care decisions may involve high-cost, complex technology and uncertainty and risk. Testing of the findings from this study in health-care information search and decision-making situations is warranted.

Instruments

Reference to information-seeking activities and decision-making preferences in the health-care literature is not found until the 1960s. These accounts are predominantly clinical anecdotes.[1] Gradually, however, more studies address various facets of information-seeking activities and decision-making preferences for consumers of health care.[1,3,14,15,21,22]

Little has been written on theories of information-seeking behaviors. Lazarus's theory of stress and coping often is used as a conceptual framework when studying the concept of information-seeking activities. He maintains that knowledge reduces stress and thereby enhances coping.[7] It seems logical, therefore, that people who actively seek information enhance their ability to cope with a particular situation.

Mills and Krantz conceptualized information as a form of cognitive control because it often results in the interpretation of an aversive event so that the threat is lessened.[23] Lenz conceptualized search as an interpersonal process with the primary sources of information being others to whom one has direct access or can be referred.[1] According to Lenz, this process contains six steps: (1) a stimulus; (2) goal setting; (3) a decision regarding whether to seek information actively; (4) search behavior; (5) information acquisition and codification; (6) decision regarding the adequacy of the information acquired; and (7) outcomes.[1]

Hopkins[3] conceptualized information search as a process that occurs throughout a series of related stressful episodes and is characterized by the polar extremes of avoidance and hypervigilance. It is defined as a coping strategy with varying levels of intensity measured quantitatively on the Information Preference Questionnaire (IPQ).

Research in the area of information-seeking activities and decision-making preferences has increased in the last 5 years. Instruments have been developed that measure search behavior, identify factors influencing information-seeking behavior, and describe situations in which individuals wish to participate in decision making.[24] Many studies have recently addressed the issues of patient information search and desire to participate in decision making, but valid and reliable standardized instruments that are clinically useful are few. Studies are now needed that strengthen instrument validity and reliability. This can be accomplished through collaborative research efforts, use of multiple instruments in the same study, and research conducted with diverse populations.

The following sections review existing scales, their testing, scoring and validity and reliability, the populations in which they have been tested, and strengths and limitations. Studies using the scales are evaluated.

Lenz Analytical Model of Information Search Episode

Lenz developed a model (Figure 27.1) that "represents the analytically distinct steps hypothesized to comprise a search episode, the flow of events which precede the initial voluntary contact (or attempted contact) with a health service provider."[1,p182] This model assumes that a person desires a health-related service or, at the least, desires information

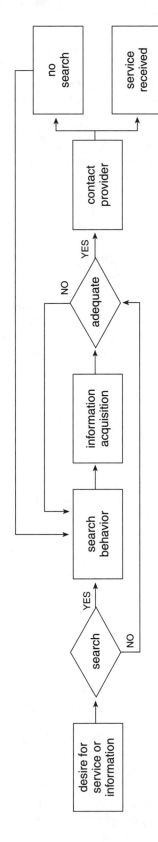

Figure 27.1 Lenz model (From Lenz, E.R. In Bowens, E., Ed., *Clinical nursing research: Its strategies and findings. II.* Indianapolis: Sigma Theta Tau, 1979, p. 183. Courtesy of Sigma Theta Tau.)

about health resources that may be used at a later time. Search commences and can vary in length and extent. There are several decision points along the continuum. Information continues to accrue until the person has acquired sufficient data according to some predetermined criterion. A person then decides whether to use the information immediately, store it for future use, or continue the search if the information acquired is insufficient. It is hypothesized that the individual follows this sequence of events each time a new search is undertaken. According to Lenz, the model can be used to describe the search process and/or generate hypotheses to predict relationships among variables in one step with variables in other steps.

To test the hypothesis underlying this model, Lenz sampled individuals who had moved at least 20 miles away to a new community within the last 8 to 12 months. The purpose of the study was to answer the following questions: How do newcomers seek and acquire information about local health services? To what extent does their search behavior relate to the information they acquire and the service they receive? What role do nurses and other health professionals play as consultants to newcomers in their information search?[25,p182]

A stratified random sample of 129 households was used. The interview focused on (1) ascertaining from whom the household members had received health services since the move; (2) describing the search process undertaken before receiving services; and (3) ascertaining information about search activities that did not result in the use of services. Retrospective household interviews were conducted using a semistructured interview technique. Lenz and others recognized the retrospective character of the study as a significant limitation.

The findings from the survey are consistent with the Lenz model of search behavior. Associations between identified variables of the search episodes are all highly significant using either Cramer's V, Pearson's product–moment correlation coefficient, or Kendall's tau. Some of the variables strongly associated include the type of stimulus and the extent of search (Cramer's V = 0.40, $p < 0.001$), the time allotted and the extent of search (Kendall's tau = 0.16, $p < 0.001$), the extent of search and the amount of information acquired (Pearson's product–moment correlation coefficient = 0.32, $p < 0.001$), and the amount of information acquired and level of satisfaction (Kendall's tau = –0.09, $p < 0.003$).

Lenz's results were consistent with other findings about search reported in the consumer literature. An interesting finding of significance to health-care providers was the fact that subjects (newcomers to the community) began their search before their actual need for services. This finding may be a result of the sample characteristics: high socioeconomic status, more than 50% of the heads of households were professionals, owners, managers, or proprietors, more than 89% were headed by people younger than 45 years of age, and 60% of the households included children. The findings might be related to some unknown behavioral attributes, such as internal versus external locus of control. Finally, some combination of factors may be at work here. Such potential biases are important if one uses this model to design health-related information sources to target groups appropriately and efficiently.

Behrmann-Hitzig[26] used the Lenz model in her exploratory, qualitative study designed to investigate subjects' reported search process prior to making decisions concerning elective surgery. The study sample included 20 males and females interviewed postoperatively about their search activities preceding their decision to undergo elective surgery. The types of surgeries included back ($n = 4$), knee ($n = 7$), cholecystectomies ($n = 4$), hysterectomies ($n = 4$), and prostatectomy ($n = 1$). Her study aimed to:

(1) describe the process of seeking and acquiring information which was instrumental to determine the health care consumer's decision to undergo hospitalization for elective surgery; (2) clarify the nature of relationships among its [sic] variable dimensions (specifically, sociodemographic, experiential, and contextual variables); (3) compare perceived needs with actual needs for information in order to determine the degree to which information seeking was misguided or on target; (4) describe problems and barriers surrounding the health care consumer's information search and acquisition activities; and (5) explore the nature of relationships between the search process and patients' perceptions of the outcomes.[26,p15]

Behrmann-Hitzig[26] developed a semistructured interview guide that contained items paralleling Lenz's model. The interviewer asked respondents to describe the search process, identify individuals from whom they sought information prior to decision making, describe past experiences that may have influenced either search or decisions, barriers to search, and outcomes of the search process.

Two findings of interest are summarized. First, individuals generally regarded obtaining information from second or third opinions as undesirable. The author suggests that the condition of the subject (i.e., one in which the subject was faced with an acute illness, may account for this finding). This finding is supported by the work of Ende et al.[15] Findings from his work suggest that severity of illness may influence the search process and desire to participate in decision making. His work is discussed in greater detail in another section. Although this finding reported by Behrmann-Hitzig is inconsistent with that reported by Lenz, it should be noted that Lenz studied well individuals seeking information about health-care providers for potential use at some future time.

Second, Behrmann-Hitzig[26] observed that "much of the consumer's process of search was predetermined by his physician's plan of care and most of the process was not conceptualized . . . nor was it within his immediate realm of awareness." This finding suggests limited input by the consumer into the information search process. One explanation accounting for this observation may be the nature of the illness. Options for the elective surgeries for which these consumers sought care are relatively standard. Therefore, once a decision was made to intervene surgically, need for additional search may not be perceived as necessary. Other sociodemographic and contextual variables, such as age, race, culture, time from symptom onset to decision to intervene, perceived severity of condition, and provider–patient relationship, may influence this finding.

Although her data do not fully support all the premises of the Lenz model, Behrmann-Hitzig concluded that the Lenz model accurately represents an individual's search behavior. The study has the following limitations: small sample size, retrospective nature of the interviews, qualitative design posing potential threats to validity and reliability, and study subjects who were hospitalized at the time of interview. The author acknowledges these limitations. Even with the stated limitations, the exploratory work of Behrmann-Hitzig advances the utility of the Lenz model as a realistic framework for studying consumer health-care search behavior.

In summary, the Lenz model is an interesting and useful conceptualization of the information search process. Her initial research documents that people carry out the search process in an organized fashion that approximates the proposed model. Lenz initially asserted that further research was needed to validate this approach in other settings and with other samples.* Identification of both demographic and psychosocial

---

*According to Lenz (personal communication, 1994), the work of Behrmann-Hitzig is the only research that she is aware of focusing specifically on testing the model.

behavioral attributes that contribute to the search process is needed to determine variation in search patterns within groups exposed to different situations. Future work
should include development of an instrument derived from the model designed to measure these variables. This model has the potential to be applied in many settings and
with diverse populations for the purpose of providing health education and illness prevention.

Miller Behavioral Style Scale (MBSS)

Individuals cope with life experiences in a variety of ways. Use of defense mechanism,
(e.g., denial) may protect and provide the person with time to adjust to stressful events
with which he or she is faced. Coping with new situations is influenced by an individual's past experiences, choice of defense mechanisms, and successful outcomes from
previous exposure to stressful events. Information has been suggested by some as a
means of coping with these stressful events. Personality psychologists have long de-
bated the question of whether individuals exhibit consistent and stable differences in
their abilities and inclinations either to seek information or to distract themselves under
stress.[27] Recognition of the complexity of information-search behavior has forced researchers to address not only information-seeking activities but also the psychologic
and behavioral profile of consumers to meet their needs better. The following discussion describes the development and use of an instrument designed to categorize individuals according to their preference for information under hypothesized stressful
situations.

Miller and Grant described the development of a scale designed to classify people in
terms of their preference for information in a stressful situation.[28] They conceptualize informational preferences under threat as a coping style or dimension. This style catego-
rizes people into monitors (information seekers) or blunters (distractors) on the basis of
their choice to deal with a threatening situation. Monitoring involves being alert for and
sensitized to the negative aspects of an event. Blunting involves distraction from and
cognitive avoidance of objective sources of danger.[4] Miller et al. have conducted considerable research designed to determine when an individual employs a certain coping
style and when and if it is stress reducing. They have demonstrated that the effectiveness with which people cope with stressful situations is determined by their coping style
and by the fit of their preferred strategy to the specific properties of the situation.[4]

Miller developed a self-report scale, the Miller Behavioral Style Scale (MBSS), an
instrument designed to measure informational preferences. This scale was not initially
developed for use in health-care situations. Specifically, the scale describes four vignettes that represent potentially stress-producing events. Each vignette has eight statements that describe different ways in which an individual might respond. Four of the
statements are monitoring responses and four are blunting responses. The following is
an example of one vignette.[4]

> Vividly imagine that you are on an airplane. Thirty minutes from your destination the
> plane unexpectedly goes into a nose dive and then suddenly levels off. The pilot an-
> nounces that everything is okay, although the rest of the ride may be rough. You are not,
> however, convinced that all is well.[4]

An example of a monitoring response is, "I would listen carefully to the engines for
unusual noises and would watch the crew to see if their behavior was out of the ordinary." An example of a blunting response would be, "I would watch the end of the
movie even if I had seen it before."

Subjects are instructed to check statements that best describe behaviors they are likely to use in a stressful situation. Two methods of scoring the MBSS have been described. The first method involves summing the number of positive responses to the "monitor" items and subtracting the sum number of positive responses to the "blunting" items.[29] This method yields a single score ranging from –20 to 20. A negative score suggests a tendency to avoid information. The second method of scoring uses separate monitor and blunter scores. Higher scores on each scale indicates more of the behavior being measured.[29] Test–retest reliability across a 4-month period has been reported for the monitor and blunter scales ($r = 0.72$ and $r = 0.75$, respectively).

The MBSS has been shown to predict preference for information versus distraction in response to threatening situations.[4] Chorney et al.[30] have used the instrument in an experimental setting to determine how monitors and blunters perform on a cold pressor task. (The cold pressor task subjectively measures an individual's tolerance level and pain threshold of the extremities to temperature.) A sample of 92 male undergraduate psychology students volunteered for this study. Monitors performed better when the experimental strategy encouraged monitoring, and blunters did better when the situation was compatible with blunting. Their results confirm those of other studies that report the importance of matching an individual's cognitive strategies with his or her coping styles. They conclude that the MBSS "appears to provide a useful, straightforward measure of an important coping style, one which here and elsewhere has been shown to predict performance differences in stress situations."[30,p7]

Miller has used the MBSS with people faced with a short-term aversive stimulus, such as a gynecologic examination, and those faced with a chronic disease, such as cancer or hypertension. She found that blunters who received a lot of information actually reported an increase in anxiety prior to colposcopy. Monitors did not report an increase in anxiety in the same situation. The investigators concluded that this increase in anxiety exhibited by the blunters was a result of receipt of information counter to their preferences.

Barsevick and Johnson[31] examined the information-seeking behaviors of 36 women undergoing colposcopy, a stressful medical procedure. The specific aims of their study were to examine the relationship between (1) preference for information and information-seeking behavior during colposcopy; (2) preference for behavioral involvement and information-seeking behavior during colposcopy; and (3) information-seeking behavior and positive and negative emotional responses during colposcopy.[31,p2]

The MBSS and Krantz Health Opinion Survey (KHOS) were the primary instruments used by the investigators. They observed that women who ask questions or request written information do not always have characteristic preferences for information or involvement in health care.[31,p6] The authors found no significant relationship between scores on the MBSS and the number of questions asked by women undergoing colposcopy or their request for an information sheet. They reported a low correlation between the MBSS and KHOS ($r(36) = 0.33, p < 0.05$). The authors suggested that according to the findings, the MBSS is not a sensitive indicator of preference for information and involvement in health-care situations.[31,p6]

Although the MBSS has been used in a number of research situations, its clinical utility is unclear. Use of hypothetical vignettes and a lengthy administration time may make it cumbersome for routine use. However, the contribution of this work is significant. It has provided a means for eliciting individual's information preferences under stress. Development of a more clinically oriented and facile instrument that incorporates the concepts of monitors and blunters seems warranted. Research is needed that expands and refines this work.

Information Styles Questionnaire (ISQ)

Cassileth et al. developed the Information Styles Questionnaire (ISQ).[6] This instrument is a self-report tool designed to ascertain the preferences of cancer patients for information about their disease and their desire to participate actively in their treatment. The questionnaire has six sections; five contain individual questions designed to obtain general data about desire for information and preference for involvement in self-care. For example, in one of the questions respondents choose from five possible response options that describe their preference for information. These options range from 1 (no more details than needed) to 5 (as many details as possible). Another question asks the person whether he or she desires other information; if the answer is yes, the person is asked to explain. The patient is asked to choose from the following statements the one that best describes his or her point of view:

"I prefer to leave decisions about my medical care and treatment up to my doctor" and "I prefer to participate in decisions about my medical care and treatment." An additional question asks the person to select one of the following statements: "I only want the information needed to care for myself"; "I want additional information only if it is good news"; "I want as much information as possible, good or bad." The sixth section contains a list of 12 items designed to elicit specific types of information needed on a scale from "absolutely need," "would like to have," to "do you want" the information. A sample of the statements used to elicit specific information follows: what all the possible side effects are; what treatment will accomplish; whether or not it is cancer; what the likelihood of cure is.

The instrument was pilot-tested with 50 people, and the items "were shown to use wording that patients found meaningful and comprehensible and were able to discriminate among patients' viewpoints."[6,p832] The issues of instrument validity and reliability were not addressed. In addition, no specific information described the development of the instrument or the rationale for item choice.

Subsequently, the ISQ has been used with 256 cancer patients from a major urban medical center[6] and 109 cancer patients from a small community hospital. Fitzpatrick compared the frequencies of information styles and participation preferences between his sample[32] and that of Cassileth et al.[6] In general, the results appear similar in both groups; however, no statistical tests were performed to determine whether significant differences existed between the responses of the two groups.[32] As the issues of validity and reliability of the instrument were not addressed, it would have been useful to compare the two groups.

Fitzpatrick[32] stated that the results of his research essentially replicate those of Cassileth et al.[6] This statement is significant, as Cassileth et al. observed that a potential source of bias was the setting from which the patients came. Unfortunately, no detailed demographic comparison was made between the two groups. Such a comparison might have provided some clues concerning the magnitude of potential bias. Fitzpatrick indicated that demographic variables may, in fact, account for some of the observed differences. Issues of the validity and reliability of the ISQ should be addressed. The instrument should be compared with other scales to determine its discriminant validity. Further, testing of the ISQ with other samples, comparing specific demographic, psychologic, and sociologic variables, will contribute to establishing the instrument's reliability.

The ISQ appears to be a comprehensive instrument designed to elicit many aspects of information preferences. Its clinical utility lies in its structure. The ISQ can be used relatively easily and yields useful information.

Krantz Health Opinion Survey (HOS)

Krantz et al. developed the Krantz Health Opinion Survey (HOS) to measure preference for health-care information, self-treatment, and active involvement in health care. The instrument has two subscales, one measuring information preference and the second measuring the degree of behavioral involvement.[33] The original instrument consisted of 40 items that addressed the issues of how informed a person wants to be and how active a role he or she desires to play in his or her health care.

Krantz et al.[33] reported that extensive testing was undertaken to determine the instrument's validity and reliability. The initial 40-item instrument was pilot-tested on 200 undergraduate students. Fourteen items were eliminated because they had a correlation of less than 0.20 with the total score or because they had a narrow distribution of response alternatives. The 26 items were retested with a sample of 159 undergraduates. Factor analysis was used to identify components of the instrument and yielded two subscales. The 10 items not correlating with these two subscales were eliminated. The two subscales are the Information Subscale (I-Scale) and the Behavior Involvement Subscale (B-Scale). The I-Scale contains seven items measuring desire to ask questions and wanting to be informed about medical decisions. The following is an example of a statement found on the I-Scale:[33] "I usually don't ask the doctor or nurse many questions about what they're doing during a medical examination."

The B-Scale contains nine items that measure attitudes toward self-treatment and active behavioral involvement of patients with their care. The following is an example of the statements found on the B-Scale:[33] "Clinics and hospitals are good places to go for help, since it's best for medical experts to take responsibility for health care." The scale then yields a total score, which is a composite of the two subscales, and individual I-Scale and B-Scale scores. The binary, agree–disagree format was designed so that high scores represent positive attitudes toward self-directed or informed treatment.[33,p980]

Discriminant validity was established by administering the HOS in conjunction with the Crowne-Marlowe Social Desirability Scale and the Health LOC Scale to a Sample of 100 male and 100 female undergraduates. A second sample consisted of 38 undergraduates who received the HOS and the Minnesota Multiphasic Personality Inventory (MMPI) Hypochondriac Scale. A third sample ($n = 87$) received the HOS and the Ullman Repression-Sensitization (R-S) Scale. A fourth sample ($n = 87$) received the HOS and the Ullman Repression-Sensitization (R-S) Scale. A fifth sample ($n = 80$) received the HOS two times during a 7-week interval to determine test–retest reliability.[33]

Application of the KR 20 test strongly confirmed the reliability of the HOS Scale and its component subscales (KR = 0.77). The authors remark that females in general tended to score higher than males on all parts of the HOS Scale. The authors do not discuss the possible significance of this finding.

The B-Scale and I-Scale were not correlated significantly with one another. The HOS and the Wallston Health Locus of Control Scale had a correlation of 0.31, and the correlations were 0.26 and 0.23 for the B-Scale and I-Scale, respectively. The authors suggest that these low correlations indicate that the two subscales are probably measuring relatively independent processes. The HOS does not show significant correlations with the R-S, the MMPI, and the Crowne-Marlowe Social Desirability Scale.

Additional studies were conducted to establish predictive, construct, and discriminant validity of the HOS. For these studies, Krantz et al. administered the HOS to a sample of 149 students, including 56 randomly selected residents of a college residence hall, 81 students reporting to a college infirmary for routine treatment of minor illnesses, and 12 students enrolled in a medical self-help course at the same school.[32] It was predicted that the criterion group, the students attending a medical self-help course, would score higher on the behavioral involvement, information, and total scores of the HOS as their involvement in such a course was believed to demonstrate greater interest in obtaining information about health.

The scores of the self-help and clinic samples were compared to those of the residence hall students using one-way analyses of variance and Dunnett's t-test. One-tailed tests were used, as directional predictions were specified. The total HOS scores and the B-Scale scores were higher for the self-help group than for the residence hall group and significant at the $p < 0.005$ level. The clinic users did not differ on the total HOS score or the I-Scale but were significantly lower on the B-Scale ($p < 0.05$). Krantz et al. established discriminant validity of the instrument in its ability to predict correctly the differences between the criterion group of high-self-care students and the general population and in the fact that the low B-Scale scores were correlated with high use of clinic facilities.

The authors reported on three studies designed to established reliability and validity of the HOS Scale. They noted that the scale is predictive of behaviors that relate to seeking routine medical care for minor illnesses that require short-term interventions. It has not been established whether the instrument is valid or reliable in predicting illness-seeking behavior in long-term chronic or traumatic illness. Results of these studies suggest that people who prefer to be more active in their own health care are more likely to care for themselves when faced with a minor illness than to seek care from a physician.

Further testing is required to ensure the validity and predictive potential of the HOS. Since its initial design, the HOS has been used in several other settings. Auerbach et al. used the scale with 40 patients scheduled for dental surgery.[34] The study attempted to provide construct validation data for the I-Scale of the HOS. The study subjects were asked to complete several measures in conjunction with the HOS (e.g., Rotter Internal Locus of Control Scale and Corah Dental Anxiety Scale). The results demonstrated that the HOS subscales are positively correlated with the total HOS scales (I-Scale = 0.73, p = 0.0001; B-Scale = 0.63, p = 0.0001), but the subscales are not related to each other or to other scales. These results are consistent with those described by Krantz et al.[33]

The appeal of the Krantz HOS instrument is its brevity, ease of scoring, and bidimensional approach in identifying a person's desire for information and relevant behavioral components. This instrument has clinical utility and could be used in a variety of settings and with different populations as part of an initial assessment. A possible limitation of this scale, recognized by the authors, is that items on the scale are related to routine aspects of medical care; the instrument has not been used in situations where the illness is traumatic, severe, or chronic. The authors recommend that, in future use of the scale, revisions may be necessary to clarify meanings and eliminate redundancy.[33]

Beisecker Desire for Medical Information and Locus of Authority in Medical Decision-Making Scales

Beisecker and Beisecker's instrument development and research is designed to expand what is known about patient's information-seeking behaviors relative to independent health-care decision making.[14] The research sought to distinguish between patient's desire for information and whether after receiving that information, the patient actually wants to use it to make independent health-care decisions. Beisecker developed the Desire for Medical Information and Locus of Authority in Medical Decision-making scales to collect data that would answer the following research questions:[14] (1) To what extent do patients desire information from physicians?; (2) To what extent do patients feel they should make medical decisions in areas in which they desire more information?; (3) To what extent do patients engage in information-seeking communication behaviors during medical encounters?; and (4) What factors influence or explain patient information-seeking behaviors during medical encounters?[14,p20]

The two scales were initially developed to be used to assess medical rehabilitative patients' desire for medical information and to ascertain their inclination actually to participate in personal medical decision making.[14-35] The scales have subsequently been revised and used in decision making by physicians, nurses, and patients who responded to a hypothetical vignette describing a woman newly diagnosed with breast cancer. The only difference in the instruments was that the professionals were asked to respond to the situation as if the vignette represented a patient and the patient responded as if she had been diagnosed with breast cancer. The following discussion focuses on the development and testing of the "Desire for Medical Information" and "Locus of Authority in Medical Decision-Making" scales.

Each scale contains 13 parallel items. The items on one scale are designed to elicit how important an individual believes it is to have information about a certain area (Desire for Medical Information Scale). The companion scale is designed to elicit who the individual believes should have the major responsibility for decision making in that same area (Locus of Authority in Medical Decision-Making Scale). This design was used to facilitate separation of items related to search from those related to assuming responsibility for actually making independent decisions. Sum scores were calculated for each scale and mean scores compared.

No validity information is provided. For a sample of 106 rehabilitative medicine patients, Cronbach's alpha coefficient for the Desire for Information scale was 0.86 and 0.73 for the Locus of Authority Scale. No Cronbach alpha coefficients are reported for the revised scales.

The instruments were initially used to study information search behaviors of a sample of rehabilitative medicine patients. The authors sought to identify variables that may influence a person's information-seeking behaviors. Such variables may include age, gender, race, marital status, education, income, medical condition, and prior experience with physician. Patients were in varying stages of rehabilitation, were seeking care for significantly different reasons, and approximately 60% of patients were being seen at the center for the first time. Tape-recorded interviews were obtained during each patient–physician interaction. The Desire for Information and Locus of Authority scales were mailed to the 125 subjects 10 days to 2 weeks after the tape-recorded interviews. Of the 125 opinion surveys mailed, 106 were returned for a response rate of 84.8%.

All patients in the study were observed to have an overwhelming desire for information. The mean score on the Desire for Information Scale was 64.9, mode 70 (range 14 to 70). The higher the score, the more information desired. Respondents indicated that, although they desired a lot of information, they preferred to have the physician make the decisions. For the Locus of Authority Scale, a low score indicates preference for physician decision-making authority. A score of 13 indicates equal authority between physician and patient, and a score of 26 indicates maximum decision-making authority assumed by the patient. A mean score of 8.6 and a mode of 9.0 were reported suggesting a strong belief by the respondents that primary decision making should be assumed by the physician.

Attitude measures did not predict observed or taped communication behaviors. Furthermore, the subjects did not exhibit consumerist type of behaviors during the taped physician–patient interactions. However, situational variables were observed to be significant predictors of increased patient communication. These variables included length of time of patient–physician interaction, diagnosis of muscular dystrophy, presence of companion, and whether this was an initial visit.

The study also examined the relationship of the respondent's age and desire for information and participation in decision making. No statistically significant differences were observed for desire for information by age. However, a significant inverse relationship was observed between age and desire to participate in medical decision-making.

Beisecker[36] studied 110 practicing oncologists, 115 oncology nurses, and 288 female non-breast-cancer patients. The purpose of the study was "to assess attitudes toward patient input in medical decisions for breast cancer."[36,p506] The Locus of Authority scale was adapted to refer to a diagnosis of breast cancer. Physicians and nurses were given a patient scenario that described either a 40-, 60-, or 75-year-old patient presenting with a probable diagnosis of breast cancer. Patients were instructed to answer the items as if they had a diagnosis of breast cancer. Although the use of scenarios has limitations, it is a generally well-accepted research method. The instrument is a self-administered scale with 15 items that refer to typical decisions made during the course of therapy for breast cancer. Some examples of statements on the scale include whether to seek further treatment, available alternatives, type of therapy, specific treatment decisions, family involvement, and second/alternative opinions. The respondents were asked to indicate whether only the physician, the physician and patient, or only the patient should make the decision. Responses were coded a 0 (physician), 1 (both), and 2 (patient). The score range for the 15 items was 0 to 30. Low scores indicated more physician decision making, and higher scores indicated more patient responsibility for decision making.

Mean physician score was 10.23; mean nurse score was 13.79; and, mean patient score was 12.49. Each score was significantly below the midpoint of 15, suggesting a belief that greater decision-making authority belongs with the physician. These findings are consistent with earlier work of the author and with those from other studies.[8,15,37]

The scales developed by Beisecker are being refined and offer researchers an instrument that is easy to use, one that can be used with physicians, nurses, and patients and provides a measure of desire to participate in the decision-making process. The ability to discriminate between desire for information and actual participation in the process is essential. The two scales developed by Beisecker attempt to do just that. Continued use of the scales with different patient populations should enhance the reliability of the instrument.[14]

Degner: Preference to Participate in Treatment Decisions

This section reports on two studies conducted by Degner and colleagues. The first study investigated roles that cancer patients might desire to play in treatment decisions.[8] The second study compared patients' preference for treatment control between a sample of actual cancer patients and a sample of the general public given a hypothetical diagnosis of cancer.[13]

Initially, a field study was conducted to elicit how decisions were made by patients with life-threatening illnesses. Four patterns of control over decision-making emerged. These patterns include:

1. *Provider-controlled decision making.* Health personnel have final control over the design of treatment, and the patient and family are involved to varying degrees in the actual implementation of treatment.

2. *Patient-controlled decision making*. The patient exercises final control over the type of treatment received.
3. *Family-controlled decision making*. The family has final control over what treatment the patient receives.
4. *Jointly controlled decision making*. Control over the design of therapy is shared by one or more of the participants in decision making.[8,p368]

The preliminary work led Degner and Russell[8] to hypothesize that people with cancer have preferences about keeping, sharing, or giving away control over treatment decisions that can be measured along a continuum. They also were interested in finding out to whom cancer patients would delegate decision-making authority, a physician or family member. Therefore, they designed a study to answer the following research question: "Do patients facing life-threatening illness such as cancer have preexisting preferences about the roles they might play in treatment decision-making?"[8,p368]

Eight vignettes were developed that described varying degrees of control over treatment decisions. The vignettes were reviewed for clarity by four oncology nurses and four oncology physicians. They were then tested on 10 patients and revised.

Sixty adult cancer patients were selected from two oncology clinics. Clinic staff were asked to identify patients that could be classified as keepers, sharers, and givers of decision-making authority. Twenty subjects were identified for each category. Subjects were equally divided by age (39 years of age or younger and 40 years of age and older).

Two alternatives for decision control were chosen from the four patterns identified from the field study. Physician and family were chosen as alternatives for decision-making authority. Four vignettes per each alternative were used. Patient preferences were elicited by having subjects examine each of the sample vignettes in pairs. For example, vignette A and B were examined against each other, one was selected as preferred, and placed on top of the other. A third card was selected and examined against the vignette that had previously been placed on top. Priority of preference was again determined. This process was continued until a preference sequence was achieved for each of the four vignettes within the two alternatives.

Degner and Russell[8] reported that most patients preferred a pattern of shared control. Patients also reported a preference for giving control to a physician rather than a family member. The authors cite the following study limitations: patients sampled were at varying points along the disease trajectory; females with breast cancer were overrepresented and lung and bowel cancers were underrepresented in the sample compared to the population of adults with cancer. Therefore, generalization of the findings is limited to the study sample.[8]

Degner and Sloan[13] conducted companion studies designed to determine "the prevalence of differing preferences about roles in treatment decision making in the context of cancer, whether these preferences differed when people anticipate having cancer versus are actually diagnosed with cancer, and which demographic and disease treatment factors were the most important predictors of these preferences."[13p,942] The authors also were interested in determining whether illness distress affected preference in treatment decisions. The symptom distress scale was the instrument used to assess the subject's degree of perceived distress.

Degner and Sloan surveyed 436 newly diagnosed cancer patients and 482 members of the general public (householders) in the Canadian province of Manitoba between January and June 1988.[13] A card-sorting method, revised as a result of findings from the previous study, was used to determine preferences in decision-making participation. There were two alternative sets, a patient–physician and a family–physician dimension. Each set consisted of five cards. Each card depicted a different role in decision making and an illustrative cartoon. The method used with the study subjects to determine preference was the same as that used in the study conducted in 1988 by the researchers, as described.

Differences in preferences were observed between patients with a diagnosis of cancer and householders. Fifty-nine percent of newly diagnosed cancer patients preferred that physicians assume responsibility for treatment decisions. The most common choice selected by cancer patient's was that physician should consider patient's opinion. Sixty-four percent of householders reported that they would want to play an active role in treatment decisions. Both groups reported a desire for physician and family to share decision making if they became too ill. This finding suggests that distress from a diagnosis of cancer may influence the desire to participate in treatment decisions. Older subjects in both groups reported wanting less control in treatment decision making. Differences between groups on education and gender variables were observed. Among the cancer patient group being more highly educated and female was associated with a preference for more control in treatment decision making. This finding was not observed among the householders.

The work of Degner and Russell[8] provides additional insight into the roles that patients diagnosed with a potentially life-threatening illness, such as cancer, desire to play in making treatment decisions. These findings are consistent with those from other studies that suggest that relationships exist between age,[35] distress of illness,[15,17,26,31] and gender and desire for control over decision making.

A limitation to this work lies in its clinical utility. The methods employed in the two studies by Degner et al. are cumbersome and time-consuming. However, this work lays the groundwork for developing a more standardized approach to patient assessment in the area of preferences for control in treatment decision making. Degner et al. also assert that because only a small percent of the variance in preferences was accounted for by sociodemographic variables, individual assessment of patients' preferences might be the preferred approach. Additional research is needed to refine and/or identify new approaches for eliciting patient preferences in treatment decisions.

Autonomy Preference Index (API)

Ende and colleagues[15] developed the Autonomy Preference Index (API) to measure "patients' preferences for two identified dimensions of patient autonomy: decision-making and the acquisition of information."[15,p23] Ende et al. observed that increased attention has been given to the provision of information to patients to facilitate independent health-care decisions. However, they note that little research has focused on whether patients actually desire to make the decisions once they have accumulated information. These observations are consistent with those made by Beisecker.[14,35] Therefore, determining why patients want information and what they actually do with it once they obtain it seem to be fertile areas for research.

The API, a 23-item questionnaire was developed using a modified Delphi technique that involved the use of 13 experts interested in patient autonomy. The experts represented medicine, sociology, and ethics. Two dimensions emerged from this process. The dimensions were patients' preferences for making decisions and patients' desire for information. The Decision-Making Preference Scale consists of 15 items, 6 of which are general and 9 of which are related to 1 of 3 clinical vignettes. Each vignette describes a clinical condition representing increasing illness severity (mild upper respiratory tract illness; moderate hypertension; and severe myocardial infarction). The Information Seeking Scale consists of eight items.

Content validity was established by field-testing and reviewing the items with patients. "Each item was then discarded, modified and retested, or retained based on feedback from patients, the item's ability to discriminate among patients, and its reliability."[15,p23] Concurrent and convergent criterion validity of the decision-making scale were established. Concurrent validity of the decision-making scale was tested by asking the respondent to choose one of five statements that best described their attitude toward medical care. The statements ranged from "patient should have complete control" to "doctor should have complete control." Patients' responses to this item correlated with the decision-making scores ($r = 0.54$, $p < 0.0001$).

Criterion validity was assessed by administering part of the instrument to a "highly" motivated group of diabetics who were adept at self-care. The authors assumed that diabetic patients possessing these characteristics would be a good comparison group with the study sample. The diabetic population scored higher on the decision-making scale than the study population ($p < 0.1$). It is suggested that the assertion that criterion validity was established should be interpreted cautiously because no attempt was made to validate the "highly" motivated characteristics of the diabetics. No validity testing was conducted on the information-seeking scale.

Instrument reliability was established through test–retest on a sample of 50 patients. Test–retest reliability scores for the decision-making scale and for the information-seeking scale were computed. Pearson's product–moment correlation was 0.84 and 0.83, respectively. Cronbach's alpha coefficient was 0.82 for each scale.

Administration of the questionnaire takes approximately 10 minutes. Each scale is scored separately. The range of scores is from 0 (very low) to 100 (very high) preference for either decision making or information seeking. The vignettes are scored on a scale of 0 to 10, where 0 represented no desire to participate in decision making, 5 represented a desire to participate that was equal to the physician's, and 10 equaled patient desire for complete control. This approach to determining the amount of decision making desired by patients is similar to that reported by Beisecker. The scores from each of the scales can be correlated with demographic variables.

Ende et al. report the findings from their research that was designed to answer the following questions:[15,p23] (1) To what extent do patients prefer to take an active role in their own care?; (2) What patient characteristics influence these preferences?; and (3) How are these preferences affected by varying disease severity?

The authors approached 803 randomly selected general medical clinic patients for inclusion in the study. Thirty-nine percent (312 patients) agreed to participate. Comparisons were made among refusers and nonrefusers on selected demographic variables to determine whether significant differences existed between these groups. No significant differences were observed. In addition, a random selection of refusers was mailed a copy of the API with a response rate of 45%. No significant differences were observed on mean decision-making and information-seeking scores between the study participants and the refusers who returned the questionnaire. Therefore, the authors believe that they had a representative sample.

No correlation was observed between patients' desire for information and their preferences for decision making. Findings from their study suggest that, in general, patients do not want to participate in medical decision making. An inverse relationship between desire to participate and severity of illness was observed. Seventy-five percent of patients reported a preference for making decisions during a minor illness (upper respiratory infection), whereas the remaining 25% reported a preference for making decisions during a major illness (high blood pressure or myocardial infarction). A positive relationship was observed between being younger and higher educational level and preference for decision making ($p = 0.001$ and $p = 0.05$, respectively). A negative relationship was observed between marital status (e.g., separated or divorced) and skilled or semiskilled occupation and medical decision making ($p = 0.10$ [level of significance set at 0.15]).

Only younger age and higher education were positively correlated with information seeking. Of particular interest is that in regression models for both scales, less than 20% of the variance was accounted for. This finding alone has significant importance for future research in this area, as well as for the clinical application of the findings. Clearly, a lot is still unknown concerning patients' desire for information and participation in decision making. The authors correctly point out that, although approaches to ascertaining individual preferences can be standardized to a point, there remains a large degree of individual variance that can be addressed only by assessing these preferences at the time of the physician–patient encounter.

Ende and colleagues[38] sought to explore additional reasons why patients may desire information but choose not to take an active role in health-care decisions. They hypothesized that, although sociodemographic variables and role disparity between physicians and patients may influence these preferences, the role of being a patient may override these reasons in influencing behavior. Therefore, the authors designed a study that sought to answer the following research questions:[38] (1) When physicians are patients, how involved in decision making do they prefer to be?; (2) To what extent are their preferences affected by the severity of illness?; (3) How do their preferences for autonomy compare with those of regular patients?

The sample consisted of 151 physicians. Ninety percent were general internists. A sample of 315 patients was selected from individuals returning to a general medicine outpatient practice. Each subject was asked to complete the 23-item API. The only difference in the scales given to the physicians and patients was that physicians were instructed to answer the questions as if they were a patient.

Both physician patients and nonphysician patients indicated a high preference for information. Interestingly, patients reported a significantly higher preference for information than physicians. Physician patients reported a significantly higher preference to participate in decision making than patients. This difference was observed in response to general desire to participate in decision making and to the three specific vignettes. Of particular interest, however, is that both groups scored less than 50 on the general decision-making scale and less than 5 on each item from the vignettes. These findings indicate that both groups prefer decisions to be made by the provider. The desire to participate in decision making decreased with the severity of illness for both the physician patients and the patients. These findings are consistent with the authors' results in earlier work.[15]

Ende and colleagues[38] contributed significantly to the body of knowledge concerning individuals' preferences for information and desire for participation in decisions. In addition, their findings suggest that "patient role" and severity of illness are significant variables influencing desire to participate in medical care decisions. This work needs to be expanded, particularly with disenfranchised populations (e.g., minorities, the poor, and the elderly).

Summary

This chapter has presented a review of the literature on consumer and health-care information-seeking behaviors and decision-making preferences. Instruments developed to measure these concepts have been discussed. This review has revealed a number of patterns. Age, gender, education level, and severity of illness have emerged as significant variables relative to the desire for information and participation in decision making.[15,17,26,31,35] Discrepancies between desire for information and desire for participation in decision making also have been observed in several studies.[8,14,15,17] Significant advancements have been made in understanding the complex nature of information-seeking behaviors and decision-making preferences. However, both Degner and Russell[8] and Ende et al.[15] observed that only about 20% of the variance had been accounted for by sociodemographic variables inserted in models designed to elicit relationships, such as variables and preferences for information seeking and decision making. Both suggest that much remains unknown in this area and that individual assessment at the time of the patient–physician encounter continues to be an important aspect of determining the amount of information desired and preference for participation in decision making.

Several directions emerge for future research in the area of information seeking and decision making. First, refinement of instruments is essential. Adaptation of the instruments to enhance their clinical utility is a high priority. Research using several instruments together will promote the establishment of discriminant validity. Reliability will be enhanced by the use of instruments in different populations. Of particular importance is to use these instruments in samples of minorities, low-income, and other special populations. More research is needed to determine the impact that situational variables, such as severity of illness or setting, have on search and decision-making behaviors. Finally, attempts should be made to determine the predictive ability of these instruments in specific individuals and groups who have similar patterns of search and decision-making preferences. Collaborative research efforts provide one approach to achieve these outcomes.

References

1. Lenz, E.R. Information seeking: A component of client decisions and health behavior. *Adv Nurs Sci*, 1984, 6(3):59-72.

2. Janis, I.L., & Mann, L. *Decision-making: A psychological analysis of conflict, choice and commitment.* New York: The Free Press, 1977.

3. Hopkins, M.B. Information seeking and adaptational outcomes in women receiving chemotherapy for breast cancer. *Cancer Nurs*, 1986, 9(5):256-262.

4. Miller, S.M., Leinbach, A.L., & Brody, D.S. Coping styles in hypertensives: Nature and consequences. *J Consult Clin Psychol*, 1989, 57:333-337.

5. Wallston, K.A., Kaplan, G.D., & Maides, S.A. Development and validation of the health locus of control (HLC) scale. *J Consult Clin Psychol*, 1976, 44(4):580-583.

6. Cassileth, B.R., Zupkis, R.V., Sutton-Smith, K., & March, V. Information and participation preferences among cancer patients. *Ann Intern Med*, 1980, 92(6):832-836.

7. Lazarus, R.S. *Psychological stress and the coping process.* New York: McGraw-Hill, 1966.

8. Degner, L.F., & Russell, C.A. Preferences for treatment control among adults with cancer. *Res Nurs Health*, 1988, 11:367-374.

9. Newman, J.W., & Lockman, B.D. Measuring prepurchase information seeking. *J Consumer Res*, 1975, 2(3):216-220.

10. Kiel, G.C., & Layton, R.A. Dimensions of consumer information seeking behavior. *J Market Res*, 1981, 18:233-236.

11. Fleckenstein, L., Joubert, P., Lawrence, R., et al. Oral contraceptive patient information: A questionnaire study of attitudes, knowledge and preferred information sources. *JAMA*, 1976, 235(13):1331-1336.

12. Faden, R.R., Lewis, C., Becke, C., et al. Disclosure standards and informed consent. *J Health Polit Policy Law*, 1981, 6(2):255-257.

13. Degner, L.F., & Sloan, J.A. Decision-making during serious illness: What role do patients really want to play? *J Clin Epidemiol*, 1992, 45(9):941-950.

14. Beisecker, A.E., & Beisecker, T.D. Patient information seeking behaviors when communicating with doctors. *Med Care*, 1990, 28(1):19-28.

15. Ende, J., Kazis, L., Ash, A., & Moskowitz, M.A. Measuring patients' desire for autonomy: Decision-making and information seeking preferences among medical patients. *J Gen Int Med*, 1989, 4(1): 23-30.

16. Blanchard, C.G., Labrecque, M.S., Ruckdeschel, J.C., & Blanchard, E.B. Information and decision-making preferences of hospitalized adult cancer patients. *Soc Sci Med*, 1988, 27(11):1139-1145.

17. Strull, W.M., Lo, B., & Charles, G. Do patients want to participate in medical decision-making? *JAMA*, 1984, 252(21):2990-2994.

18. Payne, J.W. Task complexity and contingent processing in decision-making: An information search and protocol analysis. *Organiz Behav Hum Perform*, 1976, 16:366-369.

19. Englander, T., & Tyszka, T. Information seeking in open decision situations. *Acta Psychol*, 1980, 45:169-170.

20. Fast, J., Vosburgh, R.E., & Frisbee, W.R. The effects of consumer education on consumer search. *J Consum Affairs*, 1989, 23(1):65-90.

21. Messerli, M.L., Garamendi, C., & Romano, J. Breast cancer: Information as a technique of crisis intervention. *Am J Orthopsychiatr*, 1980, 50(4):728-731.

22. Dodd, M.J., & Mood, D.W. Chemotherapy: Helping patients to know the drugs they are receiving and their possible side effects. *Cancer Nurs*, 1981, 4(4): 311-315.

23. Mills, R.T., & Krantz, D.S. Information, choice, and reactions to stress: A field experiment in a blood bank with laboratory analogue. *J Perspect Soc Psychol*, 1979, 37(4):608-620.

24. Wallston, K.A., Smith, R.A.P., King, J.E., et al. Desire for control and choice of antiemetic treatment for cancer chemotherapy. *West J Nurs Res*, 1991, 13(1): 12-23.

25. Lenz, E.R. Newcomers' search for information about health services. In E. Bowens (Ed.), *Clinical nursing research: Its strategies and findings. II*. Indianapolis: Sigma Theta Tau, 1979, p. 182.

26. Behrmann-Hitzig, H.A. *Patterns of information search and acquisition in the adult health care consumer: An exploratory investigation of an aspect of adult learning*. New York: Teachers College, Columbia University, 1992. UMI Dissertation Services Number 9306281.

27. Miller, S.M. Monitoring and blunting: Validation of a questionnaire to assess styles of information seeking under threat. *J Person Soc Psychol*, 1987, 52(2):345-353.

28. Miller, S.M., & Grant, R.P. The blunting hypothesis: A view of predictability and human stress. In P. Soden, S. Bates, & W. Dockens (Eds.), *Trends in behavior therapy*. New York: Academic, 1979.

29. Miller, S.M., & Mangan, C.E. The interacting effects of information and coping style in adapting to gynecologic stress: Should the doctor tell all? *J Person Soc Psychol*, 1983, 45:223-236.

30. Chorney, R.L., Efran, J.S., Ascher, L.M., & Lukens, M.D. *The performance of monitors and blunters on a cold pressor task*. Paper presented before the Eastern Psychological Association, 1982.

31. Barsevick, A.M., & Johnson, J.E. Preference for information and involvement, information seeking and emotional responses of women undergoing colposcopy. *Res Nurs Health*, 1990, 13:1-7.

32. Fitzpatrick, R.J. *Emotional distress, locus of control, and information preferences among cancer patients*. Unpublished doctoral dissertation, University of Tennessee, Knoxville, 1983.

33. Krantz, D.S., Baum, A., & Wideman, M.V. Assessment of preferences for self-treatment and information in health care. *J Person Soc Psychol*, 1980, 39(5):977-990.

34. Auerbach, S.M., Martelli, M.F., & Mercuri, L.G. Anxiety, information, interpersonal impacts and adjustment to a stressful health care situation. *J Person Soc Psychol*, 1983, 44(6):1284-1296.

35. Beisecker, A.E Aging and the desire for information and input in medical decisions: Patient consumerism in medical encounters. *Gerontologist*, 1988, 28(3):330-335.

36. Beisecker, A.E., Helmig, L., Graham, D., & Moore, W.P., Attitudes of oncologists, oncology nurses and patients from a women's clinic regarding medical decision-making for older and younger breast cancer patients. *Gerontologist*, 1994, 34(4):505-512.

37. Degner, L.F., & Sloan, J.A. Decision-making during serious illness: What role do patients really want to play? *J Clin Epidemiol*, 1992, 45(9):941-950.

38. Ende, J., Kazis, L., Ash, A., & Moskowitz M.A. Preferences for autonomy when patients are physicians. *J Gen Int Med*, 1990, 5(6):506-509.

IV

Instruments for Assessing Clinical Problems

28

Measuring Alterations in Taste and Smell

Roberta Anne Strohl

It has been estimated that over 2 million Americans suffer from some impairment in taste and/or smell. The study and measurements of these disorders have not reflected the frequency of their occurrence. Disturbances in these senses are difficult to measure, and easy-to-use, reliable, and valid tools do not exist. These factors, coupled with the nonlife-threatening nature of taste and smell impairment, have led them to be called "the neglected senses." Although not as debilitating as alterations in sight or hearing, taste and smell abnormalities can contribute to nutritional compromise. People who are unable or unwilling to eat because of the unpleasant tastes of foods may not tolerate the treatment they require. Nutritional compromise may contribute to increased side effects and decreased response to therapy. Particularly in individuals treated with combined modality therapy, the inability to eat may have dire consequences. To discuss the alterations of taste and smell and their measurement, it is necessary to describe the normal taste and smell responses.

Normal Taste Sensation

Ziporyn,[1] Guyton,[2] and Schiffman[3] have extensively reviewed what is known of taste sensation. Adults have approximately 10,000 taste buds located on the tongue, palate, pharynx, tonsils, epiglottis, and in some people in the mucosa of the cheek and lips. Taste buds respond to four primary sensations: sweet, sour, salty, and bitter. Sweet receptors are found on the anterior surface and tip of the tongue, sour and salty on the two lateral sides, and bitter on the circumvallate papillae of the posterior surface. Sour and bitter tastes are perceived most acutely on the palate, whereas salty and sweet tastes are most sensitive on the tongue. Each taste bud is not exclusively sensitive to a single sensation, and all respond in varying proportions to sweet, sour, salty, and bitter. It is believed that a center in the brain detects all the variations of tastes, and the sum of these stimuli produce a distinguishable taste.[1-3]

Sweet taste originates from a mostly organic group of chemicals, including sugars, alcohols, glycol, ketones, and amides, sulfonic acids, and inorganic salts of beryllium and lead. Sour taste results from acids, and salty taste results from ionized salts. Bitter taste is caused by organic substances, such as alkaloids and long-chain acids. Intense bitter taste is objectionable, often a protective mechanism, as many poisons have a bitter taste.

Taste buds consist of both gustatory receptor cells and supporting cells. Each taste bud consists of approximately 48 cells. The life span of a taste cell is about 10 days. Cell renewal is made possible by mitotic division in the surrounding epithelium. At the center of each taste bud is a taste pore. Microvilli or taste hairs protrude from the surface of the taste cells and are believed to form the receptor surface for taste. The containerlike structure of the taste bud provides a minute cup for solutions to be tasted, allowing substances to mix with saliva for tasting. Taste nerve fibers, stimulated by the taste buds, are located in the taste cells.[1-3]

When a substance in solution comes in contact with a taste bud, the taste response is initiated. Functioning as a chemical sieve, the taste bud allows the substance to stimulate the taste nerve. Various physiologic mechanisms change the diameter of a taste pore and alter its permeability, transmitting the stimulus along nerve fibers.[1-3]

Taste impulses from the anterior two-thirds of the tongue pass first into the fifth nerve then through the chorda tympani to the facial nerve and into the tractus solitarius in the brain stem. Sensations from the circumvillate papillae on the back of the tongue and posterior mouth transmit impulses through the glossopharyngeal nerve to a lower level of the tractus solitarius. The vagus nerve transmits taste signals from the base of the tongue and pharynx.[2]

All fibers synapse in the nuclei of the tractus solitarius and send second-order neurons to the thalamus. Third-order neurons transmit the signal to the lower tip of the postcentral gyrus in the parietal cortex; taste is perceived here. Neurons that travel from the pons to the lateral hypothalamus and free endings of the trigeminal nerve in the oral cavity and tongue also participate in the taste response.[2-3]

Normal Smell Sensation

The sense of smell is less well understood. The olfactory membrane is located in the superior part of each nostril and has a surface area of approximately 2.4 cm^2. Olfactory cells are derived from the central nervous system and are specialized bipolar neurons. The olfactory receptor cells renew themselves about every 30 days. Each person has about 100 million olfactory cells. The cells form an olfactory bulb, which terminates in olfactory hairs or cilia and line the mucous coating of the nasal cavity.[1-3]

The primary sensations of smell have not yet been identified although sensations are believed to be analogous to the sweet, sour, bitter, and salty stimuli of taste. The chemical process of olfactory stimulation is unknown, and no general agreement about the basic qualities and classifications of smell exist. Attempts to classify smell have been numerous, starting with Plato, who cited only pleasant and unpleasant smells. Linnaeus, in 1752, reported seven smell classifications: aromatic, fragrant, ambrosial, alliaceous (garlicy), hircine (goaty), repulsive, and nauseous. Currently, it is postulated that separate olfactory cells respond to seven primary smells: camphoraceous, musky, floral, pepperminty, etheral, pungent, and putrid. It is unlikely that this list accurately reflects all the primary smell sensations. There may be as many as 50 primary smell sensations.[1-2]

The means of olfactory cell stimulation is unclear. A substance must be volatile to reach the cells. It also must be somewhat water- and lipid-soluble to pass through the nasal mucus, the olfactory cilia, and the tips of the olfactory cells. Smell occurs in cycles and inspiration is critical for this response. It is believed that olfactory cells respond with a change in membrane potential, much like taste cells, which then stimulates the olfactory nerve. Wave theories propose that smell is triggered by direct stimulation radiating from an odorous source. Steric theories suggest that chemical reactivity occurs when particles of an odorant react with receptor cells.[1-2]

When stimulated, the nerve fibers send the smell response to larger bundles that leave the epithelium through perforations in the cribriform plate. Axons are sent to the olfactory bulb. These terminate in dendrites in the glomerulus, which is located near the bulb's surface. Some of the axons form the olfactory tract, others lead back to tufted cells that return axons to the glomerulus. This circular pathway amplifies the message.[1]

Olfactory nerve fibers terminate in two areas of the brain, the medial and lateral olfactory areas. The medial area, located in the midportion of the brain, is superior and anterior to the hypothalamus. The lateral olfactory area, in the cerebral cortex, consists of the uncus, prepyriform area, the lateral portion of the anterior perforated surface, and part of the amygdaloid nuclei. The lateral area is believed to be responsible for the association of smell with other sensations. Although taste and smell are separate sensations, they are closely related.[2] Loss of the ability to smell during a cold has taught us that the sense of taste also is diminished.

Disorders of Taste and Smell

Given the complexity of taste and smell sensations, it should not be surprising that there are myriad of situations in which taste and smell can be altered. Although it is beyond the scope of this chapter to discuss them all, the terminology used to describe taste and smell abnormalities includes:[3]

Ageusia: absence of taste	Anosmia: absence of smell
Dysgeusia: distortion of normal taste	Dysosmia: distortion of normal smell
Hypergeusia: increased sensitivity of taste	Hyperosmia: increased sensitivity of smell
Hypogeusia: lessened sensitivity of taste	Hyposmia: lessened sensitivity of smell

Schiffman[3] classifies taste and smell disorders into four causal categories: (1) disorders resulting from local atrophy of receptor sites; (2) physical damage to neural projections; (3) surgical or traumatic disturbances of cell renewal by disease, drugs, or radiation; and (4) changes in the receptor cell environment resulting from alterations in saliva or olfactory mucosa (damage due to drugs or environmental pollutants, such as benzene, carbon disulfide, or ethyl acetate). Sensory changes as a result of disease have been studied most extensively, therefore the chapter will focus on that area.

Changes in Taste and Smell Resulting from Disease States

A number of diseases, including renal disease, diabetes, anorexia, cancer, and trauma, are associated with alterations in taste and smell. More work has been done in the area of taste abnormalities than smell abnormalities, partly because of the difficulty in measuring and lack of understanding of the sense of smell. Patients with cancer have been found to report alterations in taste and smell as a result of both the disease and its treatment. As the author's clinical practice is in oncology, this area will be emphasized. A review of the literature reveals that more research in this area is needed and that there is not a singular explanation for the changes in taste and smell reported by persons with cancer. Changes related to cancer, treatment-related factors, and coexisting diseases, are presented in Table 28.1.[4-43] Changes related to aging also are common and include: taste bud epithelial thinning; zinc deficiency due to normal dietary changes and aging process; and decreased vascular supply to taste cells, number of taste buds, overall taste sensations (may improve in edentulous patients if dentures are removed), and sense of smell related to normal changes in olfactory receptors.[44-47]

Although research in both the measurement and etiology of taste and smell disturbances is needed, the complexity of these senses and the numerous ways in which responses can be altered make these difficult to investigate. Some of the currently available testing methods are quite complex, necessitating collaborative research to identify and document clinical changes.

Table 28.1   Changes in Taste and Smell Related to Various Conditions

Nature of Change	Alteration/Explanation	Reference
Cancer		
Lowered bitter threshold	Tumor may secrete substance that stimulates bitter taste buds; results in meat aversion	4-12
Increase in sucrose threshold	Depression of cell renewal by tumor; decrease in taste cell numbers; decrease in stimulus received by taste receptors	4-9, 13-16
Weight loss	Correlates with extent of tumor; taste abnormalities improve as tumor regresses; without tumor response, abnormalities increase	6,7
Increase in salt threshold	Unknown	15
Studies in which no abnormalities found		10
Alteration in smell	Unknown; patients reported unusual smell in chemotherapy and/or radiation clinic	17
Loss of smell and taste in graft vs. host disease	An unusual manifestation of graft vs. host involving the oral cavity	18
Cancer surgery		
Removal of tongue	Loss of sweet and salty receptors	19
Removal of palate	Loss of sour and bitter receptors	19
Laryngectomy	Loss of olfactory component of taste	20
Cancer chemotherapy		
Loss of taste	Stomatitis complicated by infection and coating of tongue alters receptor sites; taste cells with high mitotic index altered by drugs that halt cell growth	21
Metallic taste	Associated with Cytoxan, Vincristine, Methotrexate	21
Food aversions	Conditioned response related to the association of nausea and vomiting with chemotherapy	21,22
Loss of taste in the anterior two-thirds of the tongue in herpes zoster	Involvement of mandibular division of trigeminal nerve	23
Head and neck irradiation		
Damage to microvilli of taste cell	Taste may be partially restored 20–60 days post-treatment and return to normal 60–120 days after treatment	24-29
Loss of saliva and related salivary gland damage		
Profound taste loss	Occurs at dose > 3000 rad (sweet taste may persist longer as there are more sweet taste buds)	
Loss of smell	Related to irradiation of nasal passage and damage to olfactory receptor site	
Some hypogeusia may be permanent		
Diabetes	Taste loss evidenced by higher thresholds for all sensations except sour, which is related to the degree of peripheral neuropathy, particularly autonomic neuropathy involving taste nerve	3,30,31

Table 28.1 *continued*

Nature of Change	Alteration/Explanation	Reference
Renal disease	Hypogeusia due to low zinc levels; persistent generalized unpleasant taste; alteration in cranial nerves related to renal failure; decrease in salivary flow; change in calcium and phosphorus saliva content	32-35
Anorexia	Taste loss related to altered zinc and copper levels	36
Head trauma	Smell alteration related to fracture of cribriform plate, laceration of olfactory nerves, and hemorrhage in frontal lobe; hemorrhage into taste center of brain	37,38
Allergic rhinitis	Higher olfactory thresholds needed. Higher thresholds in patients with nasal polyps and sinusitis related to damage of receptors and decrease in air flow	39
Liver disease	Lower tolerance to bitter taste and decreased appetite; etiology unclear	40
Alcoholism	Decrease smell threshold correlated with MRI indication of decreased cortical sulcus volume	41
Depression	19 of 47 patients reported symptoms of unpleasant taste unrelated to drug use	42
Schizophrenia	A change in the functional integrity of the odor identification pathway via the limbic system to orbitofrontal cortex may be the cause	43

Measurement of Taste

Instrument selection depends on study intent. The instruments described here either document taste changes and aversions for particular foods or food groups or actually record taste and smell thresholds. Many of these instruments are complicated and may require collaborative researcher and clinician efforts.

Documenting Taste Changes

The initial assessment of taste problems should include a brief intake questionnaire. One suggestion based on my clinical experience follows:

> Have you noticed changes in the way food tastes?
> When did you notice this change?
> Have you changed the way you season food? If so, how?
> Have the tastes of any particular foods changed?
> Do any foods taste better than others?
> What foods have you stopped eating and why?
> Are the taste changes constant?

Dobell et al.[48] used a questionnaire to examine and compare the food preferences of 50 renal patients undergoing chronic hemodialysis and continuous ambulatory peritoneal dialysis with age- and sex-matched controls ($n = 30$). Two questionnaires, one assessing food preferences for 88 items and one assessing factors influencing dietary habits were administered. The 88 foods were grouped into 14 classes. Thirty-three patients received hemodialysis, and 17 peritoneal dialysis. Analysis of variance compared groups in terms of food preference and chi-square analysis compared dietary habits. The study determined that sweet foods ($p = 0.002$), vegetables ($p = 0.003$), red meats ($p = 0.010$), and fish and poultry ($p = 0.015$) were more objectionable to patients on dialysis than for controls. Red meats ($p = 0.010$), fish and poultry ($p = 0.032$), and eggs ($p = 0.005$) were less pleasant for patients receiving hemodialysis than peritoneal dialysis. Red meat was the most unpopular food for all dialysis patients. The most common factor affecting dietary intake was a loss of interest in food and/or cooking, perhaps related to fatigue.[48]

Markley et al.[49] placed foods into six categories: breads, fruits, vegetables, meats, milk and dairy, and miscellaneous, including coffee, condiments, and carbonated beverages. Dysgeusia was classified into four alterations in taste: Type I, one food or beverage in any single group; Type II, more than one food or beverage but not all items in a group; Type III, all common items in one group; Type IV, all foods and beverages.

These classifications may be useful to compare weight loss related to taste alterations due to the progression of taste cell loss that occurs with head and neck irradiation. In patients with anorexia nervosa, taste changes can be classified using this approach, and recovery documented as the patient progresses through therapy.

The Radiation Side Effects Profile (RSEP)

In a study of the self-care strategies of patients receiving radiation therapy, Hagopian[50] developed a tool to measure not only the side effects experienced but also the self-care strategies used by patients to reduce the severity of the radiation side effects. One item on the RSEP documents taste changes and related symptoms contributing to loss of appetite or sore throat or mouth. Patients first rate the severity of each symptom on a 4-point scale from 0 (none) to 3 (very bad) and then rate the effectiveness of the self-care strategies used to alleviate the symptom using the scale, from 0 (not at all helpful) to 3 (very helpful). This rating of effectiveness constituted the Helpfulness Index.

A Severity Index indicating the severity of side effects and the helpfulness of self-care measures is determined by summing the scores. Self-care measures were classified into categories, including diet modification in which persons with taste changes indicated self-care measures, such as trying different foods and seasonings and avoiding sweets, as examples of activities.[51]

The summary score for the Severity Index may be of limited usefulness as it includes symptoms other than those related to taste. Test–retest reliability was determined for both the Severity and Helpfulness Index with Pearson's product–moment correlation values obtained at 1-week intervals during the first and second week of treatment and again during the fourth and fifth week of therapy. With 56 subjects, the correlation coefficient between week 1 and week 2 on The Severity Index was 0.59 ($p > 0.001$). In the fourth and fifth week, in 28 subjects, the correlation coefficient was 0.83 ($p > 0.001$). For the Helpfulness Index in week 1 and week 2 the correlation coefficient was 0.46 ($p > 0.0007$). For weeks 4 and 5 it was 0.56 ($p > 0.001$). Content validity was obtained with a physician and clinical nurse expert to determine the representativeness of the side effects. The judges were asked to rate the clinical relevance of side effects on a scale of 1 to 4, 1 (irrelevant) and 4 (extremely relevant). The index of the content validity or proportion of items receiving a 3 or 4 was 0.84. Construct validity was obtained for the Helpfulness Index as well. This tool has been used in other studies to document side effects in persons receiving radiation therapy.[50-52]

Wall and Gabriel Checklist

Wall and Gabriel[15] compared taste alterations in children with leukemia to a group of healthy children. Children with leukemia were oriented to the four taste qualities using posters showing sweet, sour, salty, and bitter food. A checklist of 62 foods commonly eaten by children was used to determine taste preferences. This checklist was pretested with children and their parents in the community. Parents identified what foods the child preferred before the illness and how their choices had changed since diagnosis. Parents of healthy children were given the same checklist of foods. Reliability was determined for the list of preferred foods. Children were asked to respond to three questions: (1) Do you like to eat?; (2) What are your favorite foods?; (3) What foods do you not like? Parents rated each food as 0 dislike, 1 tolerate, and 2 like. For evaluation purposes, the 62 foods were divided into the four basic food groups. Scores were summed for each food group by adding the scores and dividing by the number of foods in the group. Significant differences existed only in the meat group ($p < 0.0125$).

This study is the best controlled investigation of taste changes found in this review. The methods used could be adapted to an adult population to help to determine patterns of food likes and dislikes. Repeating this study during the course of the treatment process should further elucidate patterns of taste changes and their relationships to treatment. Interviewing patients to determine the nature of any taste changes is a logical first step. Although this is subjective, it will identify changes that may significantly influence the child's eating behaviors. Listing foods from all groups may help to cue patients to a pattern in taste alterations.

Documenting Taste Response and Thresholds

Before any taste testing is done an oral cavity exam should be performed to identify other factors that can influence or impede testing, such as candidiasis, stomatitis, xerostomia, herpes zoster, and oral cavity tumors. Although these factors do not preclude testing, they must be noted. The most commonly used technique for documenting taste is the measurement of detection and recognition thresholds. Subjects are presented with two bottles, one of which is water and the other, the substance being tested.[53-55]

Three drops of varying concentrations of the test substance are placed on the subject's tongue (usually approximately 10 concentrations). The subject rinses between tests. The point at which the substance is detected as being different from water is the *detection threshold*. The point at which the substance is recognized as sweet, sour, salty, or bitter is the *recognition threshold*. The recognition threshold usually is at a slightly higher concentration than the detection threshold. Normal subjects generally are used as the comparison group. Subjects are matched by age and should be matched for other factors, such as smoking history. Loss of the recognition threshold is believed to occur as a natural process of aging in both taste and smell, where enough receptors exist to detect a stimulus but not enough to make subtle distinctions.[53]

Schecter et al.[53] used a single-blind study to investigate the effects of zinc sulfate on taste and smell dysfunction. In this trial, subjects were initially given a placebo. If no change in taste or smell occurred, the subject was given oral doses of zinc sulfate, and each subject served as his or her own control. Subjects who improved on placebo were not given zinc. In this study, patients who did not improve with placebo improved with zinc. Reliability and validity information was not presented.

Taste Scale

Henkin et al.[54] developed a scale to document taste activity using the forced-choice three-drop concentration technique. Taste detection and recognition thresholds were assessed. The measurements were transformed to a bottle-unit scale with each concentration designated as a bottle-unit and the change from one concentration to the next a bottle-unit change. Ranges at which normal subjects were able to recognize and detect substances have been determined. Patients who are expected to experience taste loss during therapy, such as those undergoing radiation, may be given the test weekly during therapy to document loss. Recovery after treatment also can be determined in this manner, recalling that it may take 3 to 6 months for taste to recover or that there may be permanent taste loss.

Using the Henkin method Wall and Gabriel[15] found significant differences in detection thresholds for sweet ($p < 0.05$) and salt ($p < 0.05$) and in recognition thresholds for all modalities: sweet ($p < 0.05$), salt ($p < 0.05$), sour ($p < 0.05$), and bitter ($p < 0.05$).

Taste testing by the Henkin method has been criticized as revealing only certain forms of sensory loss and does not control for the area tested or the number of taste buds stimulated. It is possible to test specific areas by applying taste solutions with cotton-tip swabs to identify taste loss, but not thresholds. The application of solutions to specific areas is known as spatial testing and may be valuable in elucidating specific areas of taste loss after head and neck surgery or trauma.[55]

Rodin et al.[56] studied taste abnormalities in bulimic subjects. Subjects use a computerized visual analog scale to rate the relative strength and pleasure of salty, sweet, sour, and bitter tastes in a variety of concentrations. Scores for the various concentrations were compared to deionized water. Researchers found no difference between bulimics and controls. When a Spatial Taste Test was performed to stimulate discrete areas of the mouth and tongue, differences were found. In this study bulimics had a lower sensation of all tastes on the palate. Taste receptors on the palate may have been damaged by repeated contact with stomach acids during purging. The use of specific area testing and the ability of subjects to record their own responses using a computer-generated visual analog scale are interesting attributes that could be translated into other research areas, such as testing with children.

Taste Magnitude Estimation

Citric acid in concentrations of 0.1, 0.01, and 0.001 M is used to evaluate sensitivity to the changing magnitude of a stimulus.[56] Three cups contain a small amount of citric acid in differing concentrations. Subjects take a small sip without swallowing, hold a small amount of solution in their mouth, and rate the concentrations in the proper order.[55] Patients with taste loss may require higher concentrations of solution to be able to taste them and may not be able to detect changes in the magnitude of stimuli.

Taste Magnitude Matching

Subjects are asked to judge stimuli from two sensory continua on a common intensity scale. Audible tones varying in loudness are interspersed with taste stimuli that vary in concentration. Patients are asked to assign numbers that reflect the intensities of the tastes and the tones.[55] The purpose of this is to test patients' ability to rank the strength of stimuli. Patients with taste loss may not perceive changes in intensity and will match taste concentrations with abnormally weak tones. Comparing the taste magnitude to audible sensations does not rely on patients' memory of previous sensations.

Sucrose Threshold

Sucrose solutions of 0.32, 0.1, 0.032, and 0.01 M and distilled water are used to determine the patient's sucrose threshold. A tastant and distilled water are given to the patient in separate cups. The patient is instructed to take small sips from each cup and identify which contains the tastant. The patient does not swallow any of the samples and rinses his or her mouth between trials with distilled water. Threshold is reached when the patient can identify three consecutive samples of the same concentration. The normal human threshold is 0.032 M. Reports of increased threshold for sucrose tolerance have been reported in persons with cancer.

Electrogustometry

A 5-mm stainless steel probe is used to test electric taste thresholds in the four quadrants of the tongue as well as on both sides of the soft palate. This is an excellent way to quantify the area of involvement in taste dysfunction.[56] Threshold values in these six areas are compared with standardized measurements made on normal subjects at Nihon University School of Medicine in Japan. This mean threshold value for the Japanese is 8 U.

Thresholds for electric taste do not exactly mimic those for the four chemical tastes, but they are reproducible. Additional information on taste-testing techniques for determining thresholds, and other taste and smell testing tools, such as The Henkin, Spatial Testing and Magnitude Estimation, and Magnitude Matching may be obtained from the National Institute of Health's National Institute on Deafness and other designated centers that study chemosensory disorders. These centers focus on the regeneration of sensory and nerve cells, prevention of the effects of aging, and development of new diagnostic tests, treatment and rehabilitation. The centers are:

Richard L. Doty, Ph.D.
University of Pennsylvania Smell and Taste
    Research Center
Hospital of the University of Pennsylvania
3400 Spruce Street
Philadelphia, PA 19104-4283
213-662-6580

Marion E. Frank, Ph.D.
Taste and Smell Center
Connecticut Chemosensory Clinical
    Research Center
University of Connecticut Health Center
Farmington, CT 06032
203-679-2459

Maxwell M. Mozell, Ph.D
SUNY Health Sciences Center of Syracuse
Clinical Olfactory Research Center
766 Irving Avenue
Syracuse, NY 13210
315-464-4538

Gary Beauchamp, Ph.D.
Monell Chemical Senses Center
3500 Market Street
Philadelphia, PA 19104
215-898-6666

Thomas E. Finger, Ph.D.
Rocky Mountain Taste and Smell Center,
    Box 111
University of Colorado Health
    Sciences Center
4200 East 9th Avenue
Denver, CO 80262
303-270-6464

Measurement of Smell

Interviews may help to clarify the origin and nature of smell disorders. In the author's clinical practice, the following questions have been helpful in assessing alterations in smell:

Have you noticed a change in smell?
    Can you describe the change?
    When did it occur?
    Have certain odors become unpleasant?
    Does the area where you are being treated have an odor?
    Are there smells that have become more pleasant?
    Have you noticed any loss of smell?

Smell Threshold Testing

Thresholds for smell are determined in the same manner as those for taste. A simple test frequently used to test the first cranial nerve can be used to assess the status of smell. Substances such as coffee, peanut butter, or chocolate are placed in the bottom of a small gauze-covered jar. The blindfolded patient is given both an empty jar and one containing the stimulus to smell. The subject is given a list of possibilities from which to identify the odor. Each nostril is tested separately. Some investigators have added placing the subject's head into a box containing a volatilized agent to exclude personal body odors.[2-3]

Forced Choice Three-Sniff Technique

The Forced Choice Three-Sniff Technique has been used by Henkin and other investigators.[54] Stimuli are pyridine (onion- or garliclike), nitrobenzene (bitter almond), and thiophene (burnt rubber). Measurements are transformed to the same bottle-unit logarithmic scale as the one used for taste testing. Hyposmia is defined as one bottle-unit threshold above normal. Cowart et al.[39] used a two-alternative forced-choice technique to document hyposmia in allergic rhinitis. Olfactory thresholds were significantly higher in allergic patients than in controls ($p < 0.001$) as 23.1% of subjects demonstrated a significant loss of smell.

University of Pennsylvania Smell Identification Test (UPSIT)

The most widely used test to assess smell is the UPSIT. This test has allowed convenient and accurate measurement of smell without complex equipment. It is a 40-item "scratch-and-sniff" microencapsulated odorant test. The test is commonly used in 1,500 clinics in North America and has been used to validate other instruments. It is sensitive to a wide range of smell deficits due to sinusitis, chemical exposure, Alzheimer's disease, cystic fibrosis, alcoholism, and lesions of the cerebral cortex.

The test is self-administered and may be sent to the patient by mail. It consists of four envelope-sized booklets each containing 10 "scratch-and-sniff" odorants. The stimuli are released by scratching the strip with a pencil. Above each odorant is a multiple-choice question with four alternatives for each item. For example: "This order smells most like (a) chocolate (b) banana, (c) onion, or (d) fruit punch." Age- and gender-related norms have been established. The internal consistency reliability of the UPSIT is 0.922. Fractionated versions of the test consisting of 10-, 20-, and 30-item fractionations that have been tested for internal consistency and resulted in 0.752, 0.855, and 0.898 respectively.[57]

Testing Smell in Children

Sheene and Wright[58] grouped 40 microencapsulated odorants into groups of five each and asked children to identify each odorant by selecting responses from one of five photographs. The results were used to select 5 odorants: baby powder, bubble gum, candy cane, fish, and orange. Children 3 1/2 years to 5 years 5 months identified odorants correctly 92% of the time. Most normal children age 5 and older were able to identify these odors. This study indicated that children age 5 to 12 could be tested for smell.

Summary

Tests such as the UPSIT have made it easier to study and measure smell, but the literature, and particularly the nursing literature, lacks studies measuring alterations in taste and smell. Although they are not life-threatening, these disruptions can result in significant nutritional compromise. More research is needed to document the nature and prevalence of alterations in taste and smell.

Exemplar Study

Wall, D., & Gabriel, L. Alterations of taste in children with leukemia. *Cancer Nurs*, 1983, *6*(6):447-449.

This study compares the alterations of taste in children receiving chemotherapy to a group of healthy children. The study investigated taste acuity changes, the effects of chemotherapy, the effects of relapse or remission, and changes in food preference and appetite. The Henkin method, used successfully in children and adults with a variety of disease states, was used to measure taste. The questionnaire of changes of food likes and dislikes was compiled and received content validity from pediatric dieticians. Pretesting of the questionnaire was performed with parents of healthy children with 87.8% agreement on the list of preferred food. This study is exemplary because of the validity established for the instrument and the use of children as subjects.

References

1. Ziporyn, T. Taste and smell: The neglected senses. *JAMA*, 1982, 247(3):277, 282.
2. Guyton, A. *Textbook of medical physiology*. Philadelphia: Saunders, 1986.
3. Schiffman, S. Taste and smell in disease. Part I. *N Engl J Med*, 1983, 308(21):1275-1280
4. Murray, R.G. Ultrastructure of taste receptors. In L.M. Beidler (Ed.), *Handbook of sensory physiology*. New York: Springer-Verlag, 1971, p. 31.
5. DeWys, W.D. Abnormalities of taste as a remote effect of a neoplasm. *Ann NY Acad Sci*, 1974, 230:427-432.
6. DeWys, W.D., & Walters, K. Abnormalities of taste sensation in cancer patients. *Cancer*, 1975, 36(5):1888-1896.
7. DeWys, W.D. Changes in taste sensation in cancer patients: correlation with caloric intake. In *The chemical senses and nutrition*. New York: Academic, 1977, p. 381.
8. DeWys, W.D. Nutritional care of the cancer patient. *JAMA*, 1980, 244(4):374-376.
9. Vickers, Z., Nielsen, D., & Theologides, A. Food preferences of patients with cancer. *J Am Diet Assoc*, 1981, 79(4):441-446.
10. Trant, A.S., Serin, J., & Douglass, H. Is taste related to anorexia in cancer patients? *Am J Clin Nutr*, 1982, 36(1):45-58.
11. Brewin, T. Can a tumor cause the same appetite perversion or taste change as a pregnancy? *Lancet*, 1980, 2:907.
12. Hall, J.C., Staniland, J.R., & Giles, G.R. Altered taste thresholds in gastrointestinal cancer. *Clin Oncol*, 1980, 6(2):137-142.
13. Bruera, E., Carraro, S., Roca, E., et al. Association between malnutrition and caloric intake, emesis, psychological depression, glucose taste and tumor mass. *Cancer Treat Rep*, 1984, 68(6):873-876.
14. Barale, K., Aker, S.N., & Martinsen, C.S. Primary taste thresholds in children with leukemia undergoing marrow transplantation. *J Parenter Enter Nutr*, 1982, 6(4):287-290.
15. Wall, D.W., & Gabriel, L. Alterations of taste in children with leukemia, *Cancer Nurs*, 1983, 6(6):447-449.
16. DeWys, W., Costa, A.G., & Henkin, R. Clinical parameters related to anorexia. *Cancer Treat Rep*, 1981, 65:49-53.
17. Hall, B., Hardesty, I., & Hogan, R. *Nutrition alteration in less than body requirements related to nausea and vomiting*. In J. McNally, E. Somerville, C. Miaskowski, & M. Rostad (Eds.), *Guidelines for oncology nursing practice*. Philadelphia: W.B. Saunders, 1991, pp. 173-179.
18. LeVeque, F.G. An unusual presentation of chronic graft versus host disease in an unrelated bone marrow transplantation. *Oral Surg, Oral Med, Oral Pathol*, 1990, 69(5):581-584.
19. Kashima, H., & Kalinowski, B. Taste impairment following laryngectomy. *Ear, Nose, Throat*, 1979, 58(2): 88-92.
20. Donovan, M.L., & Pierce, S.G. *Cancer Care Nursing*. New York: Appeleton-Century Crofts, 1976.
21. Bernstein, I.L., & Bernstein, I.D. Learned food aversions and cancer anorexia. *Cancer Treat Rep*, 1981, 65(5):43-47.
22. Aker, F. The role of taste and taste dysfunction in oral diagnosis. *Quintessence Int*, 1980, 11(11):81-83.
23. Garg, R.K., Agrawal, A., Nag, D., & Jha, S. Herpes zoster associated with facial, auditory and trigeminal involvement. *J Assoc Phys India*, 1992, 40(1):45-46.
24. Donaldson, S.F. Nutritional consequences of radiotherapy. *Cancer Res*, 1977, 37(7):2407-2410.
25. Shatzman, A.R., & Mossman, K.L. Radiation effects on bovine taste bud membranes. *Radiat Res*, 1982, 92(2):353-358.
26. Mossman, K.L., & Henkin, R.I. Radiation-induced changes in taste acuity. *Int J Radiat Oncol Biol Phys*, 1978, 4(7/8):663-670.
27. Johnson, C.A., Keane, T.S., & Prudo, S.M. Weight loss in patients receiving radical radiation therapy for head and neck cancer: A prospective study. *J Parenter Enter Nutr*, 1982, 6(5):399-406.
28. Bolze, M.S., Fosmire, G.J., Stryker, J.A., et al. Taste acuity, plasma zinc levels and weight loss during radiotherapy: A study of relationships. *Radiology*, 1982, 144(1):163-168.
29. Mossman, K. Long-term effects of radiotherapy on taste and salivary function in man. *Int J Radiat Oncol Biol Phys*, 1982, 8(2):991-998.
30. Hardy, S.L., Brennand, C.P., & Wyse, B.W. Taste thresholds of individuals with diabetes mellitus and of control subjects. *J Am Diet Assoc*, 1981, 79(3):286-288.
31. Abbasi, A. Diabetes: Diagnostic and therapeutic significance of taste impairment. *Geriatrics*, 1981, 36(12): 73-79.
32. Russell, R.M., Cox, M.E., & Solomons, W. Zinc and the special senses. *Ann Int Med*, 1983, 99(2):227-239.
33. Mahajan, S.K., Prasad, A.S., Lambuian, J., et al. Improvement of uremic hypogeusia by zinc: A double-blind study. *Am J Clin Nutr*, 1980, 33(7):1517-1521.
34. Zetin, M., & Stone, R.A. Effects of zinc in chronic hemodialysis. *Clin Nephrol*, 1980, 13(1):20-26.
35. Ciechanover, M., Peresecenschi, G., Aviram, A., et al. Malrecognition of taste in uremia. *Nephron*, 1980, 26(1):20-23.
36. Casper, R.C., Kirschner, B., Sandstead, H.H., et al. An evaluation of taste function in anorexia nervosa. *Am J Clin Nutr*, 1980, 33(8):1801-1807.
37. Nakajima, Y., Utsumi, H., & Takahaski, H. Ipsilateral disturbance of taste due to pointine hemorrhage, *J Neurol*, 1983, 229(2):133-139.

38. Goto, W., Yakamoto, T., & Kaneko, M. Primary pointine hemorrhage and gustatory disturbance: Clinicoanatomic study. *Stroke*, 1983, *14*(4):507-513.

39. Cowart, B., Flynn-Rodden, K., McGeady, M., & Lowry, L. Hyposmia in allergic rhinitis. *J Allerg Clin Immunol*, 1993, *91*(3):747-751.

40. Deems, R., Friedman, M., Friedman, L., et al. Chemosensory function, food preference, and appetite in human liver disease. *Appetite*, 1993, *20*(3): 209-216.

41. Ditraglia, G., Press, D., Butters, N., et al. Assessment of olfactory deficits in detoxified alcoholics. *Alcohol*, 1991, *8*(2):109-115.

42. Miller, S., & Naylor, G. Unpleasant taste, a neglected symptom in depression. *J Affect Dis*, 1989, *17*(3):291-293.

43. Kopala, L., Clark, C., & Hyrwitz, T. Olfactory deficits in neuroleptic naive patients with schizophrenia. *Schizophr Res*, 1993, *8*(3):245-250.

44. Koopman, C.F., & Coulthard, S.W. The oral cavity and aging. *Otolaryngol Clin North Am*, 1982, *15*(2): 293-300.

45. NIH. Variation in taste thresholds with human aging. *JAMA*, 1982, *247*(6):775-779.

46. Schiffman, D. Taste and smell in disease. Part II. *N Engl J Med*, 1983, *308*(22):1337-1339.

47. Prasad, A., Fitzgerald, J., Hess, J., et al. Zinc deficiency in elderly patients. *Nutrition*, 1993, *9*(3):218-224.

48. Dobell, E., Chan, M., Williams, P., et al. Food preferences and food habits of patients with chronic renal failure undergoing dialysis. *J Am Diet Assoc*, 1993, *93*(10):1129-1135.

49. Markley, E.J., Matts-Kulig, D.A., & Henkin, R. A classification of dysgeusia. *J Am Diet Assoc*, 1983, *83*(5):578-583.

50. Hagopian, G.A. Development of a radiation side effects profile. In O.L. Strickland & C.F. Waltz (Eds.), *Measurement of nursing outcomes. Vol. 4: Measuring client self-care and coping skills.* New York: Springer, 1990, pp. 45-57.

51. Norcoss-Weintraub, F., & Hagopian, G., The effect of nursing consultation sessions on patient's well-being in a radiation oncology department. *Oncol Nurs Forum*, 1990, *17*(3):31-36.

52. Hagopian, G. The effect of a radiation therapy newsletter on patient's knowledge, self-care behaviors, and side effects. *Oncol Nurs Forum*, 1991, *18*(7): 1199-1207.

53. Schecter, P.J., Friedewald, W.T., Bancert, D.A., et al. Idiopathic hypogeusia: A description of the syndrome and a single blind study with zinc sulfate. *Int Rev Neurobiol*, 1972, (suppl 1):125-129.

54. Henkin, R., Schecter, P., & Friedewald, W. A double blind study of the effects of zinc sulfate on taste and smell dysfunction. *Am J Med Sci*, 1976, *272*(3):285-289.

55. Bartoshuk, L. Clinical evaluation of taste. *Ear Nose Throat J*, 1989, *68*(5):331-337.

56. Rodin, J., Bartoshuk, L., Peterson, C., et al. Bulimia and taste: Possible interactions. *J Abnorm Psychol*, 1990, *99*(1):32-39.

57. Doty, R., Frye, R., & Agrawal, R. Internal consistency and reliability of the fractionated and whole University of Pennsylvania Smell Identification test. *Percept Psychophys*, 1989, *45*(5):381-384.

58. Sheene, P.R., & Wright, H. Olfactory performance during childhood: Development of an odorant identification test for children. *J Pediatr*, 1992, *121*(6):908-911.

29

Measuring Bowel Elimination

Susan C. McMillan and Linda Bartkowski-Dodds

A variety of instruments and methods have been developed to provide quantitative data about human bowel function. Early attempts to objectively evaluate elimination involved simple questioning. However, wide differences in health status among populations, absence of dietary considerations, and reliance on patient recall of defecation performance resulted in questionable data.[1]

By the mid-1960s, research into the effects of diet on bowel performance precipitated the development of measurement tools and techniques for quantifying the frequency of defecation, stool consistency, stool wet weight, and intestinal transit time.[2-9] Further studies of gastrointestinal motility produced methods for quantifying intraluminal pressures within the alimentary tract.[10-14] Focusing on these parameters, numerous studies were conducted on normal subjects and those with elimination problems.

Other investigators have developed questionnaires and surveys that have provided subjective data describing attitudes and behaviors related to elimination and evaluating bowel patterns among various populations.[15-18] Depending on study objectives and the population under investigation, however, both subjective and objective dimensions of bowel elimination may need to be measured.

Because bowel function can be affected by neurophysiologic, psychologic, and cultural conditions, a comprehensive approach to the measurement of the concept of elimination must include all such parameters. Bowel function not only will vary among subjects with different underlying conditions, but also can vary in the same subject at different times. Instrument selection, therefore, is critical, and it is generally believed that a thorough study will require the use of more than one instrument.

Instruments that result in quantitative data provide objective measures of bowel function, but interpretations are limited by the normal variability of colonic function[19] and the influence of multiple variables.[20] In contrast, instruments that result in qualitative data (descriptive data) provide subjective measures that attempt to identify various bowel patterns or describe the concept of elimination per se. Instrument choice ultimately is determined by research goals, populations under study (normal versus abnormal bowel function), number of subjects, and resources available.

Objective Scales Yielding Quantitative Data

Objective measures can be categorized according to the parameters considered relevant to the investigation of bowel function. The following instruments and methods have been used to investigate both normal subjects and those with problems of elimination, such as bowel syndromes, megacolon, diverticulitis, Crohn's disease, constipation related to medication, and diarrhea associated with enteral feedings.

Bowel Transit Time

Methods that have been used to measure gut transit time may be classified as radiologic, colorimetric, particulate, chemical, and isotopic.

Radiologic Measures

Hinton et al. developed a simple technique using radiopaque pellets of barium-impregnated polyethylene.[2] A known number of pellets are swallowed, usually 20, and the disappearance of the pellets from the gut or the appearance of the pellets in the stool are observed by serial radiographs. Results are expressed as the time taken for the passage of the first and of 80% of the markers. Recovery rate using 30 subjects was 99.3%. Replicate studies were performed with only descriptive data and variability in transit time up to 2 days in the same subject. Comparison studies with other markers, again using descriptive data only, were difficult to assess because of the inherent differences in the various methods. For instance, radiopaque pellets were compared to glass beads and were shown to have a shorter mean transit time; probably because the beads have a higher specific gravity than the pellets. Comparisons with chemical markers were less than optimal because some of the chemical was found in the urine as well as the stool.

Payler et al. used Hinton's method for measuring intestinal transit time while studying the effect of bran on intestinal transit and found reproducibility poor, with variability in transit times even in the same subject.[4] To provide more accurate and reproducible data, Cummings et al. compared mean transit time (MTT) using radiopaque pellets in two different ways and compared this to Hinton's method of 80% excretion as an expression of transit time (80% TT).[3] MTT was measured using a constant amount of marker fed to subjects over a period of weeks (MTT-C) and again measured by giving single doses of similar markers to the subjects (MTT-S). The MTT-S method was found to be preferable to the 80% TT if a single-dose technique was used. The MTT-S correlated more closely with the MTT-C ($r = 0.87$) than did the 80% TT ($r = 0.78$) and gave a value for transit that is more physiologic. Although the MTT-C method provided more information about transit in individuals (data that reflect the way residue passes through the gut, i.e., colon), it can be tedious and is not suitable for studies on an epidemiologic scale.

Although it has limitations, an alternative method for measuring transit time through the gut was developed and tested by Cummings and Wiggins.[5] It requires the collection of only one stool after 4 days of ingestion of markers. It is suitable for use in epidemiologic studies on an outpatient basis. This method compared favorably with MTT-C ($r = 0.78$, $p < 0.001$) and MTT-S ($r = 0.94$, $p < 0.001$) and proved a satisfactory alternative method for validating transit techniques. Once transit times begin to exceed 4 days, its accuracy falls off, and it would not be suitable for studying the constipated patient.

A 1992 study also correlated two radiologic methods, one using daily studies and one using a single radiologic study on day 7.[21] Significant positive correlations further supported the value of the single measures of both segmental and total transit time while exposing the patient to lower doses of radiation.

Defecography, also known as *proctography*, involves the insertion of a thick barium paste into the rectum and a videorecording of the expulsion. The time for rectal evacuation is calculated from the moment of first passage of barium through the anal canal until evacuation is complete. A group of 58 patients with idiopathic constipation was compared with 20 controls.[22] The significant differences in evacuation time and in the amount of barium remaining in the rectum between the patients and controls supports the validity of this method.

The usefulness of defecography was examined in fecal incontinence by using a commercially prepared barium paste inserted into the rectum.[23] The patient was seated on a specially prepared stool for defecation and the defecogram was recorded on videotape. Radiographs were taken at rest, during maximum pelvic squeeze, and during straining to defecate. Anorectal angle changes were measured and subjects were evaluated for leakage of contrast at rest, presence of rectocele, rectal intussuception or prolapse, and the completeness of rectal evacuation. Correlation of this method with anorectal manometry produced weak to moderate correlations. The investigators concluded that defecography provided little additional information about constipation over that provided by anorectal manometry unless the patient had outlet obstruction constipation symptoms.

Colorimetric Measures

Various dyes have been used to mark stool and then calculate passage through the intestinal tract. The simplicity makes this method especially attractive, and it has been used in a variety of research settings.[24-26] Two widely used dyes are brilliant blue (100 mg/capsule) and carmine (500 mg/capsule). Dosing usually requires three capsules per each experimental day. Transit time is computed as the time from ingestion of the marker until most of the color has appeared in the feces. This requires daily stool collection and careful examination of the stool, which may lend itself to misinterpretation.

Rogers et al. compared the use of radiopaque pellets and dye in measuring bowel transit time and, after rigorous analysis of variance, concluded that the two methods gave identical information.[26] This comparison supports the validity of both methods. Colorimetric measures provide mouth-to-anus transit time but cannot provide data about passage through the different parts of the gastrointestinal tract. These measures would, therefore, be limited in usefulness when studying the diseased colon or other bowel disorders to ascertain segmental function. They lend themselves well to the study of diarrhea, as the specific gravity of radiologic markers may affect the transit time in the diarrheal stool.

Particulate Measures

Particulate measures are tedious and require complex and careful analysis of stool specimens. Furthermore, complete recovery can be seriously altered by stool adsorption of the reagent secondary to dietary fiber composition. Polyethylene glycol (PEG) can be ingested by subjects (1-g doses) after dilution in water and then analyzed in stools with a spectrophotometer. The use of PEG as a transit time measure was compared to other standard measures, including dyes, pellets, and isotopes.[24] Mean recovery for 242 doses was 85.3% (±12.6%). Low recovery was attributed to binding of PEG by stool components. A separate analysis of MTT values from all markers revealed no significant differences in transit time estimates among marker types.

Chemical Measures

One of the major limitations of the use of radiopaque pellets is that total excretion may not represent pool sizes and turnover rates of unexcreted intestinal content. Thus, pellet excretion may not have any significant relationship to the usual clinical descriptions of bowel habits. Patients may report daily bowel movements, but pool sizes could be very large and turnover small, that is, a large proportion of the colonic contents may not be excreted for long periods.[7] Because chemical markers are incorporated into the food intake, their excretion can indicate the completeness of stool collections and permit corrections for variations in fecal flow. Chromic oxide (Cr-203) has been used widely in humans since 1947 for these purposes because it is nontoxic, readily measurable in the feces, and appears to be completely unabsorbable. Subjects are given 60-mg tablets of chromic oxide with meals (not to exceed 300 mg/day). Fecal collections are pooled and stored at 4°C until the collection period is completed. Although measurements demonstrated reliability (replicate demonstrations showed a coefficient of variation of 2.8% ± 1.5%), analysis is time-consuming.[8]

Dick reported on the use of cuprous thiocyanate as a continuous marker for feces that is insoluble under physiologic conditions but could be decomposed by relatively mild chemical treatments.[6] The marker is administered with each meal, with a total daily dose of 1 g; stools are collected and stored and then analyzed for copper content. Analysis requires the addition of nitric acid followed by atomic absorption spectroscopy. Copper recovery over 79 four-day periods on 14 subjects was 99.7%. Although not statistically analyzed, a histogram comparing the recoveries of cuprous thiocyanate to barium sulfate and chromium oxide demonstrated a higher percentage of recovery with cuprous thiocyanate.

In an investigation into the effects of fiber on bowel function, Wrick et al. compared various markers for transit time, one of which was Cr (III) mordanted onto isolated bran fiber, and found no significant differences in transit time estimates between Cr (III) and PEG or radiopaque pellets.[24] Chromium-mordanted bran is prepared and placed into capsules, each dose providing 35 to 45 mg Cr, and ingested daily. Fecal Cr recovery is assessed by atomic absorption spectrophotometry. Complete stool collection is required, and a lengthy preparation procedure for spectroscopy is necessary.[24] Mean fecal Cr recovery from 244 doses of Cr-mordanted bran was 84% ± 16.9%. Incomplete conversion to chromic oxide (during preparation for spectroscopy) and marker overlap between testing periods were explanations offered by these investigators for results lower than 100%. Apparently, the cellulose within the mordanted bran altered the colonic microflora so that there was a microbial interaction with the mordant, which somehow influenced the recovery of Cr. This limitation needs to be considered with subjects who may have slow turnover of intestinal pool.

Isotopic Measures

Isotopic measures have the advantage of quantifying transit rates separately through the small and large intestines, whereas other transit time measures are suitable for total mouth-to-anus assessments only. Hansky and Connell first used Cr-51 to investigate transit times by labeling sodium chromate (Na_2CrO_4).[9] A gelatin capsule filled with 0.5 g of chromic oxide with an activity of 1 to 2 microcuries (μCi) is swallowed by the subject, and a scintillation counter permits quantification according to the amount of Cr-51 present in stools. A mean percentage recovery of radioactivity of 83.5% was demonstrated, but more important, this technique permits the quantitative measurement of the rate of passage of the maximum bulk of the markers.

Waller used Cr-51 as a marker while investigating small- and large-bowel transit times in subjects with constipation and diarrhea.[27] Other markers were used concurrently, but comparative statistical analysis was not performed. Transit times for all markers were similar. However, Cr-51 provided differential measurements for colonic function in diarrheal and constipated states that would not have been ascertained using standard measures and would be useful when investigating segmental gastrointestinal transit.

Between 1990 and 1993 three studies with four different isotopic markers were conducted.[28-30] Iodine-131-cellulose, ^{99m}Tc-radiolabeled resin, ^{111}In-labeled particles, and ^{99m}Tc-labeled aluminum magnesium sulfate were used in the studies to assess gastric and bowel transit time. All three studies found significant differences between constipated patients and controls, supporting the validity of the use of isotopic markers. One team of investigators[30] also studied the validity of the use of isotopic markers by correlating it with another method of evaluating bowel motility. Although they did find a positive association (60%) between scintigraphy and anorectal manometry in the constipated group, there was an overall poor level of agreement when nonconstipated persons were included. These researchers concluded that although scintigraphy has the advantage of low radiation exposure, its inability to distinguish between patients with slow transit constipation and defecatory complaints makes its clinical value uncertain.

Stool Consistency

Penetrometer Cone

A quantitative technique for assessing stool consistency has been devised by Exton-Smith et al. that uses a penetrometer cone, which is lowered until it is touching the stool, released, and then allowed to penetrate the stool for 5 seconds.[31] Distance of penetration is measured in units of 0.1 mm. Several readings are taken along the column of the stool and are averaged. The total range of penetrometer readings is 0 to 240, with a mean of 80.6 for hard stools and 128.9 for soft stools. Further work is being carried out to refine the method and to establish a normal range of values.

Stool Ash Analysis

In a clinical study assessing lactose intolerance with tube-fed patients, Walike and Walike found that stool ash analysis validated subjective ratings of stool consistency made by nurse clinicians.[15] Stool content was analyzed for sodium, potassium, percentage of fat, nitrogen, phosphate, percentage of ash, and wet and dry weight. Stool weight, percentage of water, and sodium were significantly higher with the lactose-containing diet and correlated well with stool consistency ratings.

Frequency of Defecation

Because self-reporting has been considered unreliable by most investigators, Hinton et al. devised a collection technique that provided accurate measurements of frequency as well as a convenient way to transport specimens to the laboratory for further analysis.[2] This method continues to be used today with a few minor alterations. It entails the use of a polyethylene bag that is suspended over the toilet to collect the stool specimen while allowing the urine to pass freely. The plastic bag is then sealed with a rubber band and inserted into a specimen cup and labeled with the appropriate information. Assuming subject compliance, this method should provide objective, quantifiable data about stool frequency.

Stool Wet/Dry Weight and Volume

Numerous investigations have shown that dietary constituents, medications, and colonic function will affect fecal characteristics.[10,11,19,26] Statistical analysis of fecal measurements often includes the calculation of coefficients of variation for each subject for each measurement. Statistical comparisons of these measures to other variables (transit time, dietary fiber, medications) are then determined to explore any relationships further.[19] Although no special instruments for measuring these parameters are described in the literature, techniques for such assessments are clearly delineated.[19]

Gastrointestinal Motility Measures

Manometer

Various invasive measures have been used to assess quantitatively the motility of the alimentary tract. Early studies using miniature balloons connected through polyethylene tubing to a metal capsule optical manometer of high sensitivity provided intraluminal pressure readings in both normal patients and those with dysfunctional conditions.[10,11] The same technique has been used to compare the effects of codeine and senna on the motor activity of the left colon.[12] Any type of cardiovascular, respiratory, or somatic movement will affect the tracings and can interfere with accurate interpretations. An assessment of colonic activity is given by the product of the total duration of activity and the mean amplitude of the slow waves. Analysis for observer error initially produced a mean standard deviation of ±3.2%. This was considered to be too great an error, and therefore the standard deviations of duplicate analyses were calculated, and the mean of these standard deviations was ±1.8% ($p = 0.01$).

Prior et al.[32] used anorectal manometry to study patients with irritable bowel syndrome. A multilumen polyvinyl catheter with sideholes at 1, 4, and 14 cm from the anal verge was placed in the rectum. This was perfused with 0.4 ml water per minute and connected to water-filled transducers. A 5-cm latex balloon was attached to the catheter between 6 and 11 cm from the anus with a side hole at 8.5 cm linked to an air-filled transducer. After a basal period of 15 minutes, the rectal balloon was serially inflated with air at intervals of 1 minute in 20-ml increments to 100 ml and then in 50-ml increments up to the sensation of discomfort. Measurements taken included: (1) the balloon volumes required to elicit sensation of gas, stool, urgency, and discomfort; (2) rectal compliance calculated as the volume divided by pressure relation; and (3) the presence or absence of repetitive rectal contractions during balloon distension.

Test–retest reliability was assessed on 15 control subjects with a 9- to 12-day delay. No changes were found in rectal sensory or motor parameters; this supports the reliability of the method. Validity was assessed by comparing rectal compliance in the treatment group before and after hypnotherapy. Hypnotherapy designed to relieve bowel symptoms resulted in a significant improvement in rectal compliance both during and after hypnotherapy. This supports the validity of the method to measure rectal compliance.[32]

Thermistor Probe

Kagawa-Busby et al. studied the effects of diet temperature on the tolerance of enteral feedings and evaluated gastric motility and intragastric temperature by inserting a nasogastric feeding tube with a thermistor probe for recording temperature and a polyethylene cannula for pressure recordings.[14] No reference was made to evaluations of the validity or reliability of the instruments used. Observation periods were predetermined and identical for all subjects; thus, analysis of observer error was not relevant. However, this does not exclude the possibility of misinterpretation of readings by omission.

Subjective Scales Yielding Quantitative Data

Elimination studies frequently attempt to measure the effects of certain variables (diet, medications, bowel diseases) on stool consistency and require the quantification of subjective data. A previously mentioned study was conducted by Walike and Walike, who assessed stool consistency among tube-fed patients on lactose-containing versus lactose-free diets. Descriptive ratings were performed by nurse clinicians and validated by concurrent stool ash analysis.[15] Descriptive parameters were plotted against time and categorized between both diets (Figure 29.1). Patients on the lactose-containing tube

	DIET									
	LACTOSE-FREE					LACTOSE-CONTAINING				
Watery						XX	XXX		XX	
Liquid						XX		X		
Very loose, semiliquid	X			X				XX		XXX
Loose, very soft			X	X						
Day	2	4	6	8	10	2	4	6	8	10

Figure 29.1 Comparison of stool frequencies and consistencies on two diets for one subject. Each X represents one stool.

feedings had at least one and a half times as many stools as the lactose-free group. The lactose containing group also had predominantly loose to liquid stools compared to the soft to hard stools of the lactose-free group.

To evaluate the effectiveness of dioctyl sodium sulfosuccinate as a prophylactic measure in preventing constipation among hospitalized patients, Goodman et al. used a scale for grading stool consistency.[16] Six descriptive categories were used. Examples are: A = watery; B = soft-formed, normal stool; C = watery, hard-formed stool.

The scales used by Walike and Walike and by Goodman et al. offer ways to categorize stool consistency. However, there was no mention of interrater reliability or validity testing by either group of investigators. It is apparent that selection criteria will vary for a given population; that is, stool characteristics for subjects with tube-fed diets will differ from those of subjects who may be at risk for constipation. This makes the establishment of a standardized scale for measuring stool consistency difficult and it emphasizes the importance of selecting appropriate criteria for the population under study.

Although some subjectively reported measures may be reports of clinicians, others require reports of patients. One such self-report measure was used in concert with anorectal manometry.[32] An unnamed 3-item scale of severity of abdominal pain, distension, and bowel habit disturbance was used. These symptoms were scored on a 0 to 10 scale and summated for a severity score of 0 to 30. Evidence of validity was provided by demonstrating a decrease in subjective symptoms (from 23.5 to 9.6) following hypnotherapy. Test–retest reliability with a 9- to 12-day delay was assessed on a group of controls. No differences were found in the two measures, supporting the reliability of the self-report measure.

A more sophisticated measure, the Bowel Disease Questionnaire, was designed to differentiate among nonulcer dyspepsia, irritable bowel syndrome, organic gastrointestinal disease, and health.[33] The 46 gastrointestinal symptoms-related items were developed based on a careful review of the literature including other previously published instruments; this provided beginning evidence of construct validity. An additional 25 questions addressing past illnesses and use of the health-care system also were included. The Bowel Disease Questionnaire (BDQ) was administered to 361 subjects, 115 with functional bowel disease (either nonulcer dyspepsia or irritable bowel syndrome), 101 with organic gastrointestinal disease, and 145 healthy adults. The mean completion time for the BDQ was 17 minutes. Variables that identified nonulcer dyspepsia were found to be: (1) upper abdominal pain more than six times in a year; (2) no increase in bowel movements when pain begins; (3) stools that were not loose or watery; and (4) no doctor visits for colonic symptoms. Variables that identified functional bowel disease included:

(1) more bowel movements when pain begins; (2) more than three bowel movements daily; (3) presence of mucus; (4) frequent feeling of incomplete evacuation; (5) vomiting; and (6) heartburn. The ability of the instrument to differentiate among the groups of patients supports its validity as a diagnostic tool. Test–retest with delay using 42 subjects supports its reliability (median kappa for all questions was 0.78 with a range of 0.52 to 1).

Constipation Assessment Scale (CAS)

The Constipation Assessment Scale (CAS) is an eight-item self-report tool designed to measure the presence and severity of constipation. The CAS was developed on a careful review of the literature, which offers beginning evidence of construct validity.[34] It is a 3-point summated rating scale resulting in a total score that ranges from 0 (no constipation) to 16 (severe constipation).

Validity of the CAS was studied using contrasted groups, including a control group ($n = 32$) of healthy working adults and a patient group ($n = 32$) of adult cancer patients at risk for constipation because of morphine or vinca alkaloids. A significant difference between the two groups ($p < 0.0001$) provided evidence of construct validity. Further evidence of validity was provided by the ability of the scale to differentiate between the levels of intensity reported by the patients receiving morphine and those receiving vinca alkaloids ($p < 0.01$).[34] A later study using 30 controls and 30 cancer patients receiving morphine reconfirmed the ability of the scale to differentiate ($p < 0.0001$) between groups.[35]

The reliability of the CAS has been studied with both test–retest and internal consistency methods. Test–retest ($n = 16$) with a 1-hour delay resulted in a strong correlation ($r = 0.98$, $p = 0.000$). Internal consistency using Cronbach's alpha was evaluated twice using two groups of cancer patients with very acceptable results (alpha = 0.70 and 0.78) for such a short scale.[34-35]

Diarrhea Assessment Scale (DAS)

The Diarrhea Assessment Scale (DAS) is a newly developed scale designed for use with patients receiving radiation therapy to the pelvic area.[36] However, it appears to be a generic measure of the presence and severity of diarrhea. To provide beginning evidence of construct validity, the DAS was developed on a careful review of the literature to include four characteristics of diarrhea: (1) frequency; (2) consistency; (3) urgency; and (4) abdominal discomfort. The patient rates each of these on a 0 to 3 scale; scores are summed, providing a range of 0 (no diarrhea) to 12 (severe diarrhea).

Construct validity of the DAS was studied using the known-groups technique. The scores of a group of apparently healthy adults ($n = 20$) were compared with those of a group of men receiving radiation therapy for cancer of the prostate ($n = 20$). A significant difference ($p < 0.0001$) between groups supports the validity of the scale. The mean score for the patient group was 7.85 (SD = 1.35). Reliability was estimated with the combined sample ($n = 40$). The resulting reliability coefficient (Cronbach's alpha 0.87) was acceptably high for such a short scale.[36] Further research on this tool is warranted, but it appears promising.

Subjective Scales Yielding Qualitative Data

Andersson et al. Scale

Andersson et al. developed a scale to evaluate bowel habits while investigating the effects of dietary restriction of fat and the use of antidiarrheal agents after bowel resection in patients with Crohn's disease.[17] The bowel habits were evaluated according to the following scale:

Satisfactory or good. Three or less bowel movements/24 hours, usually after breakfast and causing no social inconvenience

Fair. Four to six movements/24 hours, mostly in relation to meals and with minor inconvenience

Poor. Seven or more bowel movements/24 hours, considerable social inconvenience and/or incapacity for work

Drossman et al. Questionnaire

Using a broader approach, Drossman et al. developed a brief, self-administered questionnaire to identify bowel patterns among the general population.[18] The questionnaire contained several areas of inquiry for comparative analysis and provided demographic data as well as information about subject attitudes and behavior related to bowel function. Based on their responses to questions about stool frequency, abdominal pain, or awareness of changes in bowel patterns, subjects could be classified into several categories. Examples are:

Category A: alternating bowel function. Subject responded affirmatively to questions about loose, frequent stools alternating with hard, infrequent stools and to similar questions

Category B: abdominal pain. Included in this category were subjects with more than six episodes of lower abdominal pain in the last year under various circumstances, such as abdominal pain relieved by bowel movement, loose stools associated with pain

Selection criteria for the categories were based on reports from other investigations into dysfunctional bowel syndromes and were both objective and subjective. Subject attitudes regarding bowel dysfunction were assessed by such questions as "Does stress affect your bowel pattern?" with response options of "never," "sometimes," and "always."

Drossman's instrument allows the researcher to identify by questionnaire a range of bowel patterns in the general population and to categorize subjects into groups with specific types of bowel dysfunction. It was administered to 789 subjects, and the results were in agreement with data reported from other investigations into comparable bowel patterns.

Summary

A variety of types of instruments and methods are available to assess bowel function. These include both objective and subjective measures. The use of several measures may be necessary to obtain data that accurately reflects the concept of elimination and human bowel patterns. Further, considering the normal variability of colonic function, interpretations of these data will need to reflect the dynamic status of this basic human process.

Exemplar Study

McMillan, S.C., & Williams, F. Validity and reliability of the Constipation Assessment Scale. *Cancer Nurs*, 1989, *12*(3):183-189.

This study exemplifies the measurement of constipation, a pervasive problem in many nursing settings. The purpose of the study was to develop and study the Constipation Assessment Scale (CAS). The authors developed the scale based on characteristics of constipation identified by a careful review of the literature. This evidence of content validity is supplemented with evidence of construct validity accomplished through comparison of known groups. These comparisons support the validity of the CAS in assessing both the presence and severity of constipation. In addition, estimates of both internal consistency and test–retest reliability are provided. Patients are able to complete the CAS in about 2 minutes, making the scale clinically useful. The readability level of the scale is at the sixth-grade level, which further supports the clinical usefulness of the CAS.

References

1. Godding, E.W. Physiological yardsticks for bowel function and the rehabilitation of the constipated bowel. *Pharmacology*, 1980, *20*(Suppl 1):88-103.
2. Hinton, J.M., Lennard-Jones, J.E., & Young, A.C. A new method for studying gut transit times using radioopaque markers. *Gut*, 1969, *10*(10):842-850.
3. Cummings, J.H., Jenkins, D.J.A., & Wiggins, H.S. Measurement of the mean transit time of dietary residue through the human gut. *Gut*, 1976, *17*(3):210-218.
4. Payler, D.K., Pomare, E.W., Heaton, K.W., & Harvey, R.F. The effect of wheat bran on intestinal transit. *Gut*, 1975, *16*(3):209-213.
5. Cummings, J.H., & Wiggins, H.S. Transit through the gut measured by analysis of a single stool. *Gut*, 1976, *17*(3):219-223.
6. Dick, M. Use of cuprous thiocyanate as a short-term continuous marker for feces. *Gut*, 1969, *10*(5):408-415.
7. Davignon, J., Simmonds, W.J., & Aherns, E.H., Jr. Usefulness of chromic oxide as an internal standard for balance studies in formula-fed patients for assessment of colonic function. *J Clin Invest*, 1968, *47*(1):127-129.
8. Bolin, D.W., King, R.P., & Klosterman, E.W. A simplified method for the determination of chromic oxide when used as an index substance. *Science*, 1952, *116*(5):634-638.
9. Hansky, J., & Connell, A.M. Measurement of gastrointestinal transit using radioactive chromium. *Gut*, 1962, *3*(2):187-193.
10. Connell, A.M. The motility of the pelvic colon. Part I. *Gut*, 1961, *2*(2):175-179.
11. Connell, A.M. The motility of the pelvic colon. Part II. *Gut*, 1962, *3*(4):342-349.
12. Waller, S.L. Comparative effects of codeine and senna on the motor activity of the left colon. *Gut*, 1975, *16*(5):407-410.
13. Meunier, P., Rochas, A., & Lambert, R. Motor activity of the sigmoid colon in chronic constipation: Comparative study with normal subjects. *Gut*, 1979, *20*(12):1095-1101.
14. Kagawa-Busby, K.S., Heitkemper, M.M., Hansen, B.C., et al. Effects of diet temperature on tolerance of enteral feedings. *Nurs Res*, 1980, *29*(5):276-280.
15. Walike, B.C., & Walike, J.W. Relative lactose intolerance. *JAMA*, 1977, *238*(9):948-951.
16. Goodman, J., Pang, J., & Bessman, A.N. Dioctyl sodium sulfosuccinate—An ineffective prophylactic laxative. *J Chronic Dis*, 1976, *29*(1):59-63.
17. Andersson, H., Bosaeus, I., Hellberg, R., & Hulten, L. Effect of a low-fat diet and antidiarrheal agents on bowel habits after excisional surgery for classical Crohn's disease. *Acta Chir Scand*, 1982, *148*(3):285-290.
18. Drossman, D.A., Sandler, R.S., McKee, D.C., & Lovitz, A.J. Bowel patterns among subjects not seeking health care: Use of a questionnaire to identify a population with bowel dysfunction. *Gastroenterology*, 1982, *83*(3):529-534.
19. Wyman, J.B., Heaton, K.W., Manning, A.P., & Wicks, A.C.B. Variability of colonic function in healthy subjects. *Gut*, 1978, *19*(2):146-150.
20. Slavin, J.L., Sempos, C.T., Brauer, P.M., & Marlett, J.A. Limits of predicting gastrointestinal transit time from other measures of bowel function. *Am J Clin Nutr*, 1981, *34*(10):2111-2116.
21. Bouchoucha, M., Devroede, G., Arhan, P., et al. What is the meaning of colorectal transit time measurement? *Dis Colon Rectum*, 1992, *35*:773-782.
22. Turnbull, G.K., Bartram, C.I., & Lennard-Jones, J.E. Radiographic studies of rectal evaluation in adults with idiopathic constipation. *Dis Colon Rectum*, 1988, *31*:190-197.
23. Rex, D.K., & Lappas, J.C. Combined manometry and defecography in 50 consecutive adults with fecal incontinence. *Dis Colon Rectum*, 1992, *35*(11):1040-1045.
24. Wrick, K.L., Robertson, J.B., Van Soest, P.J., et al. The influence of dietary fiber source on human intestinal transit and stool output. *J Nutr*, 1983, *113*(8):1464-1479.
25. Kelsay, J.L., Behall, K.M., & Prather, E.S. Effect of fiber from fruits and vegetables on metabolic responses of human subjects: Bowel transit time, number of defecations, fecal weight, urinary excretions of energy and nitrogen and apparent digestibilities of energy, nitrogen and fat. *Am J Clin Nutr*, 1978, *31*(7):1149-1152.
26. Rogers, H.J., House, F.R., Morrison, P.J., & Bradbrook, I.D. Comparison of the effect of drugs upon some commonly used measures of bowel transit time. *Br J Clin Pharmacol*, 1978, *6*(6):493-497.
27. Waller, S.L. Differential measurement of small and large bowel transit times in constipation and diarrhea: A new approach. *Gut*, 1975, *16*(5):372-378.
28. McLean, R.G., Smart, R.C., Gaston-Parry, D., et al. Colon transit scintigraphy in health and constipation using oral iodine-131-cellulose. *J Nuc Med*, 1990, *31*:985-989.
29. Stivland, R., Camilleri, M., Vassallo, M., et al. Scintigraphic measurement of regional gut transit in idiopathic constipation. *Gastroenterology*, 1991, *101*:107-115.
30. Wald, A., Farrukh, J., Rehder, J., & Holeva, K. Scintigraphic studies of rectal emptying in patients with constipation and defecatory difficulty. *Digest Dis Sci*, 1993, *38*:343-358.
31. Exton-Smith, A.N., Bendall, M.J., & Kent, F. A new technique for measuring the consistency of feces. A report in the elderly. *Age Ageing*, 1975, *4*(1):58-62.
32. Prior, A., Colgan, S.M., & Whorwell, P.J. Changes in rectal sensitivity after hypnotherapy in patients with irritable bowel syndrome. *Gut*, 1990, *31*:896-898.
33. Talley, N.J., Phillips, S.F., Melton, L.J., et al. A patient questionnaire to identify bowel disease. *Ann Int Med*, 1989, *111*(8):671-674.
34. McMillan, S.C., & Williams, F. Validity and reliability of the Constipation Assessment Scale. *Cancer Nurs*, 1989, *12*(3):183-188.
35. McMillan, S.C., & Levy, M. Reassessment of the validity and reliability of the Constipation Assessment Scale. An unpublished study, 1990. Contact address: University of South Florida College of Nursing, MDC Box 22, Tampa, FL 33617.
36. Casey, L., & Zachariah, B. A pilot study to develop a diarrhea assessment scale. Unpublished study, 1993. Contact address: James A. Haley Veterans Hospital, 118, Tampa, FL 33613.

30

Measuring Cardiac Parameters

Susan J. Quaal

There has been an upsurge of interest in physiologic research. One element that may have fostered this interest has arisen from nurses who have pursued their graduate studies in the physiologic sciences. Much of the health-care professional's assessment is focused on physiologic dimensions of health, and physiologic research questions require the measurement of these dimensions. Issues of physiologic measurement are not any different from issues related to psychosocial and behavioral measurement. There is equal concern with validity, reliability, and generalizability of findings.

Physiologic measurement is the assignment of numbers or units of measure to physiologic processes according to rules. These measures represent a correspondence between the physiologic function being measured and the number(s) assigned to it.[1]

Physiologic measurement often requires the use of instrumentation. Ideally, the instrument: (1) should be noninvasive; (2) directly measures the variable; (3) does not change or alter the variable being measured; (4) can be applied in a variety of settings; (5) provides a quantitative value; (6) provides continuous measures that are accurate and reliable; (7) has a rapid response time (frequency response) or a wide range of values; (8) is sensitive to small changes in physiologic variables; (9) maintains calibration without drift or noise; and (10) is cost-effective and easy to operate.[2]

It is critically important that physiologic measurements be carried out with rigor and consistency. Measurement characteristics should include: (1) validity or accuracy, which is the degree to which the measured value represents the actual value (*fidelity* is another term used); (2) reliability or measurement accuracy over time; (3) sensitivity or precision (the ability of the instrument to measure repeatedly the smallest degree of change; and (4) stability or the ability of an instrument to return to zero point after an input stimulus and lack of drift (ability of the instrument to remain stable at a given setting).[3] The measurement technique must be described in great detail when designing and publishing a physiologic study. This ensures exact replication of the study.

Prior to utilizing any of the measurements and associated instrumentation, the researcher must be familiar with manufacturer-recommended operation and safety instructions. It also is the responsibility of the researcher to obtain any required certification of the instrument or measurement procedure prior to data collection.

The Concept of Blood Pressure

As the left ventricle contracts, blood is ejected into the aorta. The highest pressure generated at the peak of the pulse wave is *systolic pressure*. Arterial pressure falls to a trough level at the end of diastole, which is termed *diastolic pressure*.[4] As pressure rises in the aorta, a pulse wave is generated and propagated throughout the arterial tree. Physical characteristics of the arterial system cause this pulse wave to change in contour as it propagates from the aorta to the arteries and capillaries (Figure 30.1). The upstroke becomes steeper and the pulse wave becomes more triangular. The incisura or dicrotic notch, marking the closure of the aortic valve is prominent in recordings from the aortic arch, but becomes slurred in the distal arteries. These changes occur as the high-frequency vibrations produced during aortic valve closure are quickly damped by the viscous and inertial properties of the blood and vascular wall.[5] Energy imparted to the blood by ventricular contraction is reflected back toward the heart from various sites in the circulation. These backward-pressure waves merge with the forward-moving wave to produce the characteristic arterial pressure waveform contour.

Systolic pressure in the lower extremities may be 20 to 30 mm higher than in the upper extremities.[6] The difference between systolic and diastolic pressures is termed *pulse pressure*, which is approximately 50 mm Hg. *Mean pressure* is the average pressure during the cardiac cycle and can be approximated for central arterial pressure by using the following formula: mean pressure = diastolic pressure + 1/3 pulse pressure.

Arterial pressure is regulated by two predominant mechanisms: (1) a system of rapidly acting vascular reflexes and resistances; and (2) a group of slower mechanisms that adjust the body's fluid volume and indirectly affect arterial pressure. As a result,

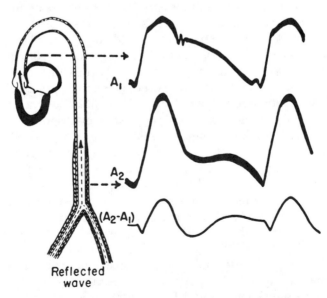

Figure 30.1 Changes in arterial pressure waveforms. The primary pulse contour (A_1) is recorded from the aortic arch. A_2 is the pulse recorded from the distal aorta. The difference between these pulses ($A_2 - A_1$) is the reflected pulse wave that travels toward the heart from the arterioles. Used by permission from Little, R.C., *Physiology of the heart and circulation* (3rd ed.). Chicago, Mosby-Yearbook Publishers, 1985, p. 243.

substantial changes in body position and level of muscular activity, as well as alterations in circulating blood volume, are tolerated without causing a significant deviation in blood pressure.[5]

Blood pressure (BP) measurement can be performed either *indirectly* with a cuff, stethoscope, and sphygmomanometer or *directly* by placing an intra-arterial catheter.

Indirect Blood Pressure Measurement

The term *indirect* is appropriate because pressure in the blood pressure cuff is measured, rather than that in the blood vessel itself. A nondistensible cuff containing an inflatable bladder is placed on the subject's arm, with the middle of the bladder placed directly over the brachial artery.

> The bladder—connected to a needle-valved rubber bulb by a piece of rubber tubing—is inflated by pumping the rubber bulb. The pressure in the cuff bladder is reflected on a mercury or aneroid manometer. Inflation of the bladder compresses the artery so that blood flow diminishes to the point of obliteration distal to the cuff. When the needle valve of the inflation bulb is released, the bladder within the cuff deflates and the cuff pressure falls. When the cuff pressure decreases to the peak pressure generated by left ventricular contraction, blood resumes flowing through the brachial artery on an intermittent basis. Sharp tapping or knocking sounds, termed *Korotkoff sounds*, are generated with each systole. The American Heart Association (AHA) describes these sounds as occurring in five distinct phases.[7]

Korotkoff sounds are named for the Russian physician who first described the auscultatory method in 1905.[8] Early investigators proposed that Korotkoff sounds were the result of a water hammer or breaker effect. Using a simulated artery of translucent latex, Sacks[9] studied the production of Korotkoff sounds in a vessel filled with colored fluid and found that the vessel was never fully occluded; some colored fluid was always present. During the production of the Korotkoff sounds the collapsed cross section of the vessel traveled longitudinally beneath the cuff, coincident with the pulse wave. Moreover, the sounds appeared to be generated when the collapsed section of the vessel arrived at the distal end of the cuff.

Such findings have led some investigators to conclude that Korotkoff sounds are the result not of turbulence within the vessel, but rather of dynamic instability of the vessel wall, which occurs when fluid oscillations imposed on it become amplified. This instability is the result of the elastic property of the artery wall. When this elastic property is diminished, as in fixed-vessel disease, a greater chance of auscultatory error is believed to exist.

In summary, consensus does not exist in the literature regarding the exact cause of Korotkoff sounds. Therefore, the AHA recommends that Phase 1, 4, and 5 pressure readings be documented when the sounds of Phase 5 extend to zero. The clinical significance of such findings is uncertain.[7] The five phases are:

> Phase 1. Pressure level at which the first faint, clear tapping sounds are heard (systolic blood pressure)
> Phase 2. Time during cuff deflation when a murmur or swishing sounds are heard
> Phase 3. Period during which sounds are crisper and increase in intensity
> Phase 4. Time when a distinct, abrupt, muffling of sound occurs. This phase reflects the diastolic pressure in children and in adults with hyperkinetic states that allow for audible sounds throughout the deflation period
> Phase 5. Pressure level when the last sound is heard and after which all sound disappears. This phase reflects the diastolic pressure in the adult[6]

Procedure for Recording an Indirect Blood Pressure

Recommendations for human blood pressure determination by sphygmomanometers are as follows:

1. Situate the individual in a quiet environment with the arm resting at heart level. Put him/her at ease and allow a 5-minute rest period.
2. Place the manometer at eye level, sufficiently close to read the calibrations marking the gauge or column.
3. Select the appropriately sized cuff. Bladder width should be at least 40% of arm circumference; bladder length should be at least 80% of arm circumference.
4. Locate the brachial artery along the inner upper arm by palpation.
5. Wrap the cuff smoothly and snugly around the arm, centering the bladder over the brachial artery. The lower margin should be 2.5 cm above the antecubital space. (Do not rely on cuff marking; find the center by folding the bladder in half.)
6. Determine the level for maximal inflation by observing the pressure at which the radial pulse is no longer palpable as the cuff is rapidly inflated (palpated systolic) and by adding 30 mm Hg. (Note presence of an irregular pulse.)
7. Rapidly and steadily deflate the cuff. Then wait 15 to 30 seconds before reinflating.
8. Position the stethoscope over the palpated brachial artery below the cuff at the antecubital fossa. Ear pieces should point forward. The bell head of the stethoscope should be applied with light pressure, ensuring skin contact at all points. Heavy pressure may distort sounds.
9. Rapidly and steadily inflate the cuff to the maximal inflation level as determined in Step 6.
10. Release the air in the cuff so that the pressure falls at a rate of 2 to 3 mm per second.
11. Note the systolic pressure at the onset of at least two consecutive beats (Phase 1) for both adults and children. Blood pressure levels should always be recorded in even numbers and read to the nearest 2 mm Hg mark on the manometer.
12. Note the diastolic pressure at muffling (Phase IV) for children and cessation of sound (Phase V) for adults. Phase V, at which the last sound is heard, is the diastolic pressure in adults. Listen for 10 to 20 mm Hg below the last sound heard to confirm disappearance, and then deflate the cuff rapidly and completely.
13. Record systolic/diastolic pressure. When Phase IV pressure is recorded, the pressure at Phase V also should be recorded. Example: 108/64/52 or 110/66/0 mm Hg.
14. Record the patient's position, cuff size, and the arm used for the measurement.
15. Wait 1 to 2 minutes before repeating the pressure measurement in the same arm to permit the release of blood trapped in the arm veins.*

Reliability, Validity, and Measurement Error

To be detected by a stethoscope, Korotkoff sounds must be at a frequency within an audible range. In low-flow states resulting from a primary reduction in cardiac output or increased peripheral vascular resistance, transmission of sounds is impaired. Sound transmission also can be decreased in obese patients or in those with severe peripheral edema.[10] Common sources of variation in blood pressure measurement are listed in Table 30.1. Indirect blood pressure measurements may be unreliable and invalid due to factors related to patient, blood pressure bladder and cuff, and the examiner.

The patient. The examiner must attempt to measure an indirect blood pressure reading that is representative of the patient's ordinary and reproducible circumstances. Ideally, blood pressure should be recorded in a quiet room at a comfortable temperature after the patient has rested for 5 minutes. Frohlich et al. state that "the patient's arm should be bared, unrestricted by clothing, with the palm of the hand exposed upward and the

*American Heart Association. Report of a special task force appointed by the steering committee. *Circulation*, 1988, 77:501A-514A. Reproduced with permission.

Table 30.1 Common Sources of Variation in Blood Pressure Measurement

Source	Cause	Effect	Remedy
Manometer	Loss of mercury	Reading impaired	Have medical equipment dealer add more mercury to zero mark
	Clogged air vent at top of manometer tube	Mercury column will respond sluggishly to pressure	Clean or replace air vent
	Loose air vent nut	Mercury column will bounce	Tighten knurled nut at top
Bladder	Too narrow	High reading	Determine bladder and cuff size
	Too wide	Low reading	Use proper technique
	Not centered over artery	High reading	Use proper technique
Cuff	Loose application	High reading	Use proper technique
	Applied over clothing	Reading impaired	Use proper technique
	Too wide	Low reading	Use pediatric cuff
Tubing	Too wide	Low reading	Check for leaks and replace
Stethoscope	Eartips not forward	Auditory impairment, low systolic, high diastolic	Use proper technique

Modified from American Heart Association of Metropolitan Chicago. *Manual for instructors in the measurement of blood pressure.* 1976. Chicago: American Heart Association, 1984, *33*:879-881.

elbow flexed at the heart level. Ideally, the person should not have eaten or smoked for 30 minutes prior to the blood pressure measurement."[6,p10]

Frohlich et al.[6] comment on the effect of arm position and measurement accuracy:

> The pressure of the arm increases as the arm is lowered from the level of the heart (phlebostatic axis); conversely, raising the arm above this position lowers the pressure measurement. The effect is largely explained by hydrostatic pressure or by the effect of gravity on the column of blood. Therefore, when measuring indirect blood pressure, the patient's arm should be positioned so that the location of the stethoscope head (preferably, the bell) is at the level of the heart. This location of the heart is arbitrarily taken to be at the junction of the fourth intercostal space and the lower left sternal border. Attention to the position of the brachial artery in relation to the heart is particularly important when the patient is standing upright. No corrections for position need to be made if the patient is lying supine on a flat surface with the head slightly raised, since the arm by the side of the body is sufficiently close to the level of the heart. When the patient is seated, placing the arm on a nearby tabletop a little above waist level will result in a satisfactory position. If the position of the arm cannot be appropriately adjusted, a correction for the hydrostatic pressure must be made: for each 1 cm of vertical height above or below the heart level, 0.8 mm Hg must be added or subtracted, respectively, to the observed pressure.

Korotkoff sounds may not always disappear but may continue to be heard until cuff pressure drops to 0 in children, patients with aortic valvular insufficiency, or high cardiac output (anemia, thyrotoxicosis, or pregnancy) and marked vasodilatation. Phase IV, during which the pitch of Korotkoff sounds changes, should then be used as the marker for diastolic pressure.

Cuff and bladder. Length and width of bladder and ratio of one to the other are known factors influencing indirect blood pressure measurement. False low blood pressure readings result if the blood pressure cuff is too small, and false high readings occur if the cuff is too large. The AHA[11] recommends a bladder width of 40% of the arm circumference, and the cuff should be long enough to encircle at least 80% of the arm in adults. The correct ratio of bladder width to arm circumference is 0:4.[11] The bladder width multiplied by 2.5 defines the ideal arm circumference of that particular cuff. Therefore the ideal arm circumference for a bladder width of 12 cm is 12.0 × 2.5, or 30 cm. Thigh cuffs should be used for obese individuals whose arm circumferences are greater than 41 cm.[7]

Banner and associate[12] determined the effect of snugness of cuff wrap on the accuracy of blood pressure measurement. The study was performed on six healthy volunteers. In both studies, control values were obtained from the right upper arm with cuffs of appropriate size and snug fit. The first study had two phases. In the first phase, cuffs of appropriate size were wrapped snugly around the upper left arm of seated subjects. The effects of two other degrees of cuff snugness were evaluated by placing a filled 250-ml intravenous fluid bag between the cuff and arm over the triceps, measuring blood pressure, then draining the same bag of half its contents and then all of its contents without rewrapping the cuff (loose and very loose fits). The second phase was identical except that the cuffs used on the left arm were one size too small. These researchers found that appropriately sized cuffs, whether wrapped tightly or loosely gave correct blood pressure readings. Cuffs snugly wrapped, but too small for the subject, gave high readings, averaging 10 mm Hg. Loose wrapping of small cuffs gave variable results in individual subjects that exaggerate systolic blood pressure from 2 to 80 mm Hg.

Direct (Invasive) Blood Pressure Measurement

Direct arterial pressure is measured via a transducer connected to a small plastic catheter, which is inserted into a peripheral artery. Transduced pressures provide systolic, diastolic, and mean values, as well as a displayed arterial waveform. Gorny[13,p68] described invasive blood pressure monitoring as follows:

> Direct blood pressure measurement is used when continuous hemodynamic monitoring for the evaluation of changing patient status, evaluation of related therapy and continuous blood sampling, such as for arterial blood gas measurement, are required. The intraarterial method is preferred to the indirect auscultation technique in patients with low cardiac output states when pulses may be poorly palpable and Korotkoff sounds may be difficult to hear.
>
> Invasive monitoring provides a moment-to-moment picture and a visual display of BP trends. During direct BP monitoring, intravascular pressure changes caused by cardiac contraction associated with the transmission of electrical impulses within the cardiac cycle are measured. An artery is cannulated with a catheter, which is connected to a fluid-filled tubing and transducer system. The transducer converts the pressure signals caused by the back and forth movement of the arterial wall sensed as the artery-catheter interface into electrical energy that is displayed as waveforms on an oscilloscope.

Arterial catheters can be placed by direct threading, the Seldinger technique, or the transfixing method. Direct technique involves inserting the catheter until arterial pressure is transmitted to the catheter, and the needle is removed while the catheter is advanced. The Seldinger technique makes use of a wire over which the catheter is threaded. The transfixation technique requires a puncture by the catheter through the posterior blood vessel wall, which is subsequently drawn into the blood vessel lumina.

Cannulation sites include the radial, brachial, axillary, femoral, dorsalis pedis, and posterior tibial arteries. The radial artery is the most commonly used peripheral site because of its easy accessibility. The indwelling arterial polyurethane catheter is then connected to a disposable transducer that converts the patient's arterial pressure to an electrical signal that is transmitted via an electrical cable to the bedside monitor that displays the blood pressure waveform and quantifies systolic and diastolic values.[14]

Reliability and Validity

Gardner and Hujcs[15,p12] point out that the "accuracy of blood pressure readings depends on establishing an accurate reference point from which all subsequent measurements are made." Zeroing a hemodynamic monitoring system is accomplished by positioning a fluid-filled stopcock at the phlebostatic axis, turning it off to the patient or open to air, and activating the bedside monitor zero function. All pressure contributions from the atmosphere are negated, and only pressure values that exist within the heart chamber or vessel are measured.[16] It is the stopcock that is opened to air, not the transducer, which is leveled to the patient's phlebostatic axis.[14,17]

Windsor and Burch[18] described the phlebostatic axis as a point of junction between a frontal and transverse chest plane located by drawing an imaginary line from the fourth sternal intercostal space and extending it around to the right side of the chest. A second imaginary line is drawn vertically from the midaxillary line down to bisect the first transverse line. Zeroing should be performed at least once a shift, after raising or lowering the head of the bed, and before implementing any treatment changes based on the invasive arterial pressure.

To measure direct invasive blood pressure accurately, the fluid-filled catheter system must be able to transit the patient's pressure with fidelity or accuracy of reproduction. Physiologic waveforms are dynamic, not static. Thus, a hemodynamic monitoring system must have excellent fidelity, termed *dynamic response*, which refers to an oscillatory response produced by the system after it is excited. This is similar to vibrations produced by striking a bell. Another example of dynamic response is the bouncing action of a tennis ball when it is thrust against a hard surface. A lesser height is reached with each successive bounce. The number of oscillations per second is referred to as its *natural frequency*.[17]

Frequency response of a catheter-plumbing hemodynamic monitoring system can be obtained by stimulating the system with high pressure and observing the system's oscillatory response. The system's in-line fast-flush device can be used to excite the system by opening and quickly closing the device. This action temporarily interrupts pressure waveform transmission and applies a step change or "square wave" pressure, followed by oscillations that revert back to the arterial pressure waveform.

Natural frequency is determined by measuring (in millimeters) the distance between two consecutive oscillatory peaks, termed a *period*, and dividing this distance by the strip recorder paper speed (25 mm/sec; Figure 30.2). Optimal natural frequency is

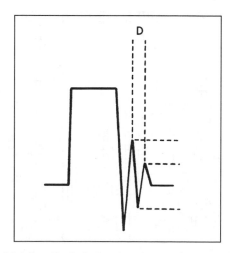

Figure 30.2 Illustration of the fast flush dynamic response (square-wave) assessment. Natural frequency is estimated by measuring the distance (D) between two consecutive peaks (the "period") and dividing by the paper speed (25 mm/sec).

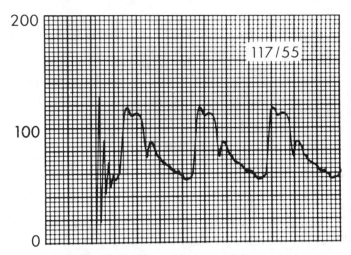

Figure 30.3 An optimal natural frequency of 25 H. There is one small box between any two successive oscillations divided by the paper speed (25 mm/sec).

about 25 H, which would be no more than 1 little box (1 mm) between each two successive vertical oscillations.[12] Figure 30.3 illustrates an optimal dynamic response of 25 H. Figure 30.4 illustrates a damped system. False low systolic and high diastolic readings occur with an overdamped system.

Because decisions regarding pharmacologic and other interventions often are contingent on the patient's blood pressure, it is imperative that direct measurement occur only after acceptable natural frequency has been validated. Measures to maximize natural frequency are: (1) to remove all air bubbles from the monitoring system; (2) to minimize the potential for clot formation at the catheter tip by using a continuous flush system; (3) to keep catheter and connecting tubing length under 5 feet; and (4) to eliminate loose-fitting connections.

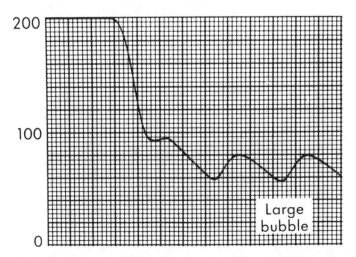

Figure 30.4 A damped response caused by a large air bubble in the software-connecting tubing.

Discrepancies between Direct and Indirect Blood Pressure Measurements

Discrepancies occur between indirect and direct methods of blood pressure measurement as the result of methodology, instrumentation, and natural physiologic causes. Research has suggested that indirect blood pressure measurement generally underestimates the systolic value and overestimates the diastolic value.[19] However, the most important contributing factor of discrepancies between these two methods can be attributed to methodology. Arm position, cuff size, obesity, and edema all can contribute to indirect measurement error.[20] It is recommended that a palpatory reading be recorded as the systolic pressure if it is found to be higher than the auscultatory reading.[7] When using the direct technique, the system must be zeroed and natural frequency assessed with correction to 25 H to achieve reliable measurements.

Thermal Dilution Cardiac Output Measurement

Cardiac output is the amount of blood ejected by the heart per unit of time and is normally 4 to 8 liters/minute.[14] Tissue viability depends on an adequate delivery of oxygen and nutrients from the circulating blood. Therefore cardiac output is an important parameter in assessing the patient with myocardial failure and as an indicator of response to therapy.

Thermal dilution technique for measurement of cardiac output was described by Fegler in 1954.[21] A specific quantity (5–10 ml) of normal saline or dextrose solution at a known temperature is injected into the bloodstream via a special pulmonary catheter with a thermistor positioned at its distal tip. The change in temperature as this bolus of fluid is warmed by the blood is recorded by the distal tip thermistor and is recorded as a temperature–time curve by a cardiac output computer that is inversely proportional to blood flow. Thermal dilution cardiac output (TDCO) determinations measure flow over only a few seconds. Therefore three to five repeated measurements are made, and the mean of these values is used to reflect the average cardiac output.

Reliability and Validity

Temperature of both blood and injectate solution must be accurate and stable. A newer closed injectate system with an in-line thermistor that measures injectate temperature as it leaves the syringe has reduced, but not eliminated, this source of measurement error. Daily and Schroeder[14] caution that heat from the injectate, whether iced or room temperature, is lost through handling the injectate syringe and throughout the catheter itself as it travels to the right atrium. A warm environment or the use of heat lamps can appreciably alter the injectate temperature. Ways to minimize injectate heat transfer or loss are listed in Table 30.2. The injectate must be administered rapidly (10 ml in ≤ 4 seconds) and evenly. Table 30.2 highlights strategies to maximize the accuracy of thermodilution-calculated cardiac output.[14]

Iced versus Room-Temperature Injectate

A total of nine studies, representing diverse patient populations, have compared 10 ml of room-temperature and iced injectate in TDCO. All but one[22] reported high correlations. Daily and Mersch[23] examined the relationship between iced and room-temperature injectates in 30 acutely ill adults. The correlation was 0.973. These observations were confirmed by Nelson and Anderson ($r = 0.970$) in 42 acutely ill adults.[24] Although Swinney et al.[25] concluded that room-temperature and iced injectates provided equivalent information ($r = 0.99$), their sample size consisted only of seven hemodynamically stable

Table 30.2   Strategies to Maximize Accuracy of Thermodilution—Calculated Cardiac Output (CO)

Strategy	Discussion
Rapid, even injection technique	Slow or uneven technique produces inaccurate data
	Cardiac output curve reveals slow or uneven upstroke
Examine each CO curve for technical adequacy	Each curve should be printed out, rather than depending solely on digital value
Delay CO computerized analysis until after injection is completed	In patients with very low stroke volumes, blood moves very slowly from the right atrium to the pulmonary artery; thus the CO computer can complete analysis before maximum temperature difference has been sensed if the analysis is begun prior to the end of the injection
Minimize injectate heat transfer or loss	
Use closed-injectate system with an in-line temperature probe	Reduces exposure to environment; minimizes hand contact with injectate. In-line temperature probe measures injectate temperature after it leaves syringe
Inject an initial volume of injectate to "cool the catheter"	Reduces heat loss of subsequent injections; do not use initial injection for CO measurement
Use room-temperature, not "iced," injectate	Similar results found between iced and room-temperature CO determinations; room-temperature injectate less likely to cause slowing of heart rate. May need to use iced injectate in hypothermic patients to ensure minimum temperature difference of 12 degrees
Keep injectate solution, tubing, and catheter away from direct sunlight or heat lamps	May cause artificial reading

patients. Vennix et al.[26] studied 27 male patients representing a broad spectrum of critically ill patients who were receiving a variety of treatments, including vasoactive pharmacologic agents and mechanical ventilation. These investigators reported a correlation coefficient of 0.989 between the use of 10 ml of room-temperature and iced injectates.

Elkayam et al.[27] observed the relationships between 10, 5, and 3 ml room-temperature injectate with 10 ml iced injectate. As the volume of room-temperature injectate decreased, reproducibility of the standard technique using 10 ml iced injectate declined. However, the error in values for cardiac outputs obtained with these techniques was not statistically significant.

Keen[28] used a sample of seven patients diagnosed with hepatic cirrhosis and compared 19 sets of cardiac outputs using iced and room-temperature injectates. The cardiac index of each patient was greater than 3.5 l/min/m^2. These results suggest that there is no difference in TDCO between using iced and room-temperature injectates in hyperdynamic patients with cirrhosis. Gawlinski[29] concluded that 5 ml iced injectate is comparable to 10 ml room-temperature and 10 ml iced injectate in most adult patients. Less than 5 ml iced temperature should not be used. Gillman[30] cautioned that a change in injectate temperature once it is measured introduces a 3% to 6% error. The associated error for inaccurate injectate volumes was found to be 1% per 0.1 ml using 10 ml injectate, and 2% per 0.1 cc using 5 cc. All crystalloid solutions were found to be acceptable.

Gardner and Hollingsworth[31] compared TDCO using iced and refrigerated

(10–15°C) injectate in 40 postop adult cardiac surgery patients. There was no statistically or clinically significant difference between the two methods. Gawlinski[29] summarized recommendations for research-based TDCO measurements.

Pulmonary Artery Wedge Pressure Measurement

Development of a flow-directed catheter has allowed indirect assessment of left ventricular function via the pulmonary artery wedge pressure (PAWP) measurement. At the tip of this catheter is a balloon that, when inflated, causes the catheter tip to become buoyant and advance in the direction of blood flow. When positioned in a capillary, forward blood flow is obstructed, and a pressure-sensing device at the distal tip reflects left atrial pressure, which is important in assessing left ventricular function when clinical signs of heart failure are present. Normal values are 6 to 12 mm Hg.

Reliability and Validity

PAWP measurement accuracy is crucial and can be obtained only through a program of excellence in quality assurance, which minimally must consist of zeroing and referencing, and dynamic response. Additional factors that ensure accuracy include confirmation of catheter location by capillary blood gases and a chest X-ray to validate placement in lung zone III.

Zeroing and Referencing

Zeroing and referencing are two independent activities performed simultaneously as the most basic quality-assurance components. Zeroing and referencing have been described as the "single most important steps in setting up a pressure measurement system" and "cause of the largest pressure measurement errors in the clinical situation."[15,p13]

Zeroing is performed by opening the system to air and therefore establishing atmospheric pressure as zero. *Referencing* is accomplished by placing the air-fluid interface (stopcock opened to air) at the right heart level to negate the weight effect of fluid (hydrostatic pressure) in the catheter tubing.[28] Windsor and Burch[18] determined that the correct reference level for PAWP was the *phlebostatic axis* located at the intersection of a frontal plane passing midway between the anterior and posterior surfaces of the chest and a transverse plane that transected the body at the junction of the fourth intercostal space and sternal margin.

The phrase "zeroing the transducer" is a misnomer that exists in our nomenclature. It is the stopcock that is opened to air, not the transducer, which is leveled to the patient's phlebostatic axis.[31] Pressure monitoring systems should be zeroed and referenced at least once per shift, after the head of the bed is raised or lowered, and before extrapolating pressure data that is used in clinical patient management decision making.

Dynamic Response Testing and Natural Frequency Assessment

Pulmonary artery wedge pressures are static and not dynamic. The catheter and connecting software's ability to transmit pressure accurately to the transducer depends on its dynamic response, which was discussed under arterial pressure measurement.

Capillary Blood Gases

Proper placement of the inflated balloon tip pulmonary artery catheter in the capillary bed can be validated by capillary (*c*) blood gases, as compared to arterial (*a*) blood gases. A properly "wedged" catheter seals off any forward blood flow. Thus a "capillary blood gas" will be higher in oxygen and lower in carbon dioxide than an arterial blood gas sample. Catheter placement in the PAWP position is validated if the following criteria are met when comparing a capillary to arterial blood gas sample:[32]

$$PcO_2 - PaO_2 \geq 19 \text{ mm Hg}$$
$$PaCO_2 - PcCO_2 \geq 11 \text{ mm Hg}$$
$$Phc - pHa \geq 0.08$$

Lung Zone Placement

Pulmonary artery wedge pressure estimates pulmonary venous or left atrial pressure only when a continuous column of blood exists from the catheter tip through the capillary bed and into the left atrium.[33] If a capillary is collapsed, patency between the left atrium and catheter tip is interrupted, a resistance is imposed, and pressure measurements are inaccurate. Capillaries are labeled as lung zone I, II, or III capillaries, depending on their horizontal reference to the left atrium. Lung zone I capillaries are above the left atrial plane. Lung zone II capillaries are horizontal to the left atrial plane, and lung zone III capillaries are below the left atrial plane (Figure 30.5). Catheter placement in a capillary located above the left atrial plane is in a lung zone I capillary. The weight of alveolar sacs transmitted from the lungs across the alveolar-capillary membrane totally collapses lung zone I capillaries. Hence a catheter positioned in a lung zone I capillary records a falsely high pulmonary artery wedge pressure. Lung zone II capillaries are located horizontal to the left atrial plane and are partially collapsed by alveolar pressure. It is only when the catheter is positioned with a capillary located below the left atrial plane (lung zone III capillary) that a continuous uninterrupted column of blood exists from the left atrium to catheter tip and therefore PAWP accurately reflects an indirect measurement of left atrial pressure.[31]

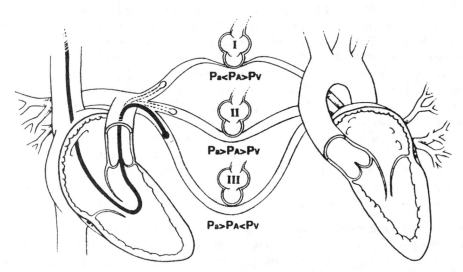

Figure 30.5 Pulmonary capillaries in reference to level of left atrium. Lung zone I capillaries are above the left atrium level. Lung zone II capillaries are horizontal to the left atrium, and lung zone III capillaries are below the left atrium. The pulmonary artery wedge pressure accurately reflects left atrial pressure only when the tip of the catheter is in a lung zone III capillary and a continuous uninterrupted column of blood exists between the left atrium and capillary. Reproduced with permission from O'Quin, R., & Marini, J.J. Occult positive end-expiratory pressure in mechanically ventilated patients with airflow obstruction. *Am Rev Respir Dis*, 1983, *128(2)*:319-326.

Exemplar Studies

Morris, A.H., & Chapman, R.H. Wedge pressure confirmation by aspiration of pulmonary capillary blood. *Crit Care Med*, 1985, *13*:736-740.

This study established criteria to confirm the placement of a pulmonary wedge pressure catheter in the capillary bed by comparing a capillary blood gas to an arterial blood gas. These findings improve the accuracy of this physiologic parameter and ensure that the pressure recorded is indeed from the pulmonary artery capillary.

Daily, E.K., & Mersch, J. Thermodilution cardiac outputs using room and ice temperature injectate: Comparison with the Fick method. *Heart Lung*, 1987, *16*:294-300.

Thermal dilution cardiac output is performed by injecting a known quality of injectate solution at a known temperature. A thermistor at the tip of the catheter measures the change in blood temperature as cooled by this injectate solution. This study suggested that use of a room-temperature injectate solution was as accurate as iced injectate, thus eliminating the need for containing the injectate solution in an ice bath at the bedside.

References

1. Heather, S.E. *Measurement of physiologic variables.* Nursing 704 course syllabus. Provo: University of Utah College of Nursing, 1990.
2. Carr, J.J., & Brown, J.M. *Introduction to biomedical equipment technology* (2nd ed.). New York: Prentice-Hall, 1993.
3. Waltz, C.F., Strickland, O.L., & Lenz, E.R. *Measurement in nursing research* (2nd ed.). Philadelphia: Davis, 1991.
4. Burton, A.C. *Physiology and biophysics of the circulation.* Chicago: Yearbook Publishers, 1972, p. 160.
5. Little, R.C. *Physiology of the heart and circulation* (3rd ed.). Chicago: Yearbook Publishers, 1985, pp. 247-269.
6. Frohlich, E.D., Grim, C., Labarthe, D.R., et al. *Recommendations for human blood pressure determination by sphygmomanometers* (vol. V). AHA publication no. 70-1005 (SA). Dallas: American Heart Association, 1987, pp. i-34.
7. Anderson, F.D., Cunningham, S.G., & Maloney, J.P. Indirect blood pressure measurement: A need to reassess. *Am J Crit Care*, 1993, *2*:272-279.
8. McCutheon, E.P., & Rusherm, R.F. Korotkoff sounds: An experimental critique. *Circ Res*, 1967, *20*:149-161.
9. Sacks, A.H. Indirect blood pressure measurements. A matter of interpretation. *Angiology*, 1979, *30*:683-695.
10. Hennaman, E.A., & Henneman, P.L. Intricacies of blood pressure measurement: Reexamining the rituals. *Heart Lung*, 1989, *18*:263-271.
11. Perloff, D., Grim, C., Flack, J., et al. Human blood pressure determination by sphygmomanometry. *AHA Medical/Scientific Statement.* Dallas: American Heart Association, 1993.
12. Banner, T.E., & Gravenstine, J.S. Comparative tightness of fit on accuracy of blood pressure measurements. *J Clin Monit*, 1991, *7*:281-284.
13. Gorny, D.A. Arterial blood pressure measurement technique. *AACN Clin Issues Crit Care Nurs*, 1993, *4*:66-80.
14. Daily, E.K., & Schroeder, J.S. *Techniques in bedside hemodynamic monitoring* (4th ed.). St. Louis: Mosby-Yearbook 1989, pp. 34-48.
15. Gardner, R.M., & Hujcs, M. Fundamentals of physiologic monitoring. *AACN's Clin Issues Crit Care Nurs*, 1993, *4*:11-24.
16. Gardner, R.M. Hemodynamic monitoring from catheter to display. *Acute Care*, 1986, *12*:3-33.
17. Quaal, S.J. Quality assurance in hemodynamic monitoring. *AACN's Clin Issues Crit Care Nurs*, 1993, *4*:197-206.
18. Windsor, T., & Burch, C.E. Phlebostatic axis and phlebostatic references levels for venous pressure measurements in man. *Proc Soc Exp Biol Med*, 1945, *58*:169-173.
19. Rebenson-Piano, M.A., Holm, K. & Powers, M. An examination of the differences that occur between direct and indirect blood pressure measurement. *Heart Lung*, 1987, *16*:285-294.
20. Chuyn, D.A. A comparison of intra-arterial and ausculatory blood pressure readings. *Heart Lung*, 1985; *14*:223-226.
21. Fegler, G. Measurement of cardiac output in anesthetized animal by thermodilution method. *Q. J Exp Physiol*, 1954, *39*:153-164.
22. Kint, P.P., van Domburg, R., & Meij, S.H. Reproducibility of thermodilution cardiac output measurements. *Circulation*, 1981, *64*(suppl IV):165-168.
23. Daily, E.K., & Mersch J. Thermodilution cardiac outputs using room and ice temperature injectate: Comparison with the Fick method. *Heart Lung*, 1987, *16*:294-300.
24. Nelson, L.D., & Anderson, H.B. Patient selection for iced versus room temperature injectate for thermodilution cardiac output determinations. *Crit Care Med*, 1985, *13*:1182-1184.
25. Swinney, R.S., Davenport, N.W., Wagers, P.W., et al.

Iced versus room temperature injectate for thermal dilution cardiac output. *Crit Care Med*, 1981, *8*:265-269.

26. Vennix, C.V., Nelson, D.H., & Pierpont, G.L. Thermodilution cardiac output in critically ill patients: Comparison of room temperature and iced injectate. *Heart Lung*, 1984, *13*:574-578.

27. Elkayam, U., Berkley, R., Azem, S., et al. Cardiac output by thermodilution technique: Effect in injectate's volume and temperature on accuracy and reproducibility in the critically ill patient. *Chest*, 1983, *83*:418-422.

28. Keen, J.H. The effect of injectate temperature on thermodilution cardiac output measurement in hyperdynamic cirrhotics. *Heart Lung*, 1985, *15*:312-315.

29. Gawlinski, A. Facts and fallacies of cardiac output measurements. *AACN's 1993 NTI Proceedings*, 1993, 50-51.

30. Gillman, P. Bolus thermodilution cardiac output: Reliable parameter or best guess? *AACN's 1993 NTI Proceedings*, 1993, 52-53.

31. Gardner, R.N., & Hollingsworth, K.W. Technology advances in invasive pressure monitoring. *J Cardiovasc Nurs*, 1988, *2*:52-55.

32. Morris, A.H., & Chapman, R.H. Wedge pressure confirmation by aspiration of pulmonary capillary blood. *Crit Care Med*, 1985, *13*:736-740.

33. O'Quin, R., & Marini, J.J. Occult positive end-expiratory pressure in mechanically ventilated patients with airflow obstruction. *Am Rev Respir Dis*, 1982, *126(2)*:166-170.

31

Measuring Physiologic Parameters in Obstetric Nursing

Jana Lauderdale

Physiologic measures are used throughout obstetric nursing to guide the management of care provided to childbearing women. As the author's professional expertise lies in the area of womens' health, this chapter examines various assessment tools used in obstetric nursing, emphasizing the strengths and limitations of each and how that in turn affects the tools' reliability and validity. The chapter assists not only nurses with maternal-child research-related interests, but also other health-care providers. Selected instruments used for antepartum, the labor and delivery, the newborn nursery, and postpartum care are discussed in light of their use to both client management and nursing research.

Antepartal Tools

Diabetes, preeclampsia, systemic lupus erythematosus, chronic hypertension, sickle cell disease, and Rh isoimmunization are all conditions that can contribute to the development of uteroplacental insufficiency (UPI). Freeman[1] reports that at least two-thirds of antepartum fetal deaths are due to UPI. Therefore, any woman who is at risk of developing UPI, previously had a stillborn child, or has noted a decrease in the amount or absence of fetal movement is considered to be a candidate for antepartum fetal assessment.

Since the 1980s a myriad of changes have taken place in obstetrical care. The use of ultrasound and increased knowledge of maternal-fetal physiology have provided physicians and nurses access to the fetus for purposes of assessment that before were never possible. Fetal assessment is one component in the process of prenatal care and involves early identification of current or potential problems. Two tools commonly used in antepartum fetal assessment, the nonstress test and the biophysical profile, are discussed.

The Nonstress Test (NST)
The Nonstress Test (NST) is one of the most widely applied tools for antepartum fetal assessment. The purpose of the test is to observe fetal heart rate (FHR) acceleration in re-

sponse to fetal movement. Accelerations of the FHR imply an intact central and autonomic nervous system that is not being affected by a decrease of oxygen to the fetus (i.e.,
intrauterine hypoxia). The NST can be administered as early as at 27 weeks of gestation
and is especially useful in the presence of pregnancy induced hypertension, diabetes, intrauterine growth retardation, multiple gestation, and spontaneous rupture of membranes. Its advantages and disadvantages are:

> Advantages of the NST
> > Noninvasive
> > Quick
> > Relatively inexpensive
> > Easy to perform
> > Easy to interpret
> > Can be performed in an outpatient setting
> > No known contraindications
> Disadvantages of the NST
> > False-positive rate for nonreactive findings resulting from fetal sleep cycles, medica
> > > tions, and fetal immaturity
> > Precise tracings inconsistently obtained
> > Woman must lie relatively still for at least 20 minutes

The woman is placed in a semi-Fowler's position, with a pillow placed under the
right hip to displace the uterus to the left and to avoid supine hypotension. An electronic
fetal monitor is used to obtain a tracing of the FHR and fetal movement. The examiner
applies belts to the woman's abdomen. One belt holds a device that detects uterine or
fetal movement. The other belt holds a device that detects the FHR. Recordings are obtained for approximately 30 to 40 minutes. Each fetal movement is documented so that
simultaneous FHR changes may be assessed.

The results of the NST are interpreted as follows:

Reactive test. Normal NST. A reactive NST shows at least two accelerations of FHR with
fetal movements, of 15 beats per minute, lasting 15 seconds or more, over 20 minutes.
Nonreactive test. Abnormal NST. The NST is considered nonreactive when fewer than
two accelerations occur over 20 to 40 minutes. If accelerations do occur, the test is considered nonreactive if their amplitude is less than 15 beats per minute, or if they do not
last 15 seconds.
Unsatisfactory test. Test yields uninterpretable data or inadequate fetal activity.

The reactive NST appears to indicate fetal well-being. A nonreactive NST indicates
the need for further testing.[2] In many cases the NST results are compared with the results of a biophysical profile or a contraction stress test to evaluate all possible parameters.[3]

Chez's[4] study was one of the first comprehensive investigations to assess the reliability of obstetric nurses' interpretations of NSTs.[4] Out of the 1,000 National Association
of American College of Obstetrics and Gynecology (NAACOG) member nurses surveyed, 412 interpreted 5 NST strips. Participants were self-identified as nurses with a
primary clinical focus of labor and delivery or antepartum. The study's three purposes
were to determine (1) whether nurses could correctly interpret NST strips; (2) to determine whether demographic variables correlated with the accuracy of interpretation; and
(3) to compare the responses of obstetric nurses to those of an obstetrician (the same
strips had been interpreted by obstetricians in a previous study).

Eighty-four to ninety-eight percent of the nurses agreed on the interpretation for
each of the five strips. Nurses' responses differed significantly from physicians' inter-

Table 31.1 Biophysical Profile: Technique and Interpretation

Variable	Normal	Abnormal
Fetal breathing movements	≥1 episode of ≥30 sec. in 30 min.	Absent or no episode of ≥30 sec. in 30 min.
Gross body movements	≥3 discrete body or limb movements in 30 min. (episodes of active continuous movement considered as single movement)	≤2 episodes of body or limb movements in 30 min.
Fetal tone	≥1 episode of active extension with return to flexion of fetal limb(s) or trunk. Opening and closing of hand considered normal tone	Either slow extension with return to partial flexion or movement of limb in full extension or absent fetal movement
Reactive Fetal Heart Rate (FHR)	≥2 episodes of FHR acceleration or of bpm lasting ≤15 sec., associated with fetal movement in 20 min.	≤2 episodes of acceleration of FHR or acceleration of ≥15 bpm in 20 min.
Qualitative amniotic fluid volume	≥1 pocket of fluid measuring ≥1 cm in two perpendicular planes	Either no pockets or a pocket ≤1 cm in two perpendicular planes

Manning, F.A. Fetal assessment based on fetal biophysical profile scoring: Experiences in 12,620 referred high-risk pregnancies. *Am J Obstet Gynecol*, 1985, *151*(3):343-350. Used with permission.

pretations of strips as reactive or nonreactive on only one strip on which 92% of the nurses concurred compared to 98% of the obstetricians. Nurses' interpretations were not related to experience, education, formal courses in electronic fetal monitoring, or other demographic variables. The findings emphasize nurses' ability and expertise in interpreting NST strips as being equivalent to that of obstetricians'.[4]

Internal validity of the Chez[4] study might be affected by the history and maturation of the participants, as the study involving physicians was already several years old at the time of the comparison study. The researchers found intraobserver (within participant) reliability in the majority of study participants.

Limitations of the NST instrument that may impact the reliability of the test include the high percentage of false-positive results (from 50% to 80%), that is, a fetus with a nonreactive NST has a normal outcome.[5] What represents normal fetal activity is under discussion and may contribute to the high false-positive rate. One approach to counteracting this limitation would be to limit testing prior to 30 weeks' gestation. This effectively reduces fetal activity variation. Studies indicate that fetal nonreactivity may be more closely associated to gestational age rather than fetal compromise.[6,7] Another means to standardize test interpretation would be to hold regular periodic joint reviews of tracings by physicians and nurses.

The Biophysical Profile (BPP)

The Biophysical Profile (BPP) utilizes ultrasound to evaluate fetal status based on multiple criteria of fetal behavior. Manning and Harman[8] indicate that the most commonly used tool evaluates five variables according to established criteria. Table 31.1 describes each variable and the criteria used for evaluation. Clinical management decisions are based on a composite of all five scores rather than a single variable. The score assists physicians and nurses in determining whether a fetus is at risk at the time of testing. A score of 0 is considered abnormal, and a score of 2 is normal. A total score of 10/10 indicates a normal BPP and a functional, nonhypoxemic fetal central nervous system. A score of 8/10 indicates a fetus not at risk of death or damage within 1 week. As the BPP score decreases to 6/10, there is an increased risk of developing perinatal complications. A score of 4/10 or less signifies fetal asphyxia and indicates the need for an immediate delivery.[3]

Manning and Harman[8] believe that an evaluation of the total score for BPP requires not only interpretive knowledge of the score but also integration of this information with the clinical situation. The evaluation of less than all pertinent data could lead to needless intervention or preventable harm.

To use this instrument in clinical antepartum assessment or in perinatal nursing research, one must be cognizant of influences that may affect outcome. Gebauer and Lowe[9] describe these influences as "endogenous" or "exogenous" variables. Endogenous variables include fetal age, fetal behavioral states, maternal or fetal infection, hypoglycemia and hyperglycemia, and postmaturity.

Gestational age and the behavior of the fetus were reported as being interdependent.[9] Fetal behavioral states include body and eye movements and heart rate patterns in relation to four states that can change from quiescence to vigorous activity. Specific parameters have been identified for fetuses beyond 35 weeks. However, for fetuses under 35 weeks, state behaviors have been found to be unstable over time. Nijhuis[10] reported that preterm fetuses were not capable of true state transitions. This suggests that to interpret a BPP score on a fetus less than 35 weeks, one must take into account the behavioral state according to fetal age.

How the fetus reacts in the presence of an infection continues to be questioned. BPP abnormalities that have thus far been associated with infection include absence of fetal heart rate reactivity and fetal breathing.[9]

Maternal hypoglycemia or hyperglycemia have been reported to affect primarily fetal breathing movements, which in turn affect the BPP score results.[11] Hypoglycemia tends to decrease fetal breathing movements, whereas hyperglycemia has been shown to increase fetal breathing movements, suggesting the importance of testing during periods of maternal normoglycemia.[12]

Additional issues to consider include the maternal presence of either therapeutic or nontherapeutic drugs. Therapeutic drugs that depress the central nervous system also decrease both fetal breathing movements and fetal heart rate variability, thus lowering the BPP score.[13]

Ingestion of nontherapeutic drugs, such as cocaine and nicotine, also have been shown to have a suppressive effect on the BPP score. Effects vary from fetal hypoxemia to reduced fetal breathing activity.[2,8-14] The final issue to be raised by Gebauer and Lowe[9] concerns postdated pregnancy and its possible effect on the BPP score. Manning[8] supports the use of the BPP to identify the compromised postdate fetus (a fetus beyond 40 weeks' gestation). However, as Gilson et al.[15] point out, although the BPP is sensitive in diagnosing a postdate fetus, the test is not sensitive enough to confirm which fetus will present with adverse perinatal effects.

All antepartum tests have some level of error in prediction. Most tests are accurate in predicting a healthy fetus, but less accurate at predicting the compromised fetus, indicating that several tests may be required to increase the validity of prediction.[16] However, according to Vintzileos,[12] the BPP has been shown to be the most accurate test for identifying a compromised fetus.

Labor and Delivery Tools

Perinatal nurses must keep constant pace with the ever-changing philosophies and new technologies of childbirth. Research in the area of labor and delivery have varied in focus. However, one proven area of research focuses on the pain of childbirth. What causes it? How to control it? These are questions that have been and are still being investigated.

According to the gate-control theory, pain occurs as a result of a mechanism in the dorsal horn of the spinal column that serves as a gate. This gate increases or reduces the flow of nerve impulses from the periphery to the central nervous system. Gates may be opened or closed by central nervous system activities, such as anxiety and excitement, or through selective localized activity.[17] The gate-control theory has implications for childbirth. Tactile stimulation can control pain. Activities to accomplish this include sacral pressure, backrub, conditioning, and distraction.

In childbirth, there is a physiologic basis for the discomfort. In the first stage of labor, pain arises from dilation or stretching of the cervix. During the second stage of labor, pain is due to hypoxia of the contracting uterine muscle cells and distention of the vagina and perineum. Pain during the third stage results from uterine contraction and cervical dilation as the placenta is expelled.[17]

Several factors can affect a woman's perception of childbirth pain. These include: cultural background, presence of a support person, fatigue and sleep deprivation, previous experience with pain, anxiety, whether she has had childbirth education, maternal position during labor, and the environment of the childbirth setting.

Women's accounts of childbirth pain are difficult to assess. The methods reported often result in conflicting information. Study results must be reviewed in light of the source of the data, that is, were the data based on the woman's perception or based on physiologic indicators of pain? One tool that has been applied to the area of assessing maternal comfort during childbirth is the Maternal Comfort Assessment Tool.

Maternal Comfort Assessment Tool

The Maternal Comfort Assessment Tool estimates the level of maternal comfort during maximum slope of labor (cervical dilation from 4 to 9 cm) while assuming one of two positions, upright or recumbent.[18] The tool measures the laboring woman's focus of attention, including eye contact, breathing pattern and vocal behavior, muscle tension and activity, and verbalizations during contractions. Vital signs, cervical changes, duration, frequency, and intensity of contractions, medications, and use of monitoring equipment also are recorded. Scores for each observable behavior are totaled, with the highest possible comfort score for each contraction being 14, the lowest 0. Comfort scores for a series of three contractions are recorded hourly.

Prestudy interrater reliability for the Maternal Comfort Assessment Tool was found to have an agreement percentage of 89%. In addition, interrater reliability was calculated by taking a series of three contractions from each of five randomly selected clients. The agreement percentage was found to be 91%.[18]

Other factors that may affect the reliability and validity of this tool include how psychologic factors such as maternal feelings of independence and control influence the tool scores. Another issue of concern is that this tool has been tested only on low-risk clients. High-risk clients may bring a different perspective to the tool's application.[18]

Electronic Fetal Monitoring (EFM)

Electronic fetal monitoring (EFM) is an auditory and visual assessment tool that provides continuous data for uterine activity and fetal heart response evaluation. Data include baseline heart rate, beat-to-beat variability, and fetal heart rate changes over time. EFM not only gathers clinical management data, but because of its self-documenting properties, it can be used to obtain research data as well in combination with direct hands-on assessment, verbal client information, and the client's vital sign assessment. All clients in labor need some form of fetal monitoring to detect potential problems. The choice of form this takes is based on multiple factors. The need for EFM has been a source of debate for years. When first introduced in the 1960s EFM's intended use was to detect the compromised fetus during labor and delivery. As Ellison et al.[19] report, EFM is fairly reliable in recognizing the dying fetus, but less reliable in identifying fetuses with hypoxia-ischemia involving the central nervous system. In a study comparing the effectiveness of EFM with periodic auscultation, it was reported that more accurate predictions about 5-minute Apgar scores (newborn assessment at birth) were made with EFM than with auscultation. This suggested that better data regarding neonatal well-being could be provided by EFM.[20] Larson goes on to suggest that one of the primary contributions of EFM may be its "ability to enable clinicians to make better predictions and judgments" regarding neonatal well-being.[20,p589] Other researchers concur with this belief, finding that EFM has significantly improved the outcome of labor and delivery by calling increased attention to the importance of fetal heart rate and to the labor process.[19]

EFM uses a tocodynamometer to record uterine contractions and a Doppler ultrasound device to monitor the fetal heart rate. Although uterine pressure measurements accurately reflect the frequency of contractions, one disadvantage to its use is that EFM does not correlate with baseline or maximum intrauterine pressure during contractions. A second disadvantage is that fetal heart rate variability obtained with external monitoring does not correlate well with the true variability obtained by the internal scalp electrode.

In internal fetal heart rate monitoring, the fetal ECG is recorded on the electronic fetal monitor. This is accomplished through the use of a fetal scalp electrode. This method provides an accurate representation of the baseline fetal heart rate variability. A fluid-filled catheter or a pressure transducer can be used in conjuction with the EFM. This catheter, or transducer, provides a quantitative measure of intrauterine pressure during a contraction.

Specific conditions that can alter or effect the reliability and validity of information obtained with electronic fetal monitoring equipment comes from a variety of sources. The labor room environment itself can affect monitor operation. Environmental specifications for proper operation include an operating temperature of 0°C to +55°C; a storage temperature of –40°C to +75°C, and a relative humidity of 5% to 95%.[21] Table 31.2 describes areas that must be considered when data from the EFM do not agree with coexisting physiologic measures.

Newborn Assessment Tools

Immediately following birth, numerous physiologic adaptations take place in the newborn. Care focuses on assessing and stabilizing the newborn. Assessment involves the collection of data from several parameters. Assessment as an ongoing process enables caregivers to compare initial findings with data obtained at a later time. Two assessment tools, the Apgar Scoring Tool and the Dubowitz Tool, are discussed in the following sections.

Table 31.2 Troubleshooting Inconsistent EFM Data

Dilemma	Possible Cause	Resolution
Poor pen tracing	Active fetus, maternal movement, loose belt, insufficient gel, maternal obesity	Readjust belt, reposition transducer, relax client, apply gel
FHR higher than normal range	Recording maternal heart rate, fetal arrhythmia or fetal death	Compare maternal pulse to signal, listen to FHR with fetoscope
Tracing burned into paper	Stylet heat too high, jammed paper	Turn stylet knob counterclockwise to lower heat, check paper feed
Tocotransducer		
No contraction	Machine recording, negative pressures	Adjust uterine waveform, activity baseline
Waveform hard to differentiate	Check placement of toco	Place toco over fundus, or where uterine movement is strongest
Inverted waveform	Maternal activity may alter toco position during contractions	Reposition toco
ECG-Spiral Electrode		
Occasional vertical lines on tracing	Faulty cable, or spiral electrode, or no ECG signal	Check leg plate and wires, apply new electrode
Equipment malfunction	Connection of leads to leg plates incorrect, connect interference, i.e., excess fetal hair can sometimes cause poor tracing	Reconnect leads or apply new electrode
Intrauterine Catheter		
Straight line on tracing	Check cable plug, pressure transducer defective	Plug in cable, replace transducer
No contraction waveform or pressure changes during contraction	Plugged catheter, uterine perforation	Flush catheter, test monitor, check uterine activity during valsalva
Tracing indicates peak of waveform	Monitor not calibrated	Calibrate monitor to zero only transducer
Waveform artifacts	Tip of catheter in uterine wall or dry area	Pull catheter out 2 to 3 cm, flush clear with normal saline

Adapted from Hewlett-Packard Medical Products Booklet, Palo Alto, CA: Hewlett-Packard, 1990.

Apgar Scoring Tool

Virginia Apgar, an anesthesiologist, first introduced the Apgar Scoring Tool in 1953.[22] The purpose of the Apgar score is to evaluate the physical condition of the newborn at birth and any potential resuscitation requirement. The score is based on five indicators of neonatal adjustment to extrauterine life: heart rate, respiratory effort, reflex irritability, muscle tone, and color. The newborn is rated 1 minute after birth, again at 5 minutes, and receives a total score ranging from 0 to 10 assessed in the following manner:

1. Heart rate is auscultated or palpated.
2. Respiratory rate is assessed by counting the number of respirations for 1 full minute.
3. Muscle tone is determined by evaluating the degree of flexion and resistance to straightening of the extremities and the rapidity with which they return to a state of flexion.
4. Reflex irritability is evaluated by rubbing the back or flicking the soles of the feet.
5. Color of the neonate's skin is evaluated for cyanosis and pallor.

Even though it has been widely accepted since the 1950s, its value has been repeatedly questioned.[23] Apgar[24] herself reminded us that the tool should in no way substitute for a careful examination or repeated observations over the first few hours of life.

Livingston[25] examined the interrater reliability of the Apgar score in both term and preterm infants. Fifty-two infants were included in the study; 11 were premature, and 41 were term. Apgar scores were assigned to each infant and then compared to scores recorded in the mother's chart.

Percentage agreement at 1 and 5 minutes for each of the five indicators was calculated. In the preterm infant group, the agreement of 1-minute scores ranged from a high of 82% for tone and respiratory rate to a low of 55% for heart rate. At 5 minutes, the agreement was highest for heart rate (100%) and lowest for reflex irritability (36%). The mean percent agreement of the five indicators was 69% at both 1 minute and 5 minutes. The poor interrater reliability estimates could be due to recall errors in recording. The Apgar scores were recorded after resuscitative efforts and were based on the recorder's memory of the infant's condition at 1 and 5 minutes.

Percentage agreement for the term infants was lowest for reflex irritability (81%) and highest for heart rate (98%). At 5 minutes, percentage agreement for heart rate, tone, and reflex irritability was 98%; for color and respiratory rate, percentage agreement was 95%. The mean percentage agreement was 89% at 1 minute and 97% at 5 minutes.

Even though the findings of this study suggest that use of the Apgar in premature infants is questionable, the score still provides valuable data on the neonate during the first few minutes of life. Reliability may be improved by periodic review and interrater checks, the use of a timing device, and education in how to use the Apgar.[25,26]

Finally, observer bias on the part of the person delivering the infant can be an issue. As Apgar scores have become equated with the quality of health care, it is recommended that the one delivering the infant not be the one to assign the Apgar score.[27]

The Dubowitz Assessment Tool

The Dubowitz assessment tool was developed by Lilly Dubowitz and coworkers in the 1960s and continues to be a reliable tool for determining the appropriate gestational age of the neonate regardless of birth weight. The tool is used to assess intrauterine growth alterations and preterm neonates by assessing physical characteristics and neuromuscular tone indices on admission to the newborn nursery.

The tool contains 21 criteria (10 neurologic and 11 external physical criteria). Each category is scored, and the scores summed to a total score. Total scores range between 0 to 69, indicating gestational ages between 26 and 46 weeks.

The original study by Dubowitz and associates[28] was carried out on 167 infants in a large metropolitan hospital. Only if an infant had an absent Moro reflex or was too ill was she or he excluded. All infant assessments were made by one investigator and within 5 days of delivery. The majority of assessments were made in the first 24 hours. The external score correlated with gestation 91% of the time. Neurologic scores correlated with gestation 89% of the time. A combined total correlation of 95% produced a stronger result than either alone.

The reliability of this tool can be increased by using it with neonates between the gestational ages of 28 and 42 weeks. Before assessing, Olds et al.[29] suggests the need to document preexisting maternal conditions that can affect the neonate assessment results. Conditions such as diabetes, which appears to accelerate fetal physical growth, may retard maturation. Also pregnancy-induced hypertension, which retards fetal physical growth, may speed maturation. Other characteristics that may affect the neuromuscular outcome scores include the active muscle tone and edema seen in neonates of women with pregnancy-induced hypertension, respiratory depression seen as the result of certain maternal analgesia and anesthesia, and the flaccid and edematous neonate that often results from respiratory distress syndrome.[29]

Postpartum Assessment Tool

The postpartum period (puerperium) is the 6 weeks between the birth of the newborn and the return of the reproductive organs to the nonpregnant state. Unfortunately, today the time spent with clients following delivery is brief, ranging from a few hours for a normal birth to 4 days for a cesarean birth. Even though the time may be short, the information shared between nurse and client can be substantial in terms of client education and research possibilities.

REEDA Tool

One tool used for postpartum assessment of episiotomy healing was developed by Davidson.[30] This tool appraises the perineum or incision for signs of *r*edness, *e*dema, *ec*chymosis, *d*ischarge, and *a*pproximation. Thus, the tool came to be known as the REEDA scale. Each category is assessed and a number assigned, for a total score range from 0 to 15. The higher the score presumably, the more tissue trauma.

Hill's[31] investigation of the psychometric properties of the REEDA evaluated interrater reliability and construct validity of the tool. A total of 94 women participated. Eighty-six women received an episiotomy, the remaining eight delivered with an intact perineum. Perineal assessments were conducted on 56% of the women during the first 24 hours following delivery, with the remaining assessments completed during the second 24 hours. During the rater training period it was discovered that the trainers had difficulty assessing redness and ecchymosis. This continued during data collection. After 39 participants were assessed, it was decided to add a sixth category, called "discoloration," so that a differentiation between redness and ecchymosis was not needed.

To determine interrater reliability between raters and for the addition of the category "discoloration" the kappa statistic was used. Correlations for the total REEDA score between raters were only moderate. Correlations using discoloration were higher than those for redness and ecchymosis, indicating higher rater agreement by using the descriptor discoloration. To evaluate construct validity of the REEDA, the known-groups technique was used. Results indicated support for the construct validity for this tool.

Hill[31] believes that with moderate interrater reliability and the problem of "redness and ecchymosis assessment," the REEDA tool may be less than reliable for research purposes. Other issues affecting reliability and validity include measurement discrepancies (i.e., the scale measures edema in terms of width, not considering length or depth), inconsistent correlations between the descriptors "edema" and "pain," and only three properties of wound healing were reported to be useful in this study. Construct validity questions have been raised regarding use of the REEDA in the immediate postpartum period. The use of the descriptor "approximation" as an index of better healing and decreased pain is questioned.[31] Further investigation is needed to determine the strengths and limitations of the use of the REEDA scale in clinical practice or research.

Summary

The chapter has examined and discussed the application of various tools used throughout the perinatal nursing area, emphasizing the strengths and limitations of each. It is hoped that the review has familiarized the reader with some of the tools available not only for clinical use but also for research. It also was our intent to stimulate critical thinking regarding the reliability and validity issues that need consideration and further investigation before a tool is appropriate for research purposes.

Exemplar Study

Andrews, C., & Chrzanowski, M. Maternal position, labor and comfort. *Appl Nurs Res*, 1990, 3(1):1-7.

Based on the knowledge we have regarding the potentially negative effects to both mother and fetus of laboring in the recumbent position, Andrews and Chrzanowski developed a study to ascertain whether women laboring in an upright position reported less discomfort and had a shorter phase maximum slope as indicated by their labor pattern. These women were compared to women laboring in the recumbent position. The study utilized the Maternal Comfort Assessment Scale.

The study findings were that women who labor in the upright position had a significantly shorter labor ($t(38) = 3.2$, $p = 0.003$). The length of the phase of maximum slope correlated positively with age and race. Young, black women indicated having shorter phases. Comfort scores were found to vary only slightly between the two groups ($t(38) = 1.42$, $p = 0.163$).

References

1. Freeman, R.K. The contraction stress test. In R. Eden and F. Boehm (Eds.), *Assessment and care of the fetus*. Norwalk, CT: Appleton & Lange, 1990.
2. Manning, F.A. Fetal assessment based on fetal biophysical profile scoring: Experiences in 12,620 referred high-risk pregnancies. *Am J Obstet Gynecol*. 1985, 151(31):343-350.
3. Gegor, C., & Paine, L. Antepartum fetal assessment techniques: An update for today's perinatal nurse. *J Perinat Neonat Nurs*, 1992, 5(4):1-15.
4. Chez, B.F., & Chez, R. Interpretations of nonstress tests by obstetric nurses. *J Gynecol Neonat Nurs*, 1990, 19(3):227-232.
5. Kisilevsky, B.S. Human fetal responses to sound as a function of stimulus intensity. *Obstet Gynecol*, 1989, 73:971-976.
6. Bishop, E. Fetal acceleration test. *Am J Obstet Gynecol*, 1981, 141:905-909.
7. Keegan, K. The nonstress test. *Clin Obstet Gynecol*, 1987, 30:921-935.
8. Manning, F.A., & Harman, C.R. The fetal biophysical profile. In R.D. Eden & F.H. Boehm (Eds.), *Assessment and care of the fetus*. Norwalk, CT: Appleton & Lange, 1990.
9. Gebauer, C., & Lowe, N. The biophysical profile: Antepartal assessment of fetal well-being. *J Gynecol Neonat Nurs*, 1993, 22(2):115-125.
10. Nijhuis, J.G. Behavioral states: Concomitants, clinical implications and the assessment of the condition of the newborn's system. *Eur J Obstet Gynecol Reproduct Biol*, 1986, 21:301-308.
11. Gabbe, S.G. Antepartum fetal evaluation. In S. Gabbe, J. Niebyl, & J. Simpson (Eds.), *Obstetrics: Normal and problem pregnancies*. New York: Churchill Livingstone, 1991, pp. 377-424.
12. Vintzileos, A.M., Campbell, W.A., Nochimson, D.J., & Weinbaum, P.J. The use and misuse of the fetal biophysical profile. *Am J Obstet Gynecol*, 1987, 157:527-533.

13. Carlan, S., & O'Brien, W.F. The effect of magnesium sulfate on the biophysical profile of normal term fetuses. *Obstet Gynecol*, 1991, 7:681-684.
14. McLeod, W., Brien, J., Loomis, C., et al. Effects of maternal ethanol ingestion on fetal breathing movements, gross body movements and heart rate at 37 to 40 weeks gestational age. *Am J Obstet Gynecol*, 1983, 145:251-257.
15. Gilson, G.J., O'Brien, M.E., Vera, R.W., et al. Prolonged pregnancy and the biophysical profile: A birthing center perspective. *J Nurs Midwifery*, 1988, 33:171-177.
16. Schifrin, B.S., & Clement, D. Why fetal monitoring remains a good idea. *Contemp Obstet Gynecol*, 1990, 35(2):70-86.
17. Bobak, I., & Jensen, M. *Maternity and gynecologic care. The nurse and the family* (5th ed.). St. Louis, MO: Mosby Year Book, 1993.
18. Andrews, C.M. & Chrzanowski, M. Maternal position, labor and comfort. *Appl Nurs Res*, 1990, 3(1):1-7.
19. Ellison, P., Foster, M., Sheridan-Pereira, M., & MacDonald, D. Electronic fetal heart monitoring, auscultation, and neonatal outcome. *J Obstet Gynecol*, 1991, 164(5):1281-1289.
20. Larson, E.B. Fetal monitoring and predictions by clinicians: Observations during a randomized clinical trial in very low birth weight infants. *Obstet Gynecol*, 1989, 74:584-589.
21. Hewlett-Packard Medical Products Booklet. Palo Alto, CA: Hewlett-Packard, 1990.
22. Apgar, V. A proposal for a new method of evaluation of the newborn infant. *Curr Res Anesthes Analges*, 1953, 32:260-267.
23. Sykes, G.S., Molloy, P.M., Johnson, P., et al. Do Apgar scores indicate asphyxia? *Lancet*, 1982, 1:494-496.
24. Apgar, V., & James, L. Further observations of the newborn scoring system. *Am J Dis Child*, 1962, 104:419-428.

25. Livingston, J. Interrater reliability of the Apgar scores in term and preterm infants. *Appl Nurs Res*, 1990, *3*(4):164-165.

26. Auld, P., Rudolph, A., Avery, M., et al. Responsiveness and resuscitation of the newborn. The use of the Apgar score. *Am J Dis Child*, 1961, *101*:69-80.

27. Apgar, V. The newborn (Apgar) scoring system. Reflections and advice. *Pediatr Clin North Am*, 1966, *13*:645-650.

28. Dubowitz, L., Dubowitz, B., & Goldberg, C. Clinical assessment of gestational age in the newborn infant. *J Pediatr*, 1970, *77*(1):1-10.

29. Olds, S., London, M., & Ladewig, P. *Maternal newborn nursing. A family centered approach* (4th ed.). Reading, MA: Addison-Wesley, 1992.

30. Davidson, N. Evaluating postpartum healing. *J Nurs Midwifery*, 1974, *19*:7-10.

31. Hill, P. Psychometric properties of the REEDA. *J Gynecol Neonat Nurs*, 1990, *35*(3):162-165.

32

Measuring Dyspnea

Mary L. Scott

Dyspnea, or shortness of breath, is a common symptom of pathologic cardiopulmonary conditions requiring clinical assessment and intervention. It may be present during exercise or at rest in acute or chronic diseases.

Dyspnea occurs most frequently in persons with primary pulmonary disease (asthma and chronic obstructive pulmonary disease [COPD]), coronary artery disease, and neuromuscular disorders affecting the respiratory muscles. This complex symptom can occur in conditions resulting in increased ventilation, alteration in the physical properties of the lung, or increased respiratory work. It may be present with pregnancy, obesity, or psychologic conditions characterized by anxiety.[1] It also has been described in persons with cancer, post-bypass surgery, congestive heart failure, cocaine addiction, rheumatoid arthritis, hyperthyroidism, and other medical-surgical conditions.[2] Carrieri-Kohlman et al.[3] enhance this description by describing dyspnea as a "multifaceted process influenced by personal, situational, health status and environmental factors."[3,p226] Furthermore, the perception of the symptom also is influenced by age, gender, personality, perceived self-efficacy, concurrent illness disease severity, and length of time the symptom has been experienced.[3] Emotions, moods, and social support can also influence dyspnea perception and the coping mechanisms of the individual who is dealing with the symptom.

Dyspnea connotes one's awareness of an excessive effort to breathe based on the level of physical exertion experienced. The neural pathways involved in the development of dyspnea are not clearly understood, and no single mechanism can account for all clinical situations in which dyspnea occurs.

Conceptual Considerations

Dyspnea has been defined as difficult, labored, and uncomfortable breathing.[4,5] The sensation is subjective and involves personal perception and reaction to the sensation. In sum, dyspnea is complex, sensory, perceived, and interpreted by the individual experiencing it,[6] indicating that it should be rated by the person experiencing it. One's degree of physical compensation may or may not reflect subjective interpretation, and any objective measurement may or may not correlate with subjective feelings. At one end of the continuum are individuals who describe severe dyspnea and demonstrate minor pathophysiologic alterations. At the other are individuals describing minimal dyspnea but demonstrating marked change in pulmonary function. This finding has been supported by investigators who have observed and attempted to quantify dyspnea in a variety of disease states.[4-8] These investigators agree that pulmonary function disturbances differ by disease and that no one measurement of lung function can define respiratory capacity. Therefore, the observation of increased respiratory rate (tachypnea) or increased depth of respiration (hyperpnea) should not be confused with dyspnea.[2] Patients with primary pulmonary disease experience abnormal breathing mechanics.[9] Diseases such as pulmonary fibrosis, asthma, and emphysema illustrate the relationship between inspiratory effort and dyspnea. In pulmonary fibrosis, the lungs and thorax are stiffer than normal and inspiratory muscles must increase their tension to produce the same tidal volume. When the thoracic volume is abnormally large, as in emphysema and chronic asthma, it is necessary for the patient to breathe near-maximum inspiratory levels and use accessory inspiratory muscles to overcome a high resistance to airflow at normal lung volumes. In acute asthma, dyspnea is correlated with sternocleidomastoid muscle retraction. In emphysema, a large lung volume is created by the loss of elastic tissue recoil at rest. Dyspnea in these patients is related to a decreased capacity to respond to the ventilatory stimulus. Improving mechanical function (using bronchodilators) and decreasing ventilatory stimulus (improved oxygenation levels) can decrease dyspnea in patients with asthma and emphysema.

In cancer patients, dyspnea may be the result of disease or treatment.[10] It may be present before a malignancy is diagnosed, or it may develop at any point during the illness. Patients with primary lung or mediastinal tumors and those with neck or central nervous system tumors involving the respiratory centers are at high risk for developing altered ventilatory patterns. Individuals with cancer who have received radiation to the chest or neck or who have received antineoplastic agents that can cause pulmonary toxicity may develop dyspnea. Complications, such as pleural effusion, ascites, pneumonia, or pulmonary emboli, also may produce dyspnea. Patients with concurrent histories of pulmonary disease, cigarette smoke exposures, congestive heart failure, environmental/occupational exposures, or anemia may exhibit dyspnea, as well as those who have had surgery of the head, neck, chest, or lung.

A study of perceived dyspnea in 30 lung cancer patients highlights the need for careful and thoughtful assessment of this sensation.[11] This study described patterns of dyspnea, identified coping and adaptive strategies used by lung cancer patients, and determined the relationship between activity and dyspnea. A convenience sample was interviewed twice over a 2-month interval. At time 1, the American Thoracic Society Questionnaire (including the Grade of Breathlessness Scale [GBS]), the Dyspnea Interview Schedule, the Dyspnea Visual Analog Scale (DVAS), and the Karnofsky Performance Scale (KPS) were completed.[12] At time 2, the GBS, KPS, and DVAS were administered.

Data were analyzed using parametric and nonparametric statistics. The American Thoracic Society Questionnaire and the Dyspnea Interview Schedule provided thematic descriptions of physical and emotional sensations experienced during episodes of dyspnea. Precipitants and patterns of dyspnea also were identified. The patients in this study reported significant dyspnea, felt extreme fatigue, and experienced losses in concentration, memory, and appetite during periods of shortness of breath. Subjects reported a high average number of self-taught coping strategies. It was felt that long-standing preexisting obstructive and restrictive disease accounted for these high levels of coping strategies. No patient identified the use of strategies previously taught by nurses.

This study demonstrated that dyspnea is a significant problem for patients with lung cancer. It also pointed to the need to evaluate dyspnea carefully with multiple instruments. The DVAS, GBS, and KPS are easy to administer, reliably measure the subjective symptoms of dyspnea, and facilitate appropriate planning for intervention.

Roberts et al.[13] report that only pain and eating problems are identified more frequently than dyspnea in late-stage cancer patients. Using self-report surveys, chart audits, and interviews with patients and the nurses caring for them, Roberts and colleagues studied the meaning of dyspnea in late-stage cancer. They concluded that, although patients appeared to be coping, they were isolated, inconsistently managed, and inadequately supported. Furthermore, they concluded that dyspnea was overlooked among late-stage cancer patients, that patients did not report their symptoms of dyspnea, and that nurses caring for these patients did not have a clear understanding of the symptom or its management. The researchers reported that medical intervention was inconsistent and narcotic use, described as beneficial in terminal dyspnea, was not utilized. Reducing physical activity was reported as the primary dyspnea control strategy.

Physical and Psychosocial Variables Correlated with Dyspnea Perception

The patient's description of the dyspnea sensation varies with diagnosis and extent of disease. Persons with obstructive disease (e.g., emphysema, chronic bronchitis) recognize that they have great difficulty moving air in and out of their lungs. Individuals with restrictive disease (e.g., pulmonary fibrosis or infiltrative disease) complain of "hard breathing"[14] with little exertion and appear to experience sensations that would be normal for a higher level of exercise. However, some of the above individuals and others with pulmonary vascular disease, heart disease, or respiratory muscle weakness may describe a feeling or sense of suffocation, which is different from the shortness of breath sensation previously described.

Efforts have been made to correlate physiologic parameters with breathing difficulty. Blood gas levels and static lung volumes do not appear to correlate with the development of dyspnea.[15-17] Blood gases, however, are affected by the level of ventilation. Although respiratory work and the oxygen cost of breathing are elevated in pulmonary disease, investigators have discovered that they do not correlate with reported dyspnea or cause perceived dyspnea.[15-17]

Pulmonary function studies have been used to try to correlate pulmonary dysfunction and severity of dyspnea with specific lung diseases. Restrictive disease decreases vital capacity and limits perfusion. Forced vital capacity and diffusing capacity have been shown to correlate moderately with the severity of dyspnea experience in restrictive diseases. In obstructive diseases, the maximal voluntary ventilation (MVV)—the largest liter volume that can be breathed per minute voluntarily—has the highest reported correlation with dyspnea.

The Dyspnea Index is a percentage of the MVV and expresses the minute ventilation at a specific level of exercise.[18] For a normal person walking 2 miles per hour on level ground, this measurement is ±12%.[18] Studies have shown that if the dyspnea index is less than 30%, shortness of breath usually does not occur. Subjects with an index greater than 50% are likely to be short of breath at abnormally low exercise levels. However,

Fishman and Leslie[19] and Gottfried et al.[20] found that patients with obstructive lung disease may not complain of dyspnea even with a dyspnea index of 50% or greater.[19]

Since testing for MVV is difficult to reproduce, the 1-second Forced Expiratory Volume (FEV_1) is the most convenient and useful measure of evaluating prolonged expiration and degree of airway obstruction. The FEV_1 is correlated slightly lower with dyspnea than the MVV and depends on individual effort and cooperation.

To determine the threshold at which dyspnea is perceived, measurements of resistive and elastic loads have been added to breathing tests to aid clinicians in understanding how some patients can experience airflow obstruction without breathlessness. Studies have shown that for patients with chronically high airway resistance, increased changes in resistance are needed to experience dyspnea. Asthmatics probably experience high thresholds for and decreased perception of dyspnea because of more frequent episodes of bronchospasm and greater responsiveness to histamine.[7]

Emotional states can profoundly affect levels of dyspnea in persons with airway constriction secondary to pulmonary disease.[11,21-24] Fatigue, depression, anxiety, helplessness, loss of vitality, preoccupation, nervousness, and fear have been reported to accompany dyspnea.[11,21-24] The presence of panic, worry, and anger can confound measurement of dyspnea as a solitary symptom. Gift[21] examined the psychologic and physiologic factors associated with acute dyspnea in patients with COPD. She concluded in an in-depth pilot study that clinical symptoms and physiologic responses change during dyspnea. Clinical symptoms included the number of respirations per minute, the depth of respirations, the presence or absence of sighing and paradoxical breathing, and the use of accessory muscles. The Vertical Visual Analogue Scale (VVAS) was used to measure dyspnea. The Spielberger State Anxiety Inventory (SAI) and Brief Symptom Inventory (BSI) also were administered. Physiologic measures included arterial blood gas and serum cortisol levels. Medication use also was recorded. This study demonstrated the coexistence of a psychophysiologic component with dyspnea. Elevated plasma cortisol levels in the pilot group validated Gift et al.'s earlier work[23] that showed higher self-reported anxiety during periods of increased dyspnea. Gift was careful to indicate that this pilot study concluded that depression (measured by the SAI) increased during high dyspnea in patients who were taking prednisone. Anxiety, plasma cortisol levels, PCO_2, and accessory muscle use increased during severe or high periods of dyspnea. Gift emphasized that the patient's emotional status needs to be given special attention, in particular, anxiety and depression. Correlations between breathlessness and various psychosocial phenomena have been studied in adult asthmatics. Gift et al.[21] have demonstrated that the dyspnea experienced by patients with asthma is generally acute in nature and that asthma-related dyspneic events are not generalizable to patients whose dyspnea is chronic and present during rest or minimal exercise.

Carrieri et al.[22] studied dyspnea in 39 children with documented asthma and episodes of wheezing. Most of the children used inhalers with bronchodilator medications, and six received periodic oral steroids. These researchers developed an interview guide for specific use in this study. It contained open-ended questions, forced-choice response formats, and three measures of dyspnea intensity. The guide explored participants' physical sensations, emotional sensations, breathing on a good and usual day, intensity of dyspnea, and coping strategies. Measures of dyspnea intensity included a word descriptor scale, a visual analog scale, and a color shade scale. These scales had been previously used to evaluate pain in children. The visual analog was adapted by using both happy and sad circular faces and easy-to-understand anchors at each end of the 100-mm line. The shaded color scale was presented to the children following a question about what color the child's breathing was when it was bad. A 4-point color shade ranged from lightest, light, medium to dark. Carrieri et al.[22] demonstrated that children with asthma were able to rate the intensity of their dyspnea and describe the asthma sensation qualitatively.

Experiments to Produce the Sensation of Dyspnea

Efforts to study the sensation of dyspnea and to understand ventilatory regulation have focused on producing unpleasant respiratory sensations resembling breathlessness. Early investigations employed breathholding and examined perceptions of additional respiratory loads.[15] Transcutaneous vagal nerve and chest wall blocks also have been performed to try to produce the sensation of dyspnea and evaluate its effect.[15] Studies with asthmatics to determine the relationship between the psychology and physiology of dyspnea have added to a basic understanding of the neural, chemical, and muscular functions of dyspnea, but their relationship to dyspnea continues to be vague.[7]

Treadmill and standardized walking tests (2, 6, and 12 minutes) have been used to produce and evaluate dyspnea as it relates to exercise.[15,24-26] Butland et al.[27] demonstrated high correlation coefficients between 2-, 6-, and 12-minute walking tests, indicating that they are similar measures of exercise tolerance (6 minutes versus 12 minutes, $r = 0.9555$; 2 minutes versus 12 minutes, $r = 0.864$; 2 minutes versus 6 minutes, $r = 0.892$). Patients are encouraged to cover as much ground as possible in the prescribed time period. Following the walk, patients must indicate their level of dyspnea using a 10-cm visual analog scale that ranges from "Extremely short of breath" to "No shortness of breath."[27] Standardized walking tests are clinically easy to perform and have been tested for validity. They may be used by clinicians to correlate pulmonary function and physical disability in patients over long periods.

More sophisticated laboratory studies have been performed to produce dyspnea. One pharmacologic approach induces bronchoconstriction with histamine or methacholine.[28] The threshold at which the patient perceives breathlessness is then determined. Other investigators have used elastic and resistive loads to breathing to determine when subjects detect the loads and are rendered breathless.[29]

Another method of assessing treatment effects on daily functions of patients with chronic airflow limitations is to measure activity and medication. Guyatt et al.[30] studied patients with chronic airflow limitation (CAL) and asked them (1) to perform a 6-minute walk test; (2) to rate their dyspnea after the walk test; and (3) to complete three questionnaires that measured dyspnea associated with daily activities. Patients received four 2-week treatments with salbutamol and oral theophylline. At the end of each treatment period, outcomes were measured by FEV_1 and forced vital capacity. Three instruments were completed, the Rand Instrument, the Oxygen Cost Diagram, and the Chronic Respiratory Disease Questionnaire. A global rating of changes in dyspnea also was assessed. This study was rigorously performed under exacting conditions. The results of the study demonstrated that the dimension of dyspnea measured by the Chronic Disease Respiratory Questionnaire was a more responsive and valid measure of shortness of breath in daily activities than the other two functional status measures. The study also indicated that dyspnea following the walk test is best measured in conjunction with the 6-minute walk. The investigators also concluded that they successfully demonstrated the feasibility and usefulness of the comparison of functional status measures in the randomized control trial setting.

Instruments

The subjective nature of dyspnea and the lack of consistent, observable signs and symptoms have made measurements difficult.[31] Verbal reports of breathlessness and psychophysiologic magnitude estimation techniques have been used to measure dyspnea.[24,32-34] Studies have measured dyspnea from a time perspective, that is, the amount of dyspnea perceived daily and the amount of dyspnea produced at a specific time in the experimental setting.[7,13]

Retrospective determinations of daily activity and associated breathing difficulty are one method of evaluating dyspnea. Scales equating dyspnea with activity have proven to be reliable and correlate well with measures of pulmonary function. Several instruments have been developed to measure dyspnea in specific time frames and the relationship between dyspnea and specific activities.

Baseline Dyspnea Index (BDI) and Transition Dyspnea Index (TDI)

Two indices have been used to correlate lung function and exercise capacity: the Baseline Dyspnea Index (BDI) and the Transition Dyspnea Index (TDI).[35-38] Tested for reliability on patients with COPD, the BDI grades the severity of dyspnea at a single point in time. The Transition Dyspnea Index documents changes in dyspnea from a baseline assessment. The Baseline Dyspnea Index and the Transition Dyspnea Index both contain three classification axes: functional impairment (activities of daily living), magnitude of task in exertional capacity (intensity of activity), and magnitude of subject effort (effort or difficulty breathing). Each main axis contains five categories, numerically rated 0 to 4. Scores are summed for a baseline score that ranges from 0 to 12. Each main axis in the Transition Index contains seven scores, ranging from –3 (major deterioration) to +3 (major impairment). These scores are summed to form a Transition Score (–9 to +9). The BDI and the TDI, along with spirometry and a 12-minute walking distance were used to measure dyspnea, lung function, and exercise capacity in patients with obstructive pulmonary disease. Mahler et al.[35] concluded that the BDI and the TDI can be used to quantify dyspnea severity and identify changes over time. Using Jaspen's multiserial correlation coefficient (m), the study demonstrated statistically significant relationships between the mean Baseline Dyspnea Score and the 12-minute walking test ($m = 0.54$) and forced vital capacity ($m = 0.63$).

In another study, the BDI and the TDI were used to assess the effects of theophylline on dyspnea, lung function, and exercise performance on 12 male ambulatory patients with nonreversible airway obstruction.[39] Arterial gas tensions, steady-state, maximal exercise performance, and the 12-minute walking distance were measured. Results demonstrated that theophylline reduced dyspnea, but did not improve lung function, gas exchange, or exercise performance.

The BDI and TDI have been used in patients with pulmonary disease and cardiac disorders. Content validity, concurrent validity, construct validity, and sensitivity for both instruments were accomplished in several studies. The BDI is easy to administer and useful for measuring baseline dyspnea levels. The TDI may be best used to measure the effects of disease progression and the outcomes of treatment.

Borg Scale of Perceived Exertion/Modified Borg Scale

The Borg Scale of Perceived Exertion is a 15-point rating scale, with content validity established from Borg's work related to exertion, fatigue, psychophysiological relationships, perceived intensity of work, and work curves.[40] Several studies established concurrent validity, test–retest reliability, and sensitivity.[7,41-44] This instrument is particularly helpful to understand perceived exertion and effort during exercise. It also assists investigators in correlating physiologic parameters of lung disease during exercise testing.

The Modified Borg Scale is a 10-item scale, revised from the original 15-point scale. It is a quantifiable rating scale that assesses dyspnea perception at one specific time point by a particular stimulus.[42] In a study of breathlessness perception in asthmatics, Burdon et al.[7] used the Modified Borg Scale to study perceived breathlessness. The patient is asked to rate words describing increasing degrees of breathlessness by numbers between 0 and 10. The 10-item scale examines perceived breathlessness as it relates to changes in specific pulmonary function studies. Exercise testing and physiologic parameters of lung disease can be assessed, but routine activities of daily living cannot be determined.

Burdon et al.[7] documented that breathlessness increased as the FEV_1 decreased. This suggested a strong close linear relationship between the two indices (mean $r = 0.88 \pm 0.15$ SD). The researchers did, however, note considerable variation in the severity of breathlessness for any degree of airflow obstruction (mean intercept 0.50 ± 0.89 SD). A significant relationship ($p < 0.01$) between bronchial responsiveness and magnitude of respiratory distress was found.

Both the Borg Scale and the Modified Borg Scale can be used for dyspnea measurement in patients with COPD and asthma. These scales are not helpful to investigators interested in understanding responses to routine activities. Additional measures are described in Appendix 32A.

Magnitude Estimation

Magnitude estimation is a psychophysiologic technique that estimates the relationship between the subjective magnitude of a sensation and the physical magnitude of the sensation.[32] Magnitude estimation is based on the subject's designating or assigning numbers to a series of stimuli. The goal is to match the perceived intensity of a physical stimulus to another perceived modality. A range of physical stimulus intensities has been used to measure dyspnea.[31,35,39,45-47] The proportional increase in dyspnea is estimated from the subject's own reference point as loads are added. Because learning is required by the patient, this testing is performed most easily on the ambulatory patient, and with more difficulty on patients who are hospitalized and more acutely ill.

One study explored the use of magnitude estimation in patients experiencing dyspnea.[7] Open magnitude scaling has been done by Killian et al.[47-49] They used externally added resistive and elastic loads to breathing to determine whether the exponent of the power function could be reliably estimated. The results indicated that both lung volume and flow contribute to the respiratory sensation that occurs with loaded breathing. Closed magnitude scaling was done by Burdon et al. by modifying the Borg Category Ratio Scale previously described.[7]

Concerns about the reliability of magnitude estimation were addressed by Nield and Kim[33] in a study of 29 outpatient subjects with chronic obstructive lung disease ($n = 15$) and chronic resistive lung disease ($n = 14$). Subjects were exposed to increasing external resistive loads during three laboratory visits 3 to 5 days apart. The study revealed significant correlations among visits ($p = < 0.01$), confirming the reliability of magnitude estimation for measuring perceptual sensitivity. The study further enhanced the concern about the reliability of magnitude estimation by presenting clear instructions to each subject. Construct validity using an open magnitude scaling was established. This study suggests that the use of magnitude estimation is a reliable method for assessing perceived sensitivity to ventilatory effort in patients who have proven pulmonary disease but are stable.

Visual Analog Scales (VAS)

As with other sensations, Visual Analog Scales (VAS) have been used to measure dyspnea.[38] The VAS is a 100-mm measured line with descriptive phrases at each end. Respondents mark a point corresponding with his or her discomfort and symptom severity. McGavin et al.[50] correlated these scales to standardized exercise tests and pulmonary function studies to aid in determining relationships between exercise and breathlessness. Harries et al.[25] studied the relationships between standardized walking tests, lung function, and the VAS. Subjects were divided into groups according to pulmonary diagnosis: 70 had been diagnosed with bronchitis, and 33 were emphysematous. A significant correlation existed between the walking test and VAS ($r = 0.7$, $p < 0.00001$) for patients with emphysema.

In a study of 16 asthmatic patients in acute respiratory distress and 30 COPD patients, Gift[51] compared a vertical visual analog scale (VVAS) as a measure of dyspnea to the standard horizontal visual analog scale. Both scales were 100 mm in length with anchor terms being "no shortness of breath" at the left or lower end of the line and "shortness of breath as bad as can be" at the right or upper end. The VVAS was found to be easier to use. Concurrent and construct validity were confirmed by two groups of patients (asthmatics and COPD patients) and comparison to peak expiratory flow rates. The VVAS appears to be easy to understand and use by patients experiencing dyspnea. It can assist the clinical evaluation and monitoring of dyspnea and assess the effectiveness of specific interventions to decrease dyspnea.[51]

The VVAS and a scale of subjective symptoms and objectively observed signs of accessory muscle use have been combined by Gift into the Dyspnea Assessment Guide (DAG).[52] To use the DAG, the patient indicates the degree of dyspnea experienced on the vertical visual analog scale and completes the subjective symptom section by circling answers from the list provided. Accessory muscle use is assessed in the semi-Fowler's position. Sternocleidomastoid muscle contraction in combination with clavicle lifting during inspiration is assessed. Gift suggests that the DAG can be useful to evaluate clinical interventions, such as position changes, anxiety-reducing techniques, and energy-conservation measures.

Conceptual Model for Dyspnea

The use of some of the previously described instruments and those presented in Appendix 32A to measure dyspnea have assisted authors in developing conceptual models for dyspnea. Both models describe dyspnea as a complex phenomenon. Gift's model[2] identifies five components of dyspnea: sensation, perception, distress, response, and reporting. *Sensation* is described as the detection of dyspnea by receptor and neural pathways. *Perception* is the individual's interpretation of dyspnea based on past experiences and current expectations. *Distress* refers to the psychologic aspects of dyspnea. *Response* is the individual's coping style and strategies. *Reporting* includes the descriptors of dyspnea and the decision to report or not report shortness of breath.

A second model, by McCord and Cronin-Stubbs,[31] focuses on a plan for operationalizing dyspnea. The authors believe that interventions to manage dyspnea can be directed toward four constructs: antecedents, mediators, reactions, and consequences or outcomes pertinent to dyspnea are identified, assessed, and evaluated.

Similarities in the two models include the realization that psychologic and physiologic components are usually present in dyspnea and need to be evaluated. The complexity of the symptom of dyspnea requires also a systematic approach to assessment and management.

Summary

Dyspnea has been studied in a wide variety of adult and pediatric patient populations. Instruments are available to measure and quantify various aspects of this symptom. Self-reports and self-report checklists, interview guides, visual analog scales, scales measuring perceived exertion and activity, and physiologic pulmonary studies now comprise the armament for dyspnea measurement. These instruments can provide investigators with data to further define and test interventions to assist patients to cope with this problem.

References

1. Carrieri, V., Janson-Bjerklie, S., & Jacobs, S. The sensation of dyspnea: A review. *Heart Lung*, 1984, *13*(4): 436-447.
2. Gift, A. Dyspnea. *Nurs Clin North Am*, 1990, *24*(4): 955-965.
3. Carrieri-Kohlman, V., Douglas, M., Gormley, J., & Stulbarg, M. Desensitization and guided mastery: Treatment approaches for the management of dyspnea. *Heart Lung*, 1993, *22*(3):226-234.
4. Comroe, J. Some theories in the mechanism of dyspnea. In J. Howell and E. Campbell (Eds.), *Breathlessness*. Oxford: Blackwell Scientific Publications, 1966, p. 1.
5. Comroe, J. *Physiology of respiration* (2nd ed.). Chicago: Yearbook Publishers, 1974.
6. Widimsky, J. Dyspnea. *Coret Vasa*, 1979, *21*(2):128-141.
7. Burdon, J., Juniper, E., Killian, K., et al. The perception of breathlessness in asthma. *Am Rev Respir Dis*, 1982, *126*(5):825-828.
8. Janson-Bjerklie, S., Ruma, E., Stulbarg, M., & Carrieri V. Predictors of dyspnea intensity in asthma. *Nurs Res*, 1987, *36*:179-183.
9. Ball, W., & Summer, W. Clinical manifestations and diagnosis of pulmonary disease. In A. Harvey, R. Johns, V. McKusick et al. (Eds.), *The principles and practice of medicine*. New York: Appleton-Century-Crofts, 1980, p. 353.
10. Krzhsko, A., Erdel, S., Griener, M., & Lawrance, A. Guidelines for nursing care of patients with altered ventilation. *Oncol Nurs Forum*, 1983, *10*(2):113-119.
11. Brown, M., Carrieri, V., Janson-Bjerklie, S., & Dodd, M. Lung cancer and dyspnea: The patient's perception. *Oncol Nurs Forum*, 1986, *13*(5):19-24.
12. American Thoracic Society. Recommended respiratory disease questionnaire for use with adults in epidemiological research. *Am Rev Respir Dis*, 1978, *118* (Appendix):7.
13. Roberts, D., Thorne, S., & Pearson, C. The experience of dyspnea in late-stage cancer: Patients' and nurses' perspectives. *Cancer Nurs*, 1993, *16*(4):310-320.
14. Carrieri, V., & Janson-Bjerklie, S. Strategies patients use to manage the sensation of dyspnea. *West J Nurs Res*, 1986, *8*(3):284-305.
15. Epler, G., Saber, F., & Gaensler, E. Determination of severe impairment disability in interstitial lung disease. *Am Rev Respir Dis*, 1980, *121*(4):647-659.
16. McDadden, E., Kiser, R., & Degroot, W. Acute bronchial asthma. *N Engl J Med*, 1973, *288*(5):221-226.
17. Morgan, W. Pulmonary disability and impairment. *Am Thorac Soc News Basis RD*, 1982, *10*(1):1-18.
18. Carrieri, V., & Janson-Bjerklie, S. Dyspnea. In V. Carrieri, A. Lindsey, & C. West (Eds.), *Pathophysiological phenomena in nursing*. Philadelphia: Saunders, 1986, p. 191.
19. Fishman, A.P., & Leslie, J.F. Dyspnea. *Bull Eur Physiol Respir*, 1979, *15*(5):789-804.
20. Gottfried, S., Altose, M., Kelson, S., & Cherniak, N. Perception of changes in airflow resistance in obstructive pulmonary disorders. *Am Rev Respir Dis*, 1981, *124*(5):566-570.
21. Gift, A., & Cahill, C. Psychophysiologic aspects of dyspnea in chronic obstructive disease: A pilot study. *Heart Lung*, 1990, *19*(3):252-257.
22. Carrieri, V., Kieckhefer, G., Janson-Bjerklie, S., & Souza, J. The sensation of pulmonary dyspnea in school age children. *Nurs Res*, 1991, *40*(2):81-86.
23. Gift, A., Plaut, S., & Jacox, A. Psychologic and physiologic factors related to dyspnea in subjects with chronic obstructive pulmonary disease. *Heart Lung*, 1989, *15*(6):595-601.
24. Gift, A., & Pugh, L. Dyspnea and fatigue. *Nurs Clin North Am*, 1993, *28*(2):373-384.
25. Harries, D., Booker, H., Rehaln, M., & Collins, J. Measurement and perception of disability in chronic airways obstruction. *Am Rev Respir Dis*, 1983, vol 127 (4) (suppl):119-120.
26. Bilman, M., Rambhatla, K., Blair, G., & Sieck, G. Breathlessness index, a simple and repeatable exercise test for patients with chronic obstructive pulmonary disease. *Am Rev Respir Dis*, 1983, vol 127 (4) (suppl):109.

27. Butland, R., Pang, J., Gross, E., et al. Two-, six-, and 12-minute walking tests in respiratory disease, *Br Med J*, 1982, *284*(6320):1607-1608.

28. Guyatt, G., Townsend, M., Keller, J., et al. Measuring functional status in chronic lung disease: Conclusions from a randomized control trial. *Resp Med*, 1991, *85*(suppl B):17-21.

29. Burki, N., Mitchell, K., & Chaudhary, B. The ability of asthmatics to detect added resistive loads. *Am Rev Respir Dis*, 1978, *117*(1):71.

30. Guyatt, G., Townsend, M., Berman, L., & Pugsley, S. Quality of life in patients with chronic airflow limitation. *Br J Dis Chest*, 1987, *81*(1):45-54.

31. McCord, M., & Cronin-Stubbs, D. Operationalizing dyspnea: Focus on measurement. *Heart Lung*, 21(2):167-179.

32. Nield, M., Kim, M., & Patel, M. Use of magnitude estimation for estimating the parameters of dyspnea. *Nurs Res*, 1989, *38*(2):77-80.

33. Nield, M., & Kim, M. The reliability of magnitude estimation for dyspnea measurement. *Nurs Res*, 1991, *40*(1):17-19.

34. Burki, N., Davenport, P., Safdar, R., & Zechman, F. The effects of airway anesthesia on magnitude estimation of added inspiratory resistive and elastic loads. *Am Rev Respir Dis*, 1983, *127*(1):2-4.

35. Mahler, D., Weinberg, D., Wells, C., & Feinstein, A. Measurement of dyspnea: Description of two new indexes, interobserver agreement, and physiologic correlations. *Am Rev Respir Dis*, 1982, *125*(suppl):138.

36. Mahler, D., & Wells, C., Evaluation of clinical methods for rating dyspnea. *Chest*, 1988, *93*(1):580-586.

37. Mahler, D., Rosiello, R., Harver, A., et al. Comparison of clinical dyspnea ratings and psychophysical measurements of respiratory sensation in obstructive pulmonary disease. *Am Rev Respir Dis*, 1987, *135*(6):1229-1233.

38. Mahler, D., Harver, A., Rosiello, R., & Daubenspeck, J. Measurement of respiratory sensation in interstitial lung disease. *Chest*, 1989, *96*(4):767-771.

39. Mahler, D., Mattay, R., Berger, H., et al. Sustained-release theophylline reduces dyspnea in non-reversible obstructive airway disease. *Am Rev Respir Dis*, 1983, *127*(suppl):87.

40. Borg, G. Perceived exertion as an indicator of somatic stress. *Scand J Rehab Med*, 1970, *2*(2-3):92-98.

41. Gottfried, S., Altose, M., Kelson, G., & Cherniak, N. Perception of changes in airflow resistance in obstructive pulmonary disorders. *Am Rev Respir Dis*, 1981, *124*(5):566-570.

42. Wilson, R., & Jones, R. A comparison of the visual analog scale and modified Borg scale for the measurement of dyspnea during exercise. *Clin Sci*, 1989, *76*(3):277-279.

43. Moody, L. Measurement of psychophysiologic response variables in chronic bronchitis and emphysema. *Appl Nurs Res*, 1990, *3*(1):36-38.

44. Moody, L., McCormick, K., & Williams, A. Disease and symptom severity, functional status and quality of life in chronic bronchitis and emphysema. *J Br Med*, 1990, *13*(3):297-306.

45. Janson-Bjerklie, S., Carrieri, V., & Hudes, D. The sensation of pulmonary dyspnea. *Nurs Res*, 1986, *35*(3): 154-159.

46. Joyce, C., Zutshi, D., Hrubes, V., & Mason, R. Comparison of fixed interval and visual analogue scales for rating chronic pain. *Eur J Clin Pharmacol*, 1975, *8*(6):415-420.

47. Killian, K., Mahutte, C., Howell, J., & Campbell, E. Effect of timing, flow, lung volume and threshold pressure on resistive load detection. *J Appl Physiol*, 1980, *49*(6):958-963.

48. Killian, K., Burens, D., & Campbell, E. Effect of breathing patterns on the perceived magnitude of added loads to breathing. *J Appl Physiol*, 1982, *52*(3): 578-584.

49. Killian, K., Campbell, E., & Howell, J. The effect of increased ventilation on resistive load discrimination. *Am Rev Respir Dis*, 1979, *120*(6):1233-1238.

50. McGavin, C., Artivinli, M., Nave, H., & McHardy, G. Dyspnoea, disability, and distance walked: Comparison of estimates of exercise performance in respiratory disease. *Br Med J*, 1978, *2*(3):241-243.

51. Gift, A., Plaut, S., & Jacox, A. Psychologic and physiologic factors related to dyspnea in subjects with chronic obstructive pulmonary disease. *Heart Lung*, 1986, *15*(6):595-601.

52. Gift, A. Dyspnea assessment guide. *Crit Care Nurs*, 1991, *9*(8):79.

53. Stoller, J., Ferranti, R., & Feinstein, A. Further specification and evaluation of a new index for dyspnea. *Am Rev Respir Disease*, 1986, *143*(2):129.

54. Comstock, G. Progress report on comparison of respiratory questionnaires in Washington County, MD. *Am Rev Respir Dis*, 1978, *118*(appendix 1):1.

55. Comstock, G., Tockman, M., Helsing, K., & Hennesy, K. Standardized respiratory questionnaires: Comparison of the old with the new. *Am Rev Respir Dis*, 1979, *119*(1):45-49.

56. Kinsman, R., Fernandez, E., Schochet, M., et al. Multidimensional analysis of the symptoms of chronic bronchitis and emphysema. *J Behav Med*, 1983, *6*(4): 339.

57. Guyatt, G., Berman, L., Townsend, M., et al. A measure of quality of life for clinical trials in chronic lung disease. *Thorax*, 1987, *42*(5):773.

Appendix

32A. Additional Measures of Dyspnea

Instrument	Description	Psychometric Indices
The Bronchitis-Emphysema Checklist (31,43,56)	Delineates symptom categories in an 89-item self-report checklist Symptoms include fatigue, helplessness-hopelessness, decathexis, poor memory, peripheral sensory complaints, sleep difficulty, irritability, anxiety, alienation, dyspnea	Content validity established (sample = 29 patients with chronic bronchitis and emphysema) (56) Internal consistency, reliability, construct validity established (sample = 146 patients with chronic bronchitis or emphysema) (56) Internal consistency and reliability supported (sample = 68 patients with pulmonary disease) (43)
Chronic Disease Assessment Tool (CDAT) (43,44)	2-part questionnaire: Part I: 5 sections containing 106 items (general health and medical history, environmental risk, health impact measurement survey, quality of life index, demographics); Part II: open-ended questions addressing physical assessment and pulmonary function Allows measurement of psychophysiologic responses, functional status, and quality of life for many chronic diseases	Content validity established Internal consistency, reliability, and concurrent validity established (sample = 45 patients with chronic bronchitis or emphysema) (44) CDAT must/does address the symptom triad of dyspnea, fatigue, depression to determine applicability to clinical practice and research
Chronic Respiratory Disease Questionnaire (28,30,57)	20-item, 7-point Likert rating scale 4 subscales examine changes in quality of life over 2-week period: dyspnea (subjects asked to specify 5 important, frequent activities that cause shortness of breath (SOB)); fatigue; emotional function; mastery or control	Content validity established (sample = 100 patients with COPD) (57), resulting in a reduction from 123 original items to 20 items Test-retest reliability and concurrent validity established (sample = 25 patients with COPD) (28)
Dyspnea Interview Schedule (14) Developed by Janson-Bjerklie	48-item semistructured interview guide Asks questions about perceived dyspnea, aggravating and alleviating factors, prodromal indicators, physiologic/psychologic/behavioral correlates Elicits data about adaptive mechanisms, social support, effects of dyspnea on activities of daily living Shorter, 9-item version (Clinic Interview) developed: items from original tool; dyspnea description, precipitants, prodromal indicators, correlates, adaptive mechanisms Provides useful insight into the sensation of dyspnea	Both instruments require replication in diverse settings
Five-Level Scale of Breathlessness (13,44) Developed by the American Thoracic Society	Included in the Standardized Respiratory Interview Guide or Self-Report Questionnaire 5-point rating scale that correlates dyspnea with activity Scale is retrospective, can be used with persons experiencing chronic SOB and aids clinicians in determining baseline dyspnea levels	Content validity established Concurrent validity confirmed (sample = 45 patients with COPD) Limitation: reliability remains to be documented; uses ambulation as a major indicator of dyspnea; does not evaluate consequences of other activities

480

Modified Baseline Dyspnea Index (MDI) Developed by Stoller et al. (53)	Developed to improve the Baseline Dyspnea Index (BDI) and to determine differences between functional impairment at work and at home Interview guide with a 5-point rating scale 3 subscales Scoring for a functional impairment subscale yields total score for functional impairment at work and at home	Content and concurrent validity established (sample = 32 patients with stable COPD) Requires documentation of reliability testing and testing with larger sample sizes to compare sensitivity of MDI with BDI Advantages: may assist clinicians in developing interventions specific to patients' problems
Oxygen Cost Diagram (37-39)	Variation of Visual Analog Scale (VAS) Determines point at which a specific activity level corresponds with the subject's perception of dyspnea 100-mm vertical line used, with everyday activities placed in proportion to their oxygen cost Point where SOB limits exercise is marked by subjects	Correlates with BDI and 12-minute walk test Content validity, interrater reliability, concurrent validity, and sensitivity established (sample of patients with pulmonary or cardiac disorders, pulmonary infiltrates, COPD, asthma, cystic fibrosis, interstitial lung disease, chronic airflow obstruction) (38,39) Limitation: emphasis on ambulation
Standardized Respiratory Disease Questionnaire (ATS-DLD-78) Developed by the American Thoracic Society (14,45,54,55)	Used to evaluate the behavioral manifestations of dyspnea; obtain data on pulmonary symptomatology; and elicit demographic data Self-report or interview guide questionnaire can be used to obtain history of pulmonary disease, environmental and occupational exposures, medication use, smoking	Concurrent validity established Reliability and concurrent validity documented (sample of 946 white males) Limitations: collects comprehensive data but not over time; rigor of psychometric testing questioned

Numbers in parentheses correspond to studies cited in the References.

33

Measuring Fatigue

Barbara F. Piper

The first challenge to measuring fatigue may be to agree on a universal definition.[1,2] Currently, no such definition exists. Contributing to this lack of definitional clarity is fatigue's complexity, its multicausal and multidimensional nature,[2] and the difficulties investigators have in differentiating between its causes (e.g., anemia, depression, or beta blockers); its signs, symptoms, or indicators (e.g., reduction in force, tired eyes, legs or whole body); its outcomes, responses, or effects (e.g., decreased activity, functional status, capacity, stamina or endurance);[1] and other signs and symptoms that may or may not be related to fatigue, such as weakness, asthenia, malaise, and exertion.[3]

The chapter defines fatigue by its psychologic or biologic character (i.e., subjective vs. neuromuscular fatigue); by its origin or cause (i.e., central vs. peripheral, pathologic vs. psychologic, and attentional fatigue); by the exclusion of all other diseases (i.e., chronic fatigue syndrome); by its response to electrical stimulation (i.e., high-frequency vs. low-frequency fatigue); and by its duration (i.e., acute vs. chronic fatigue).[2] For scientists interested in developing knowledge about fatigue in clinical populations, however, it is essential to view fatigue as a multidimensional sensation[1-4] similar to pain in its complexity,[5] but with its own unique set of perceptual (subjective), physiologic, and behavioral manifestations or indicators.

Theoretical Description

Various theories have been proposed to explain how fatigue occurs.[1,2,6-13] These theories have attributed the development of fatigue to central and peripheral neurophysiologic mechanisms;[2,10] physiologic, psychologic, and situational factors;[2,6,13-15] personality and environmental factors;[2,13] symptom and activity patterns;[2,3,12,14] developmental, social, and innate host factors;[2,13] and energy variable interactions.[12] Although these etiologic theories for fatigue are not as well developed or tested as are pain theories, a number of similarities exist between these two sensations and their explanative theories. Thus, knowledge about pain as a complex phenomenon may help to direct fatigue research as it attempts to identify underlying fatigue mechanisms, better conceptualize fatigue's dimensions, and improve its measurement and the formulation of management theories.

For example, both pain and fatigue are complex, perceptual sensations that may be explained, in part, by their underlying central and peripheral nervous system mechanisms. It is well known that the nervous system plays a significant role in the transduction, transmission, perception, modulation, and response to pain.[16] As a better understanding of the underlying neurophysiologic mechanisms for pain has emerged, so too have improved conceptualization and measurement of pain's multidimensions evolved.[5,16] The nervous system is postulated to play a significant role in the perception and modulation of fatigue,[2,10] and similar theory building for fatigue's conceptualization and measurement is expected.

For example, central nervous system mechanisms proposed for fatigue include lack of motivation, impaired recruitment of motor neurons, and inhibition of voluntary effort.[10,17,18] The action of sensory pathways on the reticular formation are thought to be critical to the understanding of these central fatigue mechanisms.[19] Chemoreceptors in fatigued muscles are thought to send feedback impulses to the reticular formation in the central nervous system. These impulses result in "the inhibition of motor pathways anywhere from the voluntary centers in the brain to the spinal motor neurons."[19] This inhibition of voluntary effort may be overridden by feedback stimuli from nonfatigued muscles that stimulate the facilitory portion of the reticular formation, resulting in decreased inhibition and decreased fatigue.[19]

Similar inhibition-facilitation mechanisms may be operant in attentional fatigue states,[1] as the ability to concentrate, focus, and direct attention involves the active inhibition of competing stimuli.[20] As mental effort is required to maintain this directed attention, prolonged mental effort can lead to fatigue of the underlying neural mechanisms that block competing or distracting stimuli.[20] Inability to think clearly; to direct attention; or to concentrate may be manifestations of this mental or cognitive fatiguing process.[9]

Peripheral nervous system mechanisms proposed for fatigue include impaired peripheral nerve function, neuromuscular junction transmission, and fiber activation.[10] Impaired neuromuscular junction transmission has been implicated in causing fatigue in myasthenia gravis patients;[21] whereas disturbances in the neurotransmitter acetylcholine have been associated with causing fatigue in botulism patients.[22]

Both central and peripheral nervous system mechanisms may be involved in the overwhelming fatigue that patients experience with chronic fatigue syndrome, cancer therapies, or multiple sclerosis.[2] For example, it has been postulated that the central and peripheral release of endogenous cytokines by leukocytes, lymphocytes, and macrophages may be responsible for fatigue in these patients because of cytokine effects on the central and peripheral nervous systems, metabolism, and other bodily functions.[23] Thus, cytokines may interact with these systems to produce many of the common manifestations seen in fatigue.

For example, cytokines have been implicated in causing fatigue in cancer patients receiving radiation[2,24] and biotherapies[23] and in patients exhibiting signs and symptoms of cognition disorders[1,23] and anemia.[25] The exogenous administration of cytokines, such as interferon in cancer patients, has been postulated to produce fatigue, anorexia, and cognition disorders through direct toxic effects on the frontal lobe, brain structural neurons, or neurotransmitters.[26] Peripheral neuropathies are reported with high-dose interferon therapies.[27] Similarly, the release of endogenous gamma interferon and tumor necrosis factor (TNF) in response to interleukin-2 administration has been implicated in causing alterations in neuroendocrine secretion,[28] brain electrical activity,[29] and blood–brain barrier permeability.[30]

In addition to their effects on the nervous system, TNF and interleukin-1 have been implicated in causing the progressive muscle wasting associated with cancer cachexia.[31] Thus, these particular cytokines may cause fatigue secondary to their effects on the body's metabolic functions.[31] Clearly, as a better understanding about these and other underlying fatigue mechanisms evolves, improved conceptualization, measurement, and interventions for fatigue will result. The history of concept derivation can be summarized as follows:

1920–1929	Poffenberger: developed first single-item measure of tiredness[32]
	Definition of concept of fatigue: controversy persisted
1921–1922	Musico: fatigue composed of multiple unrelated phenomena[33]
1940–1949	Cameron, Bartley: stated complexity makes definition difficult[7,34]
1947	First text written on fatigue[35]
1950–1959	Merton led the way: physiologic theory that fatigue is caused by central and peripheral nervous system mechanisms[36]
	Pearson and Byars: developed a tiredness scale (Fatigue Feeling Tone Checklist);[37] paved the way for nursing studies
	Dorpat and Holmes: linked occurrence of fatigue with pain[38]
	Anecdotal interventions reported[39]
1960–1961	First international conference on fatigue convened with noted fatigue theorists as speakers (Dr. Grandjean,[11,40] Yoshitake,[41-43] and members of Japanese Industrial Research Committee on Fatigue[40]
	Studies conducted using Fatigue Symptom Checklist (FSCL)[41]
1970–1979	Further studies using FSCL[42,43] including nursing studies[44-47]
	Hart found that patients with multiple sclerosis (MS) had more severe fatigue during day than normal controls and that this was related to patient's mobility status[44]
	Haylock and Hart identified fatigue indicators in patients receiving radiation therapy[45]
	Putt published first study examining relationship between an environmental stimulus (e.g., noise) and fatigue[46]
	Classic works published in other disciplines[48-50]
1980–1989	Dramatic increase in number of fatigue studies conducted and published by nurses,[51,52] physicians,[53] and other disciplines[8]
	Fatigue accepted for clinical testing as a nursing diagnosis (North American Nursing Diagnosis Association, NANDA)[54]
	Emergence of "chronic fatigue syndrome"
1990–present	Studies of fatigue enhanced through multidisciplinary collaboration;[55] improved designs addressing methodologic issues;[51,56] and interventions tailored to specific fatigue dimensions to better predict outcomes[55,57]

Dimensions of Fatigue

Most definitions of fatigue allude to its multidimensionality and include a performance or work decrement dimension, a physical/physiologic dimension, and a subjective or symptom/sensory dimension.[6,33,35,46,58,59] Several investigators stress the importance of measuring fatigue's subjective dimension.[2-4] One investigator has proposed that fatigue be defined based on an adaptation of McCaffrey's definition for pain: "fatigue is whatever the patient says it is, whenever (the person) says it is."[4]

Other dimensions that have been proposed include situational,[58] cognitive/mental,[46] psychologic,[13,58] psychosocial,[60] personality,[13] temporal/timing,[46,51] severity,[51] affective,[3,51] biochemical,[3] and behavioral.[3,51]

Unfortunately, although fatigue may be defined multidimensionally,[51,61] few instruments or studies have been able to measure it in this fashion.[46,51,62,63] Thus, the dimensions of fatigue are not as well researched or conceptualized as are the dimensions for pain, although similar dimensions have been proposed for both, such as sensory, affective, behavioral, and physiologic dimensions.[3,5,51]

Yoshitake[41-43] and other Japanese investigators[64,65] were the first to develop a scale to measure symptoms of fatigue multidimensionally. This Fatigue Symptom Checklist (FSCL) was tested initially in healthy Japanese industrial workers. Three symptom dimensions were identified using factor analytic techniques: "general feelings of incongruity" or a "dull, drowsy" factor; "mental symptoms" and "specific feelings of incongruity"; or "projection of fatigue to specific body parts." The FSCL is presented in Appendix 33B.

Piper and associates[3] were the first to propose a multidimensional measurement model for fatigue's manifestations. In this model, subjective perception was believed to be key to understanding how fatigue might vary between healthy and ill individuals. This model was strongly influenced by what was known about pain's manifestations at the time,[66] and by the clinically useful signs and symptoms model used by medicine. Thus, indicators of fatigue in this model were grouped into two major dimensions, subjective and objective manifestations, each with its own subdimensions.

The subjective dimension included perceptions about the timing of fatigue (temporal dimension); the mental, physical, and emotional symptoms of fatigue (sensory dimension); the emotional meaning attributed to the fatigue (affective dimension); and the impact and distress fatigue has on activities of daily living (severity dimension).[3,51] The objective dimension included signs of fatigue that could be validated by physiologic, biochemical, and behavioral means.[3,51] The Piper Fatigue Scale (PFS) was developed to measure the four subjective dimensions of fatigue proposed in this model[51] and is presented in Appendix 33B.

Clearly, more research is needed before the dimensions of fatigue can be agreed upon and specified. The need to dichotomize fatigue into subjective and objective dimensions, however, may have lost its perceived utility. In the past, certain disciplines and studies placed more attention and emphasis on investigations that used the more "objective" measures of fatigue in healthy populations, such as changes in adenosine triphosphate (ATP), serum lactate, and pH levels. Less attention, and thus value, was given to the development and testing of self-report scales that could be used to measure the more "subjective" dimension of fatigue, particularly in clinical populations. At the time, dichotomizing fatigue into these two broad dimensions was useful as it enabled investigators to see more clearly the "gaps" in knowledge development particularly as it related to fatigue measurement issues. As a consequence, more attention was given to the development of valid and reliable self-report scales that could be used in conjunction with physiologic or "objective" methods to measure fatigue.

Currently, this dichotomy may no longer be needed as methods designed to measure both the subjective and the objective indicators of fatigue or signs and symptoms have become more numerous, valid, and reliable. Emphasis must now be placed on using these methods in combination with one another better to measure fatigue's signs and symptoms in diverse populations; to specify fatigue's dimensions and their underlying mechanisms; and to target fatigue interventions to specific dimensions, to predict outcomes. As a consequence, the following dimensions are proposed for the study of fatigue's signs and symptoms and the tailoring of interventions: temporal, sensory, cognitive, affective, behavioral, and physiological. These dimensions are presented in Appendix 33A along with indicators and measures for each dimension.

Conflicting data exist about the relationship between depression and fatigue.[3] Some studies have found positive correlations;[51,61,62,67,68] others have not.[69-71] It can be said of pain and depression that "pain can cause depression, and . . . depression can worsen pain."[57] The directional relationships and distinctions between fatigue and depression are not clear.[2] In many cases, these relationships may defy a simple, unidirectional model of causation and may be bidirectional.[57] Treatment of one may lead to improvement in the other.[57]

For example, fatigue frequently is a presenting symptom of depression. Sleep disturbances, such as insomnia, multiple awakenings during sleep, or early waking are common in depression and may contribute to fatigue.[72] In contrast, fatigue can occur in the absence of depression or may cause depression itself because of its negative impact on perceived quality of life. Thus, depression and fatigue may be outcome indicators of one another, depending on how they are measured and conceptualized in a given study.

Methodologically, many depression inventories have been designed specifically for use in psychiatric populations and are not easily tailored to measure reactive depression in the general population. In addition, many depression scales contain items of a somatic nature, such as loss of appetite, decreased energy levels, and fatigue,[73] that make it difficult to distinguish depression from fatigue and the side effects of disease or treatment. Findings are therefore confounded by measurement redundancy. Until such methodologic issues are resolved, depression can be considered a cause, a manifestation, and/or an outcome indicator of this dimension depending on the research questions posed.

Selecting a Fatigue Instrument

Clearly, the research questions and the theoretical or conceptual framework that drive the study dictate the measurement strategies to be used. Methods selected depend on the particular dimension(s) the investigator is interested in studying, such as the selection of a battery of neurocognitive tests to measure the cognitive dimension of fatigue.

Reliability and validity of the measures are critical if the outcomes of the study are to have credibility and generalizability.[74] Single-item, self-report scales, such as one-item intensity measures, may be less reliable than are multiple-item fatigue measures.[75] Using multiple fatigue methods together in a given study, a process called triangulation,[76] can enhance the reliability and validity of the study findings. Investigators must use caution in the selection and the number of fatigue measures, however, to avoid inducing "iatrogenic fatigue" in the respondent. Methods that are too lengthy, redundant, or cumbersome can confound fatigue findings and lead to subject refusal to participate and to subject attrition over time in longitudinal studies.

The timing of measurement must be addressed and described. For example, will the time of day for measurement be held constant across all subjects to control for circadian patterns? How do the usual diurnal fluctuations of self-report and physiologic indicators covary and affect measurement strategy? Will self-report and physiologic measures be administered within a short time of one another to enhance validity? Will subjects be less compliant if asked to complete measures when they are most fatigued? Unfortunately, the issue related to the timing of fatigue measures is often not addressed in published studies.[2] When timing is mentioned, it usually is addressed in studies that have used repeated measures throughout the day to capture circadian patterns (i.e., on arising, at midday, late afternoon, and bedtime)[22,77] or in studies that control for the effects of treatment (i.e., always 2 hours after radiation therapy).[45] Ideally laboratory studies or physiologic measures should be performed concurrently or within a few hours of self-report measures.[2]

To investigate differences between healthy or control subjects and clinical populations, it is important to have an instrument that effectively discriminates fatigue between these groups (discriminant validity). In addition, an instrument needs to be sensitive to changes in fatigue patterns over time, particularly in longitudinal studies. Last, sample characteristics must be considered. Age, educational level, language, culture, visual, hearing, and motor coordination all can influence measurement strategy, subject compliance, and findings.[2,78]

Instruments available to measure fatigue can be single-item or multi-item, unidimensional or multidimensional scales. Important measures are described in Appendix 33B. Three additional scales, not included in the Appendix, have been recently reported in the literature.[79-81]

Summary of Research Findings to Date

Twenty-six studies to date have used prospective, repeated-measures designs to study fatigue. Despite the number of longitudinal studies, the ability to generalize from these studies is limited, as pertinent demographic, treatment, and disease-related factors have not been consistently reported. With these limitations in mind, however, the following findings are suggestive of fatigue patterns by diagnostic categories.

Cancer[4] and multiple sclerosis (MS) patients tend to report more fatigue than do healthy controls.[47,69] Surprisingly in MS patients, the least disabled report more fatigue symptoms and higher levels of fatigue than do their more disabled counterparts.[47] A similar relationship between a higher number of symptoms and increased levels of fatigue is found in kidney dialysis patients.[71] In cancer patients, increased distress from symptoms other than fatigue also is associated with higher levels of fatigue.[12] Fatigue is positively related to depression in systemic lupus,[69] cancer,[82] and depressed patients, but no such relationship has been documented in renal dialysis patients.[71]

From a demographic standpoint, two studies have found that younger patients with cancer have higher levels of fatigue than do older patients.[4,83] This is in contrast to healthy, pregnant women, where the reverse has been documented.[84] Only two studies have examined cultural and ethnic differences in fatigue patterns;[84,85] higher levels of fatigue were reported in non-Caucasian pregnant women in one study;[84] more gastrointestinal symptoms were attributed to fatigue by Korean women with breast cancer than their American counterparts in the other study.[85]

Consistent across studies is the finding that disturbances in sleep patterns are related to increases in severity of fatigue.[15,83,86] Similarly, increased levels of fatigue are associated with decreases in activities of daily living and performance status.[83,87,88]

From an intervention standpoint, subjects consistently report that rest and/or distraction are helpful in alleviating fatigue,[46,51,61,67,88] but what constitutes rest or distraction has not been adequately studied. Similarly, exercise may have a beneficial effect on fatigue. Studies have documented that women who report formal exercise as a lifestyle pattern have decreasing levels of fatigue.[52,83,89,90]

Unfortunately, very few of the studies have included biologic or physiologic measures in their designs. Thus, the ability to correlate perceptions of fatigue to physiologic measures is limited. Thus far, changes in oral and forehead temperatures in MS patients[47] and weight declines in cancer patients[12,45] are the only physiologic indicators that correlate with self-reports of fatigue.

Although other empiric studies have documented negative correlations between self-reports of fatigue and pH, oxygen saturation, and cardiac ejection fractions in congestive heart failure patients[91] and decreases in physical activity and grip strength behaviorally in arthritis patients,[92] the preponderance of fatigue self-report studies show no relationship to physiologic measures.[77] Similar findings are reported in studies that have examined the relationships between other symptoms and their possible physiologic indicators.[57]

Studying these relationships is complicated not only by the diurnal fluctuations that may affect the timing and measurement of these indicators,[2] but also by the complex nature of their relationships. For example, "physiological variables can be profoundly abnormal without the patient having any symptoms."[57,p60] In contrast, a wide variety of symptoms may be present, as in the case of chronic fatigue syndrome and other disorders, but no physiologic abnormality or etiology can be documented.

Because of the inconsistent relationship between symptoms and physiologic indicators, Wilson and Cleary conclude that "it is unlikely that treatments directed at biological and physiological factors alone, even if they can be identified, will be fully effective in the relief of symptoms."[57] These authors suggest that other factors, such as social, psychologic, patient expectations, and relationships to health-care providers, may need to be explored as well.[57] Whether this holds true for the study of fatigue remains to be seen.

The exemplar study at the end of the chapter illustrates how a study to measure fatigue can be designed. It was selected because of its longitudinal design, its homogeneous sample, the use of instruments with established reliability and validity estimates, and its attempt to correlate physiologic measures (i.e., hematocrit) with self-report.[61]

Summary

Research findings support the commonly held belief that fatigue is a multidimensional construct that can be positively and/or negatively influenced by activity, exercise, rest, sleep, disease, symptom, and psychologic patterns. Thus, these findings support hypothesized and inferred relationships proposed in published fatigue frameworks and theories.[1,3,12] Further research is needed to better specify the dimensions of fatigue and their underlying mechanisms; determine how specific variables may influence the signs and symptoms of these dimensions; and evaluate the effects of fatigue interventions on patient or family outcomes.

Exemplar Study

Piper, B.F. *Subjective fatigue in women receiving six cycles of adjunctive chemotherapy for breast cancer.* Unpublished doctorical dissertation, University of California, San Francisco, California, 1992.

The primary purpose of this study was to determine prospectively the incidence, timing, and intensity of subjective fatigue symptoms in women with breast cancer receiving adjuvant chemotherapy (CT). A secondary purpose was to predict risk factors (age, stage of disease, performance status, hematocrit level, length of CT cycle [21 days vs. 28 days], inclusion of Adriamycin in the regimen, mood/affective states [vigor, depression, mood disturbance], and social support) for the development of subjective fatigue over time (chronic).

Selected components of an investigator-designed and published fatigue framework integrating fatigue theories guided this study. Fatigue was measured by the Profile of Mood States' Fatigue-Inertia Subscale (POMS F/I), the Piper Fatigue Scale (PFS), and the Fatigue Symptom Checklist (FSCL) during the first three consecutive and sixth and final CT cycles, including nadirs

(Times 1–8). Mood states were measured by the POMS (Times 1–8) and social support by the Norbeck Social Support Questionnaire (Times 1, 5, and 7).

Repeated-measures analysis of variance (ANOVA), Pearson's correlations, chi-square analyses, and independent t-tests were used to determine changes over time, validity estimates, and relationships between fatigue and moderator variables. Forward stepwise multiple regression and graphic residual analyses were used to determine predictors of fatigue over time.

In this sample ($n = 37$, stage I/II disease, predominantly CMF [cytoxan, methotrexate, and fluorouracil] CT), the number and intensity of fatigue symptoms (FSCL) did not increase over time. No significant differences in fatigue were noted as a function of the length of CT cycle or of the inclusion of Adriamycin in the treatment regimen. Significant insomnia and declines in social support were documented. Study results suggest that knowledge about depression, vigor, and mood disturbance scores can enable the clinician to predict, with a 47% to 76% degree of accuracy, a woman's risk for developing fatigue over time while receiving adjuvant CT for breast cancer. If these risk factors can be confirmed by other studies, the timing and selection of fatigue interventions can be tailored to those at high risk.

Some of the limitations in the study's design are subject attrition ($n = 74$ to $n = 37$); lack of an ethnically diverse sample; lack of a comparable, healthy, age-matched control group; and the weaknesses inherent in not collecting physiologic measures in conjunction with self-report scales.

References

1. Winningham, M.L., Nail, L.M., Burke, M.B., et al. Fatigue and the cancer experience: The state of the knowledge. *Oncol Nurs Forum*, 1994, 21(1):23-36.
2. Piper, B.F. Fatigue. In V. Carrieri-Kohlman, A.M. Lindsey, & C.M. West (Eds.), *Pathophysiological phenomena in nursing: Human responses to illness* (2nd ed.). Philadelphia: Saunders, 1993, pp. 279–302.
3. Piper, B.F., Lindsey, A.M., & Dodd, M.J. Fatigue mechanisms in cancer: Developing nursing theory. *Oncol Nurs Forum*, 1987, 14(6):17-23.
4. Glaus, A. Assessment of fatigue in cancer and noncancer patients. *Support Care Cancer*, 1993, 1:305-315.
5. McGuire, D.B. Comprehensive and multidimensional assessment and measurement of pain. *J Pain Sympt Manag*, 1992, 7(5):312-319.
6. Aistars, J. Fatigue in the cancer patient: A conceptual approach. *Oncol Nurs Forum*, 1987, 14:25-30.
7. Cameron, C. A theory of fatigue. *Ergonomics*, 1973, 16:633-646.
8. Ciba Foundation Symposium 82. *Human muscle fatigue: Physiological mechanisms*. London: Pittman Medical, 1981.
9. Cimprich, B. Attentional fatigue following breast cancer surgery. *Res Nurs Health*, 1992, 15:199-207.
10. Gibson, H., & Edwards, R.H.T. Muscular exercise and fatigue. *Sports Med*, 1985, 2:120-132.
11. Grandjean, E.P. Fatigue: Its physiological and psychological significance. *Ergonomics*, 1968, 11:427-436.
12. Irvine, D., Vincent, L., Graydon, J.E., et al. The prevalence and correlates of fatigue in patients receiving treatment with chemotherapy and radiation therapy: A comparison with the fatigue experienced by healthy individuals. *Cancer Nurs*, 1994, 17(5):367-378.
13. Potempa, K., Lopez, M., Reid, C., & Lawson, L. Chronic fatigue. *Image*, 1986, 18:165-169.
14. Nail, L., & Winningham, M. Fatigue. In S.L. Groenwald, M. Frogge, M. Goodman, & C. Yarbro (Eds.), *Cancer nursing: Principles and practice* (3rd ed.). Boston: Jones and Bartlett, 1993, pp. 608-619.
15. Pugh, L.C. *Psychophysiological correlates of fatigue during childbirth*. Unpublished doctoral dissertation, University of Maryland, Baltimore, 1989.
16. National Institute of Nursing Research. *Symptom management: Acute pain (1994). A report of the NINR priority expert panel on symptom management acute pain*. Bethesda, MD: U.S. Department of Health and Human Services, NIH, 1994.
17. Maclaren, D.P.M., Gibson, H., Parry-Billings, M., & Edwards, R.H.T. A review of metabolic and physiological factors in fatigue. *Exerc Sport Sci Rev*, 1989, 17:29-66.
18. Poteliakhoff, A. Adrenocortical activity and some clinical findings in acute and chronic fatigue. *J Psychosom Res*, 1981, 25:91-95.
19. Asmussen, E. Muscle fatigue. *Med Sci Sports Exerc*, 1979, 11:313-321.
20. Kaplan, S., & Kaplan, R. *Environment and cognition*. New York: Praeger, 1982.
21. Vollestad, N.K., & Sejersted, O.M. Biochemical correlates of fatigue. *Eur J Appl Physiol*, 1988, 57:336-347.
22. Cohen, F.L., & Hardin, S.B. Fatigue in patients with catastrophic illness. In S.G. Funk, E.M. Tournquist, M.T. Champagne, L.A. Copp, & R.A. Weise (Eds.), *Key aspects of comfort: Management of pain, fatigue, and nausea*. New York: Springer, 1989, pp. 208-216.
23. Piper, B.F., Reiger, P.T., Brophy, L., et al. Recent advances in the management of biotherapy-related side effects: Fatigue. *Oncol Nurs Forum*, 1989, 16:27-34.
24. Greenberg, D.B., Gray, J.L., Mannix, C.M., et al. Treatment-related fatigue and serum interleukin-1 levels in patients during external beam irradiation for prostate cancer. *J Pain Sympt Manag*, 1993, 8(4):196-200.
25. Barlogie, B., & Beck, T. Recombinant human erythropoietin and the anemia of multiple myeloma. *Stem Cells*, 1993, 11:88-94.

26. Adams, F. Quesada, J.R., & Gutterman, J.U. Neuropsychiatric manifestations of human leukocyte interferon therapy in patients with cancer. *JAMA*, 1984, *252*(1):938-941.

27. Bernsen, P.L.J.A., Wong-Chung, R.D., Janssen, J.T. Neurologic amyotrophy and polyradiculopathy during interferon therapy. *Lancet*, 1985, *1*(8419):50.

28. Besedovsky, H.O., del Rey, A.E., & Sorkin, E. Immune-neuroendocrine interactions. *J Immunol*, 1985, *135*(suppl 2):750S-754S.

29. Krueger, J.M., Walter, J., Dinarello, C.A., et al. Sleep-promoting effects of endogenous pyrogen (interleukin-1). *Am J Physiol*, 1984, *246*(6, pt 2):R994-R999.

30. Denikoff, K.D., Rubinow, D.R., Papa, M.Z., et al. The neuropsychiatric effects of treatment with interleukin-2 and lymphokine-activated killer cells. *Ann Int Med*, 1987, *107*(3):293-300.

31. St. Pierre, B., Kasper, C., & Lindsey, A.M. Fatigue mechanisms in patients with cancer: Effects of tumor necrosis factor and exercise on skeletal muscle. *Oncol Nurs Forum*, 1992, *19*:419-425.

32. Poffenberger, A.T. The effects of continuous work upon output and feelings. *J Appl Psychol*, 1928, *12*(5):450-467.

33. Muscio, B. Is a fatigue test possible? *Br J Psychol*, 1921, *12*:31-46.

34. Bartley, S.H. What do we call fatigue? In E. Simonson & P.C. Weiser (Eds.), *Psychological aspects and physiological correlates of work and fatigue.* Springfield, IL: Charles C. Thomas, 1976, pp. 409-414.

35. Bartley, S.H., & Chute, E. *Fatigue and impairment in man.* New York: McGraw-Hill, 1947.

36. Merton, P.A. Voluntary strength and fatigue. *J Physiol*, 1954, *123*:553-564.

37. Pearson, R.G., & Byars, G.E. *The development and validation of a checklist for measuring subjective fatigue.* Report No. 56-115. Randolph Air Force Base, TX: School of Aviation Medicine, U.S. Air Force, 1956.

38. Dorpat, T.L., & Holmes, T.H. Mechanisms of skeletal muscle pain and fatigue. *Arch Neurol Psychiatr*, 1955, *74*(1):638-640.

39. Snow, E.W., Machlan, L.O., Jr., Warnell, C.E., & Utt, T.P. The tired patient. *Med Times*, 1959, *87*:1500-1504.

40. Hashimoto, K., Kogi, K., & Grandjean, E. (Eds.). *Methodology in human fatigue assessment.* London: Taylor & Francis, 1971.

41. Yoshitake, H. Rating the feelings of fatigue. *J Sci Labour*, 1969, *45*(7):422-432.

42. Yoshitake, H. Relations between the symptoms and the feeling of fatigue. *Ergonomics*, 1971, *14*:175-186.

43. Yoshitake, H. Three characteristic patterns of subjective fatigue symptoms. *Ergonomics*, 1978, *21*(3):231-233.

44. Hart, L.K. Fatigue in the patient with multiple sclerosis. *Res Nurs Health*, 1978, *1*(4):147-157.

45. Haylock, P.J., & Hart, L.K. Fatigue in patients receiving localized radiation. *Cancer Nurs*, 1979, *2*(6):461-467.

46. Putt, A.M. Effects of noise on fatigue in healthy middle-aged adults. *Commun Nurs Res*, 1977, *8*:24-34.

47. Freel, M.I., & Hart, L.K. *Study of fatigue phenomena of multiple sclerosis patients.* (Grant No. 5R02-NU-00524-2), Division of Nursing, USDHEW, 1977.

48. Kinsman, R.A., & Weiser, P.C. Subjective symptomatology during work and fatigue. In E. Simonson & P.C. Weiser (Eds.), *Psychological aspects and physiological correlates of work and fatigue.* Springfield, IL: Charles C. Thomas, 1976, pp. 336-405.

49. Meyerwitz, B.E., Sparks, F.C., & Sparks, I.K. Adjuvant chemotherapy for breast cancer. *Cancer*, 1979, *43*:1613-1618.

50. Rose, E.A., & King, T.C. Understanding postoperative fatigue. *Surg Gynecol Obstet*, 1978, *147*:97-101.

51. Piper, B.F., Lindsey, A.M., Dodd, M.J., et al. The development of an instrument to measure the subjective dimension of fatigue. In S.G. Funk, E.M. Tornquist, M.T. Champagne, L.A. Copp, & R.A. Wiese (Eds.), *Key aspects of comfort: Management of pain, fatigue, and nausea.* New York: Springer, 1989, pp. 199-208.

52. Pardue, N.H. *Energy expenditure and subjective fatigue of chronic obstructive pulmonary disease patients before and after a pulmonary rehabilitation.* Unpublished doctoral dissertation, Catholic University: Washington, DC, 1984.

53. Valdini, A.F. Fatigue of unknown etiology: A review. *Fam Pract*, 1985, *2*(1):48-53.

54. Voith, A.M., Frank, A.M., & Pegg, J.S. Nursing diagnosis: Fatigue. In R.M. Carroll-Johnson (Ed.), *Classification of nursing diagnoses: Proceedings of the eighth conference.* Philadelphia: Lippincott, 1989, pp. 453-458.

55. Schleuderberg, A., Straus, S.E., Peterson, P., et al. Chronic fatigue syndrome research: Definition and medical outcome assessment. *Ann Int Med*, 1992, *117*(4):325-331.

56. Moore, K. (1992). Integrating biological and behavioral variables in cancer nursing research. *Proceedings of the Second National Conference on Cancer Nursing Research.* Atlanta: American Cancer Society, January 1992.

57. Wilson, I.B., & Cleary, P.D. Linking clinical variables with health-related quality of life: A conceptual model of patient outcomes. *JAMA*, 1995, *273*(1):59-65.

58. Milligan, R.A., & Pugh, L.C. Fatigue during the childbearing period. In J.J. Fitzpatrick, & J.S. Stevenson (Eds.), *Annual review of nursing research* (vol. 12). New York: Springer, 1994, pp. 33-49.

59. Pugh, L.C. Childbirth and the measurement of fatigue. *J Nurs Measure*, 1993, *1*(1):57-66.

60. Fisk, J.D., Ritvo, P.G., Ross, L., et al. Measuring the functional impact of fatigue: Initial validation of the fatigue impact scale. *Clin Infect Dis*, 1994, *18*(suppl 1):S79-S83.

61. Piper, B.F., *Subjective fatigue in women receiving six cycle chemotherapy for breast cancer.* University of California, San Francisco. Unpublished doctorial dissertation, 1992.

62. Belza, B.L., Henke, C.J., Yelin, E.H., et al. Correlates of fatigue in older adults with rheumatoid arthritis. *Nurs Res*, 1993, *42*(2):93-99.

63. Belza, B.L. Comparison of self-reported fatigue in rheumatoid arthritis and controls. *J Rheumatol*, 1995, *22*(4):639-643.

64. Kogi, K., Saito, Y., & Mitsuhashi, T. Validity of three components of subjective fatigue feelings. *J Sci Labour*, 1970, *46*(5):251-270.

65. Saito, Y., Kogi, K., & Kashiwagi, S. Factors underlying subjective feelings of fatigue. *J Sci Labour*, 1970, *46*(4):205-224.

66. Melzack, R. (Ed.) *Pain measurement and assessment.* New York: Raven, 1983.

67. Dean, G.E., Spears, L., Ferrell, B.R., et al. Fatigue in patients with cancer receiving interferon alpha. *Cancer Pract,* 1995, 3(3):164-172.

68. Bruera, E., Brennis, C., Michaud, M., et al. Association between nutritional status, lean body mass, anemia, psychological status, and tumor mass in patients with advanced breast cancer. *J Pain Sympt Manag,* 1989, 4:59-63.

69. Krupp, L.B., LaRocca, N.G., Muir-Nash, J., & Steinberg, A.D. The Fatigue Severity Scale: Application to patients with multiple sclerosis and systemic lupus erythematosus. *Arch Neurol,* 1989, 46:1121-1123.

70. Pickard-Holley, S. Fatigue in cancer patients: A descriptive study. *Cancer Nurs,* 1991, 14:13-19.

71. Srivastava, R.H. Fatigue in end-stage renal disease patients. In S.G. Funk, E.M. Tournquist, M.T. Champagne, L.A. Copp, & R.A. Weise (Eds.), *Key aspects of comfort: Management of pain, fatigue and nausea.* New York: Springer, 1989, pp. 217-224.

72. Blumenthal, M.D. Depressive illness in old age: Getting behind the mask. *Geriatrics,* 1980, 35:34-43.

73. Endicott, J. Measurement of depression in patients with cancer. *Cancer,* 1984, 53(10):2243-2249.

74. Schulte, P.A. Validation of biologic markers for use in research on chronic fatigue syndrome. *Rev Infect Dis,* 1991, 13(suppl 1):S87-S89.

75. Lee, K.A., Hicks, G., & Nino-Murcia, G. Validity and reliability of a scale to assess fatigue. *Psychiatr Res,* 1991, 36:291-298.

76. Polit, D.F., & Hungler, B.P. *Nursing research: Principles and methods.* Philadelphia: Lippincott, 1987.

77. Cardenas, D.D., & Kutner, N.G. The problem of fatigue in dialysis patients. *Nephron,* 1982, 30:336-340.

78. McGuire, D.B. Measuring pain. In M. Frank-Stromborg (Ed.), *Instruments for clinical nursing research.* Norwalk, CT: Appleton & Lange, 1988, pp. 333-356.

79. Glaus, A., Crowe, R., Bohme, C. et al. Development of a Fatigue Assessment Questionnaire (FAQ) for cancer patients. *Ann Oncology,* 1996, 7(suppl 5):134.

80. Meek, P.M. Internal consistancey, reliability, and validity of a new measure of cancer treatment, and related fatigue; The General Fatigue Scale (GFS), *Oncol Nurs Forum,* in press.

81. Schwartz, A. Reliability and validity of the cancer fatigue scale. *Oncol Nurs Forum,* in press.

82. Jamar, S.C. Fatigue in women receiving chemotherapy for ovarian cancer. In S.G. Funk, E.M. Tournquist, M.T. Champagne, L.A. Copp, & R.A. Weise (Eds.), *Key aspects of comfort: Management of pain, fatigue, and nausea.* New York: Springer, 1989, pp. 224-233.

83. Piper, B.F., Dibble, S., Dodd, M.J. & Weiss, M.C. The influence of insomnia on subjective fatigue in women survivors of breast cancer. *Proceedings of the 4th National Conference on Cancer Nursing Research,* Atlanta, American Cancer Society, 1997.

84. Pitzer, M.S. Patterns of fatigue and psychological factors during pregnancy: Their relationship to preterm labor/birth. *Nursing research: Global health perspectives: Proceedings of the 1991 International Nursing Research Conference,* American Nurses' Association, Washington, DC, 1991.

85. Piper, B., Lee, H.O., Kim, O., et al. Fatigue-transcultural implications for nursing interventions. In A.P. Pritchard (Ed.), *Cancer nursing: The balance. Proceedings of the Sixth International Conference on Cancer Nursing.* London: Scutari Press, 1991, pp. 140-144.

86. Krupp, L.B., Jandorf, L., Coyle, P.K., & Mendelson, W.B. Sleep disturbances in chronic fatigue syndrome. *J Psychosom Res,* 1993, 37(4):325-331.

87. Rieger, P.A. (TRAHAN). *Interferon-induced fatigue.* Unpublished master's thesis, Houston: University of Texas Health Science Center, 1986.

88. Berger, A. Measurement of fatigue and quality of life in cancer patients receiving chemotherapy. *Oncol Nurs Forum,* 1993, 20(2):311.

89. MacVicar, M.G., & Winningham, M.L. Promoting functional capacity of cancer patients. *Cancer Bull,* 1986, 38(5):235-239.

90. Mock, V., Burke, M.B., Sheehan, P., et al. A nursing rehabilitation program for women with breast cancer receiving adjuvant chemotherapy. *Oncol Nurs Forum,* 1994, 21(5):899-906.

91. Schaefer, K.M. A description of fatigue associated with congestive heart failure: Use of Levine's conservation model. In M. Parker (Ed.), *Nursing theories in practice.* Publication No. 15-2350. New York: National League for Nurses, 1990, pp. 217-237.

92. Tack (Belza), B. *Dimensions and correlates of fatigue in older adults with rheumatoid arthritis.* Unpublished doctorial disseration, University of California, San Francisco, 1990.

93. Paul, S. The Piper Fatigue Scale: Further psychometric testing in women with breast cancer. *Oncol Nurs Forum,* in press.

94. Rodriguez, A.A., & Agre, J.C. Physiologic parameters and perceived exertion with local muscle fatigue in postpolio subjects. *Arch Phys Med Rehab,* 1991, 72:305-308.

95. Smets, E.M.A., Garssen, B., Schuster-Uitterhoeve, A.L.J., & de Haes, J.C.J.M. Fatigue in cancer patients. *Br J Cancer,* 1993, 68:220-224.

96. DeLuca, J., Johnson, S.K., & Natelson, B.J. Information processing efficiency in chronic fatigue syndrome and multiple sclerosis. *Arch Neurol,* 1993, 50(3):301-304.

97. McDonald, E., Cope, H., & David, A. Cognitive impairment in patients with chronic fatigue: A preliminary study. *J Neurol Neurosurg Psychiatr,* 1993, 56:812-815.

98. Heuting, J.E., & Sarphati, H.R. Measuring fatigue. *J Appl Physiol,* 1966, 50:535-538.

99. Arendt, D., Borbely, A.A., Franey, C., & Wright, J. The effects of chronic, small doses of melatonin given in the late afternoon on fatigue in man: A preliminary study. *Neurosci Lett,* 1984, 45:317-321.

100. Burton, R.R. Human responses to repeated high G simulated aerial combat maneuvers. *Aviat Space Environ Med,* 1980, 51:1185-1192.

101. Miller, R.G., Giannini, D., Milner-Brown, H.S., Layzer, R.B., et al. Effects of fatiguing exercise on high-energy phosphates, force and EMG: Evidence for three phases of recovery. *Muscle Nerve,* 1987, 10:810-821.

102. Friedman, J., & Friedman, H. Fatigue in Parkinson's disease. *Neurology,* 1993, 43:2016-2018.

103. Katerndahl, D.A. Differentiation of physical and psychological fatigue. *Fam Pract Res J*, 1993, *13*(1): 81-91.

104. Schwartz, J.E., Jandorf, L., & Krupp, L.B. The measurement of fatigue: A new instrument. *J Psychosom Res*, 1993, *37*(7):753-762.

105. Taphoorn, M.J.B., van Someren, E., Snoek, F.J., et al. Fatigue, sleep disturbances and circadian rhythm in multiple sclerosis. *J Neurol*, 1993, *240*:446-448.

106. Bentall, R.P., Wood, G.C., Marrinan, T., et al. A brief mental fatigue questionnaire. *Br J Clin Psychol*, 1993, *32*:375-379.

107. Lee, H.O. *Fatigue in myocardial infarction patients.* Unpublished doctorial dissertation, University of California, San Francisco, 1993.

108. Reeves, N., Potempa, K., & Gallo, A. Fatigue in early pregnancy: An exploratory study. *J Midwifery*, 1991, *36*(5):303-309.

109. Chalder, T., Berelowitz, G., Pawlikowska, T., et al. *J Psychosom Res*, 1993, *37*(2):147-153.

110. Bonner, D., Ron, M., Chalder, T., & Wessely, S. Chronic fatigue syndrome: A follow up study. *J Neurol Neurosurg Psychiatr*, 1994, *57*:617-621.

111. Walford, G.A., Nelson, W., & McCluskey, D.R. Fatigue, depression, and social adjustment in chronic fatigue syndrome. *Arch Dis Child*, 1993, *68*(3):384-388.

112. Ridsdale, L., Evans, A., Jerrett, W., et al. Patients with fatigue in general practice: A prospective study. *Br Med J*, 1993, *307*(6896):103-106.

113. Konishi, Y., Horiguchi, S., Miyama, Y., & Kawai, T. A questionnaire study on fatigue symptoms of municipal personnel. *Osake City Med J*, 1991, *37*(2):157-162.

114. Jensen, S., & Given, B.A. Fatigue affecting family caregivers of cancer patients. *Cancer Nurs*, 1993, *14*(5):181-187.

115. Barrere, C., Trotta, P., & Foster, J. The experience of fatigue in women undergoing radiation therapy for early stage breast cancer. *Oncol Nurs Forum*, 1993, *20*(2):335.

116. Silverman, S.L., Belza, B., Mason, J., & Nakasone, R. Measurement of fatigue in patients with fibromyalgia (FM) as compared to rheumatoid arthritis (RA). *American College of Rheumatology 57th Annual Scientific Meeting Proceedings*, San Antonio, TX, 1993.

117. Ray, C., Phillips, L., & Weir, W.R.C. Quality of attention in chronic fatigue syndrome: Subjective reports of everyday attention and cognitive difficulty, and performance on tasks of focused attention. *Br J Clin Psychol*, 1993, *32*:357-364.

Appendices

33A. Dimensions of Fatigue

Dimension	Indicators	Instruments Measuring This Dimension
Temporal: signs and symptoms relating to timing, onset, pattern, duration of fatigue (4,22,51,62,92)	Timing/circadian pattern (when occurs) Onset/duration (seconds to years) Pattern (brief, momentary, transient; intermittent, seldom or frequent, continuous, constant or chronic) Changes in pattern over time	Self-report scales: PFS (51); Multidimensional Assessment of Fatigue Scale (MAF), an adapted PFS (51,62,92)
Sensory: signs and symptoms and their intensities (46,51,93)	Location: signs and symptoms may be localized to specific muscle groups/fibers (e.g., tired eyes) or may be generalized to whole body (whole-body fatigue) (94) Analogous to pain model: symptoms and intensities may attenuate over time (95)	Included in most self-reports
Cognitive/mental: signs and symptoms reflecting impact of fatigue on thought processes (9,51,59,60,93)	Ability to concentrate; remember; think clearly; be alert, drowsy, or sleepy	PFS (51,93), FSCL (41-43); Modified FSCL (59); Visual Analogue Scale to Measure Fatigue's severity (VAS-F) (75); Functional Impact of Fatigue Scale (FIS) (60); Neurocognitive Measures (e.g., Forward-Backward Digit Span tests) (9,59,96,97)
Affective/emotional: reflects emotional manifestations of fatigue (51,67,92,93)	Degree of emotional distress caused by the fatigue Emotional response to fatigue (e.g., mood changes, irritability, weariness) Emotional meaning attributed to fatigue	PFS (51,93) MAF (62,92)
Behavioral: impact of symptoms on Activities of Daily Living (ADLs) (3,61, 62,63,92,93)	Impact of fatigue on ADLs and on activities related to performance Subjective observations may reveal longer time required to complete task Changes in performance (e.g., card sorting, posture, communication style)	Many exist
Physiologic: refers to biologic mechanisms of fatigue (15,43,58,59,87,89,94,95,98)	Anatomic, biochemical, genetic, metabolic, neurophysiologic, neuroendocrinologic	Studies measuring fatigue: (1) loss of force/work-generating capacity; (2) shifts in power spectrum of electromyelogram; (3) muscle slowing (conduction velocity and contractile speed) Other studies: changes in: (1) serum melatonin (99); (2) heart rate and oxygen consumption (100); (3) hematocrit levels (82) (4) temperature (47) Accumulation or depletion of metabolites (101); fluid and electrolyte shifts Noninvasive measurement of phosphate-containing compounds (101)

Numbers in parentheses correspond to studies cited in the References.

33B. Important Measures of Fatigue

Instrument	Description	Psychometric Indices
Unidimensional scales Single-item instrument Visual Analogue Scale (VAS), numeric, Likert-type scales (2)	Measure intensity of subjective fatigue Most appropriate to capture circadian patterns of fatigue requiring repeated measures during a 24-hour period Effective, time-efficient for use in clinical practice	Correlate well with other unidimensional, multiple-item measures of intensity (e.g., Profile of Mood States [POMS], Fatigue-Inertia subscale, Pearson-Byars Fatigue Feeling Tone Checklist [PBFS]) (70,71)
Multiple-item instrument Pearson-Byars Fatigue Feeling Tone Checklist (PBFS) (37)	10-item adjective rating scale Subjects asked to rate whether they feel "same as," "worse than," or "better than" each adjective; adjective is placed on continuum from "1," very peppy, to "10," ready to drop Numbers summed to give total fatigue score (8–20)	Comparable reliability and validity estimates Limitations: colloquialism, patients may have difficulty knowing how to respond to items (93) Published studies using this measure (12,22,44,45,73,76,89)
KRUPP Fatigue Severity Scale (FSS) (74)	9-item, self-report scale, originally developed to measure fatigue in patients with MS or systemic lupus erythematosus (69) Responses indicate degree of agreement with each statement (1 strongly disagree, 7 strongly agree)	Internal consistency, established Correlates well with VAS measures Discriminates between patients and controls, detects clinically predicted changes in fatigue over time Published studies using this measure: (69,86,102,103,104,105)
Mental Fatigue Inventory (MFI) (106)	9-item measure of mental fatigue symptoms (e.g., poor concentration) 5-point Likert scale (0 not at all, 4 very much) Further testing warranted	Reported to have good internal consistency, test–retest reliability and beginning discriminant validity in British patients with CFS, depression, and healthy controls
Multidimensional Fatigue Scales Visual Analogue Scale to Measure Fatigue (VAS-F) Developed by Lee et al. (75)	Measures severity of fatigue 18 items, 2 subscales: energy (5 items), fatigue (13 items) Brief, easy to administer Further testing warranted (factor analysis testing in clinical populations)	Internal consistency (Cronbach's alpha): 0.91–0.96 (fatigue); 0.94–0.96 (energy) Concurrent validity established by Pearson's correlations (VAS-F compared to Stanford Sleepiness Scale [SSS] and the POMS fatigue-inertia and vigor-activity subscales) Reliabilities (patients with myocardial infarction) 0.86 (fatigue), 0.83 (energy) (107)
Fatigue/Stamina Scale (F/ST) Developed by Reeves et al. (108)	25-item measure: fatigue (11 items) and physical stamina (14 items) Likert scale Further testing in clinical populations warranted	Cronbach's alphas: 0.89 (fatigue), 0.87 (stamina) Significant Pearson's correlations: fatigue scale and POMS fatigue/inertia scale = 0.79; stamina scale and POMS vigor/activity scale = 0.62 Stamina significantly and inversely related to fatigue

Instrument	Description	Reliability/Validity
Chalder Fatigue Scale (CHFS) (109)	11-item, self-report measure of mental and physical symptoms of fatigue Items rated on 4-point Likert scale (better than usual to much worse than usual) Further testing warranted	Confirmed 2 factors Cronbach's alpha: 0.89 Face validity established and reasonable discriminant validity in adult (110), pediatric (111), and general practice patients (112)
Fatigue Impact Scale (FIS) Developed by Fisk et al. (60)	40-item self-report measure of the impact of fatigue on function: cognition (10 items), physical (10 items), and psychosocial (20 items) in MS patients Items rated according to degree a fatigue-related problem exits (0 no problem to 4 extreme problem) Maximum score = 160	Grade 8 reading level High internal consistency reliabilities (Cronbach's alpha >0.93) Confirmatory factor analysis and additional testing warranted
Fatigue Symptom Checklist (FSCL) (41-43)	30-item self-report measure of fatigue symptoms (3 factors): (1) decline in motivation or concentration (mental fatigue); (2) general feelings of fatigue; (3) specific feelings of fatigue incongruity (e.g., stiff shoulders) Feelings (2) (e.g., want to lie down) more frequent than (1) or (3) (27,39,45,51,71) Symptoms may vary by disease or cause (e.g., thirst with patients having cancer or MS) (3,45,47,71) The more numerous the) symptoms of fatigue, the higher the fatigue intensity (41,71) Dichotomous scaling (yes-no) Modifications (MFSCL): Modified scaling has been developed (rating absence and intensity of each symptom on 1 to 4 Likert or 1 to 5 scale) (51,59,70) Items have been tailored to specific populations (46,47)	Reliability and validity estimates not always reported (must be recalculated with each study sample) Principal component analysis on modified FSCL (MFSC) in studies of pregnant and postpartum women: 6 factors extracted (subjective weariness, decreased concentration, psychologic, physical, head and neck, and physical/generalized) (59) Published studies using FSCL: (4,15,27,41-45,47,51,59,61,71,113)
Piper Fatigue Scale (PFS) (51,93)	41-item measure of 4 dimensions of subjective fatigue (temporal, severity, sensory, affective) plus 3 open-ended items (measuring perceived causes of fatigue, relief measures, and associated symptoms) Available as VAS (0-100 mm) or numeric (0-10) scale Modifications: associated symptom scale; fatigue in caregivers (114); revised for arthritic patients (62,63) Semistructured interview guide to measure subjective fatigue in biotherapy patients (23)	Excellent reliability and validity estimates in patients with cancer (51,61,67,83,93) and in pregnant women (84) Factor analyses in women with breast cancer confirmed 4 dimensions of fatigue and reduced the number of items to 22 (93) Published studies using instrument (51,67,93,114,115)

33B. Important Measures of Fatigue (*cont.*)

Instrument	Description	Psychometric Indices
Multidimensional Assessment of Fatigue Scale (MAF) (62,92)	Revised version of PFS (51) 16-item measuring 4 dimensions of fatigue (severity-2 items, distress-1, degree of interference in ADLs-11, timing-2) Scale tested in patients with rheumatoid arthritis (62,63,92), fibromyalgia (116), matched controls (62) Easy to administer and score	4 factors confirmed by factor analysis Internal consistency: Cronbach's alpha: 0.93 (rheumatoid patients) Pearson's correlations: MAF and POMS subscales of fatigue and vigor were moderate to strong Additional testing warranted
Profile of Fatigue-Related Symptoms (PFRS) (117)	54-item measure of symptoms of Chronic Fatigue Syndrome (CFS) 4 scales: emotional distress, cognitive difficulty, somatic symptoms, fatigue Each item assessed "during the past week" on 7-point rating scale (0 not at all, 6 extremely)	4 factors confirmed by factor analysis Estimates high for convergent validity, test–retest reliability, internal consistency (British subjects with CFS/postviral fatigue syndrome) Further research warranted

Numbers in parentheses correspond to studies cited in the References.

34

Measuring Mobility and Potential for Falls

Ann Marie Spellbring and Judith W. Ryan

Falls are a major cause of morbidity, immobility, and mortality. Although falls occur across the lifespan, research on falls has focused on older adults because both the risk for falling and the potential for negative sequelae increase as an individual ages. This chapter presents an approach in the conceptualization of falls, discusses methodologic issues related to measuring the incidence of falls in various settings, reviews specific measures used in falls and mobility research that identify risk factors for falls and characteristics of those who fall, and summarizes the future directions of falls and mobility research. Those who fall are referred to in this chapter as fallers.

Falls

Conceptualization

Falls among older adults are usually multifactorial in nature. They generally are a result of the underlying physiologic changes associated with aging, physical illnesses, effects of medications, social factors, and/or environmental hazards. Falls may be precipitated by any of these individually or, more often, in interaction with each other.[1] A significant contribution to the conceptualization of falls has been presented by Hogue.[2] She views falls as occurring when the performance level of an individual is inadequate for the demands of environmental tasks. This conceptualization is supported by the adaptation and aging model proposed by Lawton and Nahemow,[3] in which personal competence (a person's capacities) and environmental press (the demands of the environment that activate behavior) interact to stimulate behavior. For example, when an individual is frail (less competent), it takes very little, or perhaps no stimulation, from the environment to initiate a fall. On the other hand, if the environment is particularly demanding, such as sleet and ice on the steps, highly competent individuals will have difficulty and may be unable to prevent a fall.

Falls also can be viewed in the epidemiologic model,[4] in which the pathogenesis of a fall involves the host, environment, and inciting agent. Once the interactions that have caused a fall are identified, countermeasures to prevent falls can be implemented.

Definition

The lack of a standard definition of falls in falls research has contributed to the inability easily to compare and contrast studies. The researcher must be particularly attentive to what is or is not included in the fall definition for each study. Most definitions of a fall include the elements of a change in body position and the lack of intention to do so,[5] as well as a loss of balance that cannot be corrected.[6] In a consensus report of the Kellogg International Work Group on the Prevention of Falls by the Elderly[1] and supported by the report of the Institute of Medicine's Committee on Health Promotion and Disability Prevention for the Second Fifty Years,[7,p7] the following standardized definition of a fall has been proposed: "A fall is an event that results in a person coming to rest inadvertently on the ground or other lower level and other than as a consequence of the following: sustaining a violent blow, loss of consciousness, sudden onset of paralysis, as in a stroke, or an epileptic seizure." Although this definition has several exclusions, it is not uncommon for researchers to include subjects with drop attacks,[4] seizures, or syncopal episodes[8] as a primary focus in their research on falls.

Falls Classification Systems

In addition to the difficulties posed by the lack of a standard definition of falls, it also is important for the researcher to explore specifically the various causes of the fall. Some authors refer to the intrinsic causes (pertaining to the individual),[9] but others have reported on the situational or extrinsic causes of falls (pertaining to the environment).[10] Table 34.1 describes major classification systems developed by Isaacs,[11] Wild, Nayak,

Table 34.1 Falls Classification Systems

Author/Theory	Characteristics
Isaacs (11): The categorization of falls is based on activity in which person is engaged at time of fall	Imposed (contact with major external hazard) Judgmental error (occurring during hurried activity) Perceptual error (contact with an object that could have been avoided) Posture change (moving from lying, sitting, standing, with no external hazard) Walking (occurring during normal, unhurried walking with no external hazard) Standing (occurring while standing quietly)
Wild, Nayak, and Isaacs (12): Falls are the result of uncorrected displacement of the body from its support base	Displacements either initiated (created by the subject himself) or imposed (unexpected events) Displacements have two magnitudes, either ordinary or extraordinary
Morse, Tylko, and Dixon (13): Identified three types of falls based on study of 200 hospitalized patients	Physiologic, anticipated: most prevalent (78%), involving patients who were disoriented, had poor balance, impaired gait, or used walking aids Physiologic, unanticipated: occurring in oriented patients who experienced drug reactions, dizziness, drop attacks, or fainted Accidental: occurred in oriented patients who tripped, slipped, or rolled out of bed
Lach et al. (14): St Louis Oasis Study Fall Classification System (based on 3-year, prospective study of 1358 community elders)	Extrinsic falls: includes falls due to slips, trips, and externally induced displacements, such as collision Intrinsic falls: due to impaired balance or mobility, sensory, or cognitive impairment or impaired consciousness Nonbipedal falls: person not standing on two feet, may have fallen out of bed or chair, or had failure of assistive device Nonclassifiable falls: person unclear about what happened, no data

Numbers in parentheses correspond to studies cited in the References.

and Isaacs,[12] Morse, Tylko and Dixon,[13] and Lach et al.[14] The description of the fall event and its consequences are other areas of measurement.[15]

Methodologic Issues

In addition to the lack of standard definition for falls and the multifactorial causes of falls, Cumming, Kelsey, and Nevitt[16] have addressed several methodologic challenges in the study of falls. One such issue regarding falls in community settings is the reliance on self-report information as most of these types of falls are unwitnessed and the information about a fall most often must come from the person who fell. Falls are a fairly common event, and if no serious injury occurs, the person may forget the event and its details. Cummings, Nevitt, and Kidd[17] report that 13% to 32% of the people who fell did not report their fall when they were interviewed 3 to 12 months later about falls that had occurred during that study period.

Falls research has been conducted in a variety of settings, which has made comparisons among studies somewhat difficult. The three major arenas for falls research are acute care hospitals, long-term care settings, and the community. Characteristics of the samples differ, as would be expected, but the methodologies used often are setting-specific. In determining risk factors and causes of falls, incident reports and chart review can be used readily in the institutional settings, but more dependence on recall or memory is required in the home environment. It has been proposed that falls among healthy adult populations in the community are caused by situational and environmental threats, whereas falls in the more frail institutionalized populations often are more attributable to individual characteristics.[7]

It is important to decide the unit of measure of the research. Some studies have identified the number of individuals who have fallen, whereas others have identified the rate of falls as the outcome measure. Much of the research on falls has been done to describe the characteristics of the faller by comparing risk factor prevalence in those who fell and those who did not fall. An alternative approach is to study the rate of falls in those with specific risk factors and those without.

Determining a fall rate also is of methodologic concern. No commonly established standard for reporting fall rates has been adopted. Researchers present fall rates differently, often not indicating how the rate was determined, and this can lead to misleading conclusions or comparative problems for the reviewer. Sometimes fall rate is offered simply as a percentage of falls per number of subjects. Morse and Morse[18] have recommended that the following formula be used as the standard for determining fall rate:

$$\frac{\text{Number of Falls}}{\text{Number of Patient Days}} \times 1,000 = \text{Patient Fall Rate}$$

The number of patient days is determined by the daily total occupancy of the units for each day of the study. This formula yields a higher rate when the same subjects fall repeatedly as it uses the number of falls, not the number of fallers.[19]

Instruments to Measure Falls

Fall research has focused on identifying the characteristics of fallers and attempting to predict risk for falls. These studies have been done retrospectively and/or prospectively with various methods of data collection, such as incident reports, patient interviews, medical records, and observations. Instruments have been developed to address either the intrinsic or extrinsic factors that put a person at risk to fall.

Intrinsic Risks for Falls

Intrinsic risks pertain to those characteristics that are unique to the individual that might put him or her at risk for falls, such as changes in cognition, gait and balance, or vision. Table 34.2[20-47] includes selected intrinsic risk factors for falls as identified in various studies across clinical settings.[7]

The clinical nursing literature has been especially prolific on establishing high-risk profiles[48-50] for those at risk for falling. These risk profiles have been especially helpful in developing appropriate interventions to modify risks. Falls account for the majority of all incident reports in hospitalized patients. In an extensive review of falls, Whedon and Shedd[51] state that research on falls among hospitalized patients can be divided into two major categories, those studies that develop a risk profile of a faller and those that evaluate an intervention to decrease the fall rate. The profiles of those at risk to falling have varied from study to study, and few of these profiles have been tested for reliability and validity.

Spellbring's Assessment for High Risk to Fall
Instrument

Spellbring[52] developed a 30-item Assessment for High Risk to Fall Instrument to be used by nurses to identify elderly patients at risk of falling in the acute care setting. Categories addressed include: mental and functional health status, history of previous falls, vision, hearing and communication impairment, sleep patterns, mood fluctuation, hypotension, medications, and observation of gait and balance ability.

Interrater reliability was determined by the percentage of agreement between registered nurses administering the instrument simultaneously. Thirty elderly medical-surgical patients were assessed within 24 hours of admission to the nursing unit. The mean time for completing the instrument was 17 minutes. Reliability ranged from 0.76 to 1.00 per item, with an overall reliability of 0.90 for total categories.

Morse Fall Scale

Morse, Morse, and Tylko[53] developed a 6-item index, The Morse Fall Scale, to identify fall risk among 200 hospitalized patients. The scale consists of (1) history of falling; (2) secondary diagnosis; (3) ambulatory aids; (4) use of intravenous therapy; (5) gait; and (6) mental status. The six items are weighted with a score range of 0 to 25. A score of 16 or above identifies the individual as a high-risk fall candidate. However, the authors caution that the final selection of a high-risk-to-fall score should be a matter of judgment, not a predetermined summed score.

Interrater reliability was established with 21 nurses rating six patients for an r of 0.96. The reliability estimates were only for five of the six items ($r = 0.82–1.0$). Mental status was omitted because of difficulty in obtaining consent for confused patients. A test for internal consistency revealed weak inter-item correlations with a coefficient alpha of 0.16 indicating that the items are independent, as might be expected in a short instrument for a multifaceted problem such as falls.

Validation of the scale was established by randomly splitting the cases, obtaining scale weights from 50% of the cases and retesting the discriminatory power on the remaining 50%. The percent of patients correctly classified was 79% and not significantly different from the original. Validity also was tested prospectively on 2,689 patients in three different clinical settings (acute care hospital, long-term care, and rehabilitation hospital) with increasingly higher scores obtained for patients from acute care to long-term care to rehabilitation settings.

Table 34.2 Selected Intrinsic Risk Factors for Falls

Type of Risk Factor	Measure (Studies)	Strength of Evidence*
Demographic	Age >80 Men (20-23)	Strong
	Female (22-24)	Inconsistent
General health and functioning	ADL, IADL, mobility impairment (5,22,23,25-29)	Strong
	Reduced physical activity/Exercise (21-23)	Weak
	Past history of falls (5,21-23,30,31)	Strong
Medical conditions	Arthritis (5,22-24,28,32,33)	Moderate
	Stroke (21,22,27)	Moderate
	Parkinson's disease (21,22,33)	Strong
	Dementia (32-35)	Strong
	Incontinence (5,22,23,27,28,30)	Strong
	Postural hypotension (5,21-23,25,28)	Inconsistent
Musculoskeletal and neuromuscular	Reduced knee, hip, or ankle strength (5,21,22,28,32,36)	Strong
	Reduced grip strength (21,22,24,37)	Strong
	Foot problems (8,22-24,26)	Inconsistent
	Impaired knee/plantar reflexes (22,26,28)	Weak
	Slowed reaction time (22,26,38)	Weak
Sensory	Impaired visual acuity (5,8,21-23,25,28,39)	Strong
	Reduced depth perception (22)	Weak
	Visual perceptual error (21,40,41)	Weak
	Impaired lower extremity sensory function (5,22,23,28,32,39,42)	Inconsistent
Other neurologic signs	Frontal cortex/release (5,28)	Weak
	Cerebellar, pyramidal, extrapyramidal (22,28)	Weak
Gait, balance, physical performance	Gait "abnormalities" (5,22,23,28,31,43)	Strong
	Reduced walking speed (21,22,43,44)	Strong
	Postural sway (21,22,39,40)	Moderate
	Impaired dynamic balance (5,22,23,28,31,40,45)	Strong
	Impaired tandem gait, one leg (22,23,32)	Moderate
	Difficulty arising from chair (21-23,36)	Strong
Cognitive, psychologic	Reduced mental status test score (13,22,23,25,28,30,32,34,46)	Strong
	Depression (5,13,22,23,25,33)	Strong
Medication use	Sedatives, hypnotics, anxiolytics (5,12,22-30,33,42,46,47)	Strong
	Antidepressants (22,24,25,27,47)	Moderate
	Cardiovascular (5,22-25,28,33,46)	Inconsistent
	National Health Interview Survey Supplement on Aging, 1984 (21,33)	Weak
	Number of medications (5,21,24,32,33)	Strong

ADL = Activities of Daily Living; IADL = Instrumental Daily Living.

Numbers in parentheses correspond to studies cited in the References.

*Strong, association in multiple studies, at least two of which are prospective; moderate, association in multiple studies, only one of which is prospective (some studies are negative); weak, association in only a few studies, none of which are prospective (some studies are negative); inconsistent, generally conflicting and inconsistent findings in multiple studies.

Reprinted with permission from Berg, R.L., & Cassells, J.S. (Eds.), *The second fifty years: Promoting health and preventing disability.* Washington, DC: National Academy Press, 1990, pp. 270-271, 284-290. Courtesy of National Academy Press.

Schmid's Fall Risk Assessment Tool

Schmid[54] developed a fall risk assessment tool for hospitalized patients. It included assessment of mobility, mentation, elimination, fall history, and current medications. Content validity was verified by a task force of nurses who concurred on item selection and analysis. Criterion-related validity was established by examining risk scores on 334 patients who fell during a 5-week period. Construct validity was established by comparing patients assessed "at risk" for falls with patients assessed "not at risk." Test–retest reliability was established by a nurse assessing fall risk on admission and repeating the measure 4 hours later. Initially, weights were assigned to significant risk areas. A remanipulation of the data with different weightings of the fall risk tool increased test–retest reliability to 100%. Interrater reliability was established by comparing the percentage of agreement among the raters who independently administered the risk assessment to the same patient. The authors report an 88% agreement for the total score, but suggest that the tool needs to be tested in other populations. Interrater reliability remains to be determined.

Chenitz Fall Assessment Scale (FAS)

Chenitz, Kussman, and Stone[55] have created the Fall Assessment Scale (FAS) to assess patient fall risk. According to the authors, the FAS is "currently being tested for interrater reliability."[55,p320] The 17-item scale includes risk areas for falls, such as history of falls prior to hospitalization and in the hospital, patient compliance with activity order, and intravenous in place. Reliability has yet to be determined.

Heslin's Fall Prevention Assessment Form

Heslin and colleagues[56] conducted a retrospective review of incident reports and selected charts on 855 fall events that occurred in acute, long-term, and residential health-care settings. Factors identified that contributed to falls were: age, location of the fall, confusion, mobility deficits, generalized weakness, assistive devices, safety devices, medical diagnosis, and previous falls. An assessment was developed from the risk-factor analysis, with eight factors determined to be highly predictive for falls. The points allotted to each factor contribute to an overall risk score, from which three levels of risk were assigned (possible risk, potential fall risk, and actual fall risk). Policies and procedures were written to implement the Risk Assessment Form and interventions based on the level of risk. The authors note that the specificity of risk factors was based on the type of facility and stress the importance of targeting both intrinsic and extrinsic factors for successful fall prevention. No reliability or validity assessment of the instrument is presented.

Extrinsic Risks for Falls

The assessment of environmental hazards, or extrinsic factors, as part of a fall risk profile is well established in both the literature and clinical practice. Studies have indicated that 18% to 50% of falls are due to environmental conditions.[8,12,46,57] Common hazards cited include: scatter rugs, loose carpets, slippery surfaces, and raised door thresholds;[57] low beds and toilet seats;[58] inadequate lighting;[12] cracked sidewalks and unsafe stairs;[59] raised bed rails;[60] wheelchairs, walkers, and hemicanes.[61]

Tinetti and Speechley[62] identify three areas of general agreement when environmental factors are explored: (1) the more frail a person is, the more susceptible he/she is to even minor hazards; (2) an individual's specific disabilities are more likely to predict the amount of hazard a particular environmental condition presents; and (3) a person's experience with a specific environmental condition reduces the risk from it. Although these are commonly accepted areas among researchers on falls, controlled research studies are lacking that investigate the role of environmental hazards in falls. Most of the instruments used to measure environmental hazards are checklists constructed from the researcher's clinical experience and have not been standardized. In addition, the checklists are generally more qualitative than quantitative (e.g., "Are stairways adequately lighted?"). One such instrument, constructed by Tideiksaar,[4] is an environmental assessment useful in both the home and institutional settings.

It is rare that the environment is directly assessed by researchers, but rather subjects have described what they felt may have contributed to their falls. Conclusions about environment-related falls will remain uncertain until studies that include the environment of nonfallers as well are conducted.

The Home Environment Survey

Rodriquez[63] and colleagues have developed a home environment hazards assessment instrument for their case-controlled study of falls in the elderly. They identified six environmental areas of importance: (1) floors: surface and tripping hazards; (2) furniture: use for sitting and walking support; (3) lighting: adequacy and ease of use; (4) bathroom: grab bars and slip-resistant surfaces; (5) storage areas: height; and (6) stairway conditions. The survey uses both direct observation of the home and interview of subjects to assess the environment. This instrument was assessed for face, predictive, and concurrent validity, and internal consistency and repeatability. Although the study is not published, the authors state that the initial results from the validation study indicated that both the reliability and validity of the instrument are effective.

Near Falls

A relatively new area of investigation in research on falls is the study of near falls or events that are characterized by an unintentional loss of balance in which the person starts to go down but no fall occurs. The study of this phenomenon is challenged by subjects who don't have a clear definition of the term and the limited recall of persons who experience these events but, without a fall, have no real marker for remembering. Ryan, Dinkel, and Petrucci[64] created a 5-item measure to train elderly subjects in defining the term *near falls*. It includes common scenarios in which older persons may find themselves and requires them to distinguish between near falls, falls, and neither. Near falls may be an early predictor of high risk to fall, or they may indicate a person who is more fit and hence able to regain balance and prevent the fall.[65]

Measures of Mobility

Mobility has been defined[66] as the "ability of a person to move purposefully within the environment." This is dependent on the integration of multiple physical, cognitive, and psychologic characteristics. For the most part, the literature has been conclusive regarding the extent to which impaired mobility related to gait and balance disturbances has contributed to falls. Morse[13] indicates that changes in gait and balance that occur with advancing age are more reliable indicators of liability to fall than chronological age. Physical performance measures of gait and balance are gaining increased attention in the literature. Specific performance tests for mobility have been able to identify fall risk not apparent in routine physical examinations.[67] The following measures are used to assess gait and balance capabilities and can serve as screening tools for those at risk for falls.

Mobility Skills Scale

Hogue, Studenski, and Duncan[68] have developed a useful tool, the Mobility Skills Scale, to identify persons at high risk for falls because of physical mobility impairments. The advantage of the tool is that it can be used in a variety of settings by health-care professionals while they are routinely caring for patients.

The Mobility Skills Scale contains seven items and takes 5 to 10 minutes to administer. The physical mobility tasks include: (1) sitting balance; (2) sitting reach; (3) bending down to pick up a pencil; (4) rising from a chair; (5) standing reach; (6) gait without an assistive device; and (7) descending stairs. Scale scores range from 0 to 7, reflecting the number of items that can be performed independently. The Mobility Skills Scale was tested for reliability and validity with 69 homecare patients with a mean age of 72 in the participants' own home. The interrater reliability for the individual items on this scale was acceptable (kappa = 0.79 to 0.92). The scale discriminated nonfallers from one-time fallers and repeat fallers (Kruskal-Wallis' Analysis of Variance [ANOVA], $H \cong x^2(2) = 12.2, p = 0.005$). This instrument has a logical increase in difficulty for performing each subsequent task. This was confirmed with a coefficient of scaling reproducibility of 0.915 demonstrating that subjects who could perform the most difficult items on the scale could perform the easier tasks. The author suggests that the Mobility Skills Scale may be useful to screen for fall risk and detect mobility assistance needs.

Tinetti's Performance-Oriented Assessment of Balance and Gait

Tinetti and colleagues have developed a comprehensive 22-item assessment for mobility that reproduces the position changes, balance, and gait maneuvers required during daily activities.[36,69] Sample items of position change include: sitting down and rising from a chair. Balance measures include: immediate standing balance; one leg standing balance; reaching up; and bending over. Gait items include stability on turning and step length and height. Interrater and test–retest reliability for those items that were timed are all over 0.95. The kappa statistic for individual maneuvers which were not timed are all over 0.50.[69]

Dayhoff's Postural Control Scale

Dayhoff[70] has proposed a briefer and more clinically useful version of the Tinetti scales for hospitalized patients. Tinetti's 22-item assessment was reduced to 14 items related to three factors in postural control: automatic balance, voluntary control of balance, and gait. Subjects are scored on a 4-point scale according to their level of performance on each item. Examples of skills assessed include: sitting balance, rising from chair, and step length.

Criterion-related validity of self-report of a fall or no fall over 3 months prior to measurement reduced the 14 items to 6. Interrater reliability for each of the six items on the scale, using an ANOVA model for estimating generalizability coefficients, was acceptable with a range of 0.46 to 0.98 (mean 0.80). Internal reliability (coefficient alpha) was 0.88 for the sample.

Gait Abnormality Rating Scale (GARS)

The Gait Abnormality Rating Scale (GARS)[71] is a 16-item scale that was developed to assess stride length and walking speed among 49 nursing home residents, 27 of whom had a history of falls, and 22 controls. The subjects' gait was rated using 16 variables scored on a 4-point scale (normal to severely impaired). The scoring was based on ranking of the extent of dysfunction of a particular variable compared to the normal. Variables included: staggering, hip range of motion, shoulder elevation, and foot contact.

Interrater reliability for the qualitative gait assessment items using Spearman rank-order correlations ranged from 0.475 to 0.903 with 0.954 for the total scale. The Wilcoxon signed ranks test, used to compare ratings of items on the GARS, consistently ranked fallers as having more impairment than the controls. Validity also was assessed comparing scores on the GARS to stride length with Pearson's correlations of 0.82 for fallers and 0.79 for controls.

The Get-Up and Go Test

A functional mobility assessment, referred to as the "Get-Up and Go" test, was developed by Mathias, Nyak, and Isaacs.[72] It requires that the person being assessed rise from a straight chair, walk 10 feet, turn around, return to the chair, and sit down. Subjects are rated on a 5-point scale from normal to severely abnormal. Subjects with a score of 3 or above were considered at risk of falling.

The study was conducted on 40 elderly patients with a range of balance disturbances. Tests were recorded on videotapes and reviewed and scored by groups of observers from different medical backgrounds. The Kendall coefficient of concordance indicated agreement of ratings among physiotherapists at 0.85 and among senior doctors at 0.69. The same patients also were given laboratory tests of sway and balance. The mean scores were compared using Pearson's correlation coefficient with a mean sway path recorded from the Kistler force platform ($r = 0.50$) and gait speed ($r = 0.75$). Scores on the "Get-Up and Go" test correlated significantly not only with the total mean sway path and gait speed but also with several other gait parameters, which led the authors to conclude that the test is a satisfactory clinical measure of balance in elderly individuals. Podsiadlo and Richardson[73] evaluated a modified, timed version of this test and indicate that a timed score is reliable for interrater and test–retest reliability. Using time as a variable provides a sensitive dimension to determining small increments of change that may have clinical significance, but go unnoticed otherwise.

Roberts and Mueller Balance Scale

The Roberts and Mueller balance scale[74] was designed to reflect the two factors related to balance, base of support and visual cues, and consists of eight stances: bipedal stance with eyes open and closed, monopedal stance with eyes open and closed, and these same four stances repeated on a beam. The time, in seconds, that subjects were able to maintain each of the stances up to a maximum of 30 seconds was summed for a total score which ranged from 0 to 240. Higher scores indicate greater balance.

Validity and reliability were established with 61 persons aged 65 and above residing in the community. Construct validity was established by a factor analysis and four factors were extracted: monopedal factor, bipedal factor without visual cues, visual factor, and beam factor. Standardized alpha coefficients for the four factor scores ranged from 0.60 to 0.76 with an overall coefficient of 0.82.[75] Interrater reliability was 0.99.[76]

Roberts Balance Perception Questionnaire

Roberts[74,77] also developed a questionnaire to measure older adults' perception of balance. Subjects rated their perception of balance stability on a Likert scale for standing, walking, and arising from a chair. The score is the sum of the ratings (higher ratings indicate better stability perceptions). The questionnaire has a standardized alpha of 0.78. Subjects with depression and impaired cognition were determined to have inaccurate perceptions of their balance when compared to those participating in timed observational methods.

Summary

The research and literature on falls in the elderly clearly indicate that causes of falling and injuries from falls are multifactorial and should be considered from a biologic, psychologic, and sociologic perspective.[4,7,62,78] Researchers have identified the individual and environmental risks for falling, and because studies most often have focused on risks, there is little scientific evidence of the effectiveness of interventions to prevent falls.[2] Future research endeavors will focus on intervention studies to prevent falls and fall-related injuries.

A recent initiative of randomized controlled trials to identify interventions to reduce frailty and falls in the elderly has been sponsored by the National Institute on Aging and the National Center for Nursing Research (#U01-AG-09124).[79] This multisite cooperative study focusing on frailty and injuries among the elderly population is called FICSIT (Frailty and Injuries: Cooperative Studies of Intervention Techniques). Eight sites nationally were selected to participate in the FICSIT project and used a variety of clinical protocols to examine innovative interventions. Falls, near falls, and fall-related injury data were examined throughout the 3-year study.

The clinical determination of the person who is at risk to fall is an elusive phenomenon. Research in this area is important to the safety and well-being of the older adult. To measure the risk for falls and mobility successfully, reliable and valid instruments still need to be developed. These instruments should address both intrinsic and extrinsic risk factors for falls, impairment of mobility, and focus on prevention.

Exemplar Studies

Schmid, N.A. Reducing patient falls: A research-based comprehensive fall prevention program. *Milit Med*, 1990, *155*(5):202.

This study exemplifies the measurement of the many variables related to risk for falling. The design consisted of two phases. Phase one was a retrospective study of fallers and nonfallers in the hospital setting that differentiated characteristics that placed patients at risk to fall. A tool was developed with weighted fall risk factors and tested in phase two. Reliability and validity testing was rigorously addressed, and the measure was sturdy in predicting fall risk. Additional strengths of this measure are that it includes the prominent risk factors for falls, has attributes that make it easily usable by clinicians, and can serve as a basis for a fall-prevention program.

Mathias, S., Nayak, U.S.L., & Isaacs, B. Balance in elderly patients: The "Get-up and Go" test. *Arch Phys Med Rehab*, 1986, *67*:387.

This study exemplifies the measurement of functional mobility in elderly persons as it relates to falls. Balance is assessed on a 5-point scale from normal to severely abnormal. Reliability and validity testing was done with 40 patients with a variety of balance disturbances. Acceptable reliability was established with videotapes of subjects' performance evaluated by groups of observers from different medical backgrounds. Validity was acceptable when scores were compared with laboratory gait and balance devices. These techniques are explained in detail. It is a satisfactory proxy measure of balance and gait that can be used in any clinical setting without complex apparatus.

References

1. Gibson, M.J., Andres, R.O., Isaacs, B., et al. The prevention of falls in later life. *Danish Med Bull*, 1987, *34*(4):1-10.
2. Hogue, C.C. Managing falls: The current bases for practice. In S.G. Funk, E.M. Tornquist, M.T. Champagne, & R.A. Weise (Eds.), *Key aspects of elder care: Managing falls, incontinence and cognitive impairment.* New York: Springer, 1992, p. 41.
3. Lawton, M.P., & Nahemow, L. Ecology and the aging process. In C. Eisdorfer & M.P. Lawton (Eds.), *The psychology of adult development and aging.* Washington, DC: American Psychological Association, 1973, p. 619.
4. Tideiksaar, R. *Falling in old age: Its prevention and treatment.* New York: Springer, 1989.
5. Tinetti, M.E., Williams, T.F., & Mayewski, R. Fall risk index for elderly patients based on number of chronic disabilities. *Am J Med*, 1986, *80*(3):429-434.
6. Stone, J.T., & Chenitz, W.C. The problem of falls. In W.C. Chenitz, J.T. Stone, & S.A. Salisbury (Eds.), *Clinical gerontological nursing: A guide to advanced practice.* Philadelphia: Saunders, 1991, p. 291.

7. Berg, R.L., & Cassells, J.S. (Eds.). *The second fifty years: Promoting health and preventing disability.* Washington, D.C.: National Academy Press, 1990.

8. Perry, B.C. Falls among the elderly living in high rise apartments. *J Fam Pract,* 1982, *14*(6):1069-1073.

9. Nickens, H. Intrinsic factors in falling among the elderly. *Arch Int Med,* 1985, *14*(6):1089-1093.

10. Parsons, M.T., & Levy, J. Nursing process in injury prevention. *J Gerontol Nur,* 1987, *13*(7):36-40.

11. Isaacs, B. Are falls a manifestation of brain failure? *Age Ageing,* 1978, 7(suppl):97-111.

12. Wild, D., Nayak, U.S.L., & Isaacs, B. Description, classification and prevention of falls in old people at home. *Rheumatol Rehab,* 1981, *20*(3):153-159.

13. Morse, J.M., Tylko, S.J., & Dixon, H.A. Characteristics of the fall-prone patient. *Gerontologist,* 1987, *27*(4):516-522.

14. Lach, H.W., Reed, A.T., Arfken, C.L., et al. Falls in the elderly: Reliability of a classification system. *J Am Geriatr Soc,* 1991, *39*(2):197-202.

15. Nevitt, M.C. Ascertainment and description of falls among older persons by self-report. In R. Weindruch, E.C. Hadley, & M.G. Ory (Eds.), *Reducing frailty and falls in older persons.* Springfield, IL: Charles C. Thomas, 1991, p. 476.

16. Cumming, R.G., Kelsey, J.L., & Nevitt, M.C. Methodologic issues in the study of frequent and recurrent health problems: Falls in the elderly. *Ann Epidemiol,* 1990, *1*(1):49-56.

17. Cummings, S.R., Nevitt, M.C., & Kidd, S. Forgetting falls: The limited accuracy of recall of falls in the elderly. *J Am Geriatr Soc,* 1988, *36*(7):613-616.

18. Morse, J.M., & Morse, R.M. Calculating fall rates: Methodological issues. *Qual Rev Bull,* 1988, *14*(12):369-374.

19. Morse, J.M. The patient who falls and falls again. *J Gerontol Nurs,* 1985, *11*(11):15-19.

20. Beers, M., Avorn, J., Soumerai, S.B., et al. Psychoactive medication use in intermediate-care facility residents. *JAMA,* 1988, *260*:3016-3019.

21. Campbell, A., Borrie, M.J., & Spears, G.F. Risk factors for falls in a community-based prospective study of people 70 years and older. *J Gerontol,* 1989, *44*(4):112-117.

22. Nevitt, M.C., Cummings, S.R., Kidd, S., & Black, D. Risk factors for recurrent nonsyncopal falls: A prospective study. *JAMA,* 1989, *261*(18):2663-2667.

23. Tinetti, M.E., Speechley, M., & Ginter, S.F. Risk factors for falls among elderly persons living in the community. *N Engl J Med,* 1988, *319*(26):1701-1709.

24. Blake, A.J., Morgan, K., Bendall, M.J., et al. Falls by elderly people at home: Prevalence and associated factors. *Age Ageing,* 1988, *17*:365-369.

25. Campbell, A., Reinken, J., Allan, B., et al. Falls in old age: A study of frequency and related clinical factors. *Age Ageing,* 1981, *10*:264-269.

26. Gabell, A., Simons, M.A., & Nayak, U.S.L. Falls in the healthy elderly: Predisposing causes. *Ergonomics,* 1985, *28*(7):965-970.

27. Mayo, N.E., Korner-Bitensky, N., Becker, R., & Georges, P. Predicting falls among patients in a rehabilitation hospital. *Arch Phys Med Rehab,* 1989, *68*(3):139-143.

28. Robbins, A.S., Rubenstein, L.Z., Josephson, K.R., et al. Predictors of falls among elderly people: Results of two population-based studies. *Arch Int Med,* 1989, *194*:1628-1632.

29. Wickham, C., Cooper, C., Margetts, B.M., & Barker, D.J.P. Muscle strength, activity housing and the risk of falls in elderly people. *Age Ageing,* 1989, *18*:47-51.

30. Janken, J.K., Reynolds, B.A., & Swiech, K. Patient falls in the acute care setting: Identifying risk factors. *Nurs Res,* 1986, *35*(4):215-219.

31. Wild, D., Nayak, U., & Isaacs, B. How dangerous are falls in old people at home? *Br Med J,* 1981, *282*:266-268.

32. Buchner, D.M., & Larson, E.B. Falls and fractures in patients with Alzheimer's type dementia. *JAMA,* 1987, *257*(11):1492-1497.

33. Granek, E., Baker, S.P., Abbey, H., et al. Medications and diagnoses in relation to falls in a long-term care facility. *J Am Geriatr Soc,* 1987, *35*:503-508.

34. Buchner, D.M., & Larson, E.B. Transfer bias and the association of cognitive impairment with falls. *J Gen Int Med,* 1988, *3*:254-260.

35. Morris, J. C., Rubin, E.H., Morris, E.J., & Mandel, S.A. Senile dementia of the Alzheimer's type: An important risk factor for serious falls. *J Gerontol,* 1987, *42*:412-418.

36. Tinetti, M.E. Performance-oriented assessment of mobility problems in the elderly. *J Am Geriatr Soc,* 1986, *34*(2):119-124.

37. Whipple, R.H., Wolfson, L.I., & Amerman, P.M. The relationship of knee and ankle weakness to falls in nursing home residents: An isokinetic study. *J Am Geriatr Soc,* 1987, *35*:13-17.

38. Adelsberg, S., Pitman, M., & Alexander, H. Lower extremity factures: Relationship to reaction time and coordination time. *Arch Phys Med Rehab,* 1970, *70*:737-741.

39. Brocklehurst, J., Robertson, D., & Groom, J. Clinical correlates of sway in old age. *Age Ageing,* 1982, *11*:1-9.

40. Ring, C., Nayak, U.S.L., & Isaacs, B. Balance function in elderly people who have and who have not fallen. *Arch Phys Med Rehab,* 1988, *69*:261-264.

41. Tobis, J.S, & Reinsch, S. Postural instability in the elderly: Contributing factors and suggestions for rehabilitation. *Crit Rev Phys Rehab Med,* 1989, *1*(2):59-64.

42. Sorock, G.S., & Shimkin, E.E. Benzodiazepine sedatives and the risk of falling in a community-dwelling elderly cohort. *Arch Int Med,* 1988, *148*:2411-2417.

43. Guimaraes, R.M., & Isaacs, B. Characteristics of the gait in old people who fall. *Int Rehab Med,* 1980, *2*:177-183.

44. Imms, F., & Edholm, O. Studies of gait and mobility in the elderly. *Age Ageing,* 1981, *10*:147-151.

45. Wolfson, L.I., Whipple, R., & Amerman, P. Stressing the postural response: A quantitative method for resting balance. *J Am Geriatr Soc,* 1986, *335*:845-846.

46. Prudham, D., & Evans, J. Factors associated with falls in the elderly: A community study. *Age Ageing,* 1981, *10*:141-149.

47. Ray, W.A., Griffin, M.R., Schaffner, W., et al. Psychotropic drug use and the risk of hip fracture. *N Engl J Med,* 1987, *316*(7):363-366.

48. Fife, D.D., Solomon, P., & Stanton, M. A risk/fall program: Code Orange for success. *Nurs Manag,* 1984, *15*(11):50-53.

49. Hernandez, M., & Miller, J. How to reduce falls. *Geriatr Nurs*, 1986, *7*(2):97-102.

50. Spellbring, A.M., Gannon, M.E., Kleckner, T., et al. Improving safety for hospitalized elderly. *J Gerontol Nurs*, 1988, *14*(2):31-37.

51. Whedon, M.D., & Shedd, P. Prediction and prevention of patient falls. *IMAGE: J Nurs Scholar*, 1989, *21*(2):108-112.

52. Spellbring, A.M. Assessing elderly patients at high risk for falls: A reliability study. *J Nurs Care Qual*, 1992, *6*(3):30-35.

53. Morse, J.M., Morse, R.M., & Tylko, S. Development of a scale to identify the fall-prone patient. *Can J Aging*, 1989, *8*(4):366-371.

54. Schmid, N.A. Reducing patient falls: A research-based comprehensive fall prevention program. *Milit Med*, 1990, *155*(5):202-207.

55. Chenitz, W.C., Kussman, H.L., & Stone, J.T. Preventing falls. In W.C. Chenitz, J.T. Stone, & S.A. Salisbury (Eds.), *Clinical gerontological nursing: A guide to advanced practice*. Philadelphia: Saunders, 1991, p. 309.

56. Heslin, K., Towers, J., Leckie, C., et al. Managing falls: Identifying population specific risk factors and prevention strategies. In S.G. Funk, E.M. Tornquist, M.T. Champagne, & R.A. Wiese (Eds.), *Key aspects of elder care: Managing falls, incontinence and cognitive impairment*. New York: Springer, 1992, p. 70.

57. Morfitt, J.M. Falls in old people at home: Intrinsic versus environmental factors in causation. *Public Health J (Lond)*, 1983, *97*(2):115-120.

58. Rubenstein, L.Z., Robbins, A.S., Schulman, B.L., et al. Falls and instability in the elderly. *J Am Geriatr Soc*, 1988, *36*(3):266-269.

59. Czaja, S., Hammond, K., & Drury, C. *Accidents and aging: A final report*. Washington, DC: Administration on Aging, 1982.

60. Innes, E.M., & Turman, W.G. Evaluation of patient falls. *Qual Rev Bull*, 1983, *9*(2):30-36.

61. Lund, C., & Sheafor, M.L. Is your patient about to fall? *J Gerontol Nurs*, 1985, *11*(4):37-41.

62. Tinetti, M.E., & Speechley, M. Prevention of falls among the elderly. *N Engl J Med*, 1989, *320*(16):1055-1059.

63. Rodriquez, J.G., Sattin, R.W., Devito, C.A., et al. Developing an environmental hazards assessment instrument for falls among the elderly. In R. Weindruch, E.C. Hadley, & M.G. Ory (Eds.), *Reducing frailty and falls in older persons*. Springfield, IL: Charles C Thomas, 1991, p. 263.

64. Ryan, J.W., Dinkel, J.A., & Petrucci, K. Near falls incidence: A study of older adults in the community. *J Gerontol Nurs*, 1993, *19*(12):23-27.

65. Teno, J., Kiel, D.P., & Mor, V. Multiple stumbles: A risk factor for falls in community-dwelling elderly. *J Am Geriatr Soc*, 1990, *38*(12):1321-1326.

66. Creason, N.S. Mobility: Current bases for practice. In S.G. Funk, E.M. Tournquist, M.T. Champagne, L.A. Copp, & R.A. Wiese (Eds.), *Key aspects of recovery: Improving nutrition, rest and mobility*. New York: Springer, 1990, p. 55.

67. Guralnik, J.M., Branch, L.G., Cummings, S.R., & Curb, J.D. Physical performance measures in aging research. *J Gerontol Med Sci*, 1989, *44*(5):M141-M142.

68. Hogue, C.C., Studenski, S., & Duncan, P. Assessing mobility: The first step in preventing falls. In S.G. Funk, E.M. Tournquist, M.T. Champagne, L.A. Copp, & R.A. Wiese (Eds.), *Key aspects of recovery: Improving nutrition, rest and mobility*. New York: Springer, 1990, p. 275.

69. Tinetti, M.E., Baker, D.I., et al. Yale FICSIT: Risk factor abatement strategy for fall prevention. *J Am Geriatr Soc*, 1993, *41*(3):315-319.

70. Dayhoff, N.E. The postural control scale. In S.G. Funk, E.M. Tournquist, M.T. Champagne, L.A. Copp, & R.A. Wiese (Eds.), *Key aspects of elder care: Managing falls, incontinence, and cognitive impairment*. New York: Springer, 1992, p. 57.

71. Wolfson, L., Whipple, R., Amerman, P., & Tobin, J.N. Gait assessment in the elderly: A gait abnormality rating scale and its relation to falls. *J Gerontol Med Sci*, 1990, *45*(1):M12-M13.

72. Mathias, S., Nayak, U.S.L., & Isaacs, B. Balance in elderly patients: The "Get-up and Go" test. *Arch Phys Med Rehab*, 1986, *67*(6):387-391.

73. Podsiadlo, D., & Richardson, S. The timed "Up & Go": A test of basic functional mobility for frail elderly persons. *J Am Geriatr Soc*, 1991, *39*(2):142-146.

74. Roberts, B.L. Effects of walking on balance among elders. *Nurs Res*, 1989, *38*(3):180-184.

75. Roberts, B.L., & Mueller, M.G. The balance scale: Factor analysis and reliability. *Percept Motor Skills*, 1987, *65*(2):367.

76. Roberts, B.L. & Fitzpatrick, J.J. Improving balance: Therapy of movement. *J Gerontol Nurs*, 1983, *9*(3):151-156.

77. Roberts, B.L., & Wykle, M.L. Pilot study results: Falls among institutionalized elderly. *J Gerontol Nurs*, 1993, *19*(5):13-17.

78. Rubenstein, L.Z., Robbins, A.S., & Josephson, K.R. Falls in the nursing home setting: Causes and preventive approaches. In P.R. Katz, R.L. Kane, & M.D. Mezey (Eds.), *Advances in long-term care*. New York: Springer, 1991, p. 28-32.

79. Ory, M.G., Schechtman, K.B., et al. Frailty and injuries in later life: The FICSIT trials. *J Am Geriatr Soc*, 1993, *41*(3):283-286.

35

Measuring Nausea, Vomiting, and Retching

Verna A. Rhodes and Roxanne W. McDaniel

Although recent advances in pharmacology have improved the ability to prevent or control the symptoms of nausea, vomiting, and retching, they remain a problem for a variety of patients. Severe distress from these symptoms may decrease patients' quality of life, functional health status, and may lead them to discontinue potentially life-saving treatment.[1-3] To use the findings of the increasing number of studies attempting to minimize these symptoms, it is important that the individual symptoms be accurately and appropriately measured.

Postoperative nausea and vomiting continue to occur in 20% to 70% of patients.[4,5] More than 50% of pregnant women may experience such symptoms,[6] which significantly influence their quality of life.[7] Nausea and vomiting continue to be the most disturbing side effects of cancer chemotherapy.[8] Up to 60% of patients report post-chemotherapy nausea, and up to 50% report vomiting.[9-13] Anticipatory nausea and vomiting are problems for approximately 30% of the patients, but the figure has been reported to be as high as 57% among women receiving chemotherapy for breast cancer.[14,15] Radiation therapy patients also may experience the symptoms.[16]

Nausea, vomiting, and retching are separate concepts.[17] However, the interchangeable use of terms to describe them is confusing and diminishes the scientific knowledge base for practice, education, and research. *Nausea* is a subjective and unobservable phenomenon of an unpleasant sensation in the epigastrium and in the back of the throat that may or may not culminate in vomiting; it also is described as feeling "sick at the stomach." Nausea is an autonomic response that may have some objective elements, such as pallor, sweating, feeling cold usually known through self-report because of its intensity.[18-21] *Vomiting* is the forceful expulsion of the contents of the stomach, duodenum, and jejunum through the oral cavity as a result of changes in intrathoracic positive pressure. The vomiting center at the base of the medulla includes the chemoreceptor receptor trigger zone (CTZ) that receives input from multiple peripheral and central afferent sources.[22] *Retching* is the attempt to vomit without expelling any material; it is also called *dry heaves*. The act of retching is regulated by the respiratory center in the brainstem.[23]

The increased attention to nausea and vomiting is demonstrated by the growing number of studies including these symptoms as outcome measures. A review by Penta et al.[24] showed more published research on nausea and vomiting and on the efficacy of antiemetics during 1980–1981 (31 studies) than in the preceding 20 years (26 studies from 1960 to 1979). The past 5 years have witnessed an even more dramatic increase. A Medline search from 1990 to 1994 identified 1,706 articles, including studies related to anesthesia, postoperative status, pregnancy, psychiatric, chemotherapy, radiation therapy, nausea, vomiting, and emesis. As in the early 1980s, most of this work was done by health professionals associated with oncology. There is little doubt that this increased interest results from the high prevalence and severity of the side effects associated with cancer chemotherapy and other cancer treatments. Although oncology health professionals have led this work, researchers in other health-care areas also are examining the impact of nausea and vomiting on their patients.

Chemotherapy produces a variety of direct toxic effects on the body, and nausea and vomiting are among the most troublesome, challenging, and frequent. These problems often occur in anticipation of treatment through conditioned responses. The advent of more aggressive, multidrug, and higher-dose chemotherapy continues to make both direct (postchemotherapy) and anticipatory nausea and vomiting a significant problem. In addition to the psychologic stress caused by chemotherapy-induced nausea and vomiting, patients also may experience nutritional deficits, dehydration, electrolyte imbalance, weakness, and disruption in lifestyle.

Patients who often view the treatment and resulting discomfort as being worse than the disease may be reluctant to continue with repeated courses of treatment.[1-3] Because some patients stop or delay potentially curative treatment, nausea and vomiting could be considered a potentially fatal side effect if the disease is responsive to chemotherapy.[25]

Considering this negative impact, it is appropriate that considerable effort be placed in developing and assessing better pharmacologic and nonpharmacologic methods for controlling chemotherapy-related nausea and vomiting. Unfortunately, improvements in the assessment of nausea and vomiting have not kept pace with new interventions to alleviate the symptoms. Only very recently have investigators begun developing assessment and measurement methods that accurately reflect the range of important considerations for patients and providers.

Selecting an Instrument

Investigators should carefully select an instrument to measure nausea, vomiting, and retching and consider several dilemmas that exist in such measurement. Some of the major issues are:

1. The use of observational assessment versus self-report
2. Identification of specific symptoms and the components to be measured
3. Reliability and validity
4. Clarity, precision, and understandability of wording
5. Format (appearance and readability)
6. The time frame for symptom recall
7. Purpose for which instrument is intended (obstetrics, postoperative, postchemotherapy or anticipatory symptoms)
8. Ease of scoring

Global assessments of nausea, vomiting, and retching may have hindered the development of a scientific database. To obtain an accurate database, it is essential to have information about the individual symptoms. Interventions, both pharmacologic and nonpharmacologic, do not have uniform effects on these individual symptoms. Careful consideration of the issues listed is essential to measure accurately the individual phenomena, to determine symptom patterns, and to make comparisons.

Methods Available

The assessment of nausea and vomiting continues to evolve as an area of clinical research. Researchers and evaluators differentiate the separate symptoms, rather than take a global or synonymous approach. As information increases in this area, new issues arise. Researchers must maintain a balance of obtaining accurate data about the specific symptom without putting an undue burden on the patient or clinical environment. Researchers also must take care not to direct suggestive attention to the symptom. Caution is required to avoid focusing on the incidence of the symptom because of the possibility of associative learning or conditioned responses that can occur in patients experiencing nausea and vomiting related to pregnancy, motion sickness, medications, or other psychologic or physical causes.

Many comprehensive instruments may include one or more of the components of nausea, vomiting, and retching. Some, such as the Adapted Symptom Distress Scale, measure multiple components.[26] Others measure either a single component, such as the Symptom Distress Scale,[27] or are global measures of the concepts. In this chapter only instruments specifically assessing these symptoms will be addressed. Appendix 35A provides a summary comparison of these instruments.

Counting Episodes of Nausea and Vomiting

The measurement of vomiting has been done simply by counting the number of emetic episodes and expressing them as an absolute number or by obtaining an average mean score per time unit (e.g., x/hour) for a defined observation period.[28,29] This approach accurately reflects vomiting and retching, but is unable accurately to reflect nausea. The patients also must be able to provide accurate self-reports or must be continuously observed when this method is used.

Nausea and vomiting have been assessed by grouping the number of emetic and nausea episodes according to predefined criteria and then labeling the degree of severity of the side effect.[30] However, it is important to separate measures of nausea and vomiting because they are distinct symptoms. Nausea is a subjective experience that no objective method can measure. As it is not an observable phenomenon, nausea measurement must rely on patient self-report.

Duke Descriptive Scale (DDS)

The Duke Descriptive Scale (DDS) grades nausea and vomiting from I to IV as follows, taking into account intensity, severity, and impairment in patient activity for a 24-hour period:[31,32]

A. Nausea grades I to IV
   I: None
   II: Mild, activity not interfered with
   III: Moderate, activity interfered with
   IV: Severe, bedridden with nausea for more than 2 hours
B. Vomiting grades I to IV
   I: No vomiting 24 hours after chemotherapy
   II: Mild, vomiting less than five times in the 24 hours after chemotherapy
   III: Moderate, 5 to 10 times in the 24 hours after chemotherapy
   IV: Severe, more than 10 times in 24 hours, patient bedridden, possible dehydration

C. Response will be graded as follows
   CR (complete response): Grade I, no nausea or vomiting
   PR (partial response): Grade II–III, nausea and vomiting
   NR (no response): Grade IV, nausea and vomiting
D. Source of response data
   PI: Patient interview
   NO: Nurse observation
   HCT: Other health-care team

This easily administered scale lacks reported reliability and validity. In the highest grade (grade IV) it also has a low ceiling of 10 emetic episodes for a 24-hour period. Thus, patients who increase from 10 to 15 emetic episodes are evaluated as unchanged.[33]

Visual Analog Scales (VAS)

The visual analog scale (VAS) is a line, usually 100 mm in length (occasionally 150 or 160 mm long) with anchors at each end to indicate the extremes of the sensation under study (Figure 35.1). Traditionally, the VAS has been a horizontally oriented scale without indicators. However, more recently, it has been used as a vertical scale with or without markings.[34] The low endpoint is to the left in a horizontally oriented scale and at the base of a vertically oriented scale. Subjects indicate the point on the scale corresponding to the degree of sensation they are experiencing. Investigators score the intensity of the discomfort by measuring the millimeters from the low end of the scale to the mark.

Although the VAS avoids language descriptors to signify gradations of a subjective phenomenon, the anchor extremes require meaningful descriptors with tested reliability. For example, a vomiting VAS anchored at "none" on the low end of the continuum and at "constant retching" at the opposite end can link two different concepts. Administering analog scales generally requires additional explanation.

When used properly, the VAS is a reliable, valid, and sensitive self-report tool for studying subjective symptoms. However, a recent report found that analog scales did not appear to offer a specific advantage of sensitivity over a simple discrete scale, regardless of the dimension of nausea considered.[35] In fact, these investigators found no advantage in using an analog scale over a discrete scale. For subjective parameters such as nausea or toxicities of the antiemetics (e.g., sedation), VAS tools do not necessarily increase the quantitative accuracy of the assessment because respondents may be able to discriminate only between broad grades of a subjective sensation—none, mild, moderate, or severe.[36] Reliability is strengthened when stable phenomena are being evaluated.[37] Caution must be taken when administering a VAS because it was designed for use with a seated subject marking the scale. Variations can affect the results: responding from a supine position; when another individual marks the scale for the subject; when the subject marked a maximum rating, but later perceives the sensation to be greater; and ensuring the accuracy of scoring.

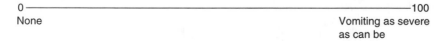

0 ——100
None   Vomiting as severe
                                                            as can be

On this line mark how much vomiting you have had in the past 4 hours. At the left is zero, none. At the right is 100, vomiting as severe as can be.

Figure 35.1   Visual analog scales (VAS) for measuring vomiting severity.

Daily Diary

Daily diaries have been used in a variety of studies to record the incidence of nausea, vomiting, and retching. The diaries have been used for periods ranging from 24 hours to 15 days.[38-40] This method requires patient self-report and has been correlated to other measures such as observation and the Functional Living Index.[41,42] Although reliability and validity are not reported, the diary card has the advantage of ease of administration and can be used in any setting. Comparison of findings among studies must be done with caution as there is no standardization of questions on the diary cards.

Morrow Assessment of Nausea and Emesis (MANE)

The Morrow Assessment of Nausea and Emesis (MANE)[25] and the Morrow Assessment of Nausea and Emesis Follow Up (MANE-FU)[43-45] are self-report, Likert scales that measure post-treatment and anticipatory aspects of nausea and vomiting separately. These instruments provide data on onset, intensity, severity, and duration of nausea and vomiting. The frequency of anticipatory nausea and anticipatory vomiting are rated on a 5-point scale from "during and after every treatment" to "never after a treatment." Post-treatment nausea and post-treatment vomiting are rated on a 5-point scale ranging from "before every treatment" to "never before a treatment." The severity rating of nausea and vomiting is rated on a 6-point, equal-interval scale ranging from "very mild" to "intolerable." The time during which nausea and vomiting are worst is measured by a 6-point scale ranging from "during treatment" to "24 or more hours after treatment." An example of an item is: "The nausea is usually the worst" with response options ranging from 1 "during treatment" to 7 "no time is any more severe than any other time." Options 2 to 6 identify time periods from 2 "0–4 hours after treatment" to 6 "24 or more hours after treatment." The MANE-FU provides information about the effectiveness of medication for controlling nausea and/or vomiting.

Test–retest reliability for the MANE was determined with 20 randomly selected cancer patients who completed the instrument after each of four consecutive chemotherapy treatments. Correlations ranged from 0.72 (post-treatment nausea severity) to 0.96 (anticipatory nausea duration and post-treatment vomiting duration). Test–retest reliability also was determined with 18 patients who completed the MANE prior to the fourth treatment and approximately 7 months later. Correlations for this group ranged from 0.61 to 0.78. Content validity of the MANE was supported by the nonsignificant relationship between patient reported anticipatory side effects and post-treatment side effects. Convergent validity was supported by the higher correlations of independent measures of nausea and vomiting than with other measures of chemotherapy side effects.[25]

Rhodes Index of Nausea and Vomiting (INV)

The Rhodes Index of Nausea and Vomiting (INV) measures the individual components of nausea, vomiting, retching, and associated distress. This 8-item, 5-point Likert pencil-and-paper tool measures patients' perceived (1) duration of nausea; (2) frequency of nausea; (3) distress from nausea; (4) frequency of vomiting; (5) amount of vomiting; (6) distress form vomiting; and (7) frequency of retching.[20,46,47] The original tool, INV-1, was developed and used by Rhodes et al. for a study to determine the reliability and validity of a self-report measure of nausea and vomiting.[19]

The INV-1 was compared to an adapted version of McCorkle and Young Symptom Distress Scale (ASDS).[19] Reliability of the INV-1 was determined employing a split-half procedure and Cronbach's alpha. Using the split-half procedure reliability estimates of 0.83 to 0.99 were obtained.[19,48] Construct and concurrent validity were assessed by comparing family members' ratings to chemotherapy patients' ratings, yielding a correlation of $r = 0.87$. Psychometric properties of the original INV have been described in detail elsewhere. The investigators reported that both the INV-1 and ASDS were reliable and valid measures of post-treatment nausea and vomiting.[19,48]

The INV-1 was refined to include the occurrence and distress of dry heaves or retching and the distress from vomiting. This revised instrument, the INV-2, includes subscales for nausea, vomiting, and retching as well as for occurrence (intensity, duration, frequency and/or amount of distress). A numerical value is assigned to each response. These range from 0 the least amount of distress, to 4 the most distress. A total experience score from nausea, vomiting, and retching is calculated by summing responses to each of the eight items on the INV-2. The score range is from 0 to 32. The potential subscale scores are: Nausea 0–12, Vomiting 0–12, and Retching 0–8. In a study of oncology patients, Cronbach's alpha for the INV-2 was 0.98.[20] Headley,[49] in a study of the influence of administration time on cisplatin-induced nausea and vomiting, reported that the three subscales were highly correlated with the total INV experience score ($p < 0.05$, $r = 0.78$–0.94).

The INV-2 was originally developed for adult oncologic populations. However, it is appropriate for use with other populations because of its conceptual development. It has been used with oncologic, obstetric, cardiovascular, and postanesthesia patients.[50-52] A pediatric form has been pilot tested with children ages 6 to 15 years. Correlations of 1.00 have been reported between the instrument and the observed and measured episodes of vomiting (M. Kachoyeamos, personal communication). An example of an item is: "During the last 12 hours, I have not felt any distress from nausea/sickness at my stomach"; "During the last 12 hours I have felt mild distress from nausea or sickness at my stomach"; "During the last 12 hours I have felt moderate distress from nausea or sickness at my stomach"; "During the last 12 hours I have felt great distress from nausea or sickness at my stomach"; "During the last 12 hours I have felt as severe distress from nausea or sickness at my stomach as can be." A new format of the INV-2, the Rhodes Index of Nausea, Vomiting, and Retching (RINVR) is currently being tested for reliability and validity. The RINVR has a more concise format.

Functional Living Index-Emesis (FLIE)

The 18-item Functional Living Index-Emesis (FLIE), developed by Lindley et al. was designed for easy, repeated patient self-administration.[53] Although modeled after the Functional Living Index-Cancer, FLIE items deal specifically with the effects of nausea and vomiting on physical activities, social and emotional function, and the ability to enjoy food. Each FLIE item is answered in a Likert format ranging from 1 to 7, with 9 items for nausea, and 9 items for vomiting. A total score is created by adding the responses to the 18 questions. The range of total scores possible is between 18 (all 1 responses on the scale) and 126 (all 7 responses on the scale). Lower scores indicate a more negative impact of nausea and vomiting. An example of an item is: "How much nausea have you had in the past 3 days?"

The validity of the FLIE is supported by the difference in mean scores of subjects experiencing vomiting and those who were not experiencing vomiting. Content- and criterion-related validity were supported in the study by Lindley et al. Cronbach's alpha correlations support the reliability of the FLIE.

Summary

Although chemotherapy-related nausea, vomiting, and retching continue to be the most frequently investigated, researchers in other clinical areas are giving increased attention to these symptoms. The earliest techniques used to measure these symptoms have been simple and direct—usually counting episodes. Self-report tools used global terms that considered these symptoms as one, rather than as individual, symptoms. Norris's[17] work in the development of these individual concepts has helped to differentiate between objective and subjective experiences with varied conditions. This information was beneficial in the development of self-report measures of nausea, vomiting, and retching.

Instruments to measure nausea, vomiting, and retching have shown increased refinement and have demonstrated reliability and validity in various trials. Although progress has been made in the measurement of these symptoms, many studies continue simply to count the number of emetic episodes, ignoring the importance of the subjective experience of nausea. Measuring the human response to the occurrence of the symptom is critical to develop appropriate interventions.

Exemplar Studies

Chin, S.B., Kucuk, O., Peterson, R., & Ezdinli, E.Z. Variables contributing to anticipatory nausea and vomiting in cancer chemotherapy. *Am J Clin Oncol*, 1992, *15*(3):262-267.

The development of anticipatory nausea and vomiting (ANV) was assessed in 40 patients receiving parenteral chemotherapy. The Morrow Assessment of Nausea and Emesis (MANE) was used to assess ANV. Sixteen patients experienced ANV. The ANV patients had greater pretreatment anxiety, post-treatment dizziness/lightheadedness, more severe postchemotherapy vomiting, and delayed onset of postchemotherapy nausea and vomiting.

Troesch, L.M., Rodehaver, C.B., Delaney, E.A., & Yanes B. The influence of guided imagery on chemotherapy-related nausea and vomiting. *Oncol Nurs Forum*, 1993, *20*(8):1179-1185.

Twenty-eight oncology patients receiving cisplatin were randomly assigned to determine whether the addition of guided imagery to a standard antiemetic regimen decreased nausea, vomiting, and retching occurrence and distress. Both groups received the same standard antiemetic regimen, but the experimental group also used a chemotherapy-specific guided-imagery audiotape. The Rhodes Index of Nausea and Vomiting Form 2 was used to measure the nausea and vomiting at five points during chemotherapy. Although no statistically significant differences were found between the two groups, the guided-imagery group indicated a significantly more positive experience ($p = 0.0001$) with chemotherapy.

Stainton, M.C. The efficacy of SeaBands for the control of nausea and vomiting in pregnancy. *Health Care Women Int*, 1994, *15*(6):563-575.

SeaBands were used in a study controlling nausea, vomiting, and retching of 27 pregnant women. SeaBands were applied between 5 and 22 weeks of pregnancy (M = 9 weeks). As measured by the Rhodes Index of Nausea and Vomiting, the occurrence of nausea, vomiting, and retching (NVR) was reduced by approximately 50%, and the distress from NVR also was reduced. Clinical implications reveal that SeaBands are more effective if applied early in the symptom experience.

Lindley, C.M., Hirsch, J.D., O'Neill, C.V., et al. Quality of life consequences of chemotherapy-induced emesis. *Qual Life Res*, 1992, *1*(5):331-340.

This study explored the impact of chemotherapy (CT)-associated nausea and vomiting on patients' and daily function quality of life and the costs associated with CT in 122 outpatients. The Functional Living Index-Emesis (FLIE) was used to assess the impact of nausea and vomiting. Approximately 56% of the subjects reported CT-induced emesis. Decline in quality of life was observed for this group. FLIE scores indicated that patients perceived that vomiting, and to a slightly lesser extent nausea, substantively influenced their ability to complete household tasks, enjoy meals, spend time with family and friends, and maintain daily function and recreation. Pearson's and Cronbach alpha correlations were used to test the reliability and validity of the FLIE. The FLIE also was correlated with actual clinical parameters and the nausea factor from another instrument. Content- and criterion-related validity were supported.

References

1. Bilgrami S., & Fallon B.G. Chemotherapy-induced nausea and vomiting. Easing patients' fear and discomfort with effective antiemetic regimens. *Postgrad Med*, 1993, *94*(5):55-58, 62-64.
2. Taylor, H., Brown, A., Butler, W., et al. Modification of VAB III in the treatment of patients with stage II and stage III nonseminomatous germ cell centre. *Proc Amer. Asso. of Cancer Research*, 1980, *21*:432.
3. Wampler, G., Schulz, J., Essig, L., et al. Virginia Oncology groups surgical adjuvant treatment Breast Carcinoma: A preliminary report. *Proc Amer. Asso. of Cancer Research*, 1980, *21*:412.
4. Bitetti, J., & Weintraub, H. Nausea and vomiting. In J. Benumof & L. Saidman (Eds.), *Anesthesia and perioperative complications*. St. Louis: Mosby Yearbook, 1992, pp. 396-412.
5. Cohen, M., Duncan, P., DeBoer, D., & Tweed, W. The postoperative interview: Assessing risk factors for nausea and vomiting. *Anesthes Analges*, 1994, *78*(1):7-16.
6. Gadsby, R., Barnie-Adshead, A., & Jagger, C. A prospective study of nausea and vomiting during pregnancy. *Br J Gen Pract*, 1993, *43*(371):245-248. [Published erratum appears in *Br J Gen Pract*, 1993, *43*(373):325].
7. O'Brien, B., Rusthoven, J., Rocchi, A., et al. Impact of chemotherapy-associated nausea and vomiting on patients' functional status and on a survey of five Canadian centres. *Can Med Assoc J*, 1993, *149*(3):296-302.
8. Morrow, G., Asbury, R., Hammon, S., et al. Comparing the effectiveness of behavioral treatment for chemotherapy-induced nausea and vomiting when administered by oncologists, oncology nurses, and clinical psychologists. *Health Psychol*, 1992, *11*:250-256.
9. Chiara, S., Conte, P., Franzone, P., et al. High-risk early-stage ovarian cancer. Randomized clinical trial comparing cisplatin plus cyclophosphamide versus whole abdominal radiotherapy. *Am J Clin Oncol*, 1994, *17*(1):72-76.
10. Du Bois, A., Meerpohl, H., Madjar, H., et al. Phase II study of pirarubicin combined with cisplatin in recurrent ovarian cancer. *J Cancer Res Clin Oncol*, 1994, *120*(3):173-178.
11. Grunberg, S., & Hesketh, P. Control of chemotherapy-induced emesis. *N Engl J Med*, 1993, *329*(24):1790-1796.
12. Love, R., Leventhal, H., Easterling, D., et al. Side effects and emotional distress during cancer chemotherapy. *Cancer*, 1989, *63*:604-612.
13. Redd, W., Jacobsen, P., & Andrykowski, M. Behavioral side effects of adjuvant chemotherapy. *Rec Results Cancer Chemother*, 1989, *115*:272-278.
14. Andrykowski, M., Jacobsen, P., Marks, E., et al. Prevalence, predictors, and course of anticipatory nausea in women receiving chemotherapy for breast cancer. *Cancer*, 1988, *62*:2607-2613.
15. Laszlo, J., & Cotanch, P. Managing chemotherapy-induced nausea and vomiting. *Cancer*, 1992, *70*(4):1007-1011.
16. Grigsby, P., Vest, M., & Perez, C. Recurrent carcinoma of the cervix exclusively in the paraaortic nodes following radiation therapy. *Int J Radiation Oncol, Biol, Phys*, 1994, *28*(2):451-455.
17. Norris, C.M. Nausea and vomiting. In C.M. Norris (Ed.), *Concept clarification in nursing*. Rockville, MD: Aspen, 1982, pp. 81-110.
18. Hogan, C.M. Advances in the management of nausea and vomiting. *Nurs Clin North Am*, 1990, *25*(2):475-497.
19. Rhodes, V., Watson, P., & Johnson, M. Development of reliable and valid measures of nausea and vomiting. *Cancer Nurs*, 1984, *7*(1):33.
20. Rhodes, V., Watson, P., Johnson, M., et al. Patterns of nausea, vomiting, and distress in patients receiving antineoplastic drug protocols. *Oncol Nurs Forum*, 1987, *14*(4):35-44.
21. Rhodes, V.A., McDaniel, R.W., Hanson, B., et al. Sensory perceptions of patients on selected antineoplastic protocols. *Cancer Nurs*, 1994, *17*:45-51.
22. Verbeuren, T.J. Synthesis storage, release and metabolism of 5-hydroxytryptamine in peripheral tissue. In J.R. Fozard (Ed.), *The peripheral actions of 5-hydroxytryptamine*. New York: Oxford University Press, 1989, p. 1.
23. Guyton, A. *A textbook of medical physiology* (6th ed.). Philadelphia: Saunders, 1980.
24. Penta, J., Poster, D., & Bruno, S. The pharmacologic treatment of nausea and vomiting caused by cancer chemotherapy: A review. In J. Laszlo (Ed.), *Antiemetics cancer chemotherapy*. Baltimore: Williams & Wilkins, 1983, p. 53.
25. Morrow, G. Assessment of nausea and vomiting: Past problems, current issues and suggestions for future research. *Cancer*, 1984, *53*(10):2267.
26. Simms, S.G., Rhodes, V.A., & Madsen, R.W. Comparison of prochlorperazine and lorazepam antiemetic regimens in the control of postchemotherapy symptoms. *Nurs Res*, 1993, *42*(4):235-239.
27. McCorkle, R. Non-obtrusive measures in clinical nursing research. In R. Tiffany (Ed.), *Cancer nursing update. Proceedings of the second international cancer nursing conference*. London: Balliere Tindall, 1981.
28. Fox, S., Einhorn, L., Cox, E., et al. Ondansetron versus ondansetron, dexamethasone, and chlorpromazine in the prevention of nausea and vomiting associated with multiple-day cisplatin chemotherapy. *J Clin Oncol*, 1993, *11*(12):2391-2395.
29. Bruera, E., Macmillan, K., Kuehn, N., et al. A controlled trial of megestrol acetate on appetite, caloric intake, nutritional status, and other symptoms in patients with advanced cancer. *Cancer*, 1990, *66*(6):1279-1282.

30. Bovbjerg, D., Redd, W., Jacobsen, P., et al. An experimental analysis of classically conditioned nausea during cancer chemotherapy. *Psychosom Med*, 1992, *54*:623-637.

31. Laszlo, J., Lucas, V., Hanson, D., et al. Levonantradol for chemotherapy-induced emesis: Phase I-II oral administration. *J Clin Pharmocol*, 1981, *21*(8, 9):515.

32. Cotanch, P. Relaxation training for control of nausea and vomiting in patients receiving chemotherapy. *Cancer Nurs*, 1983, *6*(4):277-283.

33. Cotanch, P. Measuring nausea and vomiting. In M. Frank-Stromberg (Ed.), *Instruments for clinical nursing research*. East Norwalk, CT: Appleton & Lange, 1988, pp. 313-321.

34. Bennett, B.B., & Hockenberry, M.J. An antiemetic study comparing halcion to ativan in children receiving cancer chemotherapy. *Oncol Nurs Forum*, 1989, *16*(2 suppl):175.

35. Del Favero, A., Tonato, M., & Roila, F. Issues in the measurement of nausea. *Br J Cancer*, 1992, *66*(suppl XIX):S69-S71.

36. Olver, I., Simon, R., & Aisner, J. Antiemetic studies: A methodological discussion. *Cancer Treat Rep*, 1986, *70*(5):555-563.

37. Padilla, G.V., Presant, C., Grant, M.M., et al. Quality of life index for patients with cancer. *Res Nurs Health*, 1983, *8*(1):45-60.

38. Baltzer, L., Kris, M., Tyson, L., et al. The addition of ondanstetron to the combination of metoclopramide, dexamethasone, and lorazepam did not improve vomiting prevention in patients receiving high-dose cisplatin. *Cancer*, 1994, *73*(3):720-723.

39. Buser, K., Joss, R., Piquet, D., et al. Oral ondansetron in the prophylaxis of nausea and vomiting induced by cyclophosphamide, methotrexate and 5-fluorouracil (CMF) in women with breast cancer. Results of a prospective, randomized, double-blind, placebo-controlled study. *Ann Oncol*, 1993, *4*(6):475-479.

40. Sung, Y.F., Wetchler, B.V., Duncalf, D., & Joslyn, A.F. A double-blind, placebo-controlled pilot study examining the effectiveness of intravenous ondansetron in the prevention of postoperative nausea and emesis. *J Clin Anesthes*, 1993, *5*(1):22-29.

41. Bleehen, N., Girling, D.J., Machin, D., & Stephens, R.J. A randomized trial of three or six courses of etoposide cyclophosphamide methotrexate and vincristine or six courses of etoposide and ifosfamide in small cell lung cancer (SCLC). II: Quality of life.

Medical Research Council Lung Cancer Working Party. *Br J Cancer*, 1993, *68*(6):1157-1166.

42. Clavel, M., Soukop, M., & Greenstreet, Y. Improved control of emesis and quality of life with ondansetron in breast cancer. *Oncology*, 1993, *50*:180-185.

43. Anastasio, G., Robinson, M., Little, J., et al. A comparison of the gastrointestinal side effects of two forms of erythromycin. *J Fam Pract*, 1992, *35*(5):517-523.

44. Razavi, D., Delvaux, N., Farvacques, C., et al. Prevention of adjustment disorders and anticipatory nausea secondary to adjuvant chemotherapy: A double blind placebo-controlled study assessing the usefulness of alprazolam. *J Clin Oncol*, 1993, *11*(7):1384-1390.

45. Chin, S., Kucuk, O., Peterson, R., & Ezdinli, E. Variables contributing to anticipatory nausea and vomiting in cancer chemotherapy. *Am J Clin Oncol*, 1992, *15*(3):262-267.

46. Rhodes, V.A., Watson, P.M., & Johnson, M.H. Association of chemotherapy related nausea and vomiting with pretreatment and posttreatment anxiety. *Oncol Nurs Forum*, 1986, *13*(1):41-47.

47. Rhodes, V.A., Watson, P.M., & Johnson, M.H. Patterns of nausea and vomiting in antineoplastic postchemotherapy. *Appl Nurs Res*, 1988, *1*(3):143-144.

48. Rhodes, V.A., Watson, P.M., & Johnson, M.H. A self-report tool for assessing nausea and vomiting in chemotherapy. *Oncol Nurs Forum*, 1983, *10*(1):11.

49. Headley, J.A. The influence of administration time on chemotherapy-induced nausea and vomiting. *Oncol Nurs Forum*, 1987, *14*(6):43-47.

50. Belluomoni, J. Litt, R.C., Lee, K.A., & Katz, M. Acupressure for nausea and vomiting of pregnancy: A randomized blinded study. *Obstet Gynecol*, 1994, *84*(2):159-160.

51. Troesch, L., Rodehaver, C., Delaney, E., & Yanes, B. The influence of guided imagery on chemotherapy-related nausea and vomiting. *Oncol Nurs Forum*, 1993, *20*(8):1179-1185.

52. Stainton, M., & Mesf, E. The efficacy of seabands for the control of nausea and vomiting in pregnancy. *Health Care Women Int*, 1994, *15*(6):563-575.

53. Lindley, C., Hirsch, J., O'Neill, C., et al. Quality of life consequences of chemotherapy-induced emesis. *Qual Life Res*, 1992, *1*:331-340.

Appendix

35A. Summary Comparison of Measures of Nausea, Vomiting, and Retching

Tool	Dimensions	Type	How Administered	Reliability/Validity	Strengths/Weaknesses
Duke Descriptive Scale (DDS) (31,32,33)	Nausea and vomiting with frequency, severity, and activity combined	Check scale	Patient Interview Nurse Observation Other health-care worker	Unreported	Low ceiling may limit information
Visual Analog Scales (VAS) (34,35,36,37)	May be devised for individual symptoms and their components: frequency; duration; severity; distress	A line usually 100 mm long with reliable anchor descriptors at extremes Self-report (mark when in sitting position)	Reliability is strength with stable phenomena	Unreported	Subjects' inability to discriminate between grades of sensation; Requires more administrator time; Inaccurate when marked by another or subject in supine position; Unstated time frame
Morrow Assessment of Nausea and Emesis (MANE) (25)	Post-treatment nausea and vomiting: onset; severity; intensity; duration	16-item, 5-point Likert scale (onset) 6-point Likert scale (severity-intensity)	Self-report	Test–retest reliability: 0.61–0.78 Validity: 0.72–0.96	Primarily used with antiemetic studies; Long (>24 hour) time frame
Morrow Assessment of Nausea and Emesis Follow-up (MANE-FU) (43–45)	Anticipatory nausea and vomiting (frequency)	17-item, 5-point Likert scale (severity-intensity)	Self-report	Content and convergent validity supported	Assesses anticipatory nausea
Rhodes Index of Nausea and Vomiting Form-2 (INV-2) (19,20,46,47–52)	Nausea, vomiting, retching, and the components of each symptom: frequency; amount; duration; severity; distress	8-item, 5-point Likert scale	Self-report	Split-half reliability: 0.83–0.99 Cronbach's alpha: 0.98 Validity: $r = 0.87$	12-hour time frame; Measure distress of symptom; Totals symptom experience scale; Subscales for triad and occurrence and distress; Used with varied groups
Functional Living Index Emesis (FLIE) (53)	Effects of nausea and vomiting on: physical activity; social and emotional functions; eating	18-item, 7-point Likert scale	Self-report	Content and criterion validity Internal consistency supported	Ease of use; Provides information about the effect of nausea and vomiting on functional status

Numbers in parentheses correspond to studies cited in the References.

36

Assessing the Oral Cavity

Sharon Ann Hyland

The use of chemotherapy to treat cancer patients is very familiar to the general public. More patients than ever receive intensive chemotherapy regimens combined with bone marrow transplant, and, unfortunately, the side effects of these treatments also are becoming familiar. Stomatitis is an important one of these side effects. Clinicians have for some time recognized the need for accurate clinical assessment and effective intervention measures to identify and allay the symptoms associated with stomatitis.

Stomatitis, or oral mucositis, refers to the inflammatory reaction and subsequent sequelae that can occur in the mouth and oropharynx because of the effects of radiation therapy and certain chemotherapeutic agents.[1-4] Stomatitis can present as ulceration, oral pain, and/or infection. These symptoms can significantly alter the patient's performance status and compromise nutritional intake, airway status, and vocal ability and possibly lead to systemic infection. These symptoms may require therapy dose modification or delays in further chemotherapy or radiation treatment. Ultimately, stomatitis can increase the morbidity and mortality associated with cancer therapy.[5]

Clinicians have identified the need for adequate, consistent oral assessment to measure mucosal changes and oral complications associated with cancer therapy accurately and reliably. Standardized assessment is necessary to compare the effectiveness of various agents or clinical interventions used to treat mucositis.[6] The use of intensive chemotherapy during bone marrow transplant procedures and the resulting severe stomatitis that occurs increases the need to find successful mechanisms to allay this debilitating and potentially life-threatening side effect.

Risk Factors for Stomatitis

Stomatitis is one of the most common patient complaints during chemotherapy with an incidence of 39%.[7] The likelihood of oral complications depends on the malignancy and its treatment. The incidence of stomatitis in patients with solid-tumor malignancies is about 12%; it is 33% in lymphomas, and 50% among leukemia patients.[8]

The appearance of stomatitis is the result of complex interactions with a number of factors. Patient-specific factors include type of cancer (hematologic or solid tumor); nutritional state; condition of the oral cavity, teeth, and gums prior to cancer therapy; age (younger individuals having less risk); and underlying medical conditions. Predisposing factors include pretreatment oral health, dental caries, and periodontal disease. Oral irritants include ill-fitting prostheses, exposure to irritating chemicals (tobacco, alcohol), physical exposures (coarse foods), and thermal exposures (food temperature).[9]

The most important causative factor in stomatitis is the direct effect of the therapy. Certain types of chemotherapy are known to cause stomatitis, including antimetabolites (Methotrexate, 5-FU) and antibiotics (Daunorubicin, Adriamycin®, Mitomycin C).[10-12] Head and neck radiation therapy frequently causes some degree of mucositis. The combination of both chemotherapy and head and neck radiation poses an increased risk for stomatitis.

A second treatment-related risk factor is dose of therapy. High doses are known to increase the risk and severity of stomatitis. About 75% of patients undergoing bone marrow transplant will experience significant stomatitis caused by the pretransplant chemotherapy dose.[9]

A third risk factor is prior therapy. Past and present drug therapy, including antibiotics and steroids, can affect the mucosa of the oral cavity, as can prior surgical intervention. "Recall" oral reactions from prior chemotherapy or radiation are common.

Immunocompetence significantly influences the potential for and duration of stomatitis. High-dose chemotherapy or dose intensification usually shortens the time interval before onset of stomatitis and increases the potential for infection. The degree and duration of neutropenia directly influences the probability and degree of oral complications.[13]

The drug dose, scheduling, and method of administration also may increase the frequency of occurrence of stomatitis. For example, giving a drug over a 24-hour infusion may result in stomatitis that is not experienced when the drug is given as an intravenous push. Patients with prior evidence of stomatitis are likely to experience recurrence if the same drug and dosage are administered without additional intervention. Methotrexate, even at standard dosing, can cause stomatitis. Subsequent courses at the same dose without Leucovorin® antidote or alteration in dose can result in severe stomatitis. Renal dysfunction may increase the risk of stomatitis, as drug clearance times are prolonged.

Physiologic Effects of Therapy

The oral cavity is a vulnerable environment for side effects from cancer therapy because it is an area of rapid cellular activity. There is a high rate of cell proliferation and turnover in the oral epithelium. It is one of the body's first lines of defense. Drugs act directly by interfering with the replication of epithelial cells, causing changes in the submucosal tissue. The most common histologic changes are epithelial hyperplasia and collagen degeneration.[14] The buccal and labial mucosa have the highest frequency of changes (39%), followed by the dorsum of the tongue (24%), gingiva (16%), ventral aspect of the tongue or floor of the mouth (11%), and the palate (11%).[12] These changes can lead to spontaneous or traumatic ulceration.[15] Any mucosal break can become secondarily infected. The immunocompromised patient carries the inherent risk of altered response to the large amount of microbial flora, both normal and opportunistic pathogens, present in the oral cavity, which can cause severe primary or secondary infections.[16]

Symptoms can range from a dry, painful mouth, the result of a thinning of the epithelium, to life-threatening sepsis directly caused by oral microorganisms. Stomatitis can alter the individual's ability to ingest food and fluids, ranging from avoidance of irritating foods or fluids to a total inability to swallow. Oral ulcerations in the neutropenic patient can provide a source of bacterial and fungal flora that can invade the body. Mucositis can result in local bleeding. Severe ulceration and associated edema can affect the airway as well as make it almost impossible to eat.

Stomatitis generally follows a predictable pattern. When resulting from standard-dose chemotherapy, initial oral changes occur 7 to 10 days after drug administration. Stomatitis usually corresponds to a decrease in the granulocyte count. Healing occurs by the second to third week. The severity is usually mild to moderate without associated infection. Treatment involves the use of topical combination therapy with the primary use of analgesia for symptomatic relief. The goal of therapy is to maintain nutrition and hydration.[9]

The effects of radiation therapy depend on a number of factors and are primarily local effects. The radiosensitivity of the epithelial tissue varies throughout the oral cavity. The type of radiation, fraction/dose, time between fractions, overall treatment time, cumulative dose, the type of tissue irradiated, and field size affect the probability of stomatitis. The direct effect of radiation therapy results in a change in the epithelial characteristics, as the atrophic mucosa thins, and an inflammatory reaction begins within the first week of treatment. The patient complains of a burning sensation, and there is decreased salivation in 7 to 10 days. The mucosa usually reddens and sometimes is white. The tongue may swell and develop a protective white coating. There may be isolated ulcerations. Pseudomembranes may develop within 3 to 4 weeks of therapy along with ulcerations and diminished taste sensation. Accelerated radiotherapy shortens the time to onset of mucositis by about 3 weeks. Because mucositis is more severe, treatment may need to be delayed. Healing occurs over weeks following therapy cessation.[17]

Severe stomatitis occurs commonly after bone marrow transplant conditioning regimens or extensive head and neck irradiation. Changes in the mucosal color (either red or white) occur from day 2 to 14. Mucosal atrophy is most marked between day 7 and 21. Painful, confluent ulceration results if neutropenia persists or when the adaptive resources of the patient are exhausted. With the recovery of the white blood cell count, stomatitis is self-limiting and resolves or reverses within 2 to 3 weeks. Dysphagia may be severe enough to result in an inability to swallow food and/or liquids. If there is a break in the mucosa and the blood counts are low, there is high risk for developing systemic infection. Stomatitis usually occurs near the nadir of the leukocyte count and recovery from stomatitis precedes bone marrow recovery.[14]

Because neutropenic patients are at high risk of developing oral infections such as candida or herpes simplex, it is important to differentiate whether the somatitis is a cause or effect of infection.[16] This requires direct visualization of the oral cavity on a regular basis. The patient's symptom report is not sufficient to determine accurately the cause of stomatitis. The sites of oral infections usually are the marginal, papillary, and attached gingiva. Secondary infection occurs when the leukocyte count is less than 1,000. Infection can result in opportunistic infection: bactcrial, viral, and/or fungal. The classic signs of inflammation may be absent when the patient is severely neutropenic. It is important to perform oral cultures or other diagnostic techniques regularly.

The health professional cannot assume that all oral effects are due to chemotherapy or radiation. The clinician must include all of the following in an assessment: the overall systemic status of the patient, laboratory results, vital signs, presence of graft-versus-host disease, other medications, and associated local factors.

Additional sequelae of stomatitis can be local bleeding, oral pain, and changes in the volume and consistency of the saliva. The pain can be severe enough to limit oral intake or even temporarily eliminate the ability to eat. Patients in this state require intravenous narcotics. Bleeding tends to be infrequent as long as the platelet count is adequate. Clinically, the saliva becomes more viscous.

All patients receiving chemotherapy should have an initial oral assessment, and the state of the oral cavity and teeth should be documented. The initial oral assessment includes a visual inspection with sufficient lighting to establish baseline data such as the state of the gums, the status of the teeth, and the use of any dental prostheses. Prior to bone marrow transplant, patients should have a dental consult. All patients receiving chemotherapy and head and neck radiation should have a baseline oral exam even if the treatment they receive does not cause stomatitis.

Development of Oral Assessment Guides

Historically, there have been several approaches to the assessment and evaluation of oral complications of cancer therapy. The most common guidelines grade the clinical appearance of the oral cavity with or without the addition of functional input from the patient. The oral cavity is categorized into specific areas that are scored according to the severity of stomatitis. Another approach is to stage holistically the stomatitis. Each stage includes both the functional and objective aspects of stomatitis. Both of these approaches rely on direct visualization of the stomatitis. At present, such tools are hindered by the lack of observer standardization. Complications of stomatitis (edema, infection) can further confound the observer's findings. Soliciting the patient's assessment of symptom severity also can bring quite variable results.

Early oral assessment tools lacked reliability and validity data,[6,18] and they did not specifically assess the oral effects of cancer chemotherapy. Accurate descriptions of the mouth following chemotherapy treatment were lacking as well as a systemic pattern of assessment. Although early tools were tested with noncancer patients,[19] subsequent tools were developed providing detailed descriptors of potential oral signs and symptoms appropriate for patients receiving chemotherapy. However, severity was not adequately assessed. Manifestations of stomatitis complicated mucositis assessment and influenced the reliability of comparison assessment guides. For example, the amount and degree of edema may be more important than the size and number of the oral ulcerations. Presently, most oral assessment instruments include both subjective and objective information. Instruments that include only patient-reported functional status, such as voice changes and difficulty swallowing, are an inaccurate measurement of mucositis. Patient rating of severity will be variable regardless of observed oral changes. Other factors, such as infection, also may be influencing these symptoms.

Instruments and Guides for Assessing Stomatitis

Oral Mucositis Index (OMI)

The purpose of the Oral Mucositis Index (OMI) was to assess the types, patterns, and timing or oral mucosal changes after bone marrow transplantation.[16] Specific definitions of the appearance of stomatitis were developed and are shown here:[16]

> *Erythema.* Increased redness of oral mucosa
> *Atrophy.* Clinical impression of oral mucosa appearing atrophic and thin and/or exhibiting loss of keratinization
> *Vascularity.* Clinically visible changes in apparent mucosal vascularity caused by an increase in the number of vascular elements detected and/or an increase in size of vascular elements that were seen
> *Ulceration.* Frank ulcerations and/or surface erosions; severity of ulceration is rated according to number, depth, and surface area of lesions (e.g., the greater the number of

lesions, the deeper the lesion, and/or the larger the surface area involved by the lesion, the higher the ulceration score)

Angular stomatitis. Inflammation and mucosal breakdown at the commissures of lips

Bleeding/crusted. Hemorrhage of oral cavity rated as active (bleeding) at time of examination or inactive (crusted) because of the presence of blood clots or dried blood

Saliva viscosity. Clinical impression of increased viscosity or thickness of saliva

Saliva xerostomia. Observer's impression of lack of saliva intraorally at time of evaluation

The oral cavity was divided into distinct anatomic regions: lips, labial mucosa, buccal mucosa, hard palate, soft palate, dorsal tongue, ventral tongue, and gingiva. Sites were assessed for changes from normal on a 0 to 3 rating scale (0 normal or no change, 1 mild change, 2 moderate change, 3 severe change). Tissue changes rated included mucosa, color (increased whiteness or erythema), atrophy, vascularity, and ulceration. Other parameters assessed included the presence of angular stomatitis, oral bleeding, and salivary changes. Assessment of oral pain and dryness was rated on a visual analog scale. The OMI was calculated by determining median scores of parameters that changed from baseline on specific examination days. The overall OMI score included the total of the oral mucosal changes for each anatomic region, plus the median salivary viscosity and xerostomia scores. The scores were plotted on a graph to portray oral changes over time. One examiner collected the data. Caution was advised in interpreting the data as multiple comparison tests were used.

Oral Mucosa Rating Scale (OMRS)

This tool[20] provides comprehensive measurement of a broad range of oral tissue changes that occur with cancer therapy. The goal of the tool was to quantify the type and severity of clinically evident oral mucosal changes with a scale ranging from 0 to 3 (normal to severe).

The oral cavity was divided into seven distinct anatomic regions: (1) lips; (2) labial mucosa; (3) buccal mucosa; (4) tongue; (5) floor of the mouth; (6) palate; and (7) attached gingiva. Further subdivisions were made into upper and lower (lips and labial mucosa), right and left (buccal mucosa), dorsal, ventral, and lateral (tongue), or hard and soft (palate). Descriptive categories (erythema, atrophy, hyperkeratosis, lichenoid, ulceration, and edema) included common changes in the oral cavity after bone marrow transplant. The categories were rated on a 0 to 3 scale. Erythema, atrophy, hyperkeratosis, lichenoid, and edema are rated as: 0 (normal/no change), 1 (mild), 2 (moderate), and 3 (severe). Ulceration and pseudomembrane scores were rated by estimating the involved surface area. The patient also rated mouth dryness and pain on a 1 to 10 visual analog scale (1 no dryness/pain, 10 worst possible dryness/pain).

This scale was then tested with bone marrow transplant patients with the objective to develop an overall oral mucositis index (OMI) relevant for patient care and research. The final OMI score included 34 items. Construction of the OMI was done on the basis of variance, low loading, and retention of items based on principal components analysis. Reliability was evaluated by internal consistency (Cronbach's alpha and Guttman split-half coefficient) and stability (test–retest). Validity data applied to this tool are supportive.[20] The tool is complex because of the total items assessed. It requires some training and additional time from a consistent observer, limiting its application in an ambulatory setting. The OMI uses only a partial subset of the accumulated data from the ORMS.

Mucositis with Radiation Therapy

Spijkervet scored mucositis during radiation therapy of the head and neck by using both qualitative and quantitative parameters.[17] Table 36.1 lists these parameters. Local signs of mucositis were distinguished into four categories: (0) no mucositis; (1) whitish ap-

Table 36.1 Indices for Local Mucositis Symptoms
and Indices for Length of Score Sum

Local Sign	k^*	Length (cm)	E
No mucositis	0		
White discoloration	1	<1	1
Erythema	2	1–2	2
Pseudomembranes	3	2–4	3
Ulceration	4	>4	4

*1, White appearance of oral mucosa; 2, redness more
pronounced than the red color of nonirradiated normal
mucosa; 3, white or yellow mucous plaques that are difficult
to detach; 4, local complete loss of the mucosal layer.

Spijkervet, F.K., VanSaene, H.F., Vermey, A., & Mehta, D.M.
Scoring irradiation mucositis in head and neck cancer patients.
J Oral Pathol Med, 1989, 18:167.

pearance of the oral mucosa; (2) erythema more pronounced than the red color of non-irradiated normal mucosa; (3) white or yellow plaques difficult to detach; and (4) complete loss of the mucosal layer. Mucositis was assessed at the following areas of the mouth: buccal mucosa (left and right), soft and hard palate, dorsum and border of the tongue (left and right), and mouth floor. The borders often overlapped. The degree of mucositis for each subarea was scored on an ordinal scale. The length of each subarea was measured by a modified pocket gauge and summed. The mucositis score of an area was defined as the sum of these products.

Although this assessment guide describes the local signs of mucositis, the scoring is of questionable clinical significance. There is no association with oral nutritional intake or associated oral pain. Measuring the size of oral ulceration is cumbersome and of limited clinical relevance.

WHO Index

The WHO Index is a simple, overall rating of mucositis. It often has been used as a general comparison index to other assessment scales.[21]

Grade 0. No Change
Grade 1. Soreness, erythema
Grade 2. Erythema, ulcers, can eat solids
Grade 3. Ulcers, requires liquid diet only
Grade 4. Alimentation not possible

There are no reliability or validity data on the use of this guide. The grading does not capture the variety of oral changes that occur with cancer therapy. The descriptors of the grade are too ambiguous for consistent assessment. This tool focuses only on the status of the oral cavity. The functional status of the patient is not well addressed.

Western Consortium for Cancer Nursing Research
Staging System for Stomatitis

A panel of experts from nursing, dentistry, and medicine were solicited to develop criteria to evaluate the progressive severity of chemotherapy-induced stomatitis. The Western Consortium for Cancer staging instrument was devised to measure the observable and functional dimensions of stomatitis.[22] The tool was compared with the Oral Assessment Guide (OAG) and WHO instruments. The WHO instrument was found to be ambiguous when assessing oral fluid and food intake, as lack of oral intake often could be related to nausea than mucositis. The OAG descriptive ratings 2 and 3 were not always mutually exclusive when used to assess the mucous membrane.

This assessment guide provides a general description of the commonly associated characteristics of stomatitis, as well as its effects on the patient's nutritional intake and pain status. It provides an accurate, general assessment and aims to improve observer consistency. The stages in this guide provide a complete description of the progressive severity in chemotherapy-induced stomatitis. The functional dimensions include: ability to eat, drink, and talk, which is influenced by the patient's pain perception. The observable dimensions are: erythema, edema, presence of lesions, bleeding, and infection. There is less emphasis on specific anatomic sites and more emphasis on overall oral status and deviations from normal. The guide requires assessment by a clinician rather than relying on patient report only. The tool is brief and easy to use. The ratings are simple to record, and the descriptors are consistent with the clinical situation. The holistic approach may be preferable to measuring stomatitis and its specific dimensions through combining scores by simple summation.

Oral Assessment Guide (OAG)

This tool was devised to meet the need for readily identifiable categories and easy descriptive ratings of the oral cavity in the clinical setting. The categories were consensually validated by nursing staff and through review of the literature. The categories include: voice, ability to swallow, lips, tongue, saliva, mucous membrane, gingiva, teeth, or dentures. Three levels of descriptors were identified for each of the eight categories. The descriptors were given a rating of 1, 2, or 3 (1 normal, 2 mild alteration without severe compromise of either epithelial integrity or systemic functioning, 3 definite compromise of either mucosal integrity or system function). The eight subscale scores are summed to obtain overall assessment score. The tools for assessment and methods of measurement are identified and are shown in Table 36.2. The numerical ratings have brief descriptors listed with the corresponding category to provide consistency.[23]

This assessment tool is clearly worded. The potential for consistent results among different raters is high. The OAG is useful to obtain, record, and communicate oral cavity status and to determine changes secondary to chemotherapy and/or radiation. However, it does not include functional parameters in much detail. Interrater reliability is good (0.912), but validity data have not been obtained.

Another criticism of the tool is that it assesses pain inadequately. The most pertinent clinical application for the OAG is in patients receiving high-dose radiation therapy and/or chemotherapy. The OAG would be useful when trying to identify oral care protocols or individuals at risk. Equal weight is given to the eight categories, which may not be consistent with the primary concerns of the patient. The tool combines functional performance with an objective examiner-rated evaluation.

Table 36.2 Oral Assessment Guide Example

Category	Tools for Assessment	Methods of Measurement	Numerical and Descriptive Rating		
			1	2	3
Voice	Auditory	Converse with	Normal	Deeper or raspy	Difficulty talking or painful

Eilers, J., Berger, A.M., & Peterson, M.C. Development, testing and application of the oral assessment guide. *Oncol Nurs Forum*, 1988, 15:327.

The tool is readily available from the authors. Use in the outpatient setting requires modification as it relies on nursing observation and not necessarily on patient-reported symptoms. The exquisite detail makes it cumbersome to institute on a daily basis except in a research situation.

Summary

Stomatitis is an important and common side effect of chemotherapy and radiation therapy that warrants the identification of improved health-care interventions. Developing appropriate and reliable oral assessment instruments is relevant to the evaluation of these interventions. The present tools have been primarily used in the bone marrow transplant setting because of the high incidence and severity of stomatitis. The health-care researcher now has several tools that have been tested and compared. One needs first to determine the tool most appropriate to the setting. A quick, easy grading system that provides a summary of both functional and objective data is necessary for patients in ambulatory care and can be followed up by telephone interview. Tools that describe multiple categories of location and effect of stomatitis are applicable when the patient is receiving intensive, inpatient care.

An initial, visual assessment is key to determining whether the stomatitis is related to treatment or an infection so that proper treatment can be instituted as soon as possible. The instrument should include easily recognizable descriptions of the grading or staging of stomatitis. The grading should correlate with the known pattern of stomatitis progression. The difference between grades or categories should reflect this pattern, as well as clearly correlate with distinct differences.

Finally, the grading system should include the functional status of the patient (ability to eat, drink, talk, or swallow and degree of pain). The goal of any oral assessment guide is to assist in the development of comprehensive oral care protocols to improve the patient's functional status, allay pain, promote nutrition, and quickly identify and check infection. Ultimately, proper assessments and interventions promote patient's tolerance of chemotherapy or radiation. A team approach to care in which the nurse, dentist, physician, pharmacist, and nutritionist participate is best to accomplish this goal.

References

1. Carl, W. Oral complications in cancer patients. *Am Fam Physician*, 1983, 27(2):161-170.
2. NIH. Oral complications of cancer therapy: Prevention and treatment. *NIH Consens Develop Conf Statement*, April 1989, 7(7):17-19.
3. Bruya, N., & Madiera, N. Stomatitis after chemotherapy. *Am J Nurs*, 1975, 75(8):1349-1352.
4. Chabner, B. The clinical pharmacology of antineoplastic agents. *N Engl J Med*, 1975, 292:1107-1112.
5. Wujcik, D. Current research in side effects of high dose chemotherapy. *Semin Oncol Nurs*, 1992, 8(2): 102-112.
6. Beck, S. Impact of a systemic oral protocol on stomatitis after chemotherapy. *Cancer Nurs*, 1979, 2(2): 185-199.
7. Sonis, S.T., Sonis, A.L., & Lieberman, A. Oral complications in patients receiving treatment for malignancies other than of the head and neck. *J Am Dent*, 1978, 20:468-472.
8. Nieweg, R. The validity and reliability of an oral assessment instrument. *Oncol Nurs Forum*, 1993, 20(2):349.
9. Sonis, S.T., & Clark, J. Prevention and management of oral mucositis induced by antineoplastic therapy. *Oncology*, 1991, 5(12):11-22.
10. Peterson, D.E., & Schubert, M.M. Oral toxicity. In M.C. Perry (Ed.), *The chemotherapy source book*. Baltimore: Williams & Wilkins, 1992, pp. 508-517.
11. Dreizen, T. Stomatotoxic manifestations of cancer chemotherapy. *J Prosthet Dent*, 1978, 40:650-655.
12. Lockhardt, P.B., & Sonis, S.T. Alterations in the oral mucosa caused by cancer chemotherapy. *J Dermatol Surg*, 1981, 7(12):1019-1025.
13. Guggenheimer, J. Clinicopathologic effects of cancer chemotherapeutic agents on human buccal mucosa. *Oral Surg*, 1977, 44:58-63.
14. Zerbe, N.B., Parkerson, S.G., Ortlieb, M.L., & Spitzer, T. Relationships between oral mucositis and treatment variables in bone marrow transplant patients. *Cancer Nurs*, 1992, 15(3):196-205.
15. Poland, J. Prevention and treatment of oral complications in the cancer patient, *Oncology*, 1991, 5(7):45-62.
16. Kolbinson, D.A., Schubert, M.M., Flourney, N., & Truelove, E.L. Early oral changes following bone

marrow transplantation. *Oral Surg*, 1988, *66*(1):130-138.

17. Spijkervet, F.K., VanSaene, H.F., Vermey, A., & Mehta, D.M. Scoring irradiation mucositis in head and neck cancer patients. *J Oral Pathol Med*, 1989, *18*:167-171.

18. Ginsberg, N. A study of oral hygiene nursing care. *Nursing*, 1961, *61*(10):67-69.

19. Passos, J., & Brand, L. Effects of agents for oral hygiene. *Nurs Res*, 1966, *15*:196-202.

20. Schubert, M.N., Williams, B.E., Lloid, M.E., et al. Clinical assessment scale for the rating of oral mucosal changes associated with bone marrow transplant. Development of an oral mucositis index. *Cancer*, 1992, *69*(10):2469-2477.

21. WHO. *WHO Handbook for reporting results of cancer treatment*. (Offset Publication No. 48). Geneva: World Health Organization, 1979, pp. 15-22.

22. Western Consortium for Cancer Nursing Research. Development of a staging system for chemotherapy-induced stomatitis. *Cancer Nurs*, 1991, *14*(1):6-12.

23. Eilers, J., Berger, A.M., & Peterson, M.C. Development, testing and application of the oral assessment guide. *Oncol Nurs Forum*, 1988, *15*:325-330.

37

Measuring Pain

Deborah B. McGuire

Pain is such an individual subjective experience that its measurement has long been a research challenge. Even a satisfactory definition of pain has remained elusive. Sternbach called pain "(1) a personal, private sensation of hurt; (2) a harmful stimulus which signals current or impending tissue damage; (3) a pattern of responses which operate to protect the organism from harm."[1,p12] Melzack and Casey emphasized that pain was a sensory experience with motivational and affective properties.[2] Merskey and Spear described pain as an unpleasant experience primarily associated with actual tissue damage, described in such terms, or both.[3] Because of these many definitions of pain and the complexity of pain as a phenomenon, the International Association for the Study of Pain (IASP) developed a list of pain terms and definitions.[4] Pain was defined as "an unpleasant sensory and emotional experience associated with actual or potential tissue damage or described in terms of such damage."[4,pS217] This definition encompassed pain of pathophysiologic and psychologic origin and also accounted for the sensory, affective, and motivational aspects of the experience. In this same document,[4] the IASP published a list of additional pain terms, including definitions, descriptions of chronic pain syndromes, and a classification and coding schema for the syndromes. Studies of this coding schema demonstrate reasonable reliability for body location and etiology of pain[5] and evidence of clinical utility in deriving, coding, storing, and retrieving information on characteristics of pain.[6] In the years since the IASP formulated its definitions of pain and pain-related terms, it is relatively safe to conclude that these have been accepted by most clinicians and researchers in the field of pain.

The author gratefully acknowledges Carol Newman, RN, MN, PNP, Nurse Corps, U.S. Army (graduate student, Emory University Nell Hodgson Woodruff School of Nursing, 9/93-12/94) who assisted in the preparation of this chapter.

Perception and Experience of Pain

The crucial point to remember when measuring pain is its highly subjective and unique nature. The IASP and others recognize the importance of viewing pain from the vantage point of those experiencing it.[3,4] A commonly used example of this precept is McCaffery's statement: "Pain is whatever the experiencing person says it is, existing whenever he [sic] says it does."[7] Two concepts related to the subjectivity of the pain experience are important in individuals' responses to pain. *Threshold* refers to the point at which pain is first experienced, that is, the lowest level of potential injurious sensation that produces a report of pain. *Tolerance* is the point at which an individual reports pain to be so intense that it can no longer be tolerated. These two pain response concepts are generally measured in studies of laboratory-induced pain and have had little relevance to clinical pain. Traditionally, two opposing schools of thought on the nature of pain have existed. Both are based on Descartes's seventeenth-century notion that pain is an alarm system designed to signal bodily injury. The *specificity theory* proposed that pain was a specific entity, similar to sight or smell, with its own peripheral and central components. Specific pain receptors in the skin were thought to project to a specific pain center in the brain. The *pattern theory* proposed that there were no specific fibers or endings, but that the nerve impulse pattern for pain was produced by nonspecific receptor stimulation. Several versions of the pattern theory were developed, some stressing the intensity of the painful stimuli as the critical determinant of pain and others emphasizing a central summative mechanism.

Clinicians and researchers in the twentieth century developed a new concept of pain in which the perception of pain was determined by factors such as personality, previous experience, and culture.[8,9] In 1965 Melzack and Wall challenged the adequacy of the specificity and pattern theories to provide a satisfactory general explanation of the phenomenon of pain and proposed the now-classic *gate control theory*.[10] This theory postulated that pain phenomena were determined by the interactions among three spinal cord systems. First, peripheral stimulation sent nerve impulses to the substantia gelatinosa in the dorsal horn of the spinal cord, where these cells modulated the afferent impulses (the gate control mechanism). Second, the afferent patterns in the fibers of the dorsal column acted as a central control trigger that activated selective brain processes, which in turn influenced the modulating gate control properties of the substantia gelatinosa. Third, central transmission cells in the dorsal horn activated neural mechanisms believed to be responsible for the perception of and response to pain. The gate control theory helped to explain many puzzling aspects of the phenomenon of pain and placed emphasis on the sensory and emotional components of pain perception. Although some of the proposed components of the theory have not been documented experimentally, there appears to be universal acknowledgment of the importance and value of the gate control theory in guiding pain research and clinical pain management.[11]

Following introduction of the gate control theory, a new conceptual model of pain, comprised of three dimensions, was developed by Melzack and Casey.[3] According to these authors, selection and modulation of incoming pain sensations in the neospinothalamic projection system provide the basis for the sensory/discriminative component of pain. The brain reticular formation and limbic systems drive the aversive and affective reaction to pain, forming the motivational/affective component of pain. Finally, higher central nervous system or central control activities become involved in the pain experience and response. These activities are primarily cognitive functions that selectively influence sensory processes and/or motivational mechanisms. The influences of present and past experiences are believed integral to the cognitive activities. Thus, the pain experience is believed to be a function of the interaction of all three dimensions. This notion gradually evolved into a multidimensional concept of pain.

In the early 1980s, Ahles et al. described pain as a multidimensional experience consisting of physiologic, sensory, affective, cognitive, and behavioral aspects.[12] Although their conceptualization focused on cancer-related pain, it is generalizable to other types of pain for both research and clinical activities. McGuire[13] added a sociocultural dimension to this conceptualization and described specific, measurable components for each of the six dimensions.[14] The list on p. 533 briefly describes each dimension and relevant components. A considerable body of research literature supports the existence of this multidimensional conceptualization in cancer pain as well as in other types of acute and chronic pain.[15] Researchers wishing to measure the experience of pain from this comprehensive, multidimensional standpoint should select instruments that tap dimensions relevant to their work.

Types of Pain

Pain can be arbitrarily categorized, but two commonly used methods are duration and cause. A primary distinction must be drawn between pain caused by experimental procedures in the laboratory and pain due to various organic processes (usually termed *clinical pain*). Researchers in the field of pain have long disagreed about whether both types of pain are directly comparable.[16] Experimental and clinical pain are generally not considered synonymous. The former is transient and manageable, whereas the latter may be persistent and uncontrollable.

This chapter focuses on the measurement of clinical pain for research purposes. A distinction based on duration can be made. Acute pain is associated with tissue damage. It decreases with healing and is generally of short duration, that is, days to weeks. Bonica defined acute pain as "a complex constellation of unpleasant sensory, perceptual, and emotional experiences and certain associated autonomic, psychologic, emotional, and behavioral responses."[17] He emphasized that noxious stimulation from injury to or disease involving cutaneous and deep tissues and abnormal function of visceral or musculoskeletal tissues were the two major causes of acute pain. Examples of acute pain are incisional discomfort following a surgical procedure, cholecystitis, and the unpleasant sensations that follow hitting one's thumb with a hammer.

Alternatively, chronic pain generally persists for 6 months or more. Real or impending tissue damage may or may not be a factor. Examples include inflammatory joint or degenerative disk disease, postherpetic neuralgia, and persistent cancer pain.

Some authors have developed subcategories of acute and chronic pain.[18,19] For example, acute pain may become subacute (or limited) in cases of prolonged healing, such as a crushing musculoskeletal injury. Acute pain also may be recurrent (or intermittent), such as migraine headaches or sickle cell crisis. Chronic pain can be subdivided as well. Chronic pain caused by cancer is sometimes called *intractable pain*. Another variant of chronic pain is persistent or chronic benign pain, such as low back pain or neuralgias. Finally, a classification schema for cancer pain that includes both acute and chronic pain caused by cancer, its treatment, or other causes has been developed by Foley.[20]

Measuring Pain

When considering the instruments available for measuring pain, the researcher must be deliberate in selection. The overall objective is to achieve useful and reliable data in the most expedient and sound manner possible. Several factors are important in the selection process:[14]

Research question or goal. Instrument must mesh with the researcher's measurement goals, e.g., a survey of prevalence of pain in a specific sample of patients requires a different tool than evaluation of a therapeutic intervention for pain

Dimension(s) of pain that is being measured. Once the dimension(s) of the pain experience is determined, and perhaps the component of interest within the dimension, instrument selection is narrowed considerably

Type of pain being measured. Tools used to measure acute pain may not be appropriate for measurement of chronic pain, and vice versa. Assess research that reports previous use of the instrument of interest. Some tools may be appropriate for acute and chronic pain in their original form or with minor modification. If modifications are made, psychometric re-evaluation must occur

Nature of patient population. Many individual characteristics can influence an individual's ability to complete the instrument. Consider: education or literacy level, visual and hearing ability, motor coordination, cultural background and native language, diagnosis, type of pain, clinical environment, and acuity of illness. For example, use of a long and complex instrument is inappropriate in a sample of hearing-impaired people with acute pain; a short simple pain intensity scale might be a better choice.

Ease of administration and scoring. Respondent burden is a primary concern, particularly when the person is in pain. Minimize response time and effort. Burden on the researcher should also be considered, as should data entry and analysis capability.

Available data on reliability and validity of tools being considered. Data should be carefully evaluated as to benefits and limitations of using the instrument with a given sample. For many tools described in this chapter, authors are accessible and happy to provide more current information

Regardless of the type of clinical pain to be measured, various problems will be encountered. Viewing the experience of pain from the subjective stance of the sufferer is the first major problem. Pain measurement may be influenced by individualized perceptions of and responses to pain. Thus, patients experiencing pain are not easily comparable, even when their pain has the same etiology. Verbal reports of pain may not be readily verifiable, and particular measures of pain may mean different things to different people. Finally, health professionals may differ in their responses to persons with pain, occasionally underestimating or overestimating its severity.[21-23] Despite these subjective problems, pain remains a uniquely individual experience that is private, depends on many factors, and varies between people, but is consistent in each individual. When measuring clinical pain, these perspectives must be acknowledged and incorporated into any measurement strategy.

A variety of clinical and personal issues influence the measurement of pain as well. The type of pain, its etiology, and its duration are as important as the therapy employed. Patient characteristics such as educational level, nature and acuity of physical illness, presence of affective disorders,[24] age,[13,25-27] motor coordination, visual ability, sociocultural background,[13] level of comfort or pain, hearing ability, and cognitive impairment from a variety of causes including opioid analgesics,[28] will influence not only the measurement of pain in particular populations but also the instruments selected. Situational factors also can create problems, such as the physical environment, the health-care provider, or the presence or absence of family or friends.

A third problem that occurs in measuring pain is the limited number of available instruments that are quantifiable, reliable, and valid. Some researchers have developed clinical pain measures that, although subjective, can be quantified by various experimental pain procedures that match estimates of clinical pain sensations and verbal subjective judgments.[29] These sensory matching techniques, as they are called, are based on psychophysics.[30] Because sensory matching techniques have not been used extensively in the measurement of clinical pain, they are not discussed here.

Many researchers use ordinal-level Likert-type or interval-level visual analogue scales (VASs) to measure and quantify pain, but the validity of these instruments in measuring the total experience of pain is questionable. Because pain is multidimensional, researchers must be clear which dimension of pain and which components are to be measured. They must examine the validity and reliability of appropriate tools before selecting instruments. Because much psychometric support for existing tools has been selectively gathered from specific groups, settings, and time periods, the expansion of these tools to other groups must be done cautiously and with appropriate modification and further psychometric evaluation.

Finally, an important problem in measuring clinical pain are a number of ethical issues that are addressed in some detail by Sternbach.[31] Particularly problematic in experimental research is the administration or manipulation of pain that occurs as part of the normal design of such studies. Researchers must balance goals of increasing pain-specific knowledge and its management with the potential for coercion, physical harm, mental harm, or breach of human dignity. The procedures of any study involving pain, including and especially the measurement of pain, must observe all accepted standards for the rights and protection of human subjects.

The discussion of tools for measuring pain is limited to those that have been developed or used to measure clinical pain in adults. Reviews of instruments available to measure pain in children may be found elsewhere.[25,26,32] The multidimensional conceptualization of pain described serves as this chapter's organizing framework. A number of instruments measure only one dimension of pain, others measure two dimensions, still others, more than two dimensions. Instruments are presented in two sections: unidimensional and multidimensional. Within these dichotomies, instruments are categorized by the dimension(s) they measure. Only tools that measure clinical pain from the perspective of the individual or family experience are discussed. For instruments that measure institutional quality improvement (assurance) of pain management or professionals' knowledge and beliefs about pain or their pain management practices, the reader is referred to a number of other sources.[33-39]

The instruments chosen are, for the most part, well established, have been used for research purposes, are particularly applicable or appropriate for clinical research, have been developed fairly recently (with a few exceptions), and have evidence of reliability and validity. Reviews of additional instruments may be found in other publications on pain.[40,41] The chapter presents instruments that measure both acute and chronic pain, including types of pain that are very challenging to measure, such as pain in the critically ill, verbally or cognitively impaired, or terminally ill individuals. For each tool, the discussion includes the dimension(s) measured, a brief description of the tool, available psychometric data, examples of situations in which it has been used, recommendations for appropriate use in a research context, and advantages and disadvantages. Two or three instruments in each category are discussed, and additional measures are presented in Appendices 37B–37D.

The overall focus of this chapter is on the use of these instruments for measuring pain in a clinical research setting rather than assessing pain in the clinical practice setting. However, many of the tools presented are highly appropriate for use by the clinician in both assessing and managing pain.

Unidimensional Measurement Approaches

Physiologic Dimension

Few formal measurement tools address this dimension; however, a recent review article detailed numerous sophisticated cerebral measures available to study the brain's neurophysiologic activities when clinical pain is present.[42-43] Other variables encompassed by this dimension include onset and duration of pain, type of pain, and various etiologic and anatomic aspects of pain. These can be assessed using a variety of clinical pain assessment forms and flowsheets.[44-49] Some of these tools could be used in research.

Table 37.1 Dimensions of Pain and Their Components

1. Physiologic
   a. Etiology/organic origin of pain
   b. Type of pain (duration)
   c. Endogenous opioids
   d. Psychophysiologic factors
2. Sensory
   a. Location
   b. Intensity (severity)
   c. Quality
3. Affective
   a. Emotional responses (depression, mood, anxiety, worry, helplessness, fear)
   b. Suffering
   c. Psychiatric disorders
4. Cognitive
   a. Thought processes/views of self
   b. Meaning of pain
   c. Coping strategies
   d. Attitudes, beliefs, knowledge
   e. Influencing factors
   f. Level of cognition
5. Behavioral
   a. Indicators of pain
   b. Pain control behaviors
   c. Communication of pain
   d. Associated symptoms (fatigue, sleep)
6. Sociocultural
   a. Demographic variables
   b. Cultural background
   c. Personal, family, and work roles
   d. Family factors
   e. Caregiver perspectives

Sensory Dimension

Scales are commonly used to measure this dimension, and the variable generally measured is pain intensity. Occasionally, investigators use scales to measure degree of pain relief rather than pain intensity (e.g., "no relief" to "complete relief").[50] Although quality and pattern of pain also are part of this dimension of pain, they usually are measured in the context of multidimensional instruments. Two major categories of scales are used to measure pain intensity: verbal descriptor scales and visual analogue scales.

Verbal Descriptor Scales (VDS)

VDS measure pain intensity, a major component of the sensory dimension of pain. They usually consist of three to five numerically ranked descriptors: (1) none; (2) mild; (3) moderate; (4) severe; and (5) unbearable. The number corresponding to the word chosen can be used to analyze the data on an ordinal level. The forerunner of VDS appears to have been Keele's Pain Chart, originally devised to assess responses to analgesics over a 24-hour time period[51] with descriptors ranging from agony to severe to moderate to slight to nil.

The Pain Chart displays a time-intensity curve. Keele established the reliability of the chart by administering it repeatedly to patients with various painful medical conditions. He assessed validity by administering it to patients with known painful conditions, such as angina or peptic ulcer disease, and observing increases and decreases of pain on the time-intensity curve in relation to physical activity, treatment, and other factors.

Researchers also have used simple word descriptor lists rather than an entire pain chart, although Keele makes a good case for the usefulness of the Pain Chart in clinical and experimental research.[52] Melzack's Present Pain Intensity Scale (PPI) on the McGill Pain Questionnaire (see later) is an additional type of VDS commonly found in the literature:[53]

    _____ 0   No pain
    _____ 1   Mild
    _____ 2   Discomforting
    _____ 3   Distressing
    _____ 4   Horrible
    _____ 5   Excruciating

Few authors using VDS have discussed reliability and validity, but most agree that an individual's subjective rating of the intensity of pain using word descriptors probably is a valid measurement. Keele[52] used the Pain Chart to assess patients' responses to drugs and other therapy in many conditions, including postoperatively, in angina, in cancer, and in peptic ulcer disease. Kruszewski et al.[54] used a 5-point VDS to assess discomfort in surgical patients who received dorsogluteal injections while in various positions. Appropriate uses of the Pain Chart or simple VDS would include assessing responses to therapy in patients with these conditions as well as others, provided the investigator limited the variable measured to pain intensity.

VDS are brief, easy to administer and complete, easy to score, and applicable to many types of patients and to acute or chronic pain. The data produced are probably reliable and valid. On the other hand, the word descriptors on a VDS may artificially categorize the intensity of pain and may not accurately reflect an individual's real sensory experience. Alternatively, researchers have indicated that the category words on a VDS do not divide the perceptual continuum of pain into equal segments, may lack sufficient sensitivity to measure pain intensity,[55] and require patients to "abstract an 'average' pain intensity for the requested duration."[56,p165] This latter issue can be problematic when the researcher wishes to measure pain exactly at a specific point.

Visual Analogue Scales (VAS)

VAS were first developed approximately 60 years ago to measure various subjective phenomena,[57] but the reference cited by most researchers using VAS is that of Clarke and Spear.[58] Gift[59] and Cline et al.[60] discussed a number of issues associated with using VAS to measure subjective phenomena (e.g., pain, depression, dyspnea) in research situations, including psychometric properties, advantages and disadvantages, and technical preparation and scoring. The patient is asked to place a mark through the line at the point that best describes how much pain is experienced at a particular moment. The VAS is called a Graphic Rating Scale (GRS) if descriptive words are placed along the line:[61]

No pain	Mild	Moderate	Severe	Pain as bad as it could possibly be

In pain research, VAS are generally used to measure the intensity of pain. The VAS usually consists of a 10-cm line with verbal anchors at either end:

No pain	Pain as bad as it could possibly be

Some researchers have focused on alternative formats for the VAS. One type is a mechanical format, generally described as a slide-rule type of plastic device showing a 10-cm horizontal VAS on the front with a movable tab that provides immediate feedback of numerical measures on its reverse side.[62,63] Another format is described as a "nonvisual" analogue scale[64] or a "pain intensity number" scale[65] that requests patients to score their pain on a scale from 0 (no pain) to 10 (the worst pain imaginable). The number selected by the patient, even if a fraction, is considered to be the pain intensity "score." Finally, a third VAS format is a curvilinear line (a 100-degree sector of a semicircle, 15 cm in diameter, divided into one-degree units).[66] Interval-level data are obtained on visual or graphic scales by measuring from the left end of the scale to the mark made by the patient. Price et al.[67] have validated the use of VAS as ratio-scale measures in chronic and experimental pain. VAS are considered more sensitive measures of pain intensity than VDS because they have a straight-line continuum rather than categorical responses. One report,[50] however, found no differences in sensitivity when comparing these scales. Many researchers using VAS have discussed reliability/validity issues in their published reports. Revill et al.[68] used a VAS with ten women in labor and demonstrated reliability on repeated measurements ($r = 0.95$, $p < 0.001$). Similarly, Clarke and Spear[58] found the VAS reliable and sensitive to changes in the self-assessment of well-being. Although Maxwell[57] did not study pain, he found that individuals rating sound volumes had more sensitive and accurate ratings on a VAS than did different subjects, suggesting that using VAS to compare groups might not produce reliable measures across the different groups. Dixon and Bird[69] demonstrated that subjects' ($n = 8$) ability to reproduce a set of marked scales within a given time often was inconsistent, suggesting that estimations of the same sensation could be placed at different points on the scale over time. Carlsson[70] found that in patients with chronic pain, a regular VAS was less sensitive to bias than a comparative VAS.

Liu and Aitkenhead[71] found in their study of patients with postoperative pain that repeated contemporaneous (present) pain assessments were more reliable than a single retrospective pain assessment (made for a preceding 24- or 48-hour period). Although these reliability data are somewhat varied, validity of the VAS seems to have been assumed, as with the VDS. Investigators testing mechanical and nonvisual formats of the VAS[62,63] examined concurrent validity of their new tools by comparing them to standard VAS and VDS, finding significant correlations that substantiated the validity of their newly formatted VAS. Grossman et al.[62] also examined test–retest reliability, demonstrating a high correlation ($r = 0.97$, $p < 0.001$) of repeated measures 5 minutes apart for a mechanical VAS. In general, subjective ratings of pain intensity may be considered reasonably valid regardless of the scale used.

VAS have been used to measure pain intensity in a variety of patients, including women in labor,[68] people with cancer,[72] patients with acute postoperative pain,[66,71] patients with burn pain, people with arthritis, and others. Appropriate use of the VAS would encompass any group of patients with acute or chronic pain, provided such use was restricted to the measurement of pain intensity. The evaluation of treatment outcomes, particularly pharmacologic interventions, is a popular application of VAS in clinical research.

VAS are easy to administer and score. In addition, because VAS are considered to produce interval-level data, parametric statistics may be used in analysis. VAS have several disadvantages. Although it is unclear whether people prefer horizontal or vertical VAS format,[73] some people have difficulty conceptualizing a sensory phenomenon, such as pain intensity, in a straight-line continuum. They may place their marks near the anchor words, yielding data of questionable reliability and validity. Scott and Huskisson[74] believe that patient access to previous scores is important in obtaining accurate subsequent measures when administering the VAS repeatedly because previous ratings can be used for comparison. Careful instructions to research subjects regarding how to rate pain intensity on a VAS are imperative to proper understanding and use.

Comparisons of Scales

Because both VDS and VAS measure pain intensity, many researchers have compared the two in terms of sensitivity, reliability, validity, ease of administration and patient use, and patient preference. Correlations ranging from 0.66 to 0.89 ($p = 0.01$ to 0.001) between VDS and VAS were found in several studies.[50,62,65,75-78] When Wallenstein[77] compared scores from one population of patients to another, he found a high degree of reliability in the obtained measures and no obvious or consistent response effects related to gender or age. Studies of different forms of the VDS and VAS have been performed as well. These are described in Appendix 37A.[79-85] The results of these comparative studies indicate that the scales discussed are useful for measuring perceived pain intensity and, in general, correlate reasonably well. Their reliability is relatively well established, but any researcher using such scales must consider the individual characteristics of both patients and settings before choosing specific scales. For example, the VAS may be too abstract for patients with severe acute pain, lower educational levels, or impaired motor coordination. In such instances, a VDS may be easier to use and may produce more reliable data.

Affective Dimension

This dimension involves how pain makes individuals feel and includes such variables as distress, anxiety, depression, mood, and others. Numerous instruments exist to measure these constructs, but few investigators have developed tools specifically to measure this dimension of pain, usually with VAS or VDS. Ahles et al.[86] used a 10-cm VAS to measure depression and anxiety in patients with cancer pain. The left anchor was "I am not depressed (anxious)" and the right anchor was "I am as depressed (anxious) as I can possibly imagine myself being." They found support for the validity of the VAS-depression through significant ($p = 0.05$) correlations with the Beck Depression Inventory ($r = 0.51$) and depression subscale of the Symptom Checklist-90 (SCL-90) ($r = 0.41$). The VAS-anxiety, however, was not significantly correlated with the anxiety subscale of the SCL-

90 or the State Anxiety Inventory. The VAS for depression may provide a simple, valid, and clinically practical method for measuring this component of the affective dimension.

Price et al.[87] took a different approach to this dimension, measuring the "degree of unpleasantness" associated with pain intensity using a 15-cm VAS with word anchors "not bad at all" and "the most unpleasant feeling possible for me" at either end. Patients with different types of pain (experimental, low back pain, upper back pain, myofascial pain, causalgia, cancer pain, and labor pain) were studied. These researchers hypothesized that affective ratings of pain would be higher in patients whose pain was associated with serious or life-threatening illness (e.g., cancer), given comparable levels of pain intensity. They also proposed that women in labor who focused on their impending birth rather than on labor pain itself would have lower affective (unpleasantness) ratings. Their results demonstrated that, although many patients reported a wide range of sensory and affective ratings, in general VAS affective ratings were significantly higher than VAS sensory ratings ($p < 0.01$) in cancer patients. Laboring women who focused on their babies had affective ratings approximately 50% lower than those who focused solely on their pain. The overall findings clearly indicate the importance of distinguishing between sensory and affective dimensions of pain, particularly in certain types of pain.

Finally, Jensen et al.[83] investigated the use of two verbal rating scales of pain affect, one with 11 descriptors ranging from "bearable" to "agonizing" and the other with 15 descriptors ranging from "slightly unpleasant" to "very intolerable," and compared them to eight measures of pain. Factor analyses revealed only a single factor consisting of all the intensity scales plus the two affective scales. In discussing their results, the investigators commented that the 30 correlations (covariations) of these two dimensions of pain could be attributed to their patients' acute pain, the clinical conditions under which the instruments were administered, lack of explanation to patients about the distinction between sensory and affective components of pain, or lack of usefulness of the affective scales as a measure of the affective dimension of acute clinical pain. In any case, it is clear that these scales require further evaluation.

Cognitive Dimension

As with the Physiologic Dimension, there are few pain specific unidimensional measures for the Cognitive Dimension. Some components, such as coping strategies, may be measured with tools designed for that particular construct. In general, most measures of the Cognitive Dimension are incorporated into multidimensional instruments. In addition, many components of this dimension, such as factors that exacerbate or lessen pain, can be easily assessed using some of the clinical tools cited earlier.[44,45]

Behavioral Dimension

The behavioral dimension has two major components: behaviors that are observable indicators of the presence and/or severity of pain (e.g., grimacing, nonverbal vocalizations, communication with others, guarding and splinting, fatigue), and behaviors that individuals engage in to decrease or control their pain (e.g., use of medications, positioning, sleep/rest/activity patterns). Many components of this dimension are measured within the context of multidimensional instruments such as diaries. A number of instruments, however, have been developed specifically to measure this dimension of pain in patients with acute pain who cannot complete self-report tools (such as those recovering from anesthesia) or in patients with chronic pain that affects numerous activities of daily living. Some instruments are reviewed in detail, and others are presented in Appendix 37B.[88-93]

Acute Pain

PACU Behavioral Scale. Mateo and Krenzischek[94] adapted the Chambers and Price Pain Rating Scale (Appendix 37B) to measure the behavioral manifestations of pain in patients recovering from general anesthesia with an instrument called the Post Anesthesia Care Unit (PACU) Pain Rating Scale. The purpose of their pilot study was to determine whether selected behaviors were associated with pain in PACU patients. In their adaptation of the Chambers and Price tool, they omitted attention, anxiety, nausea, and perspiration because these were deemed not relevant to the pain experienced by individuals recovering from anesthesia. They retained the behaviors of restlessness, tense muscles, frowning or grimacing, and patient sounds. Each of these four pain behavior categories was measured with a scale having a zero base and clearly defined progression through ratings of 1, 2, and 3. For example:

Patient sounds: 0 = talking in normal tone or no sound
1 = sighs, groans, moans softly
2 = groans, moans loudly
3 = cries out or sobs

In addition to these behavior categories, they used a four-point VDS (0 none, 1 mild, 2 moderate, 3 severe) for self-report of pain intensity. They ensured content validity through an expert panel: two clinical nurse researchers (one with expertise in pain assessment), a clinical nurse specialist in pain management, and several expert PACU nurses. They assessed the potential intervening variable of level of consciousness with the Glasgow Coma Scale.

In their initial validation study, the two authors observed 30 PACU patients (following gastrointestinal surgery) at two separate points, immediately after the patient's admission to the PACU, and within an hour after admission. After a pilot with five patients, they developed the following observation procedure, carried out at both timepoints: (1) the patient was verbally stimulated and level of consciousness assessed with the Glasgow Coma Scale; (2) the patient was observed by the two investigators simultaneously for 10 minutes, using the PACU; and (3) the patient was asked to complete the four-point VDS. If patients required pain medication, the researchers delayed the observation for 10 minutes to allow the medication to take effect.

The internal consistency of the PACU Behavioral Pain Rating Scale was assessed with coefficient alpha, which was 0.92. The investigators' interrater reliability across patients was measured with Pearson's correlation coefficient and ranged from 0.71 to 1.0. At the first timepoint (immediately after admission to the PACU), frowning or grimacing was significantly correlated with self-reports of pain intensity ($r = 0.69$, $p < 0.05$), but at the second timepoint (within an hour of admission), muscle tension and patient sounds ($r = 0.64$ and 0.63, respectively, $p < 0.05$) were significantly correlated with pain intensity. The VDS results indicated mild pain at time 1 and moderate pain at time 2. Glasgow Coma Scale scores remained similar across timepoints, so the relationship between level of consciousness and pain could not be adequately assessed. Mateo and Krenziscek concluded that although their scale appeared to be a reliable and valid modification of the Chambers and Price scale, it needed further testing for reliability and validity.

In a subsequent study of 50 PACU patients who had undergone gastrointestinal surgery, the instrument was used to assess pain at two timepoints.[95] At time 1 frowning/grimacing, muscle tension, and sounds were correlated with self-reports of pain intensity ($r = 0.45$–0.63; $p \leq 0.01$), and at time 2 frowning/grimacing, muscle tension, and restlessness were correlated with self-reports of pain intensity ($r = 0.42$–0.52, $p \leq 0.01$). Mateo and colleagues concluded that a sequence of pain-related behaviors occurred in patients recovering from anesthesia and that these behaviors were useful in early assessment of pain in this population.

A recent report by Webb and Kennedy[96] substantiated the reliability and validity of the PACU Behavioral Pain Rating Scale (BPRS) in a sample of 36 postoperative gynecologic surgery patients who were all receiving patient-controlled analgesia. These investigators used the BPRS in an unaltered format, but changed the pain intensity scale to 0 to 10 (to allow for more variance in pain scores), administering both scales five times to each patient within 6 hours of surgery. Their Cronbach's alphas ranged from 0.73 to 0.90. Correlations between patients' PACU BPRS and pain intensity scale scores ranged from $r = 0.56$ to 0.80 ($p < 0.05$), decreasing over time, with the highest scores within 2 hours of surgery. They stated that observations from their study indicated "that these scales used alone would not be as reliable" as when used in conjunction with others.[96,p94] In summary, the initial psychometric evidence on the PACU BPRS suggests that it has good potential applicability for research purposes in postanesthesia patients. It requires, however, further evaluation for its psychometric properties, for its ability to measure changes resulting from pain interventions, and for its applicability to other cognitively impaired patients.

Distress Checklist. This instrument was developed by Wells[97] to measure behavioral indicators of distress during painful and anxiety-producing medical procedures. Although the author defined distress as a negative emotional state in response to pain (i.e., the affective dimension of pain), she noted that emotional distress, including pain-related distress, could be observed through such behaviors as facial expression, posture, vocalization, and verbalization. Wells selected first-trimester abortion as the painful medical procedure of interest and compiled her checklist of behaviors from previous research. Her initial tool included 14 behaviors grouped into four categories of emotional distress: (1) facial expression (e.g., tension—mouth); (2) posture (e.g., flinch); (3) vocalization (e.g., audible expression); and (4) verbalization (e.g., requests termination of procedure). During the painful procedure, the instrument was used to observe patients, with behaviors scored as present or absent, then summed for a total behavioral distress score. Higher scores reflected greater distress.

Wells tested the instrument on 36 women undergoing first-trimester abortion. She obtained a preprocedure heart rate and State-Trait Anxiety Inventory, used the Distress Checklist during the procedure, and collected self-report VASs of sensation and distress and an observer-rated VAS of distress at the completion of the procedure. The McGill Pain Questionnaire was administered using an interview format after the patient was admitted to the recovery room. Wells noted that stability was not evaluated because of the transient nature of distress, but test–retest reliability assessed through interrater agreement in a subset of five patients was 100%. Internal consistency was examined using interitem correlations and the Kuder-Richardson-20. After several analyses, several items were deleted, yielding a KR-20 of 0.71 for the seven remaining. These behaviors were spread across the four categories of emotional distress as follows: (1) facial expression: tension around eyes, tension around mouth; (2) posture: flinch, fists clenched; (3) vocalization: audible expiration, pain expression; and (4) verbalization: requests termination. The summed score of these seven items was used in all subsequent analyses. No demographic or clinical variables were found to be related to behavioral distress (e.g., age, number of previous abortions or births). Wells noted that content validation was performed, but did not describe specific procedures. Concurrent validity was examined through correlational analysis, demonstrating that behavioral distress was significantly and positively correlated with self-reported ($r = 0.74, p < 0.01$) and observer-reported ($r = 0.51, p < 0.49$) distress, but not correlated with heart rate. Construct validity was evaluated in two ways, first by determining whether behavioral distress was different from state anxiety and pain intensity. Behavioral distress was significantly and positively correlated with self-reports of pain sensation on the VAS ($r = 0.66, p$ not given), but not correlated with state anxiety or pain intensity as measured by the McGill Pain Questionnaire Pain Rating Index. The second construct validation procedure was the contrasted groups approach, in which Wells hypothesized that women having an abortion with local anesthesia would have more behavioral distress than those having an abortion with intravenous sedation. This hypothesis was supported ($t[29] = 2.99, p = 0.006$), and no other potential confounding variables (e.g., pain intensity, demographic variables) were significantly different. In addition, women with previous abortions had higher mean behavioral distress scores, suggesting a sensitizing, rather than distress-reducing, effect.

In conclusion, although this instrument had adequate reliability and validity on its preliminary testing, the deletion of seven of its original items calls into question its 39 conceptual foundations. The author noted that there may be differences between distress generated by the pain of a medical procedure and distress generated by the entire situation surrounding the procedure. Nevertheless, this instrument clearly measures pain-related distress. It certainly requires further testing in various populations and with a variety of pain-producing procedures, but has potential as a useful outcome measure in clinical research.

Observations of Pain Behaviors During Sickle Cell Pain.[98] The assessment of acute pain due to sickle cell disease has received little attention from researchers and clinicians. Gil and colleagues,[98] however, tried to address this gap by assessing the utility of a brief behavioral observation tool for use during sickle cell crisis. Using literature describing behavioral indicators of pain in various patient populations, these investigators developed a checklist consisting of five behaviors (guarding, bracing, rubbing, grimacing, and sighing) with written definitions and a scoring system of 0 (absent) and 1 (present). Thirty-one patients with sickle cell disease in painful crisis were approached in the clinic and if they consented, were observed by a physician (who had received training in observing pain-related behaviors) and by the first author of the paper. The patients also completed the Short Form McGill Pain Questionnaire (SF-MPQ) (see later) and a pain intensity scale ranging from 0 (no pain) to 10 (pain as bad as it can be). In addition, the physician rated patients' pain on a scale of 0 (no pain/discomfort) to 10 (pain, discomfort as bad as it can be), and a second observer completed the same scale for 13 patients. Interrater reliability for the five behaviors overall was 0.86 and ranged from 0.69 (grimacing) to 1.0 (guarding). The two observers' ratings were significantly related ($r = 0.89, p < 0.0001$). The physician's pain ratings were lower than the patients' ratings on the Pain Rating Index (PRI) from the SF-MPQ or intensity scale and were not significantly correlated. On the other hand, the physician's ratios of patients' pain behaviors were significantly correlated with his ratings on the 0 to 10 scale ($r = 0.50–0.68, p = 0.01–0.0001$). Finally, patients' self-reports of pain intensity on the PRI and the 0 to 10 scale were not correlated with observed pain behaviors. Assessment of relationships between observed behaviors and factors thought to influence them (e.g., number of acute painful events, type of sickle cell disease) revealed no significant relationships. The authors concluded that their preliminary study provided evidence for the utility of this tool and that it possibly was sensitive to the variation of behaviors shown by patients (e.g., high incidence of guarding, sighing, and grimacing). This approach to assessing pain may be helpful in some clinical situations, but the investigators did not make a compelling case for its use over the more standard, and valid, approach of using patient subjective self-report. Researchers who want to employ this tool should take into consideration the preliminary nature of this study and its methodologic limitations, such as small sample size, single geographic location, and use of only one physician observer who was visible to patients. Although the tool holds promise, further psychometric evaluation is warranted using standard tools to determine its validity.

Chronic Pain

Some instruments are discussed in detail, and others are presented in Appendix 37C.[99-106]

Observation Method for Cancer Pain. Ahles and his colleagues[107] extended previous work on behavioral observation and tested interobserver reliability, concurrent validity, and construct validity of this approach in 19 patients with terminal cancer. Patients participated in a 10-minute videotaped recording that including sitting, standing, reclining, and walking. Videotapes were scored by two trained observers for four behaviors (sitting, reclining, standing, and movement) and five concomitant pain behaviors (guarding, bracing, rubbing, grimacing, and verbal pain behavior) over 20 observation intervals. Patients also completed a self-report VAS of pain intensity (no pain to worst pain you can imagine) and the Sickness Impact Profile (SIP), a measure of physical and psychosocial impact of an illness. A research nurse rated each patient's level of functioning on the Global Adjustment to Illness Scale (GAIS). Two nurses and three undergraduate students reviewed the videotapes and rated their perceptions of patients' pain using an 11-point numerical scale (0 no pain, 10 pain as bad as it could be), a 10-cm VAS (anchors of none to as bad as it could be), and an adjective scale comprised of 15 sensory pain descriptors. These scales were completed in a counterbalanced and independent manner by the raters, who were blind to patients' pain behavior scores.

Interobserver reliability was demonstrated through percentage agreements (occurrence versus nonoccurrence of behaviors) ranging from 96% to 99% and percentage effective agreements (occurrence divided by number of intervals with agreement and disagreement) ranging from 61% to 91%. Guarding and bracing occurred most commonly. None of the pain behavior scores correlated significantly with the VAS-Pain. The total pain behavior score ($r = 0.52$, $p < 0.05$) and guarding behaviors ($r = 0.68$, $p < 0.01$) and bracing ($r = 0.54$, $p < 0.02$) were significantly correlated with the SIP-Physical scale. The GAIS correlated negatively with guarding, verbal pain, and total pain behavior score (lower GAIS scores indicate more dysfunction). Finally, the total number of pain behaviors was highly correlated with both nurses' and students' ratings on the three pain scales ($r = 0.62$–0.80, $p < 0.01$).

The investigators concluded that their data supported the reliability of this behavioral observation method. They also noted that high correlations between pain behavior scores and the SIP-Physical and GAIS and nurses' and students' pain ratings provided evidence of validity. Differences between nurses' and students' ratings, however, suggested that professional and nonprofessional groups may use different pain behavior patterns in making judgments about pain. Lack of correlation between pain behavior scores and the VAS-Pain was thought to be due to mild to moderate levels of pain in these patients, who were all receiving morphine through an implanted pump. In addition, the VAS-Pain was completed by patients while at rest, and for many, pain occurred on movement. Despite these limitations, the investigators noted that their approach held promise as a measure of pain behavior in cancer patients. Certainly, this approach requires further evaluation, but it does have potential as an adjunct to self-report or, in some cases, a proxy measure if patients are unable to report pain.

Sociocultural Dimension

This dimension has a number of components (see list on p. 533), most notably the ethnocultural and familial-social aspects of the pain experience. Additional components included in this dimension are the beliefs, attitudes, and values about pain held by lay and professional individuals. Discussion of tools that measure these concepts is beyond the scope of this chapter, as many of them take the form of survey questionnaires, lack rigorous psychometric evaluation, and are clinically oriented. Few instruments have been developed specifically to measure this dimension of pain, although numerous tools are available that measure related concepts, such as social support.

Family Pain Questionnaire

Ferrell and colleagues developed the Family Pain Questionnaire (FPQ) in tandem with a Patient Pain Questionnaire (see later) to measure knowledge and experiences of family members caring for patients with pain.[108-110] The FPQ was originally described as a 21-item linear analogue tool with knowledge items and experience items.[108] These two areas are encompassed within the cognitive and sensory dimensions of pain, but because they are asked of family caregivers, the tool is placed in the sociocultural dimension. Examples of knowledge and experience items, respectively, are:

Patients are often given too much pain medicine.

Agre _____ Disagree

How much pain is your family member having now?

No pain _____ A great deal

The published articles provide scant information on the psychometric development and evaluation of the tool, but another publication[111] provides some detail. The tool has an overall reliability of $r = 0.92$ ($p = 0.01$), evidence of content validity by expert review, and now has 13 items (9 knowledge, 4 experience). The authors will provide on request a copy of the FPQ and its scoring criteria. Readers who desire more specific information on the psychometric testing of the FPQ are advised to contact the primary author. This tool is helpful in ascertaining knowledge and experiences of family caregivers and could provide useful baseline information prior to initiating family-oriented intervention studies. Examples of further psychometric development, or use of the tool in other published studies, are scant at present.

Multidimensional Approaches

The instruments reviewed previously measure only one dimension of pain experience and are limited in their ability to provide a comprehensive picture of pain. For a number of research projects, however, unidimensional measurement of the pain experience may be quite appropriate and even desirable. The instruments now described were devised to measure more than one dimension of pain simultaneously. Appendix 37D briefly describes additional tools.[112-144]

Short Form McGill Pain Questionnaire (SF-MPQ)

In 1987 Melzack[145] introduced a short form of the MPQ, developed to provide a shorter and quicker multidimensional measure of pain in clinical settings than the original MPQ. This tool consisted of two sections. In the first one, 11 sensory words (throbbing, shooting, stabbing, sharp, cramping, gnawing, hot-burning, aching, heavy, tender, splitting) and 4 affective words (tiring-exhausting, sickening, fearful, punishing-cruel) were listed. These descriptor words were selected because they had been chosen by 33% or more of patients with labor, menstrual, headache, phantom limb, postherpetic, dental, cancer, arthritis, and low back pain in previous studies. Each word was accompanied by 0 to 3 severity ratings (0 none, 1 mild, 2 moderate, 3 severe). Three scores were derived by summing the intensity rank values of all selected words: a sensory score, an affective score, and a total score. In the second section, two measures of pain intensity were included: the Present Pain Intensity Index (PPI) from the original MPQ, and a 10-cm VAS with anchors of "no pain" and "worst possible pain." Melzack conducted two validation studies[145] of an English version of the tool as well as a Quebec French version.

First, the Long Form (LF) MPQ was presented to postsurgical (n = 40), obstetrical (n = 20), and musculoskeletal (n = 10) patients, followed by the Short Form (SF) MPQ. Patients were tested twice, before and after medication or other treatment for pain. Second, the tools were given in random order to postsurgical (n = 31) and dental (n = 31) patients. No reliability data were reported. Concurrent validity was substantiated in analyses that demonstrated significant correlations (r = 0.51, p < 0.03) between nearly all the sensory, affective, total, and intensity scores (PPI, VAS) of the LF and SF, in all types of pain, and both before and after pain treatment. As evidence of construct validity, both the LF and SF demonstrated the significant effects of analgesics in postsurgical patients and women in labor receiving epidural blocks. Melzack also noted that these patients' selections of descriptors varied according to their type of pain, showing qualitative patterns and changes following the administration of analgesics. Melzack concluded that the SF-MPQ appeared to be a useful tool, correlating highly with the sensory, affective, and total indices on the LF-MPQ. He suggested that it might be helpful for studies in which investigators had limited time to obtain information from subjects. He reported that it took about 2 to 5 minutes to administer and was understood easily by all the subjects in his study. He also noted that further evaluation of the tool was needed to explore its use in other patient populations and clinical situations. Few subsequent validation studies have been performed on the SF-MPQ. One notable exception was a report by Dudgeon and colleagues[146] who studied the tool in 24 patients with metastatic disease and chronic pain related to their cancer. Both the LF and SF were administered to each patient on three separate occasions (3 to 4 weeks apart) and were scored according to the original instructions. Sensory, affective, total, PPI, and VAS scores were highly correlated at all measurement times (r = 0.67 to 0.91, p < 0.001). Correlations tended to be higher when the SF was given first, although generally not significantly so. The data also indicated that the SF reflected changes in pain over time (as did the LF), thus making it sensitive to therapeutic interventions for pain.

Swanston et al.[147] described a method for assessing pain using interactive computer animation and validating it by comparing it to the SF-MPQ. These investigators developed a unique way of assessing pain by having patients select colored graphic computer images representing four different types of pain: pressure, burning, throbbing, and piercing (chosen for their concreteness and their correspondence with descriptors on the SF-MPQ), and an interactive version of the VAS. Fifty-four patients attending a pain clinic for a variety of reasons comprised the initial sample; four of these did not regard interactive animation as appropriate for describing their pain, yielding a final sample size of 50. Each patient indicated whether each computer image described his or her pain and then selected a point on the range of minimum to maximum for the image. For example, pressure was depicted by a vise squeezing a round, ball-like object that ranged from a full round circle (minimum) to a narrow convex disk (maximum) as pressure increased. All correlations between the four descriptors and the VAS on the interactive animation software and the SF-MPQ were significant at $p < 0.05$, with the highest correlations being 64 between the VAS measures ($r = 0.87$, $p < 0.01$). Whether these results demonstrate validity (in part) of the SF-MPQ, or whether they demonstrate concurrent validity of the interactive assessment technique is not entirely clear; the answer is probably both. In any case, the results suggest that the SF-MPQ is acceptable to patients and performs well clinically. McGuire and colleagues[148] used the SF-MPQ to assess acute oral pain in 48 patients receiving high-dose chemotherapy and bone marrow transplantation for their malignancies. The SF was used daily to assess oral pain from the time it was initially reported by patients until it resolved. Although the study did not examine any psychometric properties of the SF, the investigators noted that the sensory component of pain appeared more germane than the affective component to these patients. The tool was not always easy to use, as patients had some difficulty considering and selecting verbal descriptors of their pain between days 5 and 6 after the transplant, when oral mucositis and pain tended to be worse. Overall, the SF was useful in this patient population and demonstrated patterns of pain that were commensurate with the development, peaking, and resolution of oral mucositis. In summary, the SF-MPQ appears to have been accepted by a number of researchers as a reliable and valid short method for measuring the sensory and affective dimensions of clinical pain. Its psychometric properties probably still need further exploration, especially in patient populations in whom it has not been used and in repeated-measure situations. Investigators who need a quick, feasible measure, particularly when testing interventions, should certainly consider using it, and if possible, should conduct concurrent validation studies.

Brief Pain Inventory

Another multidimensional instrument for measuring pain, also modeled after the McGill Pain Questionnaire, is the Wisconsin Brief Pain Questionnaire,[149] now known as the Brief Pain Inventory (BPI).[150] It is a survey instrument originally constructed to measure pain caused by cancer and other diseases, such as rheumatoid arthritis or chronic orthopedic problems. Items on the BPI address pain history, etiology, intensity, location, quality, and interference with activities. With these items, the tool addresses the sensory, affective, cognitive, behavioral, and sociocultural dimensions of pain. An example of an intensity item (sensory dimension) is:

Please rate your pain by circling the one number that tells how much pain you have right now:

	0	1	2	3	4	5	6	7	8	9	10
No Pain											Pain as bad as you can imagine

A basic stem item is used to address the interference of pain with components of the affective, cognitive, behavioral, and sociocultural dimensions. For example: the individual is asked to "Circle the one number that describes how, during the past 24 hours, pain has interfered with your general activity: 0 (does not interfere) to 10 (completely interferes)."

Additional items using this stem include mood, walking ability, normal work (inside and outside the home), relations with other people, sleep, and enjoyment of life.

Daut et al.[149] demonstrated respectable test–retest reliability over short periods. The validity of the tool was assessed with cancer patients. Differences in severity of pain were found in patients with metastatic cancer (who had more pain) and those without (who had less pain). Ratings of interference with activities increased as severity of pain increased, and the number of patients who received narcotic analgesics increased as severity ratings increased. Finally, when used in different diseases, it was found that intercorrelations among pain measurers differed, suggesting that the BPI was sensitive to different pain characteristics.

There is little additional published data on the reliability and validity of this instrument, although Cleeland[151] noted in a review article that factor analysis had been used to "uncover dimensions accounted for by our several subjective assessment measures."[151,p396] Data from a recent survey of 1,308 cancer outpatients treated in participating institutions of the Eastern Cooperative Oncology Group (ECOG)[152] have been subjected to psychometric analyses.[153] The overall group data revealed two major factors on the BPI—pain severity and pain interference. Internal consistency reliability of the severity and interference subscales on the BPI revealed alpha coefficients of 0.88 and 0.92, respectively. In a subgroup of 49 minority patients cared for in an inner-city hospital, the same two factors were observed and alpha coefficients on subscales were 0.84 for pain severity and 0.92 for pain interference.

The BPI can be used to measure pain in cancer and other conditions, although it is seen most frequently in studies of patients with cancer-related pain. The sample in the ECOG study cited included a substantial number of minority patients, some with low levels of literacy. Analysis of the BPI with several readability formulas indicates that its reading level ranges from 6.0 to 7.6 depending on the formula (D. McGuire, unpublished data, June 1994). The BPI is clearly useful for surveys of patients in which superficial information is needed. The instrument is short, easily understood, designed for self-administration, and easy to score. Its readability level and comprehensive nature make it particularly suited for clinical research. It has clinical utility as well because it was recommended as a comprehensive assessment tool in the Clinical Practice Guidelines for Management of Cancer Pain.[49] The version in the guidelines is called the Brief Pain Inventory (Short Form) and consists of 9 items total (1 pain prevalence, 1 pain location, 4 pain intensity, 2 pain treatment, and 1 pain interference [with 7 subcomponents to tap multiple dimensions]). There is little evidence to date that the BPI has been used as an outcome measure in pain intervention studies, but efforts are under way in this area.

Pain-O-Meter

The Pain-O-Meter (POM) was designed as a multidimensional measure of clinical pain[154] beginning with the exploration of verbal descriptors of painlike experiences (e.g., pain, ache, hurt) done in the mid-1980s.[155,156] The instrument is based on the gate control theory of pain and uses verbal descriptors from the McGill Pain Questionnaire. It is patented (U.S. patent #5,018,526) and is made of hard white plastic, 8 inches long, 2 inches wide, and 1 inch thick. It can be easily be held in one's hand. On one side there are two lists of words. The top half has sensory descriptors (e.g., cramping, splitting, shooting, crushing, stabbing, sharp), and the bottom half has emotional descriptors (e.g., nagging, annoying, tiring, sickening, torturing). Respondents can select the descriptors that apply to their pain. These lists include words that reflect the sensory, affective, and cognitive dimensions of pain. On the other side of the POM is a 0- to 100-mm VAS formatted vertically with anchors of no pain on the bottom and excruciating pain on top. Respondents move an adjustable tab to indicate the intensity of their pain.

Gaston-Johansson has indicated that a new model of the POM exists but is not yet in use.[154] This new model (same patent number) has several additional features. The two verbal descriptor lists now include an adjustable indicator for each descriptor that patients can use to show whether the descriptor applies to their pain or not. There also is a vertically formatted VAS with anchors of no pain and worst possible pain and a sliding indicator. On the other, there are now three items: (1) a 10-cm ruled scale with no anchors shown; (2) an item asking if pain is continuous or comes and goes; and (3) drawings of the front and back of a human figure that patients can shade to show the location of their pain (using a system of numbers on the side, letters across the top, and small squares placed directly on the figure). This model also encompasses the sensory, affective, and cognitive dimensions of pain.

The instrument was initially developed in Sweden, but an American version (A-POM) exists and has been subjected to extensive psychometric evaluation, much of it unpublished as yet.[154] In both published[157,158] and unpublished data, Gaston-Johansson details the procedures used to select descriptors for the A-POM. She used a sample of 522 subjects: 73 registered nurses, 42 physicians, 60 chronic pain patients, 40 acute pain patients, 100 lay individuals (caucasians), 75 Hispanics, 69 American Indians, and 63 African Americans to ensure that the final version of the A-POM would have applicability across cultural groups, patients, and care providers. The selected descriptors were then used to construct an instrument using the same design as the Swedish one. Although these descriptors are from the McGill Pain Questionnaire, it is important to note that in the A-POM they are not presented with intensity values; the numbers and letters corresponding to them are for recording purposes only. Thus, there appear to be no summed "sensory," "affective," or "total" scores on the A-POM, which may pose a problem in using the instrument to measure changes related to pain interventions.

Gaston-Johansson[154] describes initial psychometric validation of the instrument that included content validity of the verbal descriptors in 19 health professionals (no specific data were reported), usability in 15 patients with various types of pain including acute myocardial infarction (satisfactory), test–retest reliability in laboring multiparas (sensory $r = 0.80$, $p < 0.001$; affective $r = 0.58$, $p < 0.004$), and construct validity via hypothesis testing in laboring multiparas and patients with postoperative pain (supported). Several published articles also present supportive data on the construct- and criterion-related validity of the POM in women with labor pain[159] and patients undergoing autologous bone marrow transplantation.[160] Finally, Gaston-Johansson[154] reports additional evidence of test–retest reliability and construct validity in laboring women and postoperative automatic implantable cardioverter/defibrillator (AICD) patients gathered from master's theses conducted under her supervision at the University of Nebraska between 1987 and 1993. This instrument takes approximately 2 minutes for patients to complete. Initial work indicates that it can be used in patients ranging in age from teenagers to elderly, in patients who are acutely ill, and in the home. The A-POM appears to have excellent reliability and validity and should perform well in clinical studies. It certainly has the potential to be useful in measuring the efficacy of various interventions on clinical pain, but at this point there are no published studies documenting its use. Although the A-POM is patented, its availability to the average investigator is questionable.

Chronic Pain Experience Instrument

The Chronic Pain Experience Instrument (CPEI) was developed to assess and measure accurately persistent, nonmalignant, chronic pain.[161] Davis[161] related that this instrument extended other tools for chronic pain such as the WHYMPI by measuring personal responses to living with pain (e.g., frustration with ability to carry out activities) and provided a shorter, more feasible instrument than extensive multidimensional measures, such as the full-length, original McGill Pain Questionnaire with its clinical assessment questions.[162,163] This initial work on the assessment of chronic pain contributed to the content development of the CPEI. The instrument originally consisted of 33 items in a VAS format that were pilot-tested.[164] Following the pilot test, a 24-item CPEI was constructed, consisting of 12 items from the original instrument, and 12 new or revised items.[161] Content validity was examined by two experts (patients with rheumatic disease), resulting in a content validity index of 1.0. The 24-item version was then tested in 160 individuals with rheumatic disease. The CPEI purported to measure patient characteristics, dysphoria, and positive affect, perceived spousal response, pain-management effectiveness, and number of pain-management methods used, situational anxiety, pain intensity and pain description, and situational depression. Thus, seven other instruments were used in the psychometric evaluation: General Information Form (GIF), Multiple Affect Adjective Check List (MAACL-R), Spousal Response Scale from the WHYMPI, Pain Management Inventory (PMI), State Anxiety Inventory (SAI-Form Y), McGill Pain Questionnaire (long form), Center for Epidemiological Studies Depression Scale (CES-D).

All patients completed all instruments in paper-and-pencil format. A randomly selected subset of 36 completed the CPEI two weeks later (by mail) to test stability; 32 (89%) responded. Data analyses included Cronbach's alpha coefficients, Pearson's product–moment correlations, principal components factor analysis, theta coefficients, multiple regression analysis, Student's t-test for paired samples, the Spearman-Brown formula for reliability of tests of specified length, and descriptive statistics. These tests allowed examination of internal consistency, stability, and construct validity of the CPEI.

Davis[161] reported an alpha coefficient of 0.85 overall, but only 9 items actually met her desired criterion of 0.50 to 0.70. Additional testing reduced the instrument to 16 items, but then only 12 of these met the preset criterion for interitem correlation of 0.30 to 0.70. Eleven of the 16 items met the preset item-scale criterion of 0.50 to 0.70, and all contributed to the computed alpha of 0.89. The theta coefficient was 0.88 and was based on the principal components factor analysis with varimax rotation. Stability was $r = 0.77$. Construct validity was assessed through factor analysis and predictive modeling. Exploratory factor analysis revealed three factors with eigenvalues greater than 1.0 that accounted for 54% of the variance: (1) Distress (9 items); (2) Perceived Effects on Functioning (4 items); and (3) Rest and Sleep (3 items). These three factors resulted in further internal consistency evaluation of the three associated "scales." Distress and Perceived Effects on Functioning yielded Cronbach's alphas of 0.84 and 0.79, respectively; Rest and Sleep was 0.67. Multiple regression analysis was performed based on a four-stage theoretical model. Results indicated that significant empirical relationships were in the direction predicted, thus supporting the CPEI's external construct validity. For example, the chronic pain experience was directly influenced by pain intensity and situational depression, and the higher the pain intensity and depression, the less well the individual responded to pain. Overall, construct validity was estimated to be moderate, based on the magnitude of the various predictions ($r = 0.39$). Davis[161] concluded that the CPEI demonstrated "high internal consistency, adequate stability, and moderate construct validity" in patients with rheumatic disease. She noted that, despite the reduction of the instrument to 16 items, additional psychometric work was needed, particularly in other groups of patients with chronic pain.

In subsequent work, Davis[165] has extended the psychometric evaluation of the CPEI, but the results are not yet published. This research was conducted on 243 patients with arthritis and back pain and on 97 patients with headache. It resulted in two versions of the instrument that address two different combinations of defining characteristics for the chronic pain experience.[166] The arthritis/back pain version is called the CPEI and consists of 13 items that are accompanied by VASs with anchors of agree and disagree. An example is "I frequently get angry when I am experiencing pain."

The CPEI-H is the headache versions and consists of 10 items in an identical format. Six of the items are the same as on the CPEI, but four others are unique: (1) My pain often makes me feel helpless; (2) I feel guilty about the way in which my pain affects others; (3) I think about my pain most of the time; and (4) My pain has changed my relationship with my family.

Both versions have adequate content validity (CPEI 0.92, CPEI-H 0.89), acceptable internal consistency both overall (CPEI 0.89, CPEI-H 0.84) and for all subscales (see later), and high stability (CPEI $r = 0.86$, CPEI-H $r = 0.72$) when retested 2 to 3 weeks after initial administration. The instruments are both scored by measuring each item's VAS from the left end to the patient's mark in centimeters. Scores can then be computed for the full scales (all 13 items on the CPEI or all 10 items on the CPEI-H) and for the respective subscales on each version. The CPEI has subscales of Perceived Effects on Functioning, Distress, and Helplessness, and the CPEI-H has subscales for Self-worth and Personal and Interpersonal Stress. Little information is available on the clinical utility of these two versions, nor does there appear to be any published literature on their use as measures in intervention studies. Even so, the CPEI and CPEI-H have been subjected to extensive psychometric evaluation and have good reliability and validity.

Biobehavioral Pain Profile

The Biobehavioral Pain Profile (BPP) was developed to measure selected cognitive, behavioral, and physiologic reactions often associated with pain.[167] Using a stress-adaptation model, Dalton and colleagues[167] noted that their methodologic study was aimed at developing and testing a pain measurement instrument that incorporated physiologic, personal, and environmental factors not addressed by other existing multidimensional pain measurement instruments. These factors were assumed to modulate nociception, coping, and pain-related behaviors, and thus be important in guiding clinical treatment decisions.

The BPP was a 57-item questionnaire, with each item measured on a 0 to 7 Likert scale in which higher numbers represented more frequent or stronger influence of the item. Thus, Likert anchors included never to often, no fear to great fear, and no influence to strong influence. All items were derived from literature relevant to pain measurement, from clinical experience, and from the conceptual model. Ten items asked respondents the frequency with which they engaged in avoidance when experiencing pain (e.g., cancel a treatment appointment, avoid talking/being with family). Five items asked about physiologic sensations (e.g., increased breathing rate). Five items asked about specific thoughts related to pain, and one item asked about fear of pain. Ten items assessed environmental sources of information about pain (e.g., health professional, family experience). Finally, 26 items measured the respondent's appraisal of various situations (e.g., loss of self-esteem, loss of control, absence of pain relief, surgical experiences, knowledge about pain, and thoughts and feelings related to pain and its treatment).

Dalton et al.[167] studied three groups of patients representing different types of chronic pain: 274 persons with recurrent pain related to physical activities, such as dancing or physical education; 241 persons with chronic nonmalignant pain; and 102 persons with chronic cancer-related pain ($n = 617$). No information was given on the specific procedures used to administer the instrument or to collect the data. The analyses were quite extensive, covering construct and concurrent validity, internal consistency, and test–retest reliability. Using iterated principal factor analysis to confirm the adequacy of the proposed model, the investigators identified a 41-item, 6-factor solution that accounted for 56.3% of the total variance (and constituted six subscales): Environmental Influences; Loss of Control; Health-Care Avoidance; Past and Current Experiences; Physiologic Responsibility; and Thoughts of Disease Progression. Confirmatory factor analyses also demonstrated correlations among some of these subscales (e.g., Environmental Influence and Loss of Control [$r = 0.51$] and Loss of Control and Past and Current Experiences [$r = 0.55$, both $p < 0.001$]). Finally, the first 274 subjects also completed additional instruments that measured fear, depression, anxiety, and other psychobiologic variables, including the Fear Survey Schedule (FSS), the Beck Depression Inventory (BDI), the State-Trait Anxiety Inventory (STAI), the Body Consciousness Scale (BSS), and the Marlowe-Crown Scale of Social Desirability (MCSSD). Five of the subscales had low correlations with the FSS. Four of the subscales (Loss of Control, Environmental Influences, Past and Current Experiences, and Thoughts of Disease Progression) correlated with the STAI and the BDI, although the correlations were low. None of the subscales correlated with the BSS. All six subscales were inversely associated with the MCSSD. The six subscales demonstrated internal consistency in each of the three patient subgroups (all had alpha coefficients of 0.71 or higher). A test–retest reliability evaluation done by readministration of the BPP 2 to 3 weeks later in 146 patients with chronic recurrent pain and 30 with cancer-related pain produced correlations of 0.57 to 0.73.

The BPP was described as taking approximately 15 minutes to complete. The age range of study participants was 15 to 89 years; all were English speaking, and roughly evenly divided between males and females. No other information about the subjects was given, including educational level or cultural background. Dalton et al.[168] concluded that the BPP's six subscales represented the multidimensionality of the pain experience and were able to provide information about psychologic and environmental factors related to pain. Such information could be useful in providing patient education and clinical care. The small to moderate intercorrelations among the scales suggested possible overlap in the constructs, thus needing cross-validation in other samples of patients. The low correlations between the BPP and other measures (e.g., STAI and BDI) suggested that the BPP was measuring some aspects of these constructs. Overall, Dalton et al. noted that the BPP might permit the measurement of "biobehavioral responses to pain along universal dimensions rather than along dimensions which may be overfitted to etiological categories."[167,p104] Additional psychometric evaluation of the BPP is currently being conducted in patients with temporomandibular syndrome or dysfunction and in patients with acute pain.[168]

Summary

Although compromises must inevitably be made, a careful and deliberative selection process will help to ensure that the researcher selects appropriate instruments. The result should be reliable and valid data that assist in answering the research question(s). Given the long and painstaking process of instrument development, it may be more expedient for the researcher to use a tool that has been developed and assessed psychometrically or to revise such tools as needed. The repeated use of such instruments, with careful attention to psychometric issues, will help to refine and improve existing tools, resulting in better measures of clinical pain.

References

1. Sternbach, R.A. *Pain—A psychophysiological analysis.* New York: Academic, 1960, p. 12.
2. Melzack, R., & Casey, K.L. Sensory, motivational, and central control determinants of pain: A new conceptual model. In D. Kenshalo (Ed.), *The skin senses.* Springfield, IL: Chas. C. Thomas, 1968, pp. 423-439.
3. Merskey, H., & Spear, F.G. *Pain: Psychological and psychiatric aspects.* London: Balliere, Tindall, and Cassell, 1967.
4. International Association for the Study of Pain. Pain terms: A current list with definitions and notes on usage. *Pain,* 1986, *3*(suppl):S216-S221.
5. Turk, D.C., & Rudy, R.E. IASP taxonomy of chronic pain syndromes: Preliminary assessment of reliability. *Pain,* 1987, *30*:177-189.
6. Brose, W.G., Cherry, D.A., Plummer, J., et al. IASP taxonomy: Questions and controversies. In M.R. Bond, J.E. Charlton, & C.J. Woolf (Eds.), *Proceedings of the VIth World Congress on Pain.* Amsterdam: Elsevier, 1991, pp. 503-507.
7. McCaffery, M. *Nursing management of the patient with pain.* Philadelphia: Lippincott, 1972, p. 8.
8. Beecher, H.K. Pain in men wounded in battle. *Ann Surg,* 1946, *123*:96-105.
9. Hardy, J.D., Wolff, H.G., & Goodell, H. *Pain sensations and reactions.* Baltimore: William & Wilkins, 1952.
10. Melzack, R., & Wall, P.D. Pain mechanisms: A new theory. *Science,* 1965, *150*(3699):971-978.
11. Weisenberg, M. Pain and pain control. *Psychol Bull,* 1977, *84*(5):1008-1044.
12. Ahles, T.A., Blanchard, E.B., & Ruckdeschel, J.C. The multidimensional nature of cancer-related pain. *Pain,* 1983, *17*(3):277-288.
13. McGuire, D.B. The multidimensional nature of cancer pain. In D.B. McGuire & C.H. Yarbro (Eds.), *Cancer pain management.* Philadelphia: Saunders, 1987, pp. 1-20.
14. McGuire, D.B. Comprehensive and multidimensional assessment and measurement of pain. *J Pain Sympt Manag,* 1992, *7*:312-319.
15. National Institute of Nursing Research. *6. Symptom Management: Acute Pain: A Report of the National Institute of Nursing Research Priority Expert Panel on Symptom Management: Acute Pain.* NIH Publication No. 94-2421. Bethesda, MD: U.S. Public Health Service, National Institutes of Health, U.S. Department of Health and Human Services, 1994.
16. Wolff, B.B. Laboratory methods of pain measurement. In R. Melzack (Ed.), *Pain measurement and assessment.* New York: Raven, 1983, pp. 7-13.
17. Bonica, J.J. Definitions and taxonomy of pain. In J.J. Bonica (Ed.), *The management of pain* (ed. 2, vol. 1). Philadelphia: Lea & Febiger, 1990, p. 19.
18. Agnew, D.C., Crue, B.L., & Pinsky, J.J. A taxonomy for diagnosis and information storage for patients with chronic pain. *Bull LA Neurol Soc,* 1979, *44*:84-86.
19. Meinhart, N.T., & NcCaffery, M. *Pain: A nursing approach to assessment and analysis.* Norwalk, CT: Appleton-Century-Crofts, 1983.
20. Foley, K.M. The treatment of cancer pain. *N Engl J Med,* 1985, *313*:84-95.
21. Davitz, J.R., & Davitz, L.L. *Inferences of patients' pain and psychological distress: Studies of nursing behaviors.* New York: Springer, 1981.
22. Rankin, M.A., & Snider, B. Nurses' perceptions of cancer patients' pain. *Cancer Nurs,* 1984, *7*(2):149-155.
23. Grossman, S.A., Sheidler, V.R., Swedeen, K., et al. Correlation of patient and caregiver ratings of cancer pain. *J Pain Sympt Manag,* 1991, *6*:53-57.
24. Kremer, E.F., & Atkinson, J.H. Pain language as a measure of affect in chronic pain patients. In R. Melzack (Ed.), *Pain measurement and assessment.* New York: Raven, 1983, pp. 119-127.
25. Jeans, N.E. The measurement of pain in children. In R. Melzack (Ed.), *Pain measurement and assessment.* New York: Raven, 1983, pp. 183-189.
26. Ferrell, B.A., & Ferrell, B.R. Assessment of chronic pain in the elderly. *Geriatr Med Today,* 1989, *8*:123-134.
27. Harkins, S.W., Kwentus, J., & Price, D.D. Pain in the elderly. In C. Bendetti, C.C. Chapman, & G. Morrica (Eds.), *Advances in pain research and therapy* (vol. 7). New York: Raven, 1984, pp. 103-121.
28. Bruera, E., Macmillan, K., Hanson, J., et al. The cognitive effects of the administration of narcotic analgesics in patients with cancer pain. *Pain,* 1989, *39*:13-16.
29. Gracely, R.H. Subjective quantification of pain perception. In B. Bromm (Ed.), *Pain measurement in man: Neurophysiological correlates of pain.* Amsterdam: Elsevier, 1984, pp. 371-376.
30. Gracely, R.H. Psychophysical assessment of human pain. In J.J. Bonica, J.C. Liebeskind, & D.G. Albe-Fessard (Eds.), *Advances in pain research and therapy* (vol. 3). New York: Raven, 1979, pp. 805-824.
31. Sternbach, R.A. Ethical considerations in pain research in man. In R. Melzack (Ed.), *Pain measurement and assessment.* New York: Raven, 1983, pp. 259-265.
32. Hester, N.O. Pain in children. In J. Fitzpatrick, & J. Stevenson (Eds.), *Annual review of nursing research* (vol. II). New York: Springer, 1993, pp. 105-142.
33. American Pain Society Quality Assurance Standards for Relief of Acute Pain and Cancer Pain. In M.R. Bond, J.E. Charlton, & C.J. Woolf (Eds.), *Proceedings of the VIth World Congress on Pain.* Amsterdam: Elsevier, 1990, pp. 186-189.
34. Ferrell, B.R., Eberts, M.T., McCaffery, M., et al. Clinical decision making and pain. *Cancer Nurs,* 1991, *14*: 289-297.
35. Ferrell, B.R., McGuire, D.B., & Donovan, M.I. Knowledge and beliefs regarding pain in a sample of nursing faculty. *J Prof Nurs,* 1993, *9*:79-88.
36. Sheidler, V.R., McGuire, D.B., Grossman, S.A., et al. Analgesic decision-making skills of nurses. *Oncol Nurs Forum,* 1992, *19*:1531-1534.
37. Dalton, J.A. Nurses' perceptions of their pain assessment skills, pain management practice, and attitudes toward pain. *Oncol Nurs Forum,* 1989, *16*:225-231.
38. Ferrell, B., Wisdom, C., Rhiner, M., et al. Pain management as a quality of care outcome. *J Nurs Qual Assur,* 1991, *5*(2):50-58.
39. Ferrell, B., McCaffery, M., & Ropchan, R. Pain management a clinical challenge for nursing administration. *Nurs Outlook,* 1992, *40*:263-268.
40. Chapman, C.R., & Loeser, J.D. (Eds.). *Issues in pain measurement.* New York: Raven, 1989.

41. Donovan, M.I. A practical approach to pain assessment. In J. Watt-Watson & M. Donovan (Eds.), *Pain management: Nursing perspective*. St. Louis, MO: Mosby Year Book, 1992, pp. 59-78.

42. Chen, A.C.N. Human brain measures of clinical pain: A review. I. Topographic mappings. *Pain*, 1993, 54:115-132.

43. Chen, A.C.N. Human brain measures of clinical pain: A review. II. Tomographic imagings. *Pain*, 1993, 54:133-144.

44. McCaffery, M., & Beebe, A. *Pain: Clinical manual for nursing practice*. St. Louis, MO: Mosby, 1989.

45. McMillan, S.C., Williams, F.A., Chatfield, R., et al. A validity and reliability study of two tools for assessing and managing cancer pain. *Oncol Nurs Forum*, 1988, 15:735-741.

46. Faries, J.E., Mills, D.S., Goldsmith, K.W., et al. Systematic pain records and their impact on pain control. *Cancer Nurs*, 1991, 14:306-313.

47. Puntillo, K.A., & Wilkie, D.J. Assessment of pain in the critically ill. In K. Puntillo (Ed.). *Pain in the critically ill: Assessment and Management*. Gaithersburg, MD: Aspen, 1991.

48. Acute Pain Management Guideline Panel. *Acute Pain Management: Operative or medical procedures and trauma. Clinical practice guideline*. AHCPR Publication No. 92-0032. Rockville, MD: Agency for Health Care Policy and Research, Public Health Service, U.S. Department of Health and Human Services, 1992.

49. Jacox, A., Carr, D.B., Payne, R., et al. *Management of cancer pain. Clinical practice guideline No. 9*. AHCPR Publication No. 94-0592. Rockville, MD. Agency for Health Care Policy and Research, U.S. Department of Health and Human Services, Public Health Service, 1994.

50. Littman, G.S., Walker, B.R., & Schneider, B.E. Reassessment of verbal and visual analogue ratings in analgesic studies. *Clin Pharmacol Ther*, 1985, 38(1):16-23.

51. Keele, K.D. The pain chart. *Lancet*, 1948, 2:6-8.

52. Keele, K.D. The temporal aspects of pain: The pain chart. In R. Melzack (Ed.), *Pain measurement and assessment*. New York: Raven, 1983, pp. 205-213.

53. Melzack, R. The McGill Pain Questionnaire: Major properties and scoring methods. *Pain*, 1975, 1(3):277-299.

54. Kruszewski, A.Z., Lang, S.H., & Johnson, J.E. Effect of positioning on discomfort from intramuscular injections in the dorsogluteal site. *Nurs Res*, 1979, 28(2):103-105.

55. Heft, M.W., & Parker, S.R. An experimental basis for revising the graphic rating scale for pain. *Pain*, 1984, 19(2):153-161.

56. De Conno, F., Caraceni, A., Gamba, A., et al. Pain measurement in cancer patients: A comparison of six methods. *Pain*, 1994, 57:161-166.

57. Maxwell, C. Sensitivity and accuracy of the visual analogue scale: A psycho-physical classroom experiment. *Br J Clin Pharmacol*, 1978, 6(1):15-24.

58. Clarke, P.R.F., & Spear, F.G. Reliability and sensitivity in the self-assessment of well-being. *Bull Br Psychol Soc*, 1964, 17(55):18A.

59. Gift, A.G. Visual analogues scales: Measurement of subjective phenomena. *Nurs Res*, 1989, 38:286-288.

60. Cline, N.E., Herman, J., Shaw, E.R., et al. Standardization of the Visual Analogue Scale. *Nurs Res*, 1992, 41:378-390.

61. Huskisson, E.C. Measurement of pain. *Lancet*, 1974, 2(7889):1127-1131.

62. Grossman, S.A., Sheidler, V.R., McGuire, D.B., et al. A comparison of the Hopkins Pain Rating Instrument with standard visual analogue and verbal descriptor scales in patients with cancer pain. *J Pain Sympt Manag*, 1992, 7:196-203.

63. Price, D.D., Bush, F.M., Long, S., et al. A comparison of pain measurement characteristics of mechanical visual analogue and simple numerical rating scales. *Pain*, 1994, 56:217-226.

64. Murphy, D.F., McDonald, A., Power, C., et al. Measurement of pain: A comparison of the visual analogue scale with a nonvisual analogue scale. *Clin J Pain*, 1988, 3:197-199.

65. Wilkie, D., Lovejoy, N., Dodd, N., et al. Cancer pain intensity measurement: Concurrent validity of three tools—Finger dynamometer, pain intensity number scale, visual analogue scale. *Hospice J*, 1990, 6(1):1-13.

66. Sriwatanakul, K., Kelvie, W., Lasagna, L., et al. Studies with different types of visual analog scales for measurement of pain. *Clin Pharmacol Ther*, 1983, 34:234-239.

67. Price, D.D., McGrath, D.A., Rafii, A., et al. The validation of visual analogue scales as ratio scale measures for chronic and experimental pain. *Pain*, 1983, 17(1):45-56.

68. Revill, S.I., Robinson, J.O., Rosen, N., et al. The reliability of a linear analogue for evaluating pain. *Anaesthesia*, 1976, 31(9):1191-1198.

69. Dixon, J.S., & Bird, H.A. Reproducibility along a 10 cm vertical visual analogue scale. *Ann Rheumat Dis*, 1981, 40:87-89.

70. Carlsson, A.N. Assessment of chronic pain. 1. Aspects of the reliability and validity of the visual analogue scale. *Pain*, 1983, 16:87-101.

71. Liu, W.H.D., & Aitkenhead, A.R. Comparison of contemporaneous and retrospective assessment of postoperative pain using the visual analogue scale. *Br J Anaesth*, 1991, 67:768-771.

72. Iafrati, N.S. Pain on the burn unit: Patient vs nurse perceptions. *JCBR*, 1986, 7(5):413-416.

73. Scott, J., & Huskisson, E.C. Vertical or horizontal visual analogue scales. *Ann Rheumat Dis*, 1979, 38:560.

74. Scott, J., & Huskisson, E.C. Accuracy of subjective measurements made with or without previous scores: An important source of error in serial measurement of subjective states. *Ann Rheumat Dis*, 1979, 38:558-559.

75. Ohnhaus, E.E., & Adler, R. Methodological problems in the measurement of pain: A comparison between the verbal rating scale and the visual analogue scale. *Pain*, 1975, 1(4):379-384.

76. Scott, J., & Huskisson, E.C. Graphic representation of pain. *Pain*, 1976, 2(2):175-184.

77. Wallenstein, S.L. Scaling clinical pain and pain relief. In B. Bromm (Ed.), *Pain measurement in man: Neurophysiological correlates of pain*. Amsterdam: Elsevier, 1984, pp. 389-396.

78. Woodforde, J.N., & Merksey, H. Some relationships between subjective measures of pain. *J Psychosom Res*, 1972, 16:173-178.

79. Reading, A.E. A comparison of pain rating scales. *J Psychosom Res*, 1980, *24*:119-124.

80. Downie, W.W., Leatham, P.A., Rhind, V.M., et al. Studies with pain rating scales. *Ann Rheumat Dis*, 1978, *37*(4):378-381.

81. Kremer, E., Atkinson, J.H., & Ignelzi, R.J. Measurement of pain: Patient preference does not confound pain measurement. *Pain*, 1981, *10*:241-248.

82. Jensen, M.P., Karoly, P., & Braver, T. The measurement of clinical pain intensity: A comparison of six methods. *Pain*, 1986, *27*:117-126.

83. Jensen, M.P., Karoly, P., O'Riordan, E.F., et al. The subjective experience of acute pain: an assessment of the utility of 10 indices. *Clin J Pain*, 1989, *5*:153-159.

84. Machin, D., Lewith, G.T., & Wylson, S. Pain measurement in randomized clinical trials. *Clin J Pain*, 1994, *4*:161-168.

85. Banos, J.E., Bosch, F., Canellas, M., et al. Acceptability of visual analogue scales in the clinical setting: A comparison with verbal rating scales in postoperative pain. *Meth Find Exp Clin Pharmacol*, 1989, *11*(2): 123-127.

86. Ahles, T.A., Ruckdeschel, J.C., & Blanchard, E.B. Cancer related pain. II. Assessment with Visual Analogue Scales. *J Psychosom Res*, 1984, *28*(2):121-124.

87. Price, D.D., Harkins, S.W., & Baker, C. Sensory-affective relationships among different types of clinical and experimental pain. *Pain*, 1987, *28*:297-307.

88. Hanken, A. The measurement of pain. In M. Newton, W. Hunt, W. McDowell, & A. Hanken (Eds.), *A study of nurse action in relief of pain*. Columbus, OH: The Ohio State University School of Nursing, 1964.

89. Hanken, A., & McDowell, W. Development of a rating scale to measure pain. In M. Newton, W. Hunt, W. McDowell, & A. Hanken (Eds.), *A study of nurse action in relief of pain*. Columbus, OH: The Ohio State University School of Nursing, 1964.

90. Chambers, W.G., & Price, G.G. Influence of nurse upon effects of analgesics administered. *Nurs Res*, 1967, *16*(3):228-233.

91. Bruegel, M.A. Relationship of preoperative anxiety to perception of postoperative pain. *Nurs Res*, 1971, *20*(1):26-31.

92. Hagle, M.E. Diurnal variation in pain intensity of cancer patients. Unpublished master's thesis. University of Illinois at the Medical Center, Chicago, IL, 1980.

93. Bonnel, A.M., & Boureau, F. Labor pain assessment: Validity of a behavioral index. *Pain*, 1985, *22*(1):81-90.

94. Mateo, O.M., & Krenzischek, D.A. A pilot study to assess the relationship between behavioral manifestations and self-report of pain in postanesthesia care unit patients. *J Post Anesth Nurs*, 1992, *7*(1):15-21.

95. Mateo, O. Personal communication, July 1994.

96. Webb, M.R., & Kennedy, M.G. Behavioral responses and self-reported pain in postoperative patients. *J Post Anesth Nurs*, 1994, *9*(2):91-95.

97. Wells, N. Behavioral measurement of distress during painful medical procedures. In O.L. Strickland & C.F. Waltz (Eds.). *Measurement of nursing outcomes: Measuring client self-care and coping skills* (vol. 4). New York: Springer, 1990.

98. Gil, K.M., Phillips, G., Edens, J., et al. Observation of pain behaviors during episodes of sickle cell disease pain. *Clin J Pain*, 1994, *10*:128-132.

99. Fordyce, W.E., Lansky, T., Calsyn, D.A., et al. Pain measurement and pain behavior. *Pain*, 1984, *18*(1): 53-69.

100. Follick, M.J., Ahern, D.K., & Laser-Wolston, W. Evaluation of a daily activity diary for chronic pain patients. *Pain*, 1984, *19*:373-382.

101. Kremer, E.F., Block, A., & Gaylor, N.S. Behavioral approaches to treatment of chronic pain: The inaccuracy of patient self-report measures. *Arch Phys Med Rehab*, 1981, *62*(4):188-191.

102. Keefe, F.J., Wilkins, R.H., & Cook, W.A. Direct observation of pain behavior in low back pain patients during physical examination. *Pain*, 1984, *20*: 59-68.

103. Richards, J., Nepomuceno, C., Riles, M., et al. Assessing pain behavior: The UAB pain behavior scale. *Pain*, 1982, *14*(4):393-398.

104. Keefe, F.J., Brantley, A., Manual, G., et al. Behavioral assessment of head and neck cancer pain. *Pain*, 1985, *23*(4):327-336.

105. McDaniel, L.K., Anderson, K.O., Bradley, L.A., et al. Development of an observation method for assessing pain behavior in rheumatoid arthritis patients. *Pain*, 1986, *24*:165-194.

106. Keefe, F.J., & Block, A.R. Development of an observation method for assessing pain behavior in chronic low back pain patients. *Behav Ther*, 1982, *13*:363-375.

107. Ahles, T.A., Coombs, D.W., Jensen, L., et al. Development of a behavioral observation technique for the assessment of pain behavior in cancer patients. *Behav Ther*, 1990, *21*:449-460.

108. Ferrell, B.A., Rhiner, M., et al. Family factors influencing cancer pain. *Postgraduate Med J*, 1991, *67*(suppl):64-69.

109. Ferrell, B.R., Rhiner, N., Cohen, M.Z., et al. Pain as a metaphor for illness. Part I: Impact of cancer pain on family caregivers. *Oncol Nurs Forum*, 1991, *18*: 1303-1309.

110. Ferrell, B.R., Cohen, M.Z., Rhiner, M., et al. Pain as a metaphor for illness. Part II: Family caregivers' management of pain. *Oncol Nurs Forum*, 1991, *18*: 1315-1321.

111. Ferrell, B., Rhiner, M., & Rivera, L. Development and evaluation of the Family Pain Questionnaire. *J Psychosoc Oncol*, 1993, *10*(4):21-35.

112. Johnson, J.E. Effects of structuring patients' expectations on their reactions to threatening events. *Nurs Res*, 1972, *21*(6):499-504.

113. Johnson, E.E. Effects of accurate expectations about sensations on the sensory and distress components of pain. *J Pers Soc Psychol*, 1973, *27*(2):261-275.

114. Wells, N. The effect of relaxation on postoperative muscle tension and pain. *Nurs Res*, 1982, *31*:236-238.

115. Tursky, B. The development of a pain perception profile: A psychophysical approach. In M. Weisenberg & B. Tursky (Eds.), *Pain: New perspectives in therapy and research*. New York: Plenum, 1976, pp. 171-194.

116. Andrasik, F., Blanchard, E.B., Ahles, T., et al. Assessing the reactive as well as the sensory component of headache pain. *Headache*, 1981, *21*:218-221.

117. Urban, B.J., Keefe, F.J., & France, R.D. A study of psychophysical scaling in chronic pain patients. *Pain*, 1984, *20*:157-168.

118. Melzack, R., & Torgerson, W. On the language of pain. *Anesthesiology*, 1971, *34*(1):50-59.
119. Melzack, R., Katz, J., & Jeans, M.E. The role of compensation in chronic pain: Analysis using a new method of scoring the McGill pain Questionnaire. *Pain*, 1985, *23*(2):101-112.
120. Graham, C., Bond, T.T., Gerkovich, M.M., et al. Use of the McGill Pain Questionnaire in the assessment of cancer pain: Replicability and consistency. *Pain*, 1980, *8*(3):377-387.
121. McGuire, D.B. Assessment of pain in cancer inpatients using the McGill Pain Questionnaire. *Oncol Nurs Forum*, 1984, *11*(6):32-37.
122. Klepac, R.K., Dowling, J., Rokke, P., et al. Interview vs. paper and pencil administration of the McGill Pain Questionnaire. *Pain*, 1981, *11*:241-246.
123. Byrne, M., Troy, A., Bradley, L.A., et al. Crossvalidation of the factor structure of the McGill pain questionnaire. *Pain*, 1982, *13*:193-201.
124. Reading, A.E. The internal structure of the McGill pain questionnaire in dysmenorrhoea patients. *Pain*, 1979, *7*(3):353-358.
125. Kremer, E., & Atkinson, J.H. Pain measurement: Construct validity of the affective dimension of the McGill pain questionnaire with chronic benign pain patients. *Pain*, 1981, *11*(1):93-100.
126. Burckhardt, C.S. The use of the McGill Pain Questionnaire in assessing arthritis pain. *Pain*, 1984, *19*(3):305-314.
127. Prieto, E.J., & Geisinger, K.F. Factor-analytic studies of the McGill Pain Questionnaire. In R. Melzack (Ed.), *Pain measurement and assessment*. New York: Raven, 1983.
128. Buren, J.V., & Kleinknecht, R.A. An evaluation of the McGill Pain Questionnaire for use in dental pain assessment. *Pain*, 1979, *6*:23-33.
129. Klepac, R.K., Dowling, J., Hauge, G., et al. Sensitivity of the McGill pain Questionnaire to intensity and quality of laboratory pain. *Pain*, 1981, *10*:199-207.
130. Hunter, M., & Philips, C. The experience of headache—An assessment of the qualities of tension headache pain. *Pain*, 1981, *10*:209-219.
131. Reading, E.A. The McGill pain questionnaire: An appraisal. In R. Melzack (Ed.), *Pain measurement and assessment*. New York: Raven, 1983, pp. 55-61.
132. Reading, A.E. A comparison of the McGill Pain Questionnaire in chronic and acute pain. *Pain*, 1982, *13*:185-192.
133. Grushka, M., & Sessle, B.J. Applicability of the McGill Pain Questionnaire to the differentiation of "toothache" pain. *Pain*, 1984, *19*(1):49-57.
134. Dubuisson, D., & Melzack, R. Classification pain descriptions by multiple group discriminant analysis. *Exp Neurol*, 1976, *51*(2):480-487.
135. Reading, A.E., Everitt, B., & Sledmere, C.M. The McGill Pain Questionnaire: A replication of its construction. *Br J Clin Psychol*, 1982, *21*:339-349.
136. Turk, D.C., Rudy, T.E., & Salovey, P. The McGill Pain Questionnaire reconsidered: Confirming the factor structure and examining appropriate uses. *Pain*, 1985, *21*(4):385-397.
137. Wilkie, D.J., Savedra, M.C., Holzemer, W.L., et al. Use of the McGill Pain Questionnaire to measure pain: A metaanalysis. *Nurs Res*, 1990, *39*:36-41.
138. Vanderiet, K., Adriaensen, H., Carton, H., et al. The McGill Pain Questionnaire constructed for the Dutch language (MPQ-DV). Preliminary data concerning reliability and validity. *Pain*, 1987, *30*:395-408.
139. Kiss, I., Muller, H., & Abel, M. The McGill Pain Questionnaire—German version. A study on cancer pain. *Pain*, 1987, *29*:195-207.
140. Maiani, G., & Sanavio, E. Semantics of pain in Italy: The Italian Version of the McGill Pain Questionnaire. *Pain*, 1985, *4*:399-405.
141. De Benedittis, G., Nassei, R., Nobili, R., et al. The Italian pain questionnaire. *Pain*, 1985, *33*:53-62.
142. Fishman, B., Pasternak, T., Wallenstein, S.L., et al. The Memorial Pain Assessment Card: A valid instrument for the evaluation of cancer pain. *Cancer*, 1987, *60*:1151-1158.
143. Kerns, R.D., Turk, D.C., & Rudy, T.E. The West Haven Yale Multidimensional Pain Inventory (WHYMPI). *Pain*, 1985, *23*(4):345-356.
144. Turk, D. Personal communication, January 1994.
145. Melzack, R. The short-form McGill Pain Questionnaire. *Pain*, 1987, *30*:191-197.
146. Dudgeon, D., Raubertas, R.F., & Rosenthal, S.N. The Short-Form McGill Pain Questionnaire in chronic cancer pain. *J Pain Sympt Manag*, 1993, *8*:191-195.
147. Swanston, M., Abraham, C., Nacrae, W.A., et al. Pain assessment with interactive computer animation. *Pain*, 1993, *53*:347-351.
148. McGuire, D.B., Altomonte, V., Peterson, D.E., et al. Patterns of mucositis and pain in patients receiving preparative chemotherapy and bone marrow transplantation. *Oncol Nurs Forum*, 1993, *20*: 1493-1502.
149. Daut, R.L., Cleeland, C., & Flanery, R.C. Development of the Wisconsin Brief Pain Questionnaire to assess pain in cancer and other diseases. *Pain*, 1983, *17*:197-210.
150. Cleeland, C.S. Measurement and prevalence of pain in cancer. *Semin Oncol Nurs*, 1985, *1*(2):87-92.
151. Cleeland, C.S. Measurement of pain by subjective report. In C.R. Chapman & J.D. Loeser (Eds.), *Issues in pain measurement*. New York: Raven, 1989, pp. 391-403.
152. Cleeland, C.S., Gonin, R., Hatfield, A.K., et al. Pain and its treatment in outpatients with metastatic cancer. *N Engl J Med*, 1994, *330*:592-596.
153. Cleeland, C. Personal communication, June 1994.
154. Gaston-Johansson, F. Personal communication, June 1994.
155. Gaston-Johansson, F. Pain assessment: Differences in quality and intensity of the words pain, ache, and hurt. *Pain*, 1984, *20*:69-76.
156. Gaston-Johansson, F. & Allwood, J. Pain assessment: Model construction and analysis of words used to describe pain-like experiences. *Semiotica*, 1988, *71*(1/2):73-92.
157. Gaston-Johansson, F., Albert, M., Fagan, E., et al. Similarities in pain descriptions of four different ethnic-culture groups. *J Pain Sympt Manag*, 1990, *5*:94-100.
158. Norvell, K.T., Gaston-Johansson, F., & Zimmerman, L. Pain description by nurses and physicians. *J Pain Sympt Manag*, 1990, *5*:11-17.
159. Gaston-Johansson, F., Fridh, G., & Turner-Norvell, K. Progression of labor pain in primiparas and multiparas. *Nurs Res*, 1988, *37*:86-90.
160. Gaston-Johansson, F., Franco, T., & Zimmerman, L. Pain and psychological distress in patients under-

going autologous bone marrow transplantation. *Oncol Nurs Forum*, 1992, *19*:41-48.

161. Davis, G.C. Measurement of the chronic pain experience: Development of an instrument. *Res Nurs Health*, 1989, *12*:221-227.

162. Davis, G.C. Measuring the clinical outcomes of the patient with chronic pain. In C.F. Waltz & O.L. Strickland (Eds.), *The measurement of nursing outcomes: Measuring client outcomes* (vol. 1). New York: Springer, 1988, pp. 160-184.

163. Davis, G.C. The clinical assessment of chronic pain in rheumatic disease: Evaluating the use of two instruments. *J Adv Nurs*, 1989, *14*:397-402.

164. Davis, G.C. *Preliminary testing of an instrument for measuring the chronic pain experience*. Paper presented at the Sixteenth Annual CNR Spring Research Symposium, Ohio State University, Columbus Ohio.

165. Davis, G.C. Personal communication, April 1994.

166. Davis. G.C. Measurement of the chronic pain experience. Unpublished report, 1991. National Center for Nursing Research, Bethesda, MD.

167. Dalton, J.A., Feuerstein, M., Carlson, J. et al. Biobehavioral Pain profile: Development and psychometric properties. *Pain*, 1994, *57*:95-107.

168. Dalton, J.A. Personal communication, March 1994.

Appendices

37A. Comparison of Scales

Researchers	Scales Compared	Findings
Scott and Huskisson (76)	6 different VAS and GRS to a simple VDS	Horizontal VAS and a horizontal GRS with descriptor words placed along the length of the line produced more uniform distributions, were more sensitive to perceived pain intensity, and were easier for patients to use
Reading (79)	3 scales: PPI scale (MPQ) (53), 10-cm VAS, and a 10-point horizontal numerical scale with anchor words (none, mild, moderately distressing, very distressing, unbearable)	Patient population studies: patients with episiotomy pain Wide variability in the distribution of ratings as well as in agreement between scale differences over time and subjective comparisons Correlations between VAS and VDS were significant ($r = 0.57–0.71$) Conclusion: insufficient psychometric analyses of scales had been performed; efficacy or usefulness of these scales may vary according to patient characteristics and setting
Downie et al. (80)	VAS, VDS compared to one another as well as to a 0 to 100 numerical rating scale (NRS)	All scales correlated well and had similar loadings on factor analysis Conclusion: scales probably measured the same variable (i.e., pain intensity) 0–100 NRS preferred because it offered more choices than the VDS and was less confusing than the VAS
Kremer et al. (81)	Patient preference for VAS, NRS or 5-adjective adaptation of PPI (53)	Most patients preferred the 5-adjective scale, and all were able to complete it VAS had an 11% failure rate NRS had a 2% failure rate Conclusion: VDS, such as Melzack's PPI, may be more reliable in certain circumstances
Sriwatanakul et al. (66)	Differences between 5 VAS, (10-cm horizontal, vertical, and curvilinear scales with anchors of "no pain" <=> "pain as bad as it could possibly be") and graded horizontal and curvilinear scales with the same anchors	Normal volunteer subjects preferred the graded horizontal VAS, with the graded curvilinear scale ranked second In postoperative patients, the VAS appeared to be a more sensitive measure of pain, as significant changes in pain intensity on the VAS occurred in the absence of changes in the descriptive scales
Littman et al. (50)	VDS, VAS, and a verbal pain relief scale	1,497 patients studied with a variety of acute and chronic types of pain who were receiving analgesics All 3 measures correlated well ($r = 0.89–0.93$) No consistent differences in sensitivity between verbal and analogue scales; verbal pain relief scale was slightly more sensitive than the other 2 Conclusion: choice of scale may not be critical and should be dictated by measurement situation

37A. Comparison of Scales (*cont.*)

Researchers	Scales Compared	Findings
Jensen et al. (82)	6 scales: VAS, 100-point numerical rating scale (NRS), 11-point box rating scale (BS-11), 6-point behavioral rating scale (BRS), and 4- and 5-point verbal rating scales (VRS)	Patient sample: chronic pain Scales evaluated on (1) ease of administration and scoring; (2) rates of correct responding; (3) relative sensitivity as defined by number of response categories; (4) relative sensitivity as defined by ability to detect treatment effects; and (5) magnitude of relationship between each scale and a "best possible" combined measure of subjective pain intensity All scales similar in (2) correct responses, except for VAS (rate of incorrect responses increased with age) and in predictive validity (5), magnitude of relationship NRS surpassed all others on remaining criteria For current pain, correlation coefficients among the scales ranged from 0.65 to 0.88, ($p < 0.001$, two-tailed tests) Factor analysis: single factor for pain intensity with each scale correlating with the factor at 0.64 or above BRS correlated least, and the BS-11 and NRS the most Conclusion: scales were more similar than different, and were useful measures of pain intensity. NRS had practical advantages (ease of administration, scoring, high rate of correct response)
Jensen et al. (83)	10 scales and a linear combination of pain measures	Evaluated on (1) magnitude of relationship between them and a linear combination of pain measures; and (2) rates of incorrect response in a sample of patients with acute pain 8 scales measured pain intensity (6 from previous study, a VRS-15, and a VRS-11 for pain intensity) 2 scales measured pain affect (again on a 15- and 11-point adjectival scale) Most subjects responded correctly to all scales (VAS 7.2%, NRS 5.8% were problematic) All scales were significantly correlated ($p < 0.001$, two-tailed tests); factor analysis revealed 1 factor, with all scales loading at 0.65 or higher BRS was least related to the construct of pain intensity (patients asked to rate pain in terms of effects rather than subjective intensity) Conclusion: 11-point box rating scale was most useful clinical measure; also noted need to explore pain affect scales further as only 1 factor was extracted rather than the anticipated 2 (intensity and affect)
Machin et al. (84)	VAS and FDS as measure of treatment effects	Focused on statistical methodology used for repeated measures of these scales in a clinical trial VAS and VDS may be measuring slightly different aspects of pain Conclusion: consider using both scales in clinical trials

Banos et al. (85)	VAS and VDS	Small, Spanish study of postoperative general, gynecologic, and orthopedic patients Scores highly correlated ($p < 0.001$) and not influenced by gender, age, surgical procedure, or hospital Patient ratings compared to physician ratings: at lower levels, correlations high; as pain scores increased (pain worsened) physicians rated the pain lower VAS offered a better measure of pain intensity than the VDS because of its sensitivity and lack of verbal descriptors, which might carry different meanings for different individuals
Grossman et al. (62)	Mechanical VAS to standard VAS and VDS	High correlations between Hopkins Pain Rating Instrument and the VAS and VDS in cancer patients with pain ($r = 0.99$ and 0.85, respectively; $p < 0.0001$) M-VAS offered reliable, valid, clinically useful measures of pain intensity; also, portable, easy to score, and free of potential bias from verbal descriptors
Price et al. (63)	VDS and mechanical VAS (M-VAS) in terms of capacity to produce ratio-level measures of experimental pain	M-VAS provided consistent measures of both experimental and clinical pain intensity, was easy to administer and score M-VAS offered reliable, valid, clinically useful measures of pain intensity; also portable and free of potential bias from verbal descriptors
De Conno et al. (56)	Compared 5 scales before and after pain treatment: VAS, 0–10 NRS, Verbal Rating Scale (VRS), Italian Pain Questionnaire (PRI/Italian version of the MPQ), and the Integrated Pain Score (IPS)	Unidimensional measures (VAS, NRS, VRS) were more strongly associated with relief of pain than the multidimensional measures, but all were clinically interpretable Patients' evaluation of pain relief was a more global concept, loosely related to measures of pain intensity Conclusion: researchers must consider using pain relief scales as well as pain intensity scales when evaluating outcomes of pain treatments

Abbreviations: VAS, Visual Analogue Scale; M-VAS, Mechanical Visual Analogue Scale; VDS, Verbal Descriptor Scale; NRS, Numerical Rating Scale; VRS, Verbal Rating Scale; BRS, Behavioral Rating Scale; PPI, Present Pain Intensity (from MPQ); MPQ, McGill Pain Questionnaire.

Numbers in parentheses correspond to studies cited in the References.

37B. Additional Unidimensional Instruments to Measure the Behavioral Dimension of Acute Pain

Instrument/Study	Important Points	Psychometric Indices
Pain Rating Scale Developed by Hanken et al. (88,89) Modified by Chambers and Price (90)	Developed to measure postoperative pain 6 observable behaviors and physiologic parameters measured: attention to pain; anxiety; verbal statement of degree of pain; skeletal muscle response; characteristics of respiration; amount of perspiration Revised version (90): respiration deleted; added scales for sounds made by patient, nausea, muscle tension, and facial expression Advantages: focuses on anxiety, attention to pain, physiologic parameters; easy to administer and score Disadvantages (92): questionable construct validity; applicable to acute pain only; administration time 5–15 minutes	Construct validity: analyzed 289 nurse observations of 70 patients; correlation matrix of 6 parameters: positive relationships ($r = 0.44$–0.71) between attention, anxiety, stated degree of pain, skeletal muscle response Factor analysis (rotation): first factor was attention directed toward pain and stated degree of pain; both had highest factor loadings (89) Revised instrument (91): reported correlations between total scores and scores for verbal report of degree of pain ($r = 0.66$–0.87); validity reported: pain scores positively correlated with amount of analgesia ($r = 0.38$)
Behavioral Index for the Assessment of Labor Pain Developed by Bonnel and Boureau (93)	Study sample: 100 primiparous women Respiratory modifications, motor responses, and agitation measured Cumulative 5-point scale used (higher numbers indicated more behavioral manifestations of pain)	Validity: ratings made by obstetrician or midwife compared to patient's self-ratings to present pain intensity; global scores (entire labor period) significantly correlated ($r = 0.88$, $p < 0.001$) as were scores from different phases of labor (cervical dilations 3–10 cm, $r = 0.30$–0.50, $p < 0.01$–0.001) Further research warranted (physical parameters of labor progression and use of behavioral ratings as a potential index of self-control behaviors during labor)

Numbers in parentheses correspond to studies cited in the References.

37C. Additional Unidimensional Instruments to Measure the Behavioral Dimension of Chronic Pain

Instrument/Study	Important Points	Psychometric Indices
Pain Diaries Fordyce et al. (99) Follick et al. (100)	Initially developed as a diary form for home recording of chronic pain: measures physical act; medications; pain intensity Hourly recording over 24 hours: whether individual is sitting, standing, walking, or reclining; kind and amount of medications used; pain rating (0, no pain to 10, intolerable) Assesses functional impairment by timed activities, especially relation to consumption of pain, medications, and pain intensity Useful for home recording	Reliability studied chronic pain patients (100) Reliability coefficients for categories of daily living were positive ($r = 0.44$–0.89) and significant ($p = 0.05$–0.01) Correlations between patient and spouse ratings (standing, walking, lying down, pain intensity, pill counts); also high and significant correlation between patient reports of lying down and electromechanical monitor measurements ($r = 0.94$, $p < 0.01$) Concerns: reliability, recall bias
University of Alabama-Birmingham (UAB) Pain Behavior Scale (101–103)	Objective assessment of 10 pain-related behaviors: verbal vocal complaints; time spent lying down; facial grimaces; standing posture; mobility; body language; use of visible, supportive equipment; stationary movement; medicine Simple, easy-to-use for health personnel or patient	Good interrater reliability ($r = 0.95$, $p < 0.01$) Good test-retest reliability ($r = 0.89$, $p < 0.01$) Validity not adequately tested
Behavioral Dysfunction Index (BDI) Developed by Keefe et al. (104)	Behavioral measure of chronic pain related to head and neck cancer (clinical assessment tool) Evaluates 6 quantitative areas: (1) motor pain behaviors; (2) specific painful activities; (3) general activity level; (4) pain-relieving methods; (5) pain medication intake; (6) weight loss Measures: motor pain behaviors: observers recorded; occurrence/nonoccurrence of 4 specific behaviors (guarded movement, grimacing, rubbing, sighing) while patients sat, stood, walked, reclined, rotated their heads, swallowed, coughed Remaining 5 areas: data collected by structured interview Behavioral Dysfunction Index (BDI) developed as composite measure for each patient (from observations, interview) Scoring: 0 no dysfunction, 1–3 mild to moderate dysfunction, 4–6 extreme dysfunction	BDI scores positively and significantly ($p < 0.05$) related to pain ratings on a 0 to 10 numerical scale (0 no pain, 10 pain as bad as it can be) Warrants further psychometric evaluation Limitation: time and skill required to administer the questions
Observational Method for Rheumatoid Arthritis (RA) Pain McDaniel et al. (105,106)	Method modified from earlier work by Keefe and Block in patients with chronic low back pain (106); 4 studies conducted to determine reliability and validity of behavioral observation method Study 1: assessed interobserver reliability of method and characteristics of patients' pain behaviors $n = 20$ adult patients with rheumatoid arthritis (RA) Patients identified painful joint or body area, and were observed and videotaped for 10 minutes while sitting, walking, standing, and reclining	Observers' percentage agreements for all behaviors (96%–100%) Reliability: kappa coefficients on each behavior (0.80–1.0) Guarding and rigidity were significantly associated with patients' reports on affected body sites ($r = 0.55$ and 0.73, respectively; $p < 0.01$) Study 1: guarding and rigidity significantly correlated with one another ($r = 0.55$, $p < 0.01$); patients had similar mean numbers of pain behaviors while moving or stationary

37C. Additional Unidimensional Instruments to Measure the Behavioral Dimension of Chronic Pain (*cont.*)

Instrument/Study	Important Points	Psychometric Indices
Observational Method for Rheumatoid Arthritis *continued*	Videotapes scored by 2 trained research assistants (13 separate behaviors with operational definitions) 3 categories of behaviors recorded: (1) position: standing, sitting, reclining; (2) movement: pacing, shifting; (3) pain behavior: guarding, bracing, grimacing, sighing, rigidity, passive rubbing, active rubbing, self-stimulation Study 2: concurrent validity and objectivity of observation method examined $n = 53$ RA patients were observed and videotaped for 10 minutes during same activities as in Study 1; also completed Long form MPQ (LF-MPQ, [53]) 2 to 10-cm VAS (one, immediate pain level; one, unpleasantness of immediate pain level; anchors: "none/not at all <=> unbearable/extremely") Modified Health Assessment Questionnaire (HAQ) Depression Adjective Checklist (DAC) Trained observers viewed videotapes, recorded position, movement, pain behaviors Study 3: examined construct validity of behavioral observation method 11 psychology students reviewed 25 videotapes of RA patients engaged in described activities and made global estimates of severity or unpleasantness of patients' pain on 5 measures in counterbalanced order: 11-point categorical scale (0 no pain at all, 10 extreme pain) 10-cm VAS with anchors (no pain at all, unbearable pain) 11-point categorical scale (0 not at all unpleasant, 10 extremely unpleasant) 10-cm VAS with anchors (no unpleasantness at all, extreme unpleasantness) Verbal descriptor scale: 15 sensory intensity (SI) items, 1 descriptor of no pain Trained observer scored the 25 videotapes (as in study 1), blinded to students' ratings	Study 2: moderate and significant correlations observed between patients' pain behavior scores and the 2 VASs ($r = 0.26$, pain severity; $r = 0.32$ pain unpleasantness, both $p < 0.01$) Guarding only behavior related to VAS scores Total pain behavior scores significantly related ($r = 0.41$–0.45, $p < 0.001$) to patients' scores on certain MPQ indices: Number of words chosen (NWC), Sensory pain rating index (PRI), Affective PRI, and Total PRI Guarding most consistently related to total pain behavior scores significantly correlated with the HAQ daily function scores ($r = 0.49$, $p < 0.001$) and with DAC depression score ($r = 03.1$, $p < 0.05$) Patients' self-reports of depression correlated with the NWC and Affective and Total PRI scores (LF-MPQ) Study 3: student ratings positively and significantly correlated ($r = 0.54$–0.57, $p < 0.01$) with patients' total behavior scores Guarding and rigidity most highly associated

Study 4: tested utility of the behavioral observation method as an indicator of treatment outcome

$n = 11$ patients with RA; observed for 10 minutes before, and after a cognitive-behavioral treatment program

Completed the MPQ-LF and 2 10-cm VASs (pain severity and unpleasantness) prior to and after the intervention

Conclusion: this behavioral observation method yielded useful, objective data about RA pain

Limitation: unknown effects of the presence of observers and videotaping on patients (patients reactivity)

Further research needed particularly in other populations of patients with pain

Study 4: significant decreases in total pain behavior scores and the specific behavior of passive rubbing found pre- and post-treatment ($t = 2.31, 2.23$, respectively, $p < 0.05$)

Significant decreases found in overall number of behaviors across different times of assessment; patients' self-reports of pain also decreased

Conclusion: Study 1: reliability supported; Study 2: concurrent validity supported, functional disability scores on HAQ related to total pain behavior scores; Study 3: construct validity supported; Study 4: further evidence of construct validity through responses pre- and postintervention

Numbers in parentheses correspond to studies cited in the References.

37D. Additional Multidimensional Instruments to Measure Pain

Instrument/Study	Important Points	Psychometric Indices
Two-component Scale Developed by Johnson (112,113) Used by Wells (114)	Separate scales for measurement of sensory and reactive (affective) components Subjects experiencing experimentally induced pain rated physical sensation on a 0 to 100 scale in terms of distress (slightly to moderately, very to just bearable): high pain intensity not always accompanied by high distress simple to use	Psychometric properties not described Requires further testing
Tursky's Pain Perception Profile (PPP) Developed by Tursky (115) Used by Andrasik et al. (116) and Urban et al. (117)	Goals to enable patients to scale pain by magnitude estimation (in equal-interval stimuli as compared to a standard pain statement) 3 sets of adjectives to measure intensity, sensory, and reactive (affective) components: (1) intensity list = 15 words (e.g., excruciating); (2) sensory list = 13 words (e.g., piercing); (3) reactive list = 11 words (e.g., agonizing) Subjects select 1 word from each list Advantages over VAS: fewer constraints on responses, enables investigator to test validity of responses with known reliable relationships	Tested with 56 college undergrads without clinical pain Intensity scale appears reliable (117)
Long Form McGill Pain Questionnaire (LF-MPQ) Developed by Melzack and Torgerson (53,118) in 1975 Analysis using new scoring method (conversion of rank values to weighted-rank values) (119)	Dimensions measured by scaled portion of LF-MPQ: sensory (location, pattern, intensity); affective; cognitive (evaluative); miscellaneous Other dimensions addressed in other items: behavioral; sociocultural; diagnosis; drug intake; pain and medical history; personal history; factors increasing or decreasing pain; effects on sleep, sexual activity, and work; least and worst pain Abbreviated version: (1) 4 parts: drawing of human body on which location(s) of pain documented; (2) 20 words or descriptors (2–6 words each) to measure sensory, affective, cognitive, and miscellaneous; (3) pattern of pain (brief, transient, intermittent, continuous); (4) present pain intensity (PPI) on scale from 0 (no pain) to 5 (excruciating pain) Scoring provides 3 pain indices: (1) Total Pain Rating Index (PRI-T): sum of rank value of words chosen from list: first word of list implies least pain (= 1); 20 lists are subdivided into 4 groups, each yielding subindex of pain (lists 1–10 PRI-sensory, 11–15 PRI-affective, 16 PRI-	Repeated reliability and consistency demonstrated across many subject groups, including cancer patients (120,121), experimentally indiced pain (122), other medical, surgical diagnoses (53) Construct validity demonstrated for 3 major dimensions (sensory, affective, evaluative) in factor analytic studies of patients with low back pain (123-124), dysmenorrhea (124), chronic benign pain (125), and arthritis (126,127) Concurrent and predictive validity established in patients with dental pain (128), experimental pain (129), dysmenorrhea, headache (130), others (129,131) MPQ discriminates among groups of patients (acute and chronic pain [132]; different types of toothache pain [133], pain syndromes [134]) Reading et al. (135) attempted to replicate construction of MPQ word lists using multidimensional scaling and cluster analysis and provided evidence for reducing number of lists to 16 Turk et al. (136) confirmed 3 dimensions, but found them highly intercorrelated and without discriminant validity Metaanalysis performed (137)

	evaluative, 17–20 PRI-miscellaneous); technique available (137) to convert weighted-rank values to avoid loss of information about relative sensitivity of words chosen (2) Number of words chosen (NWC) from the 20 lists (not commonly analyzed) (3) Present Pain Intensity (PPI) or number + word combination selected from the 0 to 5 scale PRI and PPI data can be statistically analyzed Melzack considered MPQ a "rough instrument" Translated into Dutch (138), German (139), Italian (140) Italian investigators (141) developed culturally sensitive MPQ using same factor structure (3): 42 pain descriptors; 16 subclasses; quantitative data Caution in interpreting studies using MPQ (137) 5 versions, some researchers don't indicate which version used Derivation and examination of estimated normative mean scores of MPQ indices in 3,624 subjects: scores no more than 50% of maximum possible score (? skewness to left); only 19 of 78 word descriptors selected by >20% of all subjects Higher affective scores appeared related to chronic painful conditions (e.g., cancer, low back pain) Disadvantages: long and complex; can require intense concentration; takes up to 30 minutes to complete; some word descriptors may be hard to understand; scoring takes several minutes	Reliable, valid tool that can be used in a large variety of patient groups with different pain Useful in descriptive studies, evaluation of intervention outcomes, clarification of differences and similarities among pain types Wilkie (137) recommends to researchers using MPQ: (1) interpret their data in light of estimated normative scores (approach population mean); (2) report a common set of descriptive data (age, gender, ethnicity); (3) indicate version of MPQ used; (4) report percentage of sample using specific words, and look at trends by painful condition
Memorial Pain Assessment Card (MPAC) Developed by Fishman et al. (142)	Measure of cancer pain and pain relief 8.5- × 11-inch card containing a VAS measuring pain relief, pain intensity, mood, and an adaptation of Tursky's pain adjective rating scale: example, Mood Scale (worst to best mood) Card folded in middle so that 4 sides can be presented separately and quickly to patients VAS Mood Scale is a compound measure of general psychologic distress MPAC is short, simple, easy to administer and score and may be used for a variety of clinical research purposes	In a study of 50 hospitalized cancer patients strong correlation found between the VAS pain and adjective rating scales and the MPQ ($r = 0.36$–0.45, $p = 0.005$–0.001) VAS pain relief scale appeared related to VAS mood scale ($r = 0.57$, $p < 0.001$) VAS mood scale correlated at varying degrees of significance with several subscales and total score from Profile of Mood States ($r = 0.31$–0.47, $p = 0.02$–0.001) as well as with the Hamilton Depression Scale ($r = -0.41$, $p = 0.005$) and Zung Depression Scale ($r = 0.44$, $p = 0.001$) Further studies of MPAC reliability and validity needed to substantiate use in cancer and other types of pain

37D. Additional Multidimensional Instruments to Measure Pain (*cont.*)

Instrument/Study	Important Points	Psychometric Indices
West Haven-Yale Multidimensional Pain Inventory (WHYMPI) (143)	Based on cognitive/behavioral theory and developed specifically for patients with chronic pain (143) 52-item inventory divided into 3 parts: (1) perceived pain intensity and impact on various aspects of life; (2) perceptions of others' responses to pain and suffering; (3) involvement in common daily activities Patients record responses on 6-point and 7-point scales in each part (e.g., Part II: frequency with which others respond to patient's display of pain and suffering with a particular behavior [0 never to 6 very frequently]) Administration time is 15–30 minutes	Reliability and stability: coefficient alphas (internal consistency): 0.70–0.90 Pearson's product–moment correlations for test–retest reliability 0.62–0.92 Factor analysis: confirmed utility of scales within each part of the WHYMPI Factor analysis: documented construct validity Appears that WHYMPI is a reliable and valid tool for assessment of pain-related problems in a chronic pain population Cross-validation needed in other patient populations (initial sample, male veterans of U.S. Armed Services) Additional psychometric and utility data available (144)

Numbers in parentheses correspond to studies cited in the References.

38

Measuring Skin Integrity

Barbara J. Braden and Rita A. Frantz

The term *skin integrity* refers to the wholeness or intactness of the skin. For the clinical researcher, measurement issues related to skin integrity primarily revolve around etiologic factors in pressure sore development and healing of chronic and acute wounds.

Many instruments are available to the clinical researcher concerning skin integrity. Selecting one or more instruments will depend on the purpose of the inquiry. The common purposes of inquiry in this area are to identify patients at risk for skin breakdown and to determine the effectiveness of clinical modalities for preventing pressure sores and the effectiveness of treatment modalities to heal pressure sores and other wounds. Instruments available for these purposes can be divided into four categories: (1) measures of pressure and clinical determinants of pressure; (2) measures of clinical determinants of tissue tolerance for pressure; (3) measures of risk for developing pressure sores; and (4) measures of stage, size, and status of pressure sores, chronic wounds, or surgical wounds. Many instruments are discussed comprehensively, and additional measures of these categories are presented in Appendices 38A and 38B.

It is important to note that many factors contribute to the development and healing of pressure sores, and some probably remain to be discovered or adequately delineated. Certainly, many of these factors interact in ways that are not fully understood. Although it is expedient and wise to use the instruments currently available, the clinical researcher should be alert to other potentially relevant data. Furthermore, anecdotal data on a per case basis may be enlightening. Clinicians providing direct care are important sources of this type of information, and their intuitive judgments about why pressure sores develop or heal in one patient and not in others should be solicited and evaluated.

Measurement Tools

Intensity and Duration of Pressure

Instruments measuring the intensity and duration of pressure usually measure pressure at the interface between a support surface (mattress, wheelchair pad) and a body surface. Such instruments may be used in various areas of inquiry, such as investigations into the effect of positioning on specific bony prominences, the effectiveness of therapeutic mattresses or wheelchair pads in reducing interface pressure, or comparison of the effects of differing identical interface pressures on varying patient populations.

Continuous Pressure Monitor

Some studies have used relatively simple devices to measure pressure. The simplest of these, a Continuous Pressure Monitor, was used to study skin pressure measurements in cancer patients on various mattress surfaces.[1] This device has three components: (1) a pressure-sensing inflatable bladder with a 2-square-inch surface area; (2) a pump that inflates the bladder in response to internal pressures; and (3) a mercury manometer to measure the bladder pressure. The bladder is placed between the patient and the mattress at a bony prominence. The internal walls of the inflatable bladder have electrically conductive strips that are connected to the pump. When the bladder is flat, the conductive strips make contact and activate the pump. The pump inflates the bladder until the conductive strips separate. The separation occurs at a pressure that is equal to or slightly greater than the surface pressure between the patient and the mattress; this pressure is reflected on the mercury manometer. When the conductive strips separate, the pump is switched off and the bladder deflates until contact is reestablished. One group of researchers report the accuracy of this device to be ± 2 mm Hg at a pressure of 50 mm Hg mercury and below and ± 4 mm Hg from 50 to 80 mm Hg.[1] Instrument reliability is a problem, however, given that the bladder measures pressure over a very small area and the point of maximal pressure is not easily established. Positioning of the bladder and positioning of the patient (or subject) must be precisely the same if one is to obtain reliable comparisons. It is very difficult to achieve the degree of precision required to obtain reliable results with this instrument.

Texas Interface Pressure Evaluator (TIPE)

The Texas Interface Pressure Evaluator (TIPE) is more complex than the Continuous Pressure Monitor but more accurate in establishing the point of maximal pressure. Whereas the Continuous Pressure Monitor is small and has one internal contact switch, the TIPE is larger and has a 12 × 12 matrix of pneumatically activated contact switches connected to an light-emitting diode (LED) readout board. The readout board contains 144 LEDs that illuminate with pressure on the corresponding switches. As with the Continuous Pressure Monitor, the standard error using the TIPE ranged from 2.83 mm Hg to 4.49 mm Hg. However, multiple pad repositionings to determine the point of maximal pressure are not necessary with the TIPE, rendering it less vulnerable to human error. In addition to identifying the peak interface pressure at a given location, the TIPE also reveals the pressure gradient that exists across that location. This device is commercially available and has been used to evaluate patient positioning practices and wheelchair pressure-reduction cushions.[2]

A MINI-TIPE also is available. It is consists of a 4 × 4 matrix with 16 LEDs, and it is battery operated and highly portable. Like the larger version, it identifies the magnitude and location of the peak interface pressure over a bony prominence, but does not identify the pressure gradient across the area.

Purdue Pad

The Purdue Pad is the largest and most complex of the interface pressure instruments.[3] It is a full-body pressure mat that can sense pressure and subsequent changes in pressure every 5 seconds. The pressure mat is composed of two orthogonal arrays of silver-coated ribbonlike conductors, separated by open-cell natural latex foam for insulation. The points at which the horizontal and vertical conductors cross form 1,536 pressure-sensitive nodes, each representing an area of 4 cm^2, arranged in a grid of 24 × 64. The system includes the electronically fitted pressure mat, a computer to process data, and a color video that displays the results as a false color map. This allows the researcher to view all areas of interface simultaneously and over time. The color map image can be frozen and copied to disk for further analysis. Repeated measurements may be obtained with a precision of 2 to 3 mmHg. Calibration procedures can be accomplished in 30 minutes and will last for several days or until the ambient relative humidity changes. Because capacitance increases approximately 4% for every 1% change in relative humidity, the investigators are considering adding a moisture barrier, but currently recommend use in a humidity-controlled environment. The Purdue Pad was developed under a contract from Hill-Rom Company, Batesville, IN, where it has been used to measure the effectiveness of support surfaces in reducing interface pressure and the variability that occurs in patients who differ by age, height, weight, and physical condition. It is not currently available for general use, but investigators whose research goals are congruent with those of Hill-Rom may be allowed to use this instrument under certain circumstances.

Activity and Mobility

Measurement of activity and/or mobility commonly is associated with functional assessment or risk assessment tools. These tools, covered elsewhere in this book, are valuable in a number of different situations. It is important to remember, however, that the level of measurement provided by these tools is ordinal. The following instruments provide continuous data on activity/mobility and, as such, are more appropriate in certain research situations.[4]

Wheelchair Activity/Mobility

The Time-Logger Communicator (TLC) was developed by Merbitz et al.[5] to measure the number of times a patient lifts his or her body from a seated position for a period of time sufficient to relieve pressure. To prevent pressure sores, spinal cord–injured patients are taught to perform this maneuver every 15 to 20 minutes. This is referred to as "lift-off" behavior and the TLC is a pocket-sized, battery-operated, computer that is capable of continuously recording this behavior for up to 36 hours. The computer is equipped with a sensor apparatus that consists of a large, airtight vinyl bladder connected by tubing to a smaller vinyl bag. The smaller bag is inside an 8- × 13- × 26-mm box that is mounted on the frame of the wheelchair alongside the computer and a lever. The larger air-filled bladder is placed between the seat cushion and the wheelchair's sling seat, and the system is designed so that a weight greater than 20 kg over the seat cushion forces air into the smaller bladder. This in turn moves the lever, which depresses a key that enters the event and the time of occurrence into the computer. When the weight over the seat cushion is reduced to 14 kg, a spring returns the lever, and this event as well as the time and duration of the occurrence are entered into the computer. Reliability and validity data are not reported for the TLC, but further information is available from the investigator.

Bed Mobility

Schnelle et al.[6] developed an instrument for monitoring gross body movement of bedridden patients that consists of strips of Kynar brand piezoelectric plastic film. These strips are the thickness and width of electrician's tape and are placed under the bed sheets across the full width of the bed. The strips are positioned at the level of the subject's hips and shoulders and attached to two channels connected to a bedside monitor. Movement creates electrical signals transmitted to the bedside monitor and digitized from each channel over 100 times per second. The monitor then subtracts the lowest reading from the highest reading every 2 minutes, recording the peak activity for that 2-minute period. Large body moves are considered to have taken place when large moves of the hip and the shoulder are recorded in the same 2-minute interval.

Because the instrument is sufficiently sensitive to record movement from respirations and movement from extremities, investigators tested it against direct observation, using two observers. The interrater reliability (percent agreement) between these two observers for identifying large body movements (at least 45 degrees movement of body off the bed surface) was 92%. Behavioral observations (large movement, yes/no) were compared with the 424 instrument readings (large movement, other movement), and sensitivity and specificity were calculated to establish the validity (decisional accuracy) of the readings. The sensitivity for hip and shoulder movements was 83% and 84%, respectively, and the specificity was 93% and 92%. For both the hip and the shoulder, the total percent correctly classified was 92%. These investigators also used technology to detect light and sound in conjunction with body movement data, so that caregiver-initiated body turns could be distinguished from patient-initiated turns.

Sensory Perception

The intensity and duration of pressure that patients tolerate is related to their ability to perceive pain and other noxious stimuli and to respond to remove the noxious stimulus. Instruments in this section help both the clinician and the researcher develop semi-objective data related to sensory perception as it relates to the cutaneous sensation. Such instruments have been used in studies of peripheral neuropathies and might be helpful in studies of the interaction between peripheral neuropathies and other factors implicated in the etiology of chronic wounds.

Three-Point Esthesiometer

The three-point esthesiometer is a millimeter ruler with a slide placed on it. The zero end of the ruler has two spikes, one of which is placed at the end of the ruler in an axial direction that is used to apply a one-point stimulus. The second spike is placed perpendicular to the ruler below the zero line and, in conjunction with a third spike attached to a movable slide, is used to apply a two-point stimulus. Measurement of two-point discrimination is determined by applying the spikes in two trials to either one or two stimulus points and asking the subject whether two stimulus points were applied in the first or second trial. If the subject answers correctly, the distance between the two points is diminished by 1 mm and reapplied in successive trials until the subject cannot discriminate. The threshold is the smallest measurement distance between the two spikes at which the person can discriminate.

Researchers should keep in mind that inter- and intrainvestigator differences in pressure applied can influence the reliability and validity of the findings. One group of investigators found a high degree of consistency in the evaluation of five serial tests over 22 sites, but did not specify whether these measures were obtained by one person or different people.[7] They also found that the threshold for two-point discrimination increased with age, but did not differ between men and women. Reviewing the paper by Werner and Omer[8] will help potential investigators to standardize procedures and temper interpretations. See Appendix 38A for additional instruments.[7,9]

Clinical Determinants of Tissue Tolerance

Tissue tolerance refers to the ability of the skin and supporting structures to withstand the effects of pressure without adverse sequelae. The amount and duration of pressure required to damage the skin can be mediated by intrinsic and extrinsic factors that alter the ability of the tissues to tolerate pressure. The instruments covered in this section measure either the effects of varying tissue tolerance or the mediating intrinsic or extrinsic factors. See Appendix 38A for additional instruments.[10-14]

Hard Instrumented Seat to Measure Shear and Pulsatile Blood Flow

The Hard Instrumented Seat measures shear and pulsatile blood flow as well as pressure. This device consists of a hard, clear plastic seat containing flush-mounted sensors capable of monitoring all three variables. The pressure and shear sensors consist of a combination of cantilever beams and strain gauges. These sensors straddle the blood flow device at a known lateral separation that allows both average pressure and the pressure gradient over the blood flow device to be determined. The blood flow device is a photoplethysmograph, which has the disadvantage of lacking an absolute calibration procedure and limits usage to intercomparison data. It has been used to determine differences in pressure, shear, and pulsatile blood flow among paraplegic, geriatric, and normal subjects in a sitting position.[15] This device has limited applications in clinical research because it cannot be used inside soft pressure-relief mattresses or cushions and is prone to certain types of quantification errors. Nevertheless, it has several unique qualities for researchers with special interest in this area.

Magnetic Resonance Imaging and Computed Tomography Scanning

Research on the effects of external forces on soft tissue have previously been limited because of an inability to visualize adequately the deformation of these internal structures. The emergence of magnetic resonance and computer augmented x-rays has expanded the potential to analyze the anatomic changes caused by external forces imposed on bony prominences. Although the equipment needed for these measurements is expensive and often not easily accessible for clinical research, efforts to incorporate these methods in such studies could produce profound insights regarding the dynamics of pressure-induced soft-tissue injury. Magnetic resonance imaging (MRI) provides a noninvasive method of measuring tissue shapes in vivo. The technique employs magnetic energy sources to create cross-sectional images of the human anatomy without using radiation. Atomic nuclei, contained in a magnetic field created by the magnetic resonance machine and stimulated by specific radio frequencies, emit measurable radio signals that are influenced by the type and condition of tissue composed of these nuclei. The radio signals are captured and converted to a visual display on a computer monitor. By monitoring the response of atomic nuclei in magnetic fields, longitudinal and transverse views of internal tissue structures from the skin surface to underlying bony prominences can be reconstructed.[16] Reger, McGovern, and Chung[17] describe the results of using MRI to measure soft-tissue deformation in five subjects (2 normal; 3 paraplegic) seated on various support surfaces. They found distinct anatomic differences in soft tissues underlying bony prominences between the paraplegic subjects and controls. This preliminary work suggests that the measurement capability of MRI in assessing soft-tissue deformations makes it an instrument well suited to evaluating the effects of pressure on soft tissue.

Computed tomography (CT scanning) has recently been applied to in vivo study of the effects of shearing forces on soft tissue underlying bony prominences. CT scanning uses x-rays augmented with a scanning system and computer to measure the attenuation of tissue. Conner and Clarck[18] (1993) employed CT scanning to evaluate the soft tissue–skeletal relationship at the ischial tuberosity in three healthy subjects lying on various support surfaces. Using measurements derived from the pelvic CT scans, the investigators were able to calculate shear stress and shear strain. This study provides a model for future efforts to quantify the effects of external forces on the anatomic configuration of human tissue.

Skin Hydration

Recent advances in technology have enhanced the precision with which skin hydration can be measured noninvasively. Among the devices most applicable to clinical nursing research are the hydrometer (Skicon-100™), the electrical capacitance monitor (Corneometer CM 420), and the evaporimeter (Servo Med EPI™). The hydrometer measures the hydration of the stratum corneum via electrical conductance.[19] It consists of a main recorder and a probe with two concentrically arranged brass electrodes. The probe is applied to the skin, allowing high-frequency current to flow between the two electrodes. The conductance is registered and displayed digitally, expressed as reciprocal impedance in measures of 1 micro Ohm (µohm). The electrical capacitance monitor is equipped with a probe containing a circular brass grid covered with a plastic foil (Schwarzhaupt GmbH, Cologne, West Germany). The skin surface below this electrode acts as the other electrode. The probe is applied to the skin, and the capacitance is expressed digitally in arbitrary units. The evaporimeter measures water evaporation for the skin surface.[20] The probe consists of a cylindrical chamber mounted with sensors for measurement of the relative humidity and the temperature. The transepidermal water loss (TEWL) is calculated automatically and digitally displayed in terms of $g/m^2/hour$. Blichmann and Serup[20] compared the three methods of measuring skin hydration on 10 healthy subjects using test sites on the forearm and palm of the hand. They found that the hydrometer was more sensitive in measuring increased hydration, but that the electrical capacitance monitor was more highly sensitized to decreased hydration. There were no significant inter- and intraindividual variations. Reproducibility testing revealed that the electrical capacitance monitor was more accurate than the hydrometer. The investigators concluded that both the hydrometer and the electrical capacitance monitor provided valid assessments of skin hydration.

Risk for Skin Breakdown

Several instruments designed to predict the risk of skin breakdown have been reported in the literature.[21,22] These instruments use summative rating scales based on observations of factors contributing to skin breakdown and specify critical scores for identifying patients at risk. Because the panel of experts convened by the Agency for Health Care Policy and Research[23] found that only the Norton Scale and the Braden Scale had sufficient evidence of reliability and validity to warrant clinical use, discussion will be limited to these instruments.

Researchers or clinicians considering the use of these instruments should be reminded that they are designed to measure risk for skin breakdown rather than to predict with absolute accuracy the occurrence of skin breakdown. It also is important to note that these instruments were tested using almost exclusively hospitalized and institutionalized elderly subjects. It would, therefore, be unwise to expect predictive values to be similar to those previously reported when these instruments are used to study younger populations.

Norton Scale

The Norton Scale has been studied extensively. This tool consists of five parameters: physical condition, mental state, activity, mobility, and incontinence, each of which is rated from 1 to 4, with one- or two-word descriptors for each rating. The sum of the ratings for all five parameters yields a score that can range from 5 to 20, with lower scores indicating increased risk. From data collected among elderly patients, Norton concluded that a score of 14 indicated the "onset of risk" and a score of 12 or below indicated high risk for pressure sore formation.[21]

The Norton Scale was used by Roberts and Goldstone[24] in a study of 59 pressure sore–free patients over age 60 admitted to an orthopedic ward. Thirty-two patients received scores below 14, and 12 of these at-risk patients developed pressure sores deeper than Stage I. Using 14 as a cutoff score, the following values can be calculated from these data: sensitivity of 92%; specificity of 57%; a predictive value of a positive test of 37.5%; and a predictive value of a negative test of 96%. These investigators trained a team of nurses to rate the patients, but they do not report data regarding interrater reliability.

Goldstone and Goldstone[25] in a later study used only one rater in an apparent attempt to control the reliability of the scores. Among patients over age 60 admitted to an orthopedic ward, 30 of 40 were judged to be at risk, and 16 of these at risk patients developed pressure lesions. This resulted in a sensitivity of 89%, a specificity of 36%, a predictive value of a positive test of 53%, and a predictive value of a negative test of 80%. Goldstone and Goldstone do not define pressure lesions, but they likely classified skin erythema as a pressure lesion, which may account for the improvement in the predictive values.

Lincoln and her associates[26] also conducted an evaluation of the Norton Scale and reported very poor (0%) sensitivity and predictive value of a positive test. The sample size was so small, however, that these results should be considered with caution. Lincoln also tested for interrater reliability, using data from 73 patients who were rated on four separate occasions by two registered nurse investigators. They reported a low percent agreement among RN raters (39.7%). There also was disagreement among experts concerning face validity. The exact nature of these concerns was not reported, but another panel of experts convened by the Agency for Health Care Policy and Research found this scale to have enough validity and reliability to recommend it for clinical use.[23]

Braden Scale

The Braden Scale was developed in 1983 to predict the risk for pressure sore development.[22] The Braden Scale is composed of six subscales that conceptually reflect degrees of sensory perception, skin moisture, physical activity, nutritional intake, friction and shear, and ability to change and control body position. All subscales are rated from 1 to 4, with the exception of the friction and shear subscale, which is rated from 1 to 3. Each rating is accompanied by a brief description of criteria for assigning the rating to facilitate consistency in rating. Potential scores range from 4 to 23, and lower scores indicate higher risk.

This instrument has undergone extensive testing. Content validity has been established by expert opinion. Two studies of reliability have been carried out in two extended care facilities.[22] The purpose of the first study was to estimate interrater reliability between a graduate student research assistant and registered nurses trained in the use of the tool. The Pearson's product–moment correlation among 84 pairs of observation scores was $r = 0.99$ ($p < 0.001$) and the percent agreement was 88%. In no case did the total score assigned by the two raters differ by more than a 1-point difference. The purpose of the second study was to determine the reliability of the scale when used by licensed practical nurses and nurse aides who were not trained in the use of the tool. Pearson's product–moment correlations among 53 pairs of scores ranged from $r = 0.83$ to $r = 0.87$ ($p < 0.001$), but percent agreement ranged from 11% for those on the day shift to 19% for those on the evening shift.

Studies of predictive validity have been conducted using patient populations admitted to a general nursing unit, a critical care stepdown unit, and an adult intensive care unit, all in tertiary care settings. In the two studies conducted outside the intensive care unit[30] ($n = 99, n = 100$) adult subjects were heterogeneous with regard to age, and the tool demonstrated 100% sensitivity and predictive value of a negative test in both groups and 90% and 64% specificity respectively at a cutoff score of 16. However, the predictive value of a positive test diminished to 50% and 19%, respectively, in these two studies.

In the study of predictive validity among 60 subjects admitted to an adult intensive care unit,[27] a critical cutoff score of 16 or below demonstrated a sensitivity of 83%, a specificity of 64%, a predictive value of positive test of 61%, and a predictive value of a negative test of 85%. Preliminary results of a related study of subjects admitted to a skilled nursing facility indicate that a score of 18 produced a sensitivity of 79%, a specificity of 74%, a 54% predictive value of a positive test, 90% predictive value of a negative test, and 75% correct classification rate.[28]

The differences in predictive validity when using the tool in different settings probably occur as a result of variances in age and severity of illness among subjects, as well as the variance in caregiver-to-patient ratios in all three settings. For example, in areas that have low caregiver-to-patient ratios, patients who are identified as "at risk" may receive more attention to preventive strategies and some pressure sores are thus prevented. This could result in lower levels of specificity and this may have been occurring in the step-down and intensive care units as the primary nurses participated in rating the patients.

Other investigators have tested the Braden Scale with various degrees of rigor and differing results. Salvadalena, Snyder, and Brogdon[29] reported significantly lower indices of predictive validity, but the method for identifying Stage I ulcers may have led to the discrepancy with previous results.[30] Hergenroeder, Mosher, and Sevo[31] found that nurses' judgment was as reliable in predicting pressure sore risk (yes–no answer) as the Braden Scale. The wide difference in mean Braden Scale score between those patients at risk (14.45) and those patients not at risk (20.24) leaves open the question of whether nurses would be able to discriminate among patients who were more homogeneous in relation to risk or differed less in degree of risk. Xakellis et al.[32] found that the nurses base their judgments of risk on patients' diminished mobility and increased exposure to friction and shear. Although diminished mobility and increased friction and shear may identify those most obviously at risk, other factors measured in both the Norton Scale and the Braden Scale have been found to improve prediction.[33,34]

Xakellis et al.[32] also compared the Norton Scale and the Braden Scale to determine whether these tools would predict the same patients to be at risk. The Cohen's kappa for agreement between the two tools was 73. The Norton Scale identified 38% of the patients as being at risk, and the Braden Scale predicted 27% of the patients to be at risk. Because this study was cross-sectional rather than prospective, one cannot draw conclusions concerning which tool was more accurate. It could be said, however, that the Braden Scale was more conservative than the Norton in identifying patients at risk.

Pressure Sore Status

Staging

Many staging systems have been proposed, but one four-stage classification has achieved the highest degree of consensus among professionals:[35,p56]

Stage I. Nonblanchable erythema of intact skin, that heralds lesion of skin ulceration.

Stage II. Partial thickness skin loss involving epidermis and/or dermis. The ulcer is superficial and presents clinically as an abrasion, blister, or shallow crater.

Stage III. Full-thickness skin loss involving damage or necrosis of subcutaneous tissue that may extend down to, but not through, underlying fascia. The ulcer presents clinically as a deep crater with or without undermining of adjacent tissue.

Stage IV. Full-thickness skin loss with extensive destruction, tissue necrosis, or damage to muscle, bone or supporting structures (for example, tendon or joint capsule).

The clinical researcher should know that wound staging cannot be confirmed when the wound is covered with eschar or full of necrotic tissue. This staging system provides only a gross assessment of the severity of a pressure sore. It is sufficient for studies of the epidemiology of pressure sores, but it is too global to be of use for wound healing studies. Tools are somewhat more helpful in describing the severity of pressure sores are presented in Appendix 38B.[36-39]

Pressure Sore Surface Area

Meticulous and accurate measurement of pressure sore surface area is probably most important in studies related to the effectiveness of therapeutic modalities in enhancing healing. Several methods are reported in the literature, some requiring more sophisticated equipment than others.

Acetate Tracings

Three common methods of using acetate tracings to determine pressure sore surface area have been described by Bohannon and Pfaller.[40] The materials for tracing are sterilized transparency film and a fine-tip transparency marker. To obtain the tracing, the investigator places the sterilized transparency film over the sore and traces the perimeter with the transparency marker. The tracing then is cut from the transparency film and quantified by one of three methods. The first method used by Bohannan and Pfaller involved placing the tracing over metric graph paper and counting the square millimeters within the perimeter, the second method consisted of weighing the tracing on a gram balance scale, and the third method required the edges of the tracing to be retraced with an electronic planimeter.

To determine the accuracy of each method in their study, Bohannon and Pfaller used multiple tracings of the same sore obtained by two different clinicians, resulting in 10 pairs of tracings. Mean differences in the area mass identified by each of the three methods were then calculated in the 10 pairs. The mean difference with the weighing technique was 4.4%, 3.9% with the counting technique, and 3.6% with the planimetry. According to these investigators, the greatest percentage differences were found in the tracings of small wounds, but were of no greater magnitude than the difference between larger tracings. They reported that the greatest difference found in the calculated areas of tracings of the same wound by two different clinicians was 8.8%, or 0.81 cm^2.

Thomas and Wysocki[41] compared acetate tracing to methods involving photography and the Kundin Wound Gauge, a measurement device involving length and width rulers placed at right angles to each other with a recommended formula for calculating surface area. Both the photographs and the acetate tracings were digitally analyzed by an image analysis system (Zeiss Interactive Digital Analysis System). These investigators found that the results of all three methods were strongly correlated, but the acetate tracing reportedly resulted in the most accurate measure of surface area. No information was given on the image analysis system regarding standard error for readings.

Photography

Photography has been used for clinical documentation of wounds and wound progress, but quantification problems can occur that may be unacceptable in measurement of certain outcomes. Many variables, including distance from the wound, lighting for the photograph, the type of lens, the f-stop of the lens aperture, and the type of film, must be optimized and held constant.

Thomas and Wysocki[41] used a 35 mm camera (Nikon, FE2) equipped with a 120-mm medical lens (Nikkor) with built-in ring flash and reproduction ratio imprinting feature. They used color slide film (EKtachrome, ASA 100) and calculated wound area from the slide film image by placing the image on a digitizing tables and using a stylus to trace the wound margins. They found a strong correlation ($r = 0.99$, $p = < 0.0001$) between measurements obtained by the photography and acetate tracings. A significant difference between surface areas obtained by these methods was found using a repeated-measures analysis of variance, however, and these investigators concluded that acetate tracings were more accurate.

Pressure Sore Volume

Measures of surface area of pressure sores have become more sophisticated but, as two-dimensional measures, are not sensitive to progression or regression of deeper wounds. Three-dimensional measures are necessary to accurately estimate more wound volume and changes in deeper wounds. These measures are useful in testing the effectiveness of various treatments (e.g., topical applications, pressure-reducing or -relieving surfaces) in promoting wound healing. They are shown in Appendix 38B.

Status of Surgical Wounds

Measuring wound status in closed surgical wounds requires tools that are different from those used to describe pressure sores or other open, chronic wounds. Siddall[47] outlines nine criteria for external assessment of the surgical wound as follows: (1) apposition; (2) capillary fill; (3) temperature; (4) healing ridge; (5) scab; (6) drainage; (7) discoloration; (8) swelling; and (9) pain. These characteristics seem to describe the most relevant attributes of a surgical wound, but no tool could be found that offered a realistic or replicable method for quantifying these characteristics. Some measured only a few of these characteristics, and others were designed to measure internal markers of healing. Instruments used to measure surgical wounds are shown in Appendix 38B.[48-53]

Exemplar Studies

Bergstrom, N., & Braden, B. A prospective study of pressure sore risk among institutionalized elderly. *J Am Geriatr Soc*, 1992, *40*(12):747-752.

This study exemplifies measurement of many of the variables related to the etiology of one disturbance in skin integrity, pressure sores. The design is prospective, and most of the variables associated with the development of pressure sores are measured with particular attention to nutritional variables. The methods are rigorous and explained in detail. The instruments used had been previously tested for reliability and validity, and procedures were used to ensure continued reliability and validity throughout the 3 years of the study. One of these instruments, the Braden Scale, is described in this chapter, and the computer program, Nutritionist III, is described in the chapter on nutritional measures. Because the etiology of pressure sores is multivariate, appropriate multivariate analyses were used to determine the relative contribution of multiple factors in predicting pressure sore development.

Allman, R., Walker, J., Hart, M., et al. Air-fluidized beds or conventional therapy for pressure sores. *Ann Int Med*, 1987, *107*(5):641-649.

This study exemplifies measurement of treatment outcomes for one disturbance in skin integrity, pressure sores. This is a randomized clinical trial comparing healing rates of persons nursed on two different support surfaces. The methods are rigorous and described in excellent detail. The Norton Scale was used to recognize the fact that the same factors that contribute to etiology of pressure sores can contribute to maintenance and degeneration of that wound. Other factors related to pressure sore etiology, regeneration, or degeneration also were measured. The measures used to determine healing rate were acetate tracings and serial color photographs. The investigators used rigorous methods to ensure the reliability of this outcome measure. Usual care was controlled, observed, and described.

References

1. Berjian, D., Douglass, H., Holyoke, E., et al. Skin pressure measurements on various mattress surfaces in cancer patient. *Am J Phys Med*, 1983, 62(5): 217-226.

2. Garber, S., Campion, L., & Krouskop, T. Trochanteric pressure in spinal cord injury. *Arch Phys Med Rehab*, 1982, 63(11):549-553.

3. Babbs, C., Bourland, J., Graber, G., et al. A pressure-sensitive mat for measuring contact pressure distributions of patients lying on hospital beds. *Biomed Instrument Technol*, 1990, 24(6):363-369.

4. Merbitz, C., Morris, J., & Grip, J. Ordinal scales and foundations of misinference. *Arch Phys Med Rehab*, 1989, 70(4):308-312.

5. Merbitz, C.T., King, R.B., Bleiberg, J., & Grip, J.C. Wheelchair push-ups: Measuring pressure relief frequency. *Arch Phys Med Rehab*, 1985, 66(7):433-438.

6. Schnelle, J., Ouslander, J., Simmons, S., et al. Nighttime sleep and bed mobility among incontinent nursing home residents. *J Am Geriatr Soc*, 1993, 41(9):910-914.

7. Halar, E., Hammond, M., LaCava, E., et al. Sensory perception threshold measurement: An evaluation of semiobjective testing devices. *Arch Phys Med Rehab*, 1987, 68(8):499-507.

8. Werner, J., & Omer, G. Evaluating cutaneous pressure sensation of the hand. *Am J Occup Ther*, 1970, 24(5):347-356.

9. Arezzo, J., Schaumburg, H., & Laudadio, C. Thermal Sensitivity Tester: Device for quantitative assessment of thermal sense in diabetic neuropathy. *Diabetes*, 1986, 35(5):590-592.

10. Shepherd, A., Riedel, G., Kiel, J., et al. Evaluation of an infrared laser-Doppler blood flowmeter. *Am J Physiol Gastrointest Liver Physiol*, 1987, 252(6):G832.

11. Holloway, G., & Watkins, D. Laser Doppler measurement of cutaneous blood flow. *J Invest Dermatol*, 1977, 69(3):306-312.

12. Huch, R., Lubbers, D., & Huch, A. Quantitative continuous measurement of partial oxygen pressure on the skin of adults and newborn babies. *Pflugers Arch*, 1972, 337:185-192.

13. Bader, D., & Grant, C. Changes in transcutaneous oxygen tension as a result of prolonged pressures at the sacrum. *Clin Phys Physiol Meas*, 1988, 9(1):33-37.

14. Coleman, L., Dowd, G., & Bentley, G. Reproducibility of tcO^2 measurements in normal volunteers. *Clin Phys Physiol Meas*, 1986, 7(3):259-263.

15. Bennett, L., Kavner, D., Lee, B., et al. Skin stress and blood flow in sitting paraplegic patients. *Arch Phys Med Rehab*, 1984, 65(4):186-190.

16. Crooks, L.E. An introduction to magnetic resonance imaging. *IEEE Engineer Med Biol*, 1985, 4(3):8-12.

17. Reger, S., McGovern, T., & Chung, K. Biomechanics of tissue distortion and stiffness by magnetic resonance imaging. In D.L. Bader (Ed.), *Pressure sores: Clinical practice and scientific approach*. London: Macmillan, 1990.

18. Conner, L., & Clack, J. In vivo CT scan comparison of vertical shear in human tissue caused by various support surfaces. *Decubitus*, 1993, 6(2):20-26.

19. Tagami, H., Ohi, M., Iwatsuki, K., et al. Evaluation of the skin surface hydration in vivo by electrical measurement. *J Invest Dermatol*, 1980, 75(6):500-507.

20. Blichmann, C. & Serup, J. Reproducibility and variability of transepidermal water loss measurement: Studies on the Servo Med evaporimeter. *Acta Dermatol Venereol (Stockh)*, 1987, 67(3):206-210.

21. Norton, D., McLaren, F., & Exton-Smith, A. An investigation of geriatric nursing problems in hospital. Edinburgh: Churchill Livingston, 1975.

22. Bergstrom, N., Braden, B., Laguzza, A., & Holman, V. The Braden Scale for predicting pressure sore risk. *Nurs Res*, 1987, 36(4):205-209.

23. Panel for the Prediction and Prevention of Pressure Ulcers in Adults. *Pressure ulcers in adults: Prediction and prevention. Clinical practice guideline, No. 3*. AHCPR Publication No. 92-0047. Rockville, MD: Agency for Health Care Policy and Research, Public Health Service, U.S. Department of Health and Human Services, 1992.

24. Roberts, B.V., & Goldstone, L.A. A survey of pressure sores in the over sixties on two orthopaedic wards. *Int J Nur Stud*, 1979, 16(5):355-359.

25. Goldstone, L.A., & Goldstone, J. The Norton score: An early warning of pressure sores? *J Adv Nurs*, 1982, 1(5):419-425.

26. Lincoln, R., Roberts, R., Maddox, A., et al. Use of the Norton pressure sore risk assessment scoring system with elderly patients in acute care. *J Enterostomal Ther*, 1986, 13(4):17-23.

27. Bergstrom, N., Demuth, P.J., & Braden, B. A clinical trial of the Braden Scale for predicting pressure sore risk. *Nurs Clin North Am*, 1987, 22(2): 417-421.

28. Braden, B., & Bergstrom, N. Predictive validity of the Braden Scale for Pressure Sore Risk in a nursing home population. *Research in Nursing & Health*, 1994, 17(6):459-470.

29. Salvadalena, G., Snyder, M., Brogdon, K. Clinical trial of the Braden Scale on an acute care medical unit. *J Enterstomal Ther Nurs*, 1993, 19(5):160-165.

30. Bergstrom, N. Braden Scale and clinical judgement. *J Enterstomal Ther Nurs*, 1993, 20(3):133-136.

31. Hergenroeder, P., Mosher, C., Sevo, D. Pressure ulcer risk assessment—simple or complex. *Decubitus*, 1992, 5(7):47-49.

32. Xakellis, G., Franz, R., Arteaga, M., et al. A comparison of patient risk for pressure ulcer development with nursing use of preventive interventions. *J Am Geriatr Soc*, 1992, 40(12):1250-1253.

33. Bergstrom, N., & Braden, B. A prospective study of pressure sore risk among institutionalized elderly. *J Am Geriatr Soc*, 1992, *40*(8):747-758.

34. Goldstone, L.A., & Roberts, B.V. A preliminary discriminant function analysis of elderly orthopaedic patients who will or will not contract a pressure sore. *Intl J Nurs Stud*, 1980, *17*(1):17-23.

35. Bates-Jensen, B. New Pressure Ulcer Status Tool. *Decubitus*, 1990, *3*(3):14-17.

36. Bates-Jensen, B., Vredevoe, D., & Brecht, M. Validity and reliability of the Pressure Sore Status Tool. *Decubitus*, 1992, *5*(6):20-25.

38. Ferrels, B., Artinian, B.M., & Sessing, D. The Sessing Scale for assessment of pressure ulcer healing. *J Am Geriatr Soc*, 1995, *43*(1):37-40.

39. Knighton, D., Fiefel, V., Austin, L., et al. Classification and treatment of chronic nonhealing wounds. *Ann Surg*, 1986, *204*(3):323-325.

40. Bohannon, R.W., & Pfaller, B.A. Documentation of wound surface area from tracings of wound perimeters. *Phys Ther*, 1983, *63*(10):1622-1624.

41. Thomas, A., & Wysocki, A. The healing wound: A comparison of three clinically useful methods of measurement. *Decubitus*, 1990, *3*(1):18-23.

42. Kundin, J. A new way to size up a wound. *Am J Nurs*, 1989, *89*(2):206-208.

43. Eriksson, G., Eklund, A.E., Torlegard, K., & Dauphin, E. Evaluation of leg ulcer treatment with stereophotogrammetry. *Brit J Dermatol*, 1979, *101*(2):123-125.

44. Bulstrode, C.J.K., Goode, A.W., & Scott, P.J. A prospective controlled trial of topical irrigation in the treatment of delayed cutaneous healing in human leg ulcers. *Clinical Science*, 1988, *75*(6):637-640.

45. Franz, R., & Johnson, D. Stereophotography and computerized image analysis: A three-dimensional method of measuring wound healing. *Wounds*, 1992, *4*(2):58.

46. Resch, C., Kerner, E., Robson, M., et al. Pressure sore volume measurement: A technique to document and record wound healing. *J Am Geriatr Soc*, 1988, *36*(5):444-449.

47. Siddall, S. Wound healing: An assessment tool. *Home Healthcare Nurse*, 1983, *5*:35-37.

48. Holden-Lund, C. Effects of relaxation with guided imagery on surgical stress and wound healing. *Research in Nursing & Health*, 1988, *11*(4):235-241.

49. Wilson, A., Treasure, T., Sturridge, M., & Gruenenberg, R. A scoring method (ASEPSIS) for postoperative wound infections for use in clinical trials of antibiotic prophylaxis. *Lancet*, 1986, *1*(8476):311-313.

50. Viljanto, J. Assessment of wound healing speed in man. In A. Barbul (Ed.), *Clinical and experimental approaches to dermal and epidermal repair*. New York: Wiley-Liss, 1991, p. 279.

51. Raekallio, J, & Viljanto, J. Regeneration of subcutaneous connective tissue in children. A histological study with application of the Cellstic device. *J Cutan Pathol*, 1975, *2*:191-197.

52. Viljanto, J. Cellstic: A device for wound healing studies in man. Description of the method. *J Surg Res*, 1976, *20*(2):115-119.

53. Goodson, W., & Hunt, K. Development of a new miniature method for the study of wound healing in human subjects. *J Surg Res*, 1982, *33*(5):39-43.

Appendices

38A. Additional Instruments to Measure Skin Integrity

Instrument	Description	Psychometric Indices
Measures of Intensity and Duration of Pressure		
Semmes-Weinstein Pressure Aesthesiometer Measures sensory perception	Used to establish the threshold of light touch to deep pressure Investigator uses a series of 20 calibrated nylon monofilaments that exert pressure ranging from 1.65 to 6.65 mg of pressure Pressure exerted is a function of the length and diameter of each monofilament Calibration of the monofilaments provides quantification of cutaneous sensibility	Reliability established by 5 serial measurements made over 22 sites without significant differences in sensory perception thresholds (7) Instrument relatively impervious to error when used to obtain quantifiable results; requires skilled investigator in eliciting and interpreting patient responses in qualitative determinations
Thermal Sensitivity Tester Measures sensory perception	Measure of skin temperature and thermal perception thresholds at the distal portion of upper and lower limbs providing quantifiable measurement of small-fiber nerve function Portable device consisting of two 25-cm^2 nickel-coated copper plates, each connected to separate power units and perfused with water in series Temperature of each plate can be changed at a rate >1°C/sec over a 50.0°C range (accurate to within 0.1°C) Thresholds determined by a series of trials where subject contacts each plate for 2 seconds and indicates which plate is colder Temperature of finger or toe should be maintained between 28°C and 34°C Plate contact should blanch the nail	Thermal threshold means ($n = 100$, normal subjects) (9): index finger: 0.67 C (SD, 0.31°C); great toe: 1.01°C (SD, 0.61°C); both threshold and variance increase with age Repeatability tested with varied results (7,9)
Optacon Tactile Tester Measures sensory perception	Portable device used to determine vibration thresholds as an index of large-fiber nerve function Stimulator pad consists of 144 miniature rods organized into a 24 × 6 matrix Subjects positioned so rods come into contact with ventral surface of index finger pad Rods have a 2-mm horizontal and 1-mm vertical interrod spacing and protrude through a contoured plastic plate Rods vibrate continuously at 230 Hz; amplitude varies as a function of voltage During testing, vibration is manipulated and interspersed with sham stimuli	100 normal subjects studied: mean vibratory threshold: 4.54 V (SD, 1.09 V); thresholds and variance increased with age Test–retest reliability (1-week interval, 5 subjects tested for 3 trials): no significant difference in threshold (7)

38A. Additional Instruments to Measure Skin Integrity (*cont*)

Instrument	Description	Psychometric Indices
	Subjects wear earphones (continuous white noise) and eye shielding to mask changes in voltage (accompanied by noise and movement in the area of intensity knob/voltimeter) Testing period is <5 minutes	
Measurements of clinical determinants of tissue tolerance		
Laser Doppler velocitometry	Measure of physiologic consequences of compressive pressure on tissue Consists of central unit containing a laser diode light source, photodetector, electronic signal filter board, microprocessor, continuous LED digital display, probe connected to central unit by optical fiber (Vasamedics Inc, St. Paul, MN) Laser light emitted from the probe penetrates the skin to a 1-mm depth Light is scattered by soft-tissue components Scatter produced by flowing red blood cells is Doppler shifted relative to that produced by stationary soft tissue Frequencies of returned light collected by probe sensor are analyzed and expressed in mL/min/100 g of tissue	Reliability established in animal studies (linear relationship between total flow and laser Doppler blood flow on liver surface ($r = 0.98$) and gastric mucosa ($r = 0.98$) (10) Comparative measurements of cutaneous blood flow obtained by (133) Xenon clearance technique and laser Doppler; Y on X linear regression coefficient of 0.89 ($p < 0.001$, $n = 16$) (11) Artifact eliminated by preventing movement and stimulation
Skin oxygen sensor	Transcutaneous oximetry measures partial pressure of oxygen at skin surface, providing indirect indication of tissue tolerance Uses Clark polarographic electrode with oxygen-permeable membrane containing a heating element and thermistor Electrode attached to skin by adhesive ring and gel Electrode heated to present temperature (43–45°C) Stimulates maximal vasodilation, increased skin pore opening, and release of oxygen from hemoglobin molecule, producing oxygen tensions at skin surface Approximates arterial oxygen tension (12) Novametrix Medical Systems Inc, Wallingford, CT Used in studies (13)	Reliability is a function of accurate system calibration and application of the electrode; requires frequent recalibration All bubbles must be removed when applying electrode to skin 15-minute calibration is needed after electrode application to ensure maximal vasodilitation Inaccurate measure of tissue oxygen values, especially in poor perfusion states Variations of 10% from the mean in average daily measurement can be avoided by consistent placement of electrode in same anatomic location (14)

Numbers in parentheses correspond to studies cited in the References.

38B. Measurement of Pressure Sore Status

Instrument	Description	Psychometric Indices
Measures of pressure sore status		
Pressure Sore Status Tool	Measure of the status of pressure sores (35) that is composed of 13 subscales, each rated from 1 to 5 Subscale represents a physical attribute of pressure sore (e.g., size, depth, color) Scores range from 13 to 65; lower scores associated with lesser severity and improved healing; higher scores associated with greater severity and problems with healing	Delphi process involving expert clinicians used in tool development and refinement Content validity established: index 0.91 Interrater reliability (20 pairs of observations made by 2 enterostomal therapists at 2 separate observations): $r = 0.91$ and 0.92 ($p < 0.001$), respectively; rater 1: $r = 0.99$; rater 2: $r = 0.96$ ($p < 0.001$) (36)
Sessing Scale	Measure of pressure sore status Ratings range from 0 (normal skin) to 6 (severe, heavily infected) Ratings accompanied by description of wound characteristics After initial rating, wound progress described with gain scores Charts progress of wound healing in testing of pressure sore treatments (37)	Content validity index: 100% (38) Test–retest validity: 0.90 (weighted kappa) (38) Interrater reliability: 0.8. (weighted kappa) (38) Additional validity tests conducted (38)
Wound Severity Score	Quantifiable measure of severity of chronic nonhealing cutaneous wounds (39) Measures 3 groups of variables (1) Clinical: rated none (0), mild (2), or marked (4); edema, wound purulence, wound fibrin, limb pitting edema, limb brawny edema, wound granulation Wound purulence and limb brawny edema more heavily weighted (mild = 3, marked = 6) Wound granulation is reversed scored (none = 4, marked = 0) (2) Anatomic Exposed to bone (yes = 10, no = 0) Exposed tendon (yes = 7, no = 0) Dorsalis pedis and post tibial pulses (0–1+ = 5; 2+ = 2; 3–4+ = 0)	Correlation between initial wound severity score and time to 80% healing ($r = 0.29$, $p = 0.03$); time to 100% healing ($r = 44$, $p = 0.002$) No tests of interrater reliability performed includes observations of periwound erythema, periwound

38B. Measurement of Pressure Sore Status (*cont.*)

Instrument	Description	Psychometric Indices

	(3) Measured wound, patient variables
	    Size (cm^2), scored 1–10 for sizes ranging to >30 cm^2
	    Depth (mm), scored 1–10 for depths ranging to >20 mm
	    Undermining: scored 3–8 for depth ranges to >5 mm
	    Duration, scored 1–10 for duration up to >10 years
	    Wound severity score: total range 0–97; found to decline over time in relation to wound healing, declining sharply as healing approaches 100%	

Measures of pressure sore volume		
Kundin Wound Gauge	Measures wound on either 2 (length, width) or 3 (length, width, depth) dimensions (42) Ruler used to measure depth and is placed in center (flat wound) or deepest part of crater Length and width rulers slide down until edges of wound reached; distances recorded Must use same positions for all measurements Formulae used to determine surface area or wound volume Single-use item (sterile), costing approximately $2.00	Validity of wound surface area obtained using gauge compared to acetate tracings and photography (41) Highly correlated when wounds small, circular or elliptically shaped Kundin consistently underestimated surface area of large or irregularly shaped wounds No validation testing of wound volume or interrater reliability Difficulties in exact placement of gauge make repeated measurements subject to error

Stereophotography	Designed to overcome distortion in measurement of 3-dimensional multiplanar surfaces
	Method of applying optical triangulation to produce 3-dimensional photographs
	Noninvasive method to document topical surface and internal configuration of ulcer
	3 systems
	  (1) 2 cameras on a supporting bar (43)
	    Light beam projected along optical axis of each camera, and beam intersection establishes camera positioning in in relation to ulcer surface (slightly < 2 meters)
	    Measurements made of surface area, perimeter, volume, maximum depth
	    Utility limited by distance between cameras and ulcer, so inadequate for full-thickness ulcers, and wound edge determination subject to error
		Initial testing of remote stereophotogrammetry system as in (3), using sample of 144 pairs of pressure ulcers
		Technical error of measurements range: +1.00 mm (depth) and +5.6 mm^2 (surface area)
		Interrater reliability: 0.99 (circumference); 0.96 (depth)

	(2) Stereophogrammetric camera apparatus linked to computer (44) Focus and field of view remain constant More accurate than direct tracing or simple photography Useful only for ulcers on flat surfaces that can be positioned under camera frame, and smaller surfaced area ulcers so as to require no magnification adjustment (3) Remote 3-dimensional measurement by 2 simultaneously taken photographic slides (45) Lighting system projects grid on ulcer surface that accommodates to the contours of the wound surface, establishing points of reference for computer Slides scanned and converted to PICT image and analyzed by image analysis software Generates circumference, surface area, volume, maximum depth Able to monitor full-thickness wound repair	
Wounds Volume Molds	Dental mold substance specifically formulated for moist tissues used as a rapid, safe, and simple measurement Alginate compound mixed with water to form liquid plaster (Jeltrate Alginate Impression, L.D. Caulk Co, Div of Dentply Internat'l, Milford, Delaware) Wound quickly filled using syringe for craters, spatula for flat surfaces Molds removed, rinsed, placed in airtight container Mold weighed, volume estimated by dividing weight by density (1.13 g/cc) (46)	Potential sources of error: excessive dessication of the mold prior to weighing; variations in leveling procedure (error in shallow wounds); may disrupt healing process (injure fragile epithelial cells in wound base)

Measure of the status of surgical wounds

Wound Assessment Inventory	Developed for use in a study of effects of relaxation on postoperative wound healing (48) Summated rating scale: 3 subscales: edema, erythema, exudate, each rated 0 (absent) to 3 (marked) Primarily a measure of local tissue inflammation in early surgical wounds	Content validity established Interrater reliability 0.70 (2 graduate nurses in 12 pairs of ratings)
ASEPSIS	Measure of wound healing developed for use in clinical trial comparing efficacy of antibiotics (49)	Scoring; >40 agree with findings of other investigators when severe infection present; intermediate scores: provides information other tests do not

581

38B. Measurement of Pressure Sore Status (*cont.*)

Instrument	Description	Psychometric Indices
ASEPSIS (*cont.*)	Points alloted for: A: **Additional** treatment (antibiotics, 10 points) S: **Serous** discharge (drainage of pus, 5 points) E: **Erythema** (rated 1–5 depending on size, amount) P: **Purulent** exudate (same as E) S: **Separation** of deep tissues (same as E) I: **Isolation** of bacteria (10 pts) S: duration of inpatient **Stay** (>14 days, 5 points)	Interrater reliability not tested
Cellstic	Measure of healing rate Small, silastic catheter with internal jaws holds viscose cellulose sponge to collect wound cells Catheter placed in one end of surgical incision and later removed to monitor events in healing cascade Harvested wound cells analyzed histologically, biochemically, or cytologically	Developed through years of animal and human studies Demonstrates differences in healing rates with aging and shift in collagen types with wound maturation (50) Testing has involved 1,766 subjects to determine ideal procedures and materials (51,52)
PTFE tubing	Developed to evaluate healing potential of preoperative patients (53) Insertion of small tube of expanded polytetrafluoroethylene (PTFE) in lower lateral portion of upper arm; tube interstices become filled with connective tissue; tube removed after 7 days, and amounts of hydroxyproline/cm of tubing analyzed	Animal studies conducted to determine complication rates, optimal tube, and pore size Appears to be a safe, minimally invasive method for measuring healing potential; has high patient acceptability

Numbers in parentheses correspond to studies cited in the References.

39

Assessing Vaginitis

Marcia M. Grant and Sue B. Davidson

Vaginitis is a common and distressing health problem experienced by women. Three separate, but overlapping, perspectives on this problem are held by (1) the bedside, office, or clinic nurse; (2) the advanced practice nurse, whether a nurse practitioner, nurse midwife, or clinical nurse specialist; and (3) the nurse researcher. The bedside, office or clinic nurse is interested in instructing patients about preparation for vaginal examinations and the application of medications for efficacy. Advanced practice nurses are concerned about diagnostic accuracy, helping patients manage the distressing symptoms of vaginitis (such as pruritis or discharge), evaluating treatment effectiveness, and suggesting additional or alternative modes of symptom relief. The nurse researcher, on the other hand, selects specific and reliable methods and measurement approaches to explore causal relationships, test alternative or innovative interventions, and identify meaningful outcomes or experiences pertinent to the study of vaginitis. The authors' perspective is primarily that of researchers of a problem that is embedded in the clinical nursing care of women with diabetes mellitus. We became interested in vaginitis as a recurrent and distressing clinical problem for women with diabetes and were interested in testing the effectiveness of a noninvasive and nonpharmacologic approach to symptom management.[1]

Because of our combined clinical and research perspectives, our approach blends practice with research, and it should have meaning for the bedside, advanced practice, and research nurse. In this chapter, the following definitions of selected terms related to vaginitis assessment are important:

Sensitivity. The probability that test results will be reactive if the specimen is truly positive

Specificity. The probability that test results will be nonreactive if the specimen is truly negative

Precision or accuracy. The degree of accuracy of a microscope

Incidence. The number of new cases that develop in a given population during a defined period

Prevalence or point prevalence. The number of cases present in the population at risk at a specific time

Scope of the Problem

Vaginitis and vaginal discharge are among the 25 most common reasons for which women seek health care in the United States.[2] In 1983, there were 8 million office visits to physicians in the United States because of vaginal infections; in 1992, vaginitis accounted for over 10 million office visits to health-care professionals in both primary care and the specialties.[3] Three common vaginal infections have been identified: bacterial vaginosis (BV); vulvovaginal candidiasis (VVC), and trichomoniasis. In family, private practice and student health clinic settings, BV is the most common form (40%–50%), and VVC (20%–25%) and trichomoniasis are less common (15%–20%).[2,4]

Vaginitis is a costly problem. Reimbursement by Blue Cross Blue Shield for one year in North Carolina totaled $300 million for vaginitis visits to physicians.[5] These charges do not reflect the cost of medication for treatment, or earnings lost by working women. Today, women in the United States with vaginal symptoms can now buy over-the-counter antifungal treatment for vaginitis; no published estimates of the dollars spent in these purchases were found.

Appreciation of the serious problems that can result from nontreatment is emerging. For example, women with BV also tend to develop urinary tract infections. If women are untreated for BV before abdominal and gynecologic surgeries, cuff infections and other postoperative infections may occur. Anaerobic organisms from BV can precipitate pelvic inflammatory disease. Pregnant women with BV experience preterm rupture of membranes, preterm labor, and about one-third may have postpartum endometritis.[6,7] Clearly, this particular vaginal infection is a significant source of morbidity, unless treated.

Vaginitis can be difficult to diagnose and treat. Providers should, but often do not, use a systematic or thorough process for evaluating subjective symptoms and objective data for the causative organism. As many as 50% of women will experience symptoms of vaginal infection without corresponding objective evidence. Some women may have no subjective symptoms, but will have objective evidence of vaginitis. Diagnostic methods to analyze vaginal secretions vary in sensitivity and specificity. Treatment difficulties may result from the presence of an infection caused by several different organisms, the presence of resistant strains, or local topical reaction to the treatment. Alternative interventions, sometimes less costly than traditional therapy, have been explored to treat vaginitis, but their efficacy is unknown. For example, ingestion or vaginal instillations of yogurt have been cited as a way of improving lactobacilli levels.[8-10] Others have debunked this recommendation[2] or have found it has no effect.[11-16] Few research studies have been published to support or refute these options.[15]

The recurrence of vaginitis is common. Many factors can influence adherence and treatment outcomes. These include a woman's knowledge of her anatomy and the treatment, the timing and frequency of drug administration, length of the course of treatment, dosage form, and ease or difficulty of the regimen in relation to daily routines.[16] If these are not part of the decision making and planning of therapy for women with vaginitis, the infection may recur. In two of the major vaginal infections, BV and candidiasis, recurrence is a significant problem. For example, within 9 months of treatment, recurrence occurs in 30% to as many as 80% percent of the women experiencing bacterial vaginosis.[2] Fifteen to twenty percent of women with candida also have recurrence.[17] Numerous theories exist about the mechanisms of these phenomena.

In a few instances, nurses have published research dealing with some aspects of vaginitis. For example, Deitch and Smith[18] evaluated 30 women with chronic vaginitis to see whether the use of colposcopy would clarify why the infection was not responding. Although there are conceptual, sampling, and methodologic issues of concern in this study, it is important to note that these advanced practice nurses were using research processes to answer a very difficult clinical problem. Others have tested new approaches to the diagnosis of vaginal and cervical infections.[19]

Nurses in advanced practice also have published protocols for the management of vaginitis.[20-22] The advanced practice nurse (APN) role is expected to expand with healthcare reform. It may be that additional research focusing on strategies to increase treatment compliance, identify effective alternative interventions, and reduce the risk of or prevent vaginitis, will emerge as APNs assume greater role in the care of women.

Definition and Theoretical Description

Vaginitis is an inflammation of the vulvar and vaginal tissues. It usually is associated with changes in the vaginal environment and in the usual distribution of microbes and/or the presence of abnormal pathogenic organisms. Vaginosis describes vaginal changes that are not accompanied by inflammation of vaginal tissues or leukocytosis. This term is applied most frequently to bacterial vaginosis. The definition and theoretical description of vaginitis are understood within the framework of the physiology of the vaginal environment.

Vaginal Environment

A great variety of microorganisms coexist in the vagina. Particular groups of organisms are found in different areas (e.g., vaginal flora differ from cervical flora). In addition, the relationship among these organisms (the vaginal ecosystem) is complex. This ecosystem is sensitive and responsive to changes in a woman's physiologic status. When physiologic status changes, the numbers and types of organisms change, and these, in turn, change the vaginal environment. For a number of years, efforts to describe the vaginal flora and the relationships between microorganisms have been reported by researchers. Some of that research is flawed because researchers did not recognize differences between the various sites in the vagina, subjects were not homogeneous, specimen collection techniques were imperfect, and specimen transport and culture techniques varied widely.[13] Armed with this knowledge and more sophisticated identification techniques, Brown, Sautter, and Pickrum (as cited in Redondo-Lopez et al.)[13] sampled a cohort of healthy women nine times over three menstrual cycles. They found that there were four major groups of vaginal organisms. The first and most common group were gram-positive rods, of which the *Lactobacillus* species were most frequent, followed by *Corynebacterium* (in 37% of healthy women), and finally the *Propionibacterium*, *Bifidobacterium*, and *Eubacterium* species. The second most frequently observed microorganisms are gram-positive cocci such as *Staphylococcus epidermidis*, which was isolated in 62% of the healthy women. Anaerobic forms of gram-positive cocci also are found in 20% to 80% of healthy women. Gram-negative rods (*Gardnerella vaginalis*, the mobiluncus species, and the bacteroides species) also may be cultured from vaginas of healthy women (rates of 14%–40%).[23] The last group, yeasts such as *Candida albicans* and *Torulopsis glabrata*, are detected vaginally in 15%–20% of healthy women.

The vaginal epithelium is renewed from the basal toward the luminal layer. The outermost cells are sloughed along with the microorganisms that are attached to them. The vaginal epithelium is nourished by nutrients, derived from the circulation to this area of the body and intercellular channels in the vaginal epithelium. Some intracellular nutrients of vaginal epithelium become available for microorganism growth by the enzymatic degradation of sloughed cells and menstrual blood and from secretions of glands in the vagina. The vaginal environment has a pH of 4.0 to 4.5.

The thickness of the vaginal epithelium is regulated by levels of estrogen. When estrogen levels are increased, glycogen deposition in the vaginal epithelium is promoted. The lactobacilli produce acid from glycogen fermentation, which maintains a low pH and thereby fosters the growth of acid-tolerant vagina microorganisms. Fatty acids and the production of hydrogen peroxide by lactobacilli also may help to keep vaginal pH low.

Interactions occur among the normal flora inhabiting the vaginal environment. A complimentary interaction occurs when the product of metabolism of one organism is used by another for growth; an antagonistic interaction occurs when the products of metabolism of one species retard the growth of another. For example, prevalence studies of microorganisms have shown that in pregnancy, conditions that favor the presence of lactobacillus in the vagina also favor the presence of vaginal candida colonization.[12] This could be the result of a synergistic interaction. This information makes it difficult to interpret studies that focus on single microorganisms that may cause symptoms of vaginitis. Future research needs to consider synergistic interactions between flora.

Basal and laminal layers of the vaginal epithelium and the cervix contain cells that provide immune functions. Macrophages, lymphocytes, mast cells, Langerhans cells, and eosinophils can be found in the laminal layer. The levels of these may fluctuate, depending on the phase of the menstrual cycle. For example, lymphocytes located between vaginal epithelium cells increase during the luteal phase.[24] The presence of these lymphocytes and of immunoglobulin (Ig)G- and IgA-producing cells located in the vaginal epithelium strongly suggests that the vagina is able to produce antibodies.[25] The vagina can absorb substances, including drugs and/or other proteinlike materials, such as sperm, potentially producing overt or subacute inflammatory responses. As Witkin suggests, it seems very likely that vaginal T cells present antigens that are formed in response to inflammation caused by vaginal Langerhans cell activity.[24] If vaginal T cells were activated chronically, this process could be an underlying mechanism of increased risk to develop vaginal infections.

Vaginal flora may be altered. When this occurs, it can change the way the vaginal flora express virulence. A cascade of events is hypothesized, although the order in which these occur is not known. It is assumed that one of the first events is a change in vaginal pH. When this occurs, microorganism adherence is increased, possibly because of an increase in the numbers of receptors on vaginal epithelial cells or through changes in cell surface charge that create a gradient between the host and the bacterial cell surface.[13] As more microorganisms adhere, colonization is likely to occur. It does not always follow that colonization leads to symptoms.

Three common factors can alter vaginal flora, although the research base for these factors is by no means clear: (1) damage to mucosal barriers resulting from self-care practices such as douching or unusual sexual practices; (2) presence of foreign bodies such as a diaphragm, intrauterine device (IUD), certain tampons, and use of spermicides, especially those containing nonoxynol-9;[24,25] and (3) alterations in immune status, for example patients on steroids or individuals with diabetes. These changes may exist alone or, more frequently, in combination. When these alterations occur, specific varieties or combinations thereof may result. The three most common are BC, VC, and trichomoniasis. A description of each of these provides the basis for examining how vaginitis is assessed.

Bacterial Vaginosis

Bacterial vaginosis is characterized by an overgrowth of several species of facultative anaerobic bacteria. A unique characteristic of BV is that it represents a disturbance of the vaginal microbial flora versus being a tissue-based infection. In the past it has been known variously as nonspecific vaginitis, *Gardnerella vaginalis*, anaerobic vaginitis, or anaerobic vaginosis. The incidence (new cases that appear in a specific period of time) of BV varies in different populations. For example, Thomason et al.[7] indicate that in sexually transmitted disease (STD) clinics the incidence of BV is between 33% and 64%; in family planning and obstetrics clinics, the incidence is around 23% to 29%. In contrast, the incidence of BV is lowest in asymptomatic college populations (4%). The prevalence (total number of active cases, new and already existing) also varies by populations. In the United States, it is 17%–19% in family practice and student health clinics; 24% to 37% in STD clinics; and between 16% and 29% among pregnant women. Prevalence estimates of BV in STD clinics in Scandinavia in the mid-1980s have ranged between 15% and 33%.[26]

Thomason et al.[7] offer the following explanation of the mechanism by which BV occurs. Vaginal pH increases because of a reduction of lactic acid and hydrogen peroxide–producing species of lactobacilli, replacing them with species of lactobacilli or other flora that cannot maintain low vaginal pH. Growth of organisms that are usually repressed begin to flourish and produce aminopeptidases, enzymes that break down peptides into various amino acids. Part of this chain reaction involves the formation of amines, substances that produce strong odors, especially when they come in contact with alkaline substances. Amines also raise the vaginal pH. Epithelial cells slough off, and numerous bacteria attach to their surfaces (clue cells).

The most typical subjective symptoms that women with BV will note is a mild vulvar itch, possibly some burning, and a fishy vaginal odor (Table 39.1). This odor may be more noticeable right after intercourse because the alkaline semen reacts with the vaginal secretion to produce amines. Approximately 50% of women with BV are asymptomatic.

Since the mid-1980s, a system for increased accuracy of diagnosis of BV has been proposed, tested, and is now accepted as a standard of care. This system focuses on four objective signs of BV: thin vaginal secretions, vaginal pH above 4.5, presence of clue cells when vaginal secretion is examined under a microscopic, and positive potassium hydroxide odor findings. Three of the four signs must be present for the diagnosis to be confirmed.[27,28] The pH of vaginal secretions in women with BV is nearly always greater than 4.5 or 5.0. Thus, a vaginal pH of over 5.0 is a very specific indicator of BV, but it has weak sensitivity because vaginal pH can also be altered by the presence of blood, semen, and alkaline douches or creams. The vaginal discharge of a women with BV is usually present at the introitus, is malodorous, gray appearing, and has a thin, homogenous consistency. It adheres to, but can be easily wiped from, the vaginal wall. Samples of secretions should be taken from the mucosa along the vaginal walls and vault. The "whiff" test can be done on vaginal secretion that pools in the speculum or is put on a glass slide. Several drops of 10% potassium hydroxide solution are added to the secretion and the sample is smelled for the development "whiff" of a fishy odor. Vaginal secretion, mixed with normal saline, is then examined under microscopy (10X and 40X objectives and subdued light). Two particular forms should be visible. Clue cells, sloughed epithelial cells with fuzzy or ill-defined borders, must be found. The indistinct borders of these cells are caused by the collection of bacteria clinging to the cell borders. Another form that may be seen are curved rods with corkscrew motility; these signify the presence of *Mobyluncus*, another of the causitive organisms of BV. Gram stain can provide

Table 39.1   Symptom Patterns in Three Vaginal Infections

Symptoms and Signs	Bacterial Vaginosis	Vulvovaginal Candidiasis	Trichomoniasis
Subjective			
Itch	Mild	Intense, especially at night	Mild
Discharge	Mild to moderate	Scant to moderate	Mild
Odor	Fishy; stronger after intercourse	Minimal	Present
Vulvar excoriation	Absent	Present, can be severe	Absent
Dysuria	Mild	Present	Present
Dyspareunia	Not usual	Present	Present
Objective/vaginal inspection			
pH of secretions	>4.5–5.0	4.0–4.5	>4.5; usually 5–6
Discharge	Thin, homogenous, gray	Varies, thin to curdlike	Yellow-green; gray
Odor	Fishy	Not usually present	Very mild
Vulva and labia	No inflammation	Edema and redness	Cervical erythema
Vaginal vault	No inflammation	May see white plaques	Cervical erythema
Objective/laboratory			
Whiff test	Positive	Negative	Negative
Gram stain	Positive	Negative	Negative
Cells that will be seen on saline or KOH microscopy	Clue cells or motile curved rods	Budding hyphae; a few WBCs; no protozoa and no clue cells	Pear-shaped cells with flagellae; PMNs no clue cells
Culture	Not recommended	Recommended	Recommended
Papanicolaou test	Not recommended	Not recommended	Recommended

more definitive identification and reveals many small coccobacilli sticking to the clue cell's surface. Unlike other vaginal infections, culture of vaginal secretion is not recommended, because it will add little additional information. Two separate studies have shown that two criteria (presence of clue cells and a positive amine odor test) can accurately predict BV 99% of the time.[29]

The main risk factor that has a clear association with BV is use of an intrauterine device for contraception. A weaker relationship between BV and sexual activity also exists, but has not been fully confirmed.

Vulvovaginal Candidiasis

Vulvovaginal candidiasis (VVC) is a vaginal infection caused mostly by *Candida albicans*, but also by other organisms, such as *Torulopsis glabrata* or *Candida tropicalis*. Most (80%–85%) of VVC is caused, however, by *C. albicans*. This form of vaginitis has two other characteristics. One is that sometimes women with vaginitis have symptoms, but no corresponding positive findings on microscopic examination or by culture; conversely, the woman can have positive findings and not be symptomatic. The second characteristic is that there is a small, but important, group of women who have repeated episodes of VVC. Whether this is caused by chronic VVC, recurrence, relapse, or a recalcitrant episode may be difficult to clarify. Clinicians struggle to identify women in this group and to find effective treatment for them.[9]

The overall incidence (point prevalence) of VVC in the United States is 25%. World-wide, the incidence varies from around 15% in Scandinavia to between 28% and 37% in England. Incidence is higher in tropical and subtropical areas. In the United States and England, incidence of VVC has increased as much as by 42%.[26] In England, VVC is the major cause of vaginitis.

The physiologic mechanisms whereby VVC occurs are not fully defined. The contemporary view is that *C. albicans* is a commensal (normal resident) *and* a pathogen; *Candida* can and does exist in low levels among the vaginal flora of many women. What appears to tip the balance in the direction of VVC is a change in the host or in the host environment. When the balance is changed, the yeast is able to adhere to vaginal tissue and germination of the yeast and development of hyphae will occur, leading to colonization. *Candida* is then able to engage in a process of "switching," whereby cell strains that are less pathogenic are switched into more pathogenic strains through replication and division; in short, the virulence of the yeast is enhanced.[30,31] The final result of switching is that a cell strain is produced that penetrates tissue, probably via proteases or other enzymes. Once this occurs, even blastophores, the early, nonbudding form of *Candida*, can penetrate tissue, which signals a loss of local defenses in the vaginal tissue.

Generally, the most common symptom of VVC is perianal and vulvar itching (pruritis), usually more intense at night (Table 39.1). In addition, women with VVC may have dysuria, or postvoiding dysuria from urine spreading on the surface of the perianal skin where scratching has occurred. There may be vaginal discharge, although this is not a usual symptom, or it may be very minimal. There is minimal odor, and it is not offensive. There may be dyspareunia (pain upon vaginal penetration during sexual intercourse). The mechanism of these symptoms includes a yeast overgrowth with an inflammatory response in the walls of the vagina. At the same time, yeast interacts with glucose that may be present in several forms: in the form of glycogen in vaginal tissue that is converted to glucose or in the form of glucose in urine and vaginal secretion if the woman has diabetes. Either way, the yeast combines with glucose to produce an alcohol, which, when it spreads over the skin, is irritating and initiates the redness and inflammation commonly seen.

Unfortunately for the clinician and researcher, the typical subjective symptoms that women with VVC present are highly variable. One author indicates that even though pruritis is the most consistently found symptom of VVC, this symptom only predicts 38% of patients with VVC.[17]

Upon examination for objective signs of VVC, the clinician or researcher will find vulvar and labial edema and redness; these signs may extend to the groin and thighs (Table 39.1). When examining the vaginal introitus, canal, and vault, vaginal plaques may be seen. The vaginal discharge varies: it may be thin, clear, and watery or thick, white, and curdlike (20%–25% of the time). The curds, if seen, may be white or yellow and are usually adherent. These curds consist of clumps of sloughed vaginal epithelium and parts of the hyphae of the yeast. Red satellite lesions may be seen on the thighs; sometimes these red lesions have a scalloped outer edge. The vaginal pH is usually lower than 5.0 (e.g., 4.0 to 4.5).

Other objective signs may be seen during the wet-mount slide examination by using 10% potassium hydroxide (KOH) and normal saline (Table 39.1). After the vaginal pH is checked, KOH is added to the vaginal smear or secretion. In VVC, when the slide or secretion is smelled, there should be no fishy odor, meaning that the woman does not have BV. The addition of KOH to the slide serves to alter the shape of the yeast cells, making their borders more visible. What should be seen, if the woman has VVC, is budding hyphae of the yeast cells, few, if any, leukocytes, and no trichomonads or clue cells. Because noncandidal varieties can cause vaginitis, the presence of a large number of spores with no hyphae should raise the index of suspicion that vaginitis was caused by *Torulopsis glabrata*. Another slide made from a mixture of the vaginal secretion and normal saline should then be viewed. According to two nurse practitioners, the viewing of both slides can produce a 70% to 80% sensitive in detecting vaginitis caused by candida.[9]

Because as many as 50% of women with yeast infections may have negative microscopy, cultures are recommended as the last step in diagnosing VVC (Table 39.1). The following culture media can be used to detect vaginal pathogens:[32]

> *Candida albicans*
> > *Transport:* Nickerson's medium; Sabouraud's dextrose medium
> > *Culture:* Sabouraud's aga with chloramphenicol; culture enriched with broth; blood agar; Mycosel agar/Microstick-Candida
> Organisms causing bacterial vaginosis
> > *Transport:* Amies; Stuart
> > *Culture:* Human blood agar (HBT)
> *Trichomonas vaginalis*
> > *Transport:* Feinberg-Whittington medium; Diamond's TYM calf serum medium
> > *Culture:* Diamond's; Hollander's; Feinberg's

A variety of predisposing host factors have been identified for VVC. A recent course of antibiotic therapy with agents such as tetracycline, ampicillin, and/or oral cephalosporins, can predispose to VVC by eliminating the protective anaerobic and aerobic lactobacilli. The use of high-estrogen birth control pills or corticosteroids also can predispose to VVC. Uncontrolled diabetes is a risk factor, although the mechanism has never been clearly described. Another predisposing factor is pregnancy, especially the third trimester; between 30% and 40% of women in this phase of pregnancy have asymptomatic colonization. Increased frequency of sexual intercourse, or anal/oral/genital sexual intercourse is linked with predisposition to VVC. Finally, women who have had a transplant and take immunosuppressive drugs, have HIV, or are stressed for other reasons may be predisposed to VVC because of a reduction of T lymphocytes and increased levels of T-cell suppressors. Anecdotally, some clinicians believe that tight, restrictive clothes or nylon underwear, the use of commercial douches, perfumed toilet paper, or feminine hygiene sprays, and swimming in chlorinated pools are predisposing factors for VVC. Two reservoirs for recurrent VVC are the gut and/or sexual partners who carry yeasts. Research studies attempting to confirm these two factors have been inconclusive.

Trichomoniasis

Trichomoniasis, an STD, is a vaginal infection caused by an anaerobic protozoaon. It causes urethritis in men. It is considered by some[33] to be the most prevalent cause of STD. Approximately 2.5 to 3 million women are infected with this form of vaginitis annually. The prevalence varies with setting and the frequency of sexual activity. For example, the prevalence of trichomoniasis is estimated to be 5% in family planning clinics, 39% to 40% in STD clinics, and between 50% and 75% among prostitutes.[2] In the United States, the highest trichomoniasis frequency is found in the South, the lowest in Western regions. The National Disease and Therapeutic Index survey found that African American women were treated for trichomoniasis about four times more frequently than white women, even though about 60% of physician visits for this infection occurred in white females. These particular facts illustrate the complex patterns of women seeking help for vaginitis and some of the health policy issues involved in targeted treatment of groups of women at high risk for vaginitis. Both of these issues may be of interest to nurse researchers and nurse epidemiologists.

The prevalence of trichomoniasis in the United States and worldwide is decreasing.[26] Moi analyzed the incidence and prevalence of vaginitis in Scandinavian countries.[34] He believes that the decreasing incidence of trichomoniasis in Sweden is related to a 20-year policy of treating without diagnosis partners of women infected with trichomoniasis. In addition, reduced sexual activity due to fear of contracting AIDS and increased condom use may have contributed to this reduced prevalence.[34]

A picture of the pathogenesis of trichomoniasis is emerging. At first contact, these protozoa swim over the cell, layering, clumping, and then adhering by means of microfilaments to its surface. As the filaments adhere, the cells retract and lyse, possibly because of the production of free lactic or acetic acid by the protozoa themselves. The trichomonad requires multiple nutrients, such as carbohydrates, amino acids, and fatty acids. These macronutrients may be supplied by macromolecules, such as plasminogen or fibrinogen, and other molecules, such as ferritin, albumin, and transferrin, which bind to the parasite's surface. Other in vivo mechanisms that enable the trichomonad to live include interaction with growth-stimulating factors in the tissue of the host. This mechanism may account for the vaginal epithelial hyperplasia seen in trichomoniasis.[33,35]

In symptomatic women, the most typical symptoms of trichomoniasis are vulvo-vaginal irritation and pruritus (~50%) and pain on intercourse (~50%) (Table 39.1). Symptoms may occur during or right after menstruation. The reason for this may be that the trichomonad flourishes in an iron-rich mileu, such as would occur during a menstrual period. In men there may be urethral discharge or urethral inflammation. On examination, vaginal discharge may be yellow/green[4,36] or gray.[2] The vaginal pH generally is above 4.5 and usually is between 5.0 and 6.0 Under colposcopy, a procedure that enables the magnification of tissues being examined, as much as 45% to 50% of women with trichomoniasis will demonstrate a reddened and inflamed "strawberry" cervix.[2]

Other objective signs may be seen upon wet-mount examination of vaginal discharge (Table 39.1). Once a sample has been obtained from the posterior vaginal fornix, the sample should be mixed with normal saline (KOH will kill the protozoa). Identification of the organism may be assisted by keeping the sample warm (having the patient hold the specimen tube in her hand) and by reducing sources of lighting that affect the field of view. What is seen are pear-shaped cells with flagellae; some of the cells may be moving, or the cells may be stationary, but the flagellae are moving. A concentration of 10^4 or 10^5 of the organism is needed in the vaginal discharge; if this is not found, visualization may be compromised. Other methods of increasing visualization of the trichomonad are to view at least 10 microscopic fields or to focus on clumps of white blood cells where the protozoa tend to cluster.[37] Gram staining is not used in diagnosing trichomoniasis.

As with the diagnosis of other vaginitis by microscope, time, skill, and well-maintained equipment increase diagnostic accuracy. Cultures also can be used to diagnose trichomoniasis; Diamond's medium and Feinberg-Whittington medium have been shown to have the same sensitivity and specificity in identifying the organism.[38] Finally, the Papanicolaou smear is a method that has fairly high sensitivity in detecting trichomoniasis.

In summary, in symptomatic women, microscopic methods and the Papanicolaou smear have a sensitivity of around 60% to 70% in diagnosing women with trichomoniasis; cultures (read at 46 to 98 hours) have a sensitivity of 90% to 95%.[38,39] As with other vaginitis, there are multiple considerations in choosing a diagnostic method for trichomoniasis that affect both the practitioner and the researcher. Sensitivity and specificity, cost, skill at microscopy, and time influence decision making. Lossik's editorial[40] illustrates the various trade-offs that may be made by practitioners and researchers in the case of trichomoniasis. Cultures for trichomoniasis are not a perfect "gold standard," as the media currently available do not support all known species. Cultures have an estimated sensitivity of between 86% and 97%. However, the Papanicolaou smear is the most cost-effective method to diagnose trichomoniasis, but its sensitivity is similar to that of wet mounts, it has low specificity and produces too many false positives. Lossick recommends that, in the average patient population with a 5% prevalence of trichomoniasis, it would be wise to augment diagnosis on Pap smear with another more specific test such as a repeated wet mount, culture, or perhaps diagnosis by one of the newer methods.

Several factors emerge as risk factors for trichomoniasis.[33,36] As with VVC, sexual activity (more rather than less) and multiple sexual partners increase the likelihood of developing trichomoniasis. Women (gender) are more susceptible to trichomoniasis than men. Only a small number of men become symptomatic after exposure, and spontaneous resolution of trichomoniasis in men does occur. Other less clear risk factors for trichomoniasis include race (African Americans are more likely to develop it); previous history of STD; coexistent gonorrhea; use of contraceptive agents other than the barrier/hormonal type; postmenopausal; and use of moist cloths to clean the perineal area, have been cited in the literature.[33,39]

These three common vaginal infections represent some distinct, but many overlapping, subjective and objective symptoms. For the nurse in advanced practice, this represents an issue in diagnosis accuracy. Using sensitivity and specificity characteristics to decide on a diagnostic approaches improves the accuracy of diagnosis and the care delivered (Table 39.2). For the nurse researcher, selecting an approach for accurate assessment and monitoring should be based on the anticipated type of vaginitis and the nature of intervention being tested.

Table 39.2 Comparison of Sensitivity and Specificity of Diagnostic Methods for Vaginitis

Method	Sensitivity (%)	Specificity (%)
Vulvovaginitis		
KOH (microscopic examination)	19	98
Culture (Nickerson's medium)		
24 hours	31	99
48 hours	72	97
Culture (Microstix-CA)		
24 hours	51	97
48 hours	83	96
Trichomoniasis		
Microscopic examination		
Symptomatic women	60–80.9	100
Asymptomatic women	40–50	
Culture	90–98.5	95
Papanicolaou test	60–70	95
Monoclonal antibody tests	86	99

Other Vaginal Infections

Women may contract other serious vaginal infections, such as chlamydia, gonorrhea, and/or herpes. The causative pathogens and locus of infection may differ from the vaginal infections that have just been described. However, issues related to measurement and/or diagnosis for nurses in advanced practice and nursing research are much the same for nearly all kinds of vaginitis.

Other Techniques to Diagnose Vaginitis

A variety of approaches have been developed that augment wet-mount, gram stain, and culture techniques to identify organisms. The following new techniques are emerging as valuable measures in the assessment of vaginitis:

> *Plastic envelope method.* Developed to increase shelf life of media, reasonable cost
> *Latex agglutination test.* Low specificity and reactivity, valuable only in screening non-symptomatic patients
> *Gas liquid chromatography.* High specificity (93.6%), but expensive
> *Enzymatic reaction.* High specificity and sensitivity, but time-consuming and expensive
> *Antigen or antibody tests.* Includes fluorescein-tagged monoclonal antibodies and ELISA. High sensitivity, but need high-quality microscope and trained personnel

These methods, their sensitivity and/or specificity, and other related conditions are reviewed in Appendix 39A.[41-45] Methodologies for diagnosing vaginitis such as enzyme-linked immunosorbent assay (ELISA) offer greater specificity in populations with high rates of a particular type of vaginitis. They offer potential to the nurse researcher because of their high sensitivity and specificity. Drawbacks are cost and the need for special equipment and trained personnel.

Issues Related to Instrument Selection

In most studies on vaginitis the purpose is to examine the incidence of the problem in the population in general or to test specific approaches to prevention and treatment. The development of an instrument to measure vaginitis has been the focus of few publications. Some studies, however, have compared incidence rates using different methods for identification of organisms and different sets of signs and symptoms. These have been described in relation to specific infections.

Information used to assess vaginitis can be classified into three groups: (1) identification of pathogenic organisms; (2) complaints of subjective symptoms; and (3) observation of objective signs. For each group, clinicians and investigators may select different methods and different parameters, depending on sensitivity and reliability as well as cost and availability.

Identification of Pathogenic Organisms

Two major approaches are used to identify pathogenic organisms associated with vaginitis. The wet mount, or immediate microscopic examination, is done right after the vaginal examination and collection of vaginal secretions. A slide is prepared and examined under the microscope for characteristics of suspected pathogens. In the second method, secretions obtained during the vaginal examination are transferred onto various culture media. They are incubated for at least 48 hours, after which pathogenic organisms are identified.

Because the organism associated with vaginitis may be a yeast, a bacterium, or a protozoan, different methods must be used. A typical procedure involves both wet mount and culture.[42] Performing the vaginal examination to obtain exudate and conducting the wet-mount examination are technologies done generally by the health practitioner, either medical or nursing. Nurses in advanced practice roles carry out these procedures. Culture media used varies depending on the organism to be identified. Recommended media are listed on p. 590.

Validity and reliability of the various methods of identifying the microbes involve comparing results across the various methods and various preparations and comparing results obtained among different investigators. When comparing immediate wet-mount and microscopic examination versus culture and subsequent examination, results show that additional identification of organisms occurs when culture data are added to data obtained from immediate microscopic examination only. In practical terms, treating patients without culture confirmation of pathogenic organisms usually is based on expediency; that is, the patient has acute symptoms that are typical and treatment is not held up for 3 days to await culture results. In addition, costs (cultures using various media and requiring laboratory identification procedures) can be prohibitively expensive.[42]

Subjective Symptoms

The second group of parameters used to assess vaginitis are the subjective symptoms obtained during patient interview. They generally included pruritis, discharge, odor, dyspareunia, dysuria, and vaginal pressure, soreness, or burning.[2,4,7,42] These symptoms may be continuous or intermittent. Symptom patterns can be used to differentiate specific vaginal infections (Table 39.1). However, use of symptoms, alone or combined with historical data, is of limited value in the accurate diagnosis of vaginal infections.[46,47] Approximately half of the patients presenting with vaginal symptoms generally are given a specific microbiologic diagnosis, as occurs when subjective symptoms are combined with examination for specific organisms as well as objective signs.[47]

Observation of Objective Signs

The third group of parameters used to assess vaginitis includes the objective signs obtained during patient examination. The external genitalia may be examined for erythema, secretions, and lesions. Secretions can be tested for pH and glucose. Typical signs for each type of vaginitis are described in Table 39.1. The standard procedure for clinical diagnosis is to accept three typical signs (e.g., pH, discharge characteristics, and odor) as acceptable evidence of disease. This method, however, still results in a sensitivity of 60% to 72%.[47] Combining culture, objective, and subjective information to assess vaginitis clearly is the best current way to obtain the most accurate diagnosis.

Assessment Tools and Treatment Protocols

With the development of the advanced practice role of the nurse and the increased use of the physician's assistant, assessment tools and treatment protocols have been developed to assist in the diagnosis and differentiation of the various kinds of vaginitis. Several of these are highlighted in Appendix 39A.[1,4,12,14,22,48]

Summary

Assessment of vaginitis may involve three kinds of information: identification of pathogenic organisms, subjective symptoms, and objective signs. Different combinations of information are useful depending on whether the nurse, the practitioner, or the researcher is involved in the assessment. Most studies dealing with the validity and reliability of the variables have focused on methods for organism identification. Continuing issues in assessment of vaginitis include testing predisposing factors, the problem of mixed infections, the recurrence of the problem, how to manage symptoms, and the need for increased specificity and sensitivity of organism identification methods. These issues illustrate the need for a more thorough assessment of the patient to explain the problem further. For researchers, the variables used in assessment often are most valuable when they are standardized and understood. For the nurse working with patients clinically, management of symptoms is an important focus. One way to enrich this clinical practice would be to supplement the tools already developed for assessing vaginitis with some qualitative information; for example, what relationships occur between vaginitis and sexual function, personal hygiene, and clothing styles. In this way, tools developed via a qualitative methodology could be used to assess, measure, and diagnose the responses of women to vaginitis and help to identify additional variables to be explored in other research projects.

References

1. Grant, M., & Davidson, S. *Effects of perineal care on diabetic vulvovaginitis: Final report of project.* Washington, DC: Division of Nursing, Bureau of Health Manpower, Health Resources Administration, Department of Health and Human Resources, 1984.
2. Sobel, J.D. Vaginitis in adult women. *Obstet Gynecol Clin North Am*, 1990, 17(4):851-879.
3. Centers for Disease Control and Prevention. CDC Surveillance Summaries, August 13, 1993. *MMWR*, 1993, 42:583.
4. Eschenbach, D.A., & Mead, P.B. Managing problem vaginitis. *Patient Care*, 1992, 26(14):137-141.
5. Gwyther, R.E., Addison, C.A., Spottswood, S., et al. An innovative method for specimen autocollection in the diagnosis of vaginitis. *J Fam Pract*, 1986, 23: 487-488.
6. Biswas, M.K. Bacterial vaginosis. *Clin Obstet Gynecol*, 1993, 36(1):166-176.
7. Thomason, J.L., Gelbart, S.M., & Scaglione, N.J. Bacterial vaginosis: Current review with indications for asymptomatic therapy. *Am J Obstet Gynecol*, 1991, 165:1210-1217.
8. Fredriccson, B., Englund, K., Weintraub, L., et al. Ecological treatment of bacterial vaginosis. *Lancet*, 1987, 1:276.
9. Carcio, H.A., & Secor, R.M.C. Vulvovaginal candidiasis: A current update. *Nurse Pract Forum*, 1992, 3(3):135-144.
10. Weinhouse, B. Women doctors' own remedies. *Redbook*, 1994, 182(6):100-101.
11. Kaufman, R.H., & Hammill, H.A. Vaginitis. *Primary Care*, 1990, 17(1):115-125.
12. Larsen, B. Vaginal flora in health and disease. *Clin Obstet Gynecol*, 1993, 36(1):110-121.
13. Redondo-Lopez, V., Cook, R.L., & Sobel, J.D. Emerging role of lactobacilli in the control and maintenance of the vaginal bacterial microflora. *Rev Infect Dis*, 1990, 12(5):856-872.
14. Summers, P.R., & Sharp, H.T. The management of obscure or difficult cases of vulvovaginitis. *Clin Obstet Gynecol*, 1993, 36(1):206-214.
15. Hilton, E., Isenberg, H.D., Alperstein, P., et al. Ingestion of yogurt containing *Lactobacillus acidophilus* as prophylaxis for candidal vaginitis. *Ann Int Med*, 1992, 116:353.
16. Nixon, S.A. Vulvovaginitis: The role of patient compliance in treatment success. *Am J Obstet Gynecol*, 1991, 165:1207-1209.
17. Odds, F.C. Candidosis of the genitalia. In F.C. Odds (Ed.), *Candida and candidosis* (2nd ed.). London: Balliere Tindal, 1988, p. 124.
18. Deitch, K.V., & Smith, J.E. Symptoms of chronic vaginal infection and microscopic condyloma in women. *JOGNN*, 1990, 19(2):133-138.
19. Knud-hansen, C.R., Dallabetta, G.A., Reichart, C., et al. Surrogate methods to diagnose gonococcal and chlamydial cervicitis: Comparison of leukocyte esterase dipstick, endocervical gram stain, and culture. *Sex Transm Dis*, 1991, 18(4):211-216.
20. Gietl, K.A. Role of the nurse practitioner in the management of vaginitis. *Am J Obstet Gynecol*, 1988, 158:1009-1111.
21. Bennett, E.J. Vaginitis: Its diagnosis and treatment. *Health Care Women Int*, 1987, 8:65-73.
22. Schodde, G. A vaginitis protocol that helps teach. *Nurse Practitioner*, 1975, 1(2):64.
23. Levison, M.E., Corman, L.C., Carrington, G.R., & Kaye, D. Quantitative microflora of the vagina. *Am J Obstet Gynecol*, 1977, 127:80-85.
24. Witkin, S.S. Immunology of the vagina. *Clin Obstet Gynecol*, 1993, 36(1):122-128.
25. Mardh, P.A. The vaginal ecosystem. *Am J Obstet Gynecol*, 1991, 165:1163-1168.
26. Kent, H.L. Epidemiology of vaginitis. *Am J Obstet Gynecol*, 1991, 165:1168-1176.
27. Gardner, H.L., & Dukes, C.D. Haemophilus vaginalis vaginitis: A newly defined specific infection previously classified as "nonspecific vaginitis." *Am J Obstet Gynecol*, 1955, 68:962-976.
28. Amsel, R., Totten, P.A., Spiegel, C.A., et al. Nonspecific vagnitis. *Am J Med*, 1983, 74:14-22.
29. Thomason, J.L., Gelbart, S.M., Anderson, R.J., et al. Statistical evaluation of diagnostic criteria for bacterial vaginosis. *Am J Obstet Gynecol*, 1990, 162:155-160.
30. Robertson, W.H. Mycology of vulvovaginitis. *Am J Obstet Gynecol*, 1988, 158(4):989-991.
31. Sobel, J.D. Candidal vulvovaginitis. *Clin Obstet Gynecol*, 1993, 36(1):153-165.
32. Horowitz, B.J. Mycotic vulvovagnitis: A broad overview. *Am J Obstet Gynecol*, 1991, 165:1188-1192.

33. Heine, P., & McGregor, J.A. *Trichomonas vaginalis*: A reemerging pathogen. *Clin Obstet Gynecol*, 1993, *36*(1):137-144.

34. Moi, H. Epidemiologic aspects of vaginitis and vaginosis in Scandinavia. In B.J. Horowitz & P.A. Mardh (Eds.), *Vaginitis vaginosis*. New York: Wiley-Liss, 1991, p. 85.

35. Graves, A., & Gardner, W.A. Pathogenecity of *Trichomonas vaginalis*. *Clin Obstet Gynecol*, 1993, *36*(1): 145-152.

36. Reed, B.D., Huck, W., & Zazove, P. Differentiation of *Gardnerella vaginalis*, *Candida albicans*, and *Trichomonas vaginalis* infections of the vagina. *J Fam Pract*, 1989, *28*(6):673-680.

37. Havens, C.S., Summers, P., Tilton, R.C., & Wolner-Hanssen, P. Diagnosing gynecologic infections. *Patient Care*, 1990, *24*(8):74-79.

38. Krieger, J.N., Tam, M.R., Stevens, C.E., et al. Diagnosis of trichomoniasis: Comparison of conventional wet-mount examination with cytologic studies, cultures, and monoclonal antibody staining of direct specimens. *JAMA*, 1988, *259*(8):1223-1227.

39. McCue, J.D. Evaluation and management of vaginitis. *Arch Int Med*, 1989, *149*:565-568.

40. Lossick, J.G. The diagnosis of vaginal trichomoniasis. *JAMA*, 1988, *259*(8):1230.

41. Beal, C., Goldsmith, R., Kotby, M., et al. The plastic envelope method, a simplified technique for culture

42. Eschenbach, D.A., & Hillier, S.L. Advances in diagnostic testing for vaginitis and cervicitis. *J Reproduct Med*, 1989, *34*(suppl 8):555-565.

43. Thomason, J.L., Gelbart, S.M., & Broekhuizen, F.F. Advances in the understanding of bacterial vaginosis. *J Reproduct Med*, 1989, *34*(suppl 8):581-587.

44. Thomason, J.L., Gelbart, S.M., Wilcoski, L.M., et al. Proline aminopeptidase activity as a rapid diagnostic test to confirm bacterial vaginosis. *Obstet Gynecol*, 1988, *71*:607-611.

45. Schoonmaker, J.N., Lunt, B.D., Lawellin, D.W., et al. A new proline aminopeptidase assay for diagnosis of bacterial vaginosis. *Am J Obstet Gynecol*, 1991, *165*:737-742.

46. Bergman, J.J., & Berg, A.O. How useful are symptoms in the diagnosis of candida vaginitis? *J Fam Pract*, 1983, *16*(3):509-511.

47. Schaaf, V.M., Perez-Stable, E.J., & Borchardt, K. The limited value of symptoms and signs in the diagnosis of vaginal infections. *Arch Int Med*, 1990, *150*: 1929-1933.

48. Greenfield, S., Friedland, G., Scifers, S., et al. Protocol management of dysuria, urinary frequency, and vaginal discharge. *Ann Int Med*, 1974, *81*(4):452.

diagnosis of trichomoniasis. *J Clin Microbiol*, 1990, *30*(9):2265-2268.

Appendices

39A. Assessment Tools and Treatment Protocols for Vaginitis

Instruments	Description	Psychometric Indices
Assessment tools		
Vaginitis Assessment Form (1)	Designed for diabetic patients Tests effectiveness of a perineal care technique on prevention and management of vaginitis Subjects followed for 1 month Form includes: subjective symptoms; objective signs; laboratory findings	Content validity established by a panel of nurse practitioner experts familiar with assessing vaginitis Sensitivity and reliability by random, weekly exam assessment of 143 subjects Cronbach's alpha: history: 0.78; external exam: 0.97; internal vaginal exam: 0.82; total of all variables: 0.92 Some consistency within subscale and total scale Relationship between occurrence of vulvovaginal symptoms and positive cultures Comparison of 90 subjects having positive vulvovaginal symptoms at beginning of study (64%) vs. 90 subjects with positive cultures for *Candida, Trichomonas,* and/or *Gardnerella* (13%) High incidence of patients with positive symptoms and negative cultures leads to need for assessment tool that includes signs/symptoms plus culture data
Sumners and Sharp Vaginitis History Form (12)	Targets information needed for obscure or difficult cases Data elicited: occurrence of symptoms; medications; other symptoms (e.g., rashes, dry skin, painful joints); sexual history General guidelines described, including situations to refer to a dermatologist	Reliability and validity reports not included
Treatment protocols		
Schodde Protocol (22)	Includes: subjective symptoms (e.g., odor, burning after urination); objective physical exam (e.g., vulvar inflammation, vaginal discharge); laboratory tests; area for interpreting the assessment data and planning the follow-up treatment	None reported
Greenfield et al. Protocol (48)	Used in the management of dysuria, urinary frequency, and vaginal discharge Uses branching logic format, including: history; physical exam; laboratory criteria	Logic format validated by medical consultants Effectiveness tested on 146 patients: group 1 (patient seen by nurse using the protocol form, then by physician using usual medical approach); group 2 (patient seen by physician using usual medical approach)

39A. Assessment Tools and Treatment Protocols for Vaginitis (*cont.*)

Instruments	Description	Psychometric Indices
Greenfield et al. Protocol. (*cont.*)		Agreement: Medical history: 139/146 (6/7 discrepancies = physician error); physical exam: 137/146; lab data: similar Criteria validated by demonstrating that patients receiving protocol-directed treatment obtained same high degree of symptom relief as those treated by physician Reliability of nurse identification of *Candida* under microscopic determined by nurse results with lab technician results: lab failed to identify *Candida* in 9/39 positive cases Summary: tool criteria has initial reliability and validity and includes parameters relative to dysuria, frequent urination, vaginitis
Eschenbach and Mead Protocol (4)	Branching patient flowchart leading practitioner through steps needed: begins with patient's reported signs/symptoms; pH of vaginal secretions; gram staining Treatment based on findings; includes first-line therapy as well as recommendations for persistent infections or recurrences	No reliability or validity reported
Summers and Sharp Protocol (14)	Organized approach to treatment of obscure or difficult cases: history form; physical exam approaches; subjective symptoms; objective signs; therapeutic options	No reliability or validity reported

Numbers in parentheses correspond to studies cited in the References.

39B. Other Techniques to Diagnose Vaginitis

Diagnostic Test/ Microorganism	Description	Psychometric Indices/ Advantages/Disadvantages
Plastic Envelope Method (PEM) (41) Culture for trichomoniasis	Easy process for culture Soft, transparent plastic pouch with 2 equal size sections and a small, plastic frame to prevent buckling; sections interconnected by a small channel Dry PEM medium diluted by adding 4 ml water into the uppersection, mixing, and forcing all but a little medium into the lower section of the pouch Small amount of medium is then innoculated with vaginal fluid, mixed, then directed down into lower section Pouch is hung vertically for incubation Results of growth on medium read by looking through the plastic pouch with a microscope	PEM results compare favorably with other culture media (41) Overcomes problem of limited shelf-life of liquid or jellylike media Less expensive than other methods
Latex Agglutination Test Diagnostic test for VVC	Polystyrene latex particles, coated with purified immunoglobulins, are exposed to purified derivatives of the cell wall of C. albicans (serotypes A, B) and Torulopsis glabrata Vaginal swab added to the sensitive latex on a black cardboard slide and mixed Swab washings are added to a latex cardboard, which does not contain immunoglobulins (control) Positive reaction is a coarse clumping within prescribed time (antigen/antibody reaction to the organism)	Sensitivity 72.7% in study with 137 symptomatic and asymptomatic women with C. albicans (lower than sensitivity of KOH method, 90%) (2,42)
Gas Liquid Chromatography (GLC) (43) Defines bacterial microorganisms in BV	Microorganisms produce short-chain organic acid byproducts Each genus has unique "signature" pattern (e.g., GLC of vaginal fluid of women with BV have increased amounts of succinic acid and decreased amounts of lactic acid) Vaginal fluid collected with saline-moistened cotton swabs, swished in sterile water to produce a washing with vaginal matter suspended in it Fluid introduced to GLC, which by heat and a carrier gas passes the sample over an analytical column Organic acids reach a detecting and recording device, and the particular wave form is captured on a readout	Sample, 500 women, of which 70% had some type of vaginitis: sensitivity 54.3%; specificity 93.6% Advantages: has highest specificity of any diagnostic test for BV Disadvantages: time-consuming, expensive
ProLine Aminopeptidase Method Bacteria, candida	Detects enzyme proline aminopeptidase, which is produced in vitro by wide wide variety of bacteria (e.g., lactobacillus, Mobiluncus), and Candida Vaginal washing samples combined with L-proline b napthylamide or L-proline p nitroanilide, which acts as a color developer Enzyme reaction measured by color intensity, either visually or by spectrophotometer	Compared to other methods (e.g., culture, gram stain) (44): sensitivity 81%; specificity 96% Another study found (45): sensitivity 93%; specificity 91–93% Advantages: batches of samples can be done, works better than GLC Disadvantages: time-consuming, expensive

39B. Other Techniques to Diagnose Vaginitis (*cont.*)

Diagnostic Test/ Microorganism	Description	Psychometric Indices/ Advantages/Disadvantages
Enzyme-Linked Immunosorbent (ELISA) Identifies monoclonal antibody specific to microorganism (42)	Basis for a number of tests measuring the response of vaginal fluid to test antigen or antibody systems Vaginal fluid is mixed with specific antibody, and antigens are formed; another substance is added (e.g., antigen-enzyme sensitive to antibody/ antigen reaction); the substance interacts with original antibody-antigen complex; then dyes attached to the enzyme develop color indicating positive response ELISA may be used with monoclonal antibodies, direct or indirect immuno-fluorescence, and sometime with fluoresceintagged monoclonal antibodies	Sensitivity: 91–96% (38) Sample of 60 patients, with an incidence of trichomoniasis of 13% (38): sensitivity 86%; specificity 99%; positive predictive value 96% Advantages: require little time to perform, standard prep for cytologic evaluations (38) Disadvantages: requires special reagents, high-quality microscopes, trained personnel; predictive value drops when used on low-risk populations

Numbers in parentheses correspond to studies cited in the References.

Index